Myocardial Ischaemia

Edited by Kristian Thygesen
and John Kjekshus

OXFORD

BLACKWELL SCIENTIFIC PUBLICATIONS

LONDON EDINBURGH BOSTON

MELBOURNE PARIS BERLIN VIENNA

Editorial Offices:
Osney Mead, Oxford OX2 0EL
25 John Street, London WC1N 2BL
23 Ainslie Place, Edinburgh EH3 6AJ
3 Cambridge Center, Cambridge
Massachusetts 02142, USA
54 University Street, Carlton
Victoria 3053, Australia

Other Editorial Offices:
Arnette SA
2, rue Casimir-Delavigne
75006 Paris
France

Blackwell Wissenschaft
Meinekestrasse 4
D–1000 Berlin 15
Germany

Blackwell MZV
Feldgasse 13
A–1238 Wien
Austria

First published 1990
Reprinted 1991

Printed and bound in Great Britain at the University Press, Cambridge

DISTRIBUTORS

Marston Book Services Ltd
PO Box 87
Oxford OX2 0DT
(*Orders*: Tel: 0865 791155
Fax: 0865 791927
Telex: 837515)

USA
Mosby–Year Book, Inc.
200 North LaSalle Street
Chicago, Illinois 60601
(*Orders*: Tel: 312 726–9733)

Canada
Mosby–Year Book, Inc.
5240 Finch Avenue East
Scarborough, Ontario
(*Orders*: Tel: 416 298–1588)

Australia
Blackwell Scientific Publications
(Australia) Pty Ltd
54 University Street
Carlton, Victoria 3053
(*Orders*: Tel: 03 347–0300)

ISBN 0–632–03055–0

Contents

Coronary syndromes

Arrhythmias and sudden death

Late management, therapeutic approach

Epidemiological aspects

Preface

Ischaemic heart disease is a plague of our times and a scourge of industrialized society. It is essential that knowledge arising from the extensive research into the cause, development and treatment of the condition be passed on to a wider forum. Therefore, we have taken the opportunity of presenting some of the more recent advances in this field, covering a wide spectrum from the ischaemic cell to manifest ischaemic heart disease.

Naturally, as the editors are from Denmark and Norway many of the contributions originate from these countries. However, a number of Swedish authors have been kind enough to write about subjects in which they are particularly knowledgeable. Associate professor *Karl Swedberg*, M.D. has willingly helped in arranging contributions from Sweden.

We would like to thank *Niels-Bo Jensen*, M.Sc. and *C. N. Harris*, B.Sc, Ph.D. for their assistance. Without the assistance and financial support of Astra Cardiovascular Denmark, we would have been unable to publish this book.

Kristian Thygesen *John Kjekshus*

Contributors

Henning Rud Andersen, M.D., Department of Cardiology, Skejby University Hospital, Aarhus.

Kai Andersen, M.D., Head of Department of Clinical Physiology, Haukeland Hospital, University of Bergen, Bergen.

Harald Arnesen, M.D., Head of Department of Medicine, Ullevål Hospital, Oslo.

Jens Peder Bagger, M.D., Lecturer, Department of Cardiology, Skejby University Hospital, Aarhus.

Petter C. Borchgrevink, M.D., Head of Department of Anaesthesiology, University Hospital of Trondheim, Trondheim.

Hans Erik Bøtker, M.D., Department of Cardiology, Skejby University Hospital, Aarhus.

Peter Clemmensen, M.D., Department of Medicine and Cardiology, Rigshospitalet, University of Copenhagen, Copenhagen.

Ragnar Danielsen, M.D., Department of Clinical Physiology, Haukeland Hospital, University of Bergen, Bergen.

Kenneth Egstrup, M.D., Lecturer, Department of Clinical Physiology, Odense University Hospital, Odense.

Gunnar Erikssen, M.D., Department of Clinical Physiology, Ullevål Hospital, Oslo.

Jan Erikssen, M.D., Head of Department of Medicine, Central Hospital of Akershus, Nordbyhagen.

Erling Falk, M.D., Associate Professor, Institute of Forensic Medicine, Odense University, Odense.

Ole Færgeman, M.D., Associate Professor, Head of Department of Medicine and Cardiology, Aarhus County and University Hospital, Aarhus.

Niels Gadsbøl, M.D., Department of Medicine and Cardiology, Rigshospitalet, University of Copenhagen, Copenhagen.

Willie Gerhardt, M.D., Head of Department of Clinical Chemistry, Helsingborg Hospital, Helsingborg.

John Godtfredsen, M.D., Head of Section of Cardiology, Herlev Hospital, University of Copenhagen, Copenhagen.

Peer Grande, M.D., Department of Medicine and Cardiology, Rigshospitalet, University of Copenhagen, Copenhagen.

Gotfried Greve, M.D., Department of Anatomy, University of Bergen, Bergen.

Ketil Grong, M.D., Associate Professor, Surgical Research Laboratory, Haukeland Hospital, University of Bergen, Bergen.

Torben Haghfelt, M.D., Associate Professor, Head of Department of Cardiology, Odense University Hospital, Odense.

Stig Haunsø, M.D., Professor, Head of Department of Medicine and Cardiology, Rigshospitalet, University of Copenhagen, Copenhagen.

Per Henningsen, M.D., Professor, Head of Department of Cardiology, Skejby University Hospital, Aarhus.

Steen Elkjær Husted, M.D., Lecturer, Department of Cardiology, Skejby University Hospital, Aarhus.

Poul Flemming Høilund-Carlsen, M.D., Head of Section of Clinical Physiology, Holbæk Central Hospital, Holbæk.

Mogens Hørder, M.D., Professor, Head of Department of Clinical Chemistry, Odense University Hospital, Odense.

Gorm Jensen, M.D., Head of Department of Medicine, Section of Cardiology, Hvidovre Hospital, University of Copenhagen, Copenhagen.

Harald G. Jodalen, M.D., Department of Anatomy, University of Bergen, Bergen.

Karl-Arne Johannessen, M.D., Department of Clinical Physiology, Haukeland Hospital, University of Bergen, Bergen.

Per Jynge, M.D., Professor, Department of Pharmacology and Toxicology, University of Trondheim, Trondheim.

John Kjekshus, M.D., Head of Department of Medicine and Cardiology, Baerum Hospital, Oslo.

Ib Christian Klausen, M.D., Department of Medicine and Cardiology, Aarhus County and University Hospital, Aarhus.

Synnøve Fønnebø Knutsen, M.D., Department of Medicine, University Hospital of Tromsø, Tromsø.

Ole Kromann, M.D., Head of Department of Cardiovascular Surgery, Skejby University Hospital, Aarhus.

Jon Lekven, M.D., Professor, Surgical Research Laboratory, Haukeland Hospital, University of Bergen, Bergen.

Erling Birk Madsen, M.D., Lecturer, Department of Medicine and Cardiology, Rigshospitalet, University of Copenhagen, Copenhagen.

Jan Kyst Madsen, M.D., Lecturer, Department of Medicine and Cardiology, Rigshospitalet, University of Copenhagen, Copenhagen.

John Gunnar Mæland, M.D., Associate Professor, Research Center for Health Promotion, Environment and Lifestyle, University of Bergen, Bergen.

Mogens Møller, M.D., Director of Department of Cardiology, Odense University Hospital, Odense.

Hans Kræmmer Nielsen, M.D., Lecturer, Department of Cardiology, Skejby University Hospital, Aarhus.

Torsten Toftegaard Nielsen, M.D., Lecturer, Head of Department of Cardiology, Skejby University Hospital, Aarhus.

Jan Erik Nordrehaug, M.D., Department of Medicine, Cardiology Section, Haukeland Hospital, University of Bergen, Bergen.

Peter Kildeberg Paulsen, M.D., Professor, Head of Department of Cardiovascular Surgery, Skejby University Hospital, Aarhus.

Terje R. Pedersen, M.D., Head of Department of Medicine, Cardiac Division, Aker Hospital, Oslo.

Peter Pless, M.D., Department of Cardiology, Odense University Hospital, Odense.

Klaus Rasmussen, M.D., Head of Department of Cardiology, Aalborg Hospital, Aalborg.

Jan Ravkilde, M.D., Department of Medicine and Cardiology, Aarhus County and University Hospital, Aarhus.

Åsmund Reikvam, M.D., Head of Department of Medicine, Central Hospital of Sogn and Fjordane, Førde.

Svein Rotevatn, M.D., Associate Professor, Department of Anatomy, University of Bergen, Bergen.

Kari I. Saunamäki, M.D., Head of Laboratory of Cardiology, Rigshospitalet, University of Copenhagen, Copenhagen.

Pål Smith, M.D., Department of Cardiology, Ullevål Hospital, Oslo.

Jesper Hastrup Svendsen, M.D., Department of Medicine and Cardiology, Rigshospitalet, University of Copenhagen, Copenhagen.

Karl Swedberg, M.D., Associate Professor, Head of Department of Medicine, Section of Cardiology, Östra Hospital, Gothenburg University, Gothenburg.

Erik Thaulow, M.D., Head of Department of Clinical Physiology, Ullevål Hospital, Oslo.

Per Thayssen, M.D., Lecturer, Head of Department of Cardiology, Odense University Hospital, Odense.

Dag S. Thelle, M.D., Professor, National Health Screening Service, Oslo.

Anne Rahbek Thomassen, M.D., Lecturer, Department of Medicine and Cardiology, Aarhus County and University Hospital, Aarhus.

Poul Erik Bloch Thomsen, M.D., Associate Professor, Head of Department of Cardiology, Skejby University Hospital, Aarhus.

Kristian Thygesen, M.D., Associate Professor, Head of Department of Medicine and Cardiology, Aarhus County and University Hospital, Aarhus.

Jarle Vaage, M.D., Professor, Head of Department of Surgery, Division of Thoracic and Cardiovascular Surgery, University Hospital of Tromsø, Tromsø.

Edvardas Varnauskas, M.D., Professor, Head of Cardiology Division, Sahlgrenska Hospital, Gothenburg University, Gothenburg.

Lars Wallentin, M.D., Associate Professor, Head of Department of Medicine, Division of Cardiology, University Hospital of Linköping, Linköping.

Jørgen Westby, M.D., Surgical Research Laboratory, Haukeland Hospital, University of Bergen, Bergen.

Knut Westlund, M.D., Professor, Institute of Community Medicine, University of Tromsø, Tromsø.

Kirsti Ytrehus, M.D., Associate Professor, Department of Physiology, Institute of Medical Biology, University of Tromsø, Tromsø.

Coronary flow and myocardial perfusion

1

Myocardial blood flow regulation

STIG HAUNSØ,
JESPER HASTRUP SVENDSEN

Anatomy and function of the coronary circulation

The normal coronary system can, in simplified terms, be described as 1) *large epicardial* vessels that normally offer little intrinsic resistance to myocardial flow, 2) *intramyocardial arteries and arterioles* (10-200 μm) that due to their small diameter and a media layer packed with smooth muscle cells have the capacity to alter profoundly the resistance to coronary flow, 3) a high density network of *capillary vessels* (5 μm) which is uniform throughout the left ventricular wall, and 4) *native* thin-walled *collaterals* which link the large conduit vessels to each other. The ratio of capillaries to muscle fibres is very close to 1:1 and the intercapillary distance is about 15 μm (1). There are twice as many venous as arterial channels and they interconnect far more than the arterials. The coronary arteries are well innervated by autonomic nerves and fine unmyelinated nerve fibres running in close association with the coronary vessels, and naked varicose nerve endings are often seen close to capillaries (2).

The function of the coronary circulation is to supply the continuously working, energy demanding myocardium with oxygen and nutrients and eliminate waste products. This is done 1) *by convection,* i.e., by the movement of blood and its containing substances through the capillaries and 2) *by diffusion*, i.e., the movement of substances across the capillary wall and through the interstitium or vice versa along a concentration gradient. The exchange of oxygen and nutrients between blood and myocytes during normal conditions is a quite fast process probably because of a relatively large capillary surface area available for diffusion, short diffusion distances, and a relatively high level of concentration gradient from blood to myocytes.

Relationship between myocardial metabolism and blood flow

The myocardium relies on an ability to increase myocardial blood flow (MBF) during increased metabolic demand since it cannot sustain an oxygen debt and has a very high oxygen extraction, resulting in a coronary venous oxygen saturation in the range of 20-30% (3). This unusual, close and parallel relationship between myocardial metabolism and blood flow is described by the equation:

$$MVO_2 = (A-V)O_2 \times MBF$$

where MVO_2 represents the total myocardial oxygen uptake primarily determined by wall stress, contractility and heart rate (4). The arterio-venous oxygen difference, $(A-V)O_2$, is near maximum at rest. MBF can be increased from about 100 $ml \times (100g \times min)^{-1}$ to about 300-400 $ml \times (100g \times min)^{-1}$.

The moment to moment regulation of local myocardial blood flow in response to changing metabolic needs is a function of the intramural resistance vessels. The influence of arteriolar resistance and driving pressure on myocardial flow can be defined by the equation:

$$Q = \Delta P/R$$

where Q is blood flow, ΔP is the driving pressure across the coronary vascular bed (usually considered to be the difference between aortic and right atrial pressure), and R is the coronary arteriolar resistance (4).

Relationship between coronary vascular tone and perfused capillaries

A secondary effect of dilatation of resistance vessels is opening (perfusion) of previously non-perfused capillaries, called *capillary recruitment*. Such a response, demonstrated in canine myocardium (5, 6), improves the supply of substrates to the myocardium, since this is mainly accomplished by diffusive processes. It also allows a larger regional oxygen extraction without a substantial change in overall vascular resistance.

In ischaemic heart disease, a special problem is present, dealing with spatial as well as transmural local area with 1) low capillary density (i.e., *derecruitment)*, 2) increased inter-capillary distance because of low perfusion pressure and blood flow, and 3) interstitial fibrosis. Under these circumstances transport of oxygen and nutrients by diffusion may be too slow to meet the variations in local metabolic demand.

Distribution of coronary blood flow across the free left ventricular wall

Experimental evidence is accumulating that the contracting left ventricle uses energy unevenly, with the subendocardial layers using more per unit weight (7, 8). Electron microscopy has demonstrated that subendocardial sarcomeres are longer in diastole and shorten more in systole than subepicardial fibres, an indication of greater subendocardial work and energy demand (7, 8). The observed lower oxygen tension of blood in the subendocardial veins and tissue compared to that of the subepicardial veins and tissue is likely to be due to an increased oxygen extraction by the subendocardial tissue which in turn may be due to a greater work and a marked underperfusion during systole (9, 10). Due to compressive forces from myocardial contractility during systole, perfusion of the subendocardial layers decreases or ceases. During diastole an excess of blood flow is directed to this layer making the left ventricular free wall of the myocardium homogeneously perfused during a cardiac cycle. Consequently blood flow to the inner layers of the left ventricle is strongly related to the diastolic perfusion pressure and the duration of diastole (4, 10, 11).

Coronary reactive hyperaemia

When an epicardial coronary artery is transiently occluded, perfusion pressure is reduced to a minimum and the myocardium distally to the occluded artery becomes ischaemic. Intramural resistance vessels dilate within a few seconds of ischaemia. When the occlusion is released, perfusion pressure rises rapidly to the pre-ischaemic blood pressure level and local MBF increases with a factor 3 to 4 and then gradually returns to pre-occlusive values. This phenomenon of *reactive hyperaemia* has been used in several experimental approaches to study factors determining coronary vascular tone (12-14). Such data have gained from quantification of the reactive hyperaemia by measurement of maximum blood flow (MBFmax) and cumulative excess blood flow ($V_B$excess) during hyperaemia and repayment of flow debt following periods of vascular occlusion.

In man and in canine myocardium, MBFmax during reactive hyperaemia increases with increasing length of vascular occlusion up to about 20 seconds (Fig. 1 A). Prolongation of ischaemia does not increase maximum blood flow any further, indicating that the resistance vessels in the coronary vascular bed are maximally dilated following about 20 seconds of ischaemia. The cumulative excess blood flow ($V_B$excess) in the myocardium increases with increasing duration of the occlusion time, but the increment in $V_B$excess per

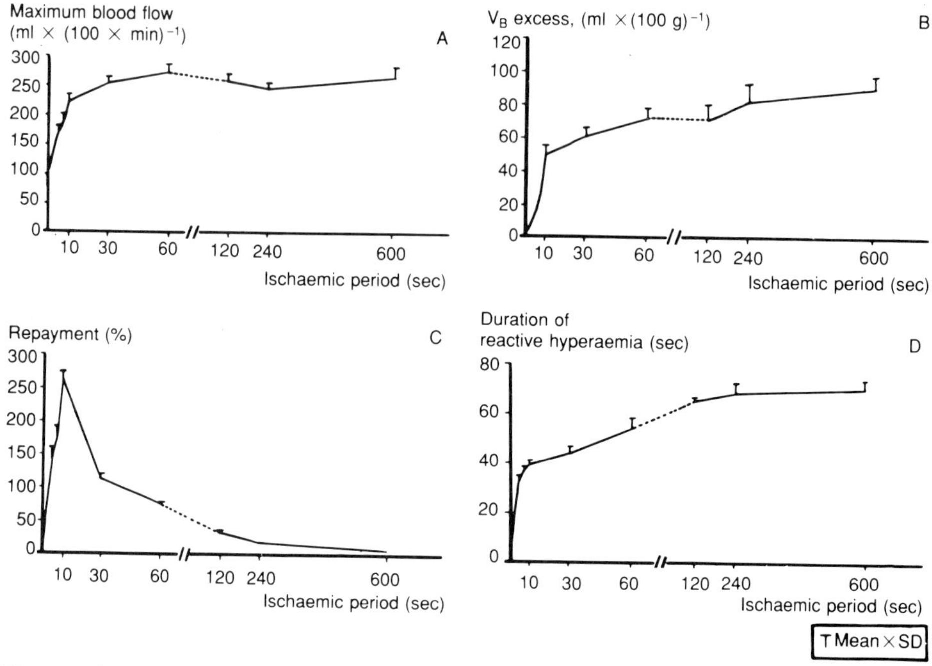

Fig. 1. *The relationship between the duration of regional myocardial ischaemia (x-axis) and a) maximum myocardial blood flow rate (Fig. A), b)* V_B*excess (i.e., the integral of blood flow during the reactive hyperaemic period minus the integrated preocclusive blood flow in a period which equals the duration of the reactive hyperaemia (in: ml* $\times$ *100g*$^{-1}$*)) (Fig. B), c) repayment (Fig. C) and d) the duration of reactive hyperaemia (Fig. D), respectively (from reference 14).*

unit extension of the occlusion time declined considerably (Fig. 1 B). These events of maximum blood flow and $V_B$excess may be due to accumulation of vasodilator metabolites in the tissue, approaching an upper concentration with increasing duration of occlusion time. These metabolites are eliminated during hyperaemia by washout, cellular uptake and/or metabolic conversion at a concentration dependent rate (14, 15).

The high value of repayment, about 300% (Fig. 1 C), found in the canine myocardium and human hearts (14) has not yet been clarified. In other tissues, metabolic repayment of flow debt does not exceed about 100% (16). It is suggested that the high value for repayment following brief coronary occlusions displays a fast rate of accumulation of vasodilator metabolites shortly after an occlusion, an accumulation that may be enhanced in the post-occlusion period by the transient increase in contractility force in the myocardium induced by ischaemia of short duration (17, 18).

A myogenic response of the smooth muscle cells in the coronary resistance vessels may play a role in the over-payment of flow debt, at least following very short periods of vascular occlusion. However, in the in-vivo working heart this response is difficult to separate from the metabolic mechanisms.

On the other hand, it is possible that vasodilator metabolites are formed at a reduced rate as myocardial contraction in the ischaemic area ceases when the arterial occlusion exceeds a certain duration (Fig. 2) (18). If this holds true, it may at least contribute to the marked fall in repayment observed with increasing duration of ischaemia above some 60 seconds as illustrated in Fig. 1 C. Thus, the magnitude of reactive hyperaemia in the myocardium demonstrates a prompt and profound metabolic mechanism for regulation of MBF. Furthermore, the observation that $V_B$excess increases considerably more in the subendocardial layer than in the subepicardial layer following more than 40-60 seconds of ischaemia (Fig. 3) strongly suggests a local metabolic control of the resistance vessels in the left ventricular free wall (19).

Autoregulation of myocardial blood flow in the left ventricle

Changes in coronary vascular resistance are the basis for the phenomenon of autoregulation: the dynamic process of keeping the myocardial blood flow constant despite abrupt changes in arterial perfusion pressure. According to the metabolic hypothesis described above, MBF and tissue metabolism are tightly coupled in such a way that any reduction in arterial inflow causes a temporary hypoxia and a build-up of vasodilator metabolites in the tissue. The resistance vessels will then dilate and blood flow is restored to a

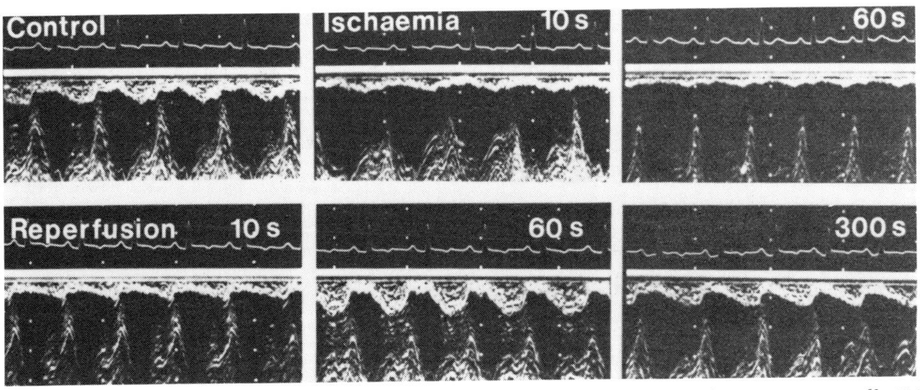

Fig. 2. *Epicardial echocardiographic recording of the left ventricular anterior wall (50 mm×sec⁻¹) in dog experiments with 120 sec of regional myocardial ischaemia. At 10 sec of ischaemia impaired wall motion is noticed and at 60 sec systolic thinning is observed. Hyperkinetic wall thickening is visualised following 60 sec of reperfusion and return to pre-occlusive amplitude of systolic thickening is seen at 300 sec of reperfusion (from reference 18).*

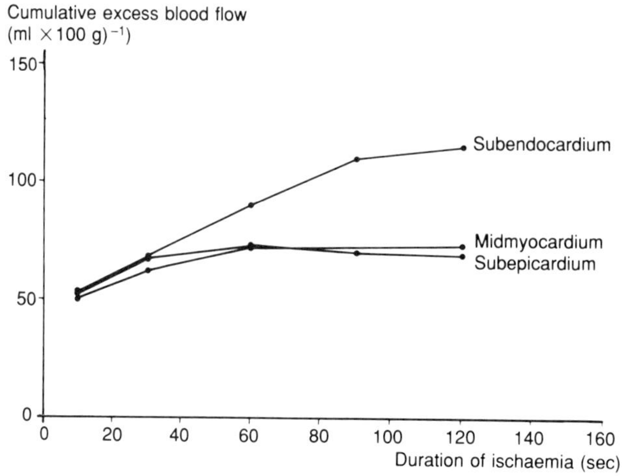

Fig. 3. *Dependence of cumulative excess blood flow on duration of ischaemia, in the subendocardial, midmyocardial and subepicardial layers of the canine myocadium (from reference 19).*

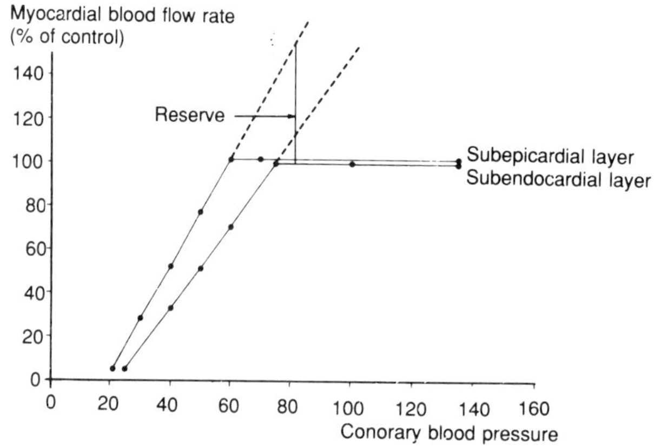

Fig. 4. *Autoregulation in the left ventricle of the dog heart. The ordinate gives blood flow expressed as per cent flow during unrestricted control conditions. The abscissa shows the mean pressure in the left anterior descending coronary artery distally to the site of constriction (from reference 10).*

value very near to that of a higher pressure level. One way of demonstrating this is shown in Fig. 4, which diagrammatically presents the results of experiments in which myocardial blood flow in the subepicardial and the corresponding subendocardial layers of the left ventricular free wall were measured by the local ^{133}Xenon washout method (10). Left ventricular pressure and cardiac work are kept constant and coronary perfusion pressure is varied. When regional coronary artery blood pressure is lowered from its normal value of 100 mmHg, the two horizontal lines show that steady state flow remains constant in the two layers until a mean pressure of about 75 mmHg. A reduction in perfusion pressure to 60-74 mmHg induced a significant reduction in blood flow to the subendocardium by about 32%, whereas blood flow remained unchanged in the epicardial layers. When perfusion pressure was lowered further, myocardial blood flow was decreased significantly, indicating that vasodilation of the resistance vessels can no longer compensate for a decreased pressure. This event occurs first in the inner layers of the left ventricle, i.e., the lower end of the autoregulatory range is reached and the resistance vessels are maximally dilated while there is still some vasodilator reserve of the vessels in the mid- and subepicardial layers. Similarly, raising the perfusion pressure does not alter MBF until a pressure of about 140 mmHg (9, 10).

The oblique, dashed lines to the left of the autoregulatory lines in Fig. 4 are the pressure-flow relationships when the resistance vessels in subepicardial and subendocardial layers are maximally dilated. The vertical distance between the autoregulated and maximally vasodilated curves at any perfusion pressure is a measure of the reserve for further vasodilation (9).

The vulnerability of the subendocardial region to decreased perfusion pressure may be due to the above mentioned inhomogeneity of the compressive pressure exerted upon intramyocardial vessels during myocardial contraction (9). This vulnerability of the inner layers of the left ventricle to ischaemia and necrosis is a well-known clinical observation both when coronary arteries are normal and when they are narrowed by atheroma. It is enhanced in severe left ventricular hypertrophy as seen in patients with hypertension and aortic stenosis (9, 20).

Determinants of coronary vascular tone

The major factors regulating coronary vascular tone and thereby MBF are illustrated in Fig. 5. The main determinant of this delicate regulation is

Metabolic factors
Adenosine (–)
ATP (–)
O_2 (+)
CO_2 (–)
H^+ (–)
K^+ (–)

Neural factors
Sympathetic nervous system
α-receptor stimulation (+)
β-receptor stimulation (–)
Vagus (–)
Central control and reflex control (+/–)
Neuropeptide Y (+)
Calcitonin gene-related peptide (–)

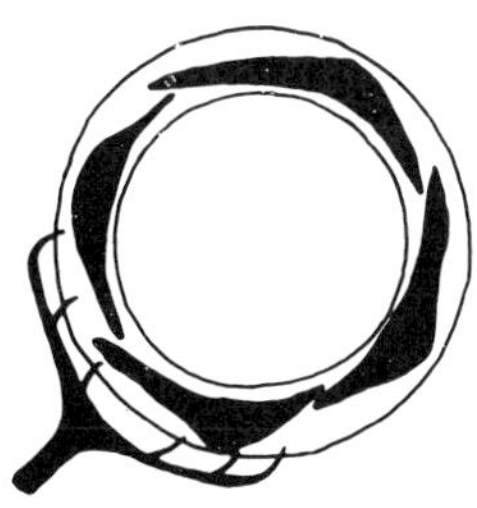

Humoral factors
Catecholamines (+)
Angiotensin (+)
Thyroid hormones (+)
Antidiuretic hormone (+)

Endothelial factors
Prostaglandins (–)
EDRF (–)
Endothelin (+)

Myogenic factor
?

Miscellaneous
Tromboxane (+)
Serotonin (+)

Symbols for effects:
(+) vasoconstriction
(–) vasodilatation

Fig. 5. *Determinants of coronary vascular tone.*

the metabolic mechanism. Neural control, humoral regulation, and the endothelial factors are of intermediate importance. The myogenic mechanism remains unproven. Of the physical factors that influence MBF, blood viscosity is of minor importance. Extravascular compression during contraction can alter MBF, however, particularly in respect of the distribution of blood flow across the left ventricular free wall as earlier described. Physical factors as well as small increases in sympathetic tone may have considerable effects on myocardial blood flow in the presence of a severe stenotic lesion in an epicardial coronary artery.

Mediators of metabolic regulation of MBF

Several "metabolic" mediators have been suggested as being the link between increased metabolic activity and increased MBF: adenosine, ATP, oxygen, carbon dioxide, pH, potassium, calcium, and osmolality. The most important of these substances will be discussed below.

Adenosine and adenine nucleotides

ATP and ADP are equipotent as coronary vasodilators and about 4 times more effective than AMP and adenosine. Adenosine can readily cross cell membranes and has a very short life time in blood ($T_{1/2}$ at 37°C: 10 sec). Consequently, adenosine produced by degradation of ATP within the ischaemic myocyte can reach the coronary vasculature. Adenosine induces a dose-dependent increase in MBF (21). A close parallelism between MBF, adenosine release (from tissue to blood), and myocardial adenosine content with changes in perfusate oxygen content have been demonstrated in isolated guinea pig hearts (22). Dipyridamole, which blocks re-uptake of released adenosine, potentiates the vasodilator effect of adenosine (23, 24). Thus, adenosine appears to play a major role in the metabolic control of coronary resistance vessels. Despite the higher vasodilatory effect of ATP, this substance cannot cross the cell membranes, and its physiological importance on vascular tone is therefore probably minimal.

Oxygen, carbon dioxide, pH and potassium

Hypoxia, below a certain limit, induces coronary vasodilation and an inverse relationship between MBF and coronary venous oxygen levels (6, 25). The effect of oxygen on smooth muscle cells in the resistance vessels is believed to be indirect, through an action on the myocytes with release of vasoactive mediators.

Hypercapnia in the dog heart seems to decrease the coronary vascular resistance (26) and hypocapnia increased the vascular resistance (27). Whether this effect is direct or indirect remains unproven. The effect of a decrease in pH induces a moderate coronary vasodilation. Furthermore, decreasing pH can enhance the vasodilator effect of adenosine (28).

Although potassium ions can modulate coronary resistance, the interstitial concentration that accompanies alterations in myocardial metabolism seems inadequate to explain the accompanying alterations in coronary vascular resistance (29).

Neural factors regulating coronary vascular tone

Autonomic nervous system

Coronary arteries have α-1, α-2, β-1 and β-2 receptors. Isolated strips of large and small canine coronary arteries have shown different responses to catecholamines indicating a predominance of β-receptors in the smaller arteries and an equal distribution of α- and β-receptors in the larger arteries (30). Stimulation of the cardiac sympathetic nerves (ganglion stellate) elicits coronary vasodilation, increased heart rate and contractility. Several experimental studies have been performed to assess if increased MBF was a direct effect of sympathetic nervous stimulation or an indirect effect to increased metabolic demand. Sympathetic stimulation seems to induce a very early decrease in MBF (activation of alpha-l receptors) before any changes in heart rate and contractility followed by a profound coronary vasodilation. This biphasic response occurs because direct metabolic coronary vasodilation after a few seconds completely overrides the direct vasoconstrictor effect of alpha-l receptor stimulation (31).

Stimulation of the vagus nerve and intracoronary infusion of acetylcholine both produce a small to moderate increase in MBF (32). Thus, the physiological role of the autonomic nervous system on regulation of MBF is probably modest.

Central control and reflexes

Stimulation of the lateral hypothalamus can induce an increase in coronary vascular resistance. The injection of the opiate antagonist fentanyl, into the lateral ventricles of dogs also induces coronary vasoconstriction which may be mediated by vasopressin. These results indicate that a central mechanism is indeed operating although its quantitative importance in regulating MBF is still unknown.

Four reflexes influence coronary vascular tone: 1) the baroreceptor reflex, 2) the chemoreceptor reflex, 3) the pulmonary inflation reflex and 4) the Bezold-Jarisch reflex (33). The baroreceptor reflex is mediated to the coronary arteries through the cardiac sympathetic nerve fibres, whereas the chemoreceptor reflex communicates to the coronary vessels through both cardiac sympathetic and parasympathetic fibres. The pulmonary inflation reflex, which is actually a component of the chemoreceptor reflex, mediates an increased MBF by hyperinflation of the lungs. The increase in MBF is caused by inhibition of alpha adrenergic tone on the coronary resistance vessels. The Bezold-Jarish reflex, which is a coronary-to-periphery directed reflex, is characterized by reflex hypotension and bradycardia. Experimental data suggest that this reflex operates during coronary occlusion, although further investigations of the significance of the reflex during myocardial ischaemia in the human heart are needed.

Neuropeptide Y and calcitonin gene-related peptide

Neuropeptide Y (NPY) is found in central and peripheral sympathetic neurones, often co-stored with norepinephrine. The NPY innervation of the coronary arteries is dense as compared with other organs. NPY is a potent vasoconstrictor in several organs including the myocardium (34). It has been demonstrated that exogenous NPY can decrease maximum blood flow and excess blood flow during reactive hyperaemia to a significant extent (35). The effect seems more pronounced on intramyocardial arterioles than epicardial arteries (35).

Calcitonin gene-related peptide (CGRP) like NPY is a 37 aminoacid neuropeptide present in the central nervous system and in nerve fibres in blood vessels of several organs including the heart. The presence of CGRP in vascular walls and its co-location with substance P, a neurokinin with potent vascular effects, suggests a role in regulating vascular tone. In the porcine heart CGRP has been shown to have pronounced vasodilator effects (34, 36).

Humoral factors regulating vascular tone

Catecholamines, thyroid hormones, angiotensin, antidiuretic hormone all have vasoconstrictor effects on coronary vessels (37). Knowledge of this effect on MBF is of clinical importance in the treatment of cardiogenic shock and dysfunction of endocrine glands, especially with concomitant ischaemic heart disease.

Endothelial factors regulating vascular tone

Previously, the endothelial lining of the vasculature was considered a passive barrier interposed between the blood and the interstitial space. But within the last 15 years the endothelial cell is considered to be a "pluripotent cell" able to synthesize and secrete a number of substances. These substances include several that can modify the tone of the coronary resistance vessels (38).

Prostaglandins (PG; Prostacyclin), formed from arachidonic acid, have a half-life in plasma of 1-2 min. PG are released from endothelial cells both to the luminal (blood) side of the cell and to the abluminal side of neighbouring smooth muscle cells in the arterioles. The vasodilator effects of PG are mediated through the second messenger cyclic AMP. PG have an anti-aggregatory effect on platelets in addition to the effect on the coronary vessels (39). PG are released from myocardium subjected to hypoxia and the reactive hyperaemic response following hypoxia is attenuated by prior administration of indomethacin, a potent inhibitor of prostaglandin synthesis.

The conflicting results from previous studies concerning the effect of vasoactive substances during in-vitro and in-vivo experimental conditions can be partly explained by the existence of an *endothelial derived relaxing factor (EDRF)* (40). EDRF has a half-life of only a few seconds. Several forms of EDRF may exist, of which one is the simple compound nitric oxide (NO). Canine and porcine arteries release at least one EDRF that is not NO. EDRF induces vasodilation through the same second messenger as that for organic nitrates, i.e., cyclic AMP, and can therefore be said to be an endogenous nitrate. EDRF and PG can interact synergistically to cause pronounced vasodilation. Dietary fish oil has been shown to increase the production of EDRF in normal and in atherosclerotic porcine arteries (40).

In 1988 it was discovered that endothelial cells produced a 21-aminoacid peptide called *endothelin* (41). This peptide is the most potent naturally occurring vasoconstricting substance known. Its physiological importance with regard to regulation of vascular tone remains to be elucidated.

The coronary collateral circulation

The collateral circulation of the heart is of vital importance in protecting and maintaining viable myocardium in local areas of the heart. The thin-walled *native* collaterals have a resistance to blood flow several times higher than the minimal resistance of the normal coronary vessels. The amount of blood carried by these small vessels is therefore insufficient to prevent ischaemia or necrosis in case of acute occlusion of a larger coronary artery. *Mature or developed* coronary collaterals can be quite large-lumen, thick-walled vessels which under ideal conditions have a maximal flow of about 60% of what can be achieved in the normal coronary vasculature (42). The development of such collaterals is a slow process induced by ischaemia due to progressive narrowing of a major coronary artery. As for normal microvessels, blood flow through collaterals occurs almost entirely during diastole (43), except in the superficial (epicardial) collaterals, since myocardial systole compresses these small vessels (44). The rate of flow is also dependent on the pressure gradient between the two ends of the collateral vessel. It is therefore difficult to separate effects of vasoactive drugs on collaterals per se versus the proximal and the distal vasculature when measurements of blood flow are employed. The flow potentials of most collaterals in the human heart are adequate for regional myocardial function at lower myocardial work but are clearly inadequate for most, if not all, conditions of increased demand.

Summary

A substantial knowledge of the mechanism regulating myocardial blood flow is available from experimental studies, whereas data from the human heart are relatively sparse at present. New technology such as Positron Emission Tomography (PET) has the impact of performing noninvasive studies of regional blood flow and metabolism in the same unit of tissue mass. Such studies have already supported some of the experimental data and will in the future undoubly bring new insight in the pathophysiology of ischaemic heart disease (45).

In conclusion, myocardial blood flow is regulated by numerous extrinsic and intrinsic factors as presented above. A local metabolic mechanism is the major determinant of the tone in the smooth muscle cells of the resistance vessels. In fact, changes in myocardial metabolism produce changes in MBF that completely override other regulatory factors.

References

1. Honig CR, Bourdeau-Martini J. Extravascular component of oxygen transport in normal and hypertrophied hearts with special reference to oxygen therapy. Circ Res 1974; 34-5 (suppl. II): 97-103.

2. Abraham A. Microscopic innervation of the heart and blood vessels in vertebrates including man. New York, Pergamon, 1969.
3. Bache RJ, Dymek DJ. Local and regional regulation of coronary vascular tone. Progr Cardiovasc Dis 1981; 24: 191-211.
4. Klocke FJ, Mates RE, Copley DP, Orlick AE. Physiology of the coronary circulation in health and coronary artery disease. In: Yu PN, Goodwin JF, eds. Progress in cardiology. Philadelphia: Lea & Febiger, 1976.
5. Rose PC, Goresky CA, Bélanger P, Chen M-J. Effect of vasodilation and flow rate on capillary permeability surface product and interstitial space size in the coronary circulation. Circ Res 1980; 47: 312-28.
6. Haunsø S. Effects of regional hypoxia and blood flow on capillary permeability in canine myocardium. Acta Physiol Scand 1982; 114: 59-65.
7. Gamble WJ, LaFarge CG, Fyler DC, Weisul J, Monroe RG. Regional coronary venous oxygen saturation and myocardial oxygen tension following abrupt changes in ventricular pressure in the isolated dog heart. Circ Res 1974; 34: 672-81.
8. Weiss HR, Neubauer JA, Lipp JA, Sinha AK. Quantitative determination of regional oxygen consumption in the dog heart. Circ Res 1978; 42: 394-401.
9. Hoffman JIE. A critical view of coronary reserve. Circulation 1987; 75 (suppl I): 1-6.
10. Haunsø S. Lower limits of blood flow autoregulation in different myocardial layers of the left ventricular free wall of dogs. Acta Physiol Scand 1981; 112; 349-50.
11. Bache RJ, Cobb FR, Greenfield JC. Effects of increased myocardial consumption on coronary reactive hyperaemia in the awake dog. Circ Res 1973; 33: 588-96.
12. Olsson RA. Myocardial reactive hyperaemia. Circ Res 1975; 37: 263-70.
13. Marcus M, Wright C, Doty D, et al. Measurements of coronary velocity and reactive hyperaemia in the coronary circulation of humans. Circ Res 1981; 49: 877-91.
14. Haunsø S & Amtorp O. Regional blood flow during reactive hyperaemia in canine myocardium as determined by local washout of Xenon-133. Acta Physiol Scand 1980; 110: 285-93.
15. Berne RM, Rubio R. Adenine nucleotide metabolism in the heart. Circ Res 1974; 34-35 (suppl. III): 109-18.
16. Kristensen JK, Henriksen O. Excess cumulative blood flow and repayment during reactive hyperaemia in human cutaneous tissue. Acta Physiol Scand 1980; 108: 1-6.
17. Theroux P, Franklin D, Ross J, Kemper WS. Regional myocardial function during acute coronary artery occlusion and its modification by pharmacological agents in the dog. Circ Res 1974; 35: 896-908.
18. Egeblad H, Haunsø S, Amtorp O. Regional dynamic behaviour of the canine myocardium following brief ischemia: wall thickness, wall thickening and blood flow. Cardiovasc Res 1982; 16: 249-55.
19. Haunsø S. Distribution of coronary blood flow across the canine left ventricular free wall during reactive hyperemia. Acta Physiol Scand 1981; 112: 225-32.
20. Strandgaard S, Haunsø S. Why does antihypertensive treatment prevent stroke but not myocardial infarction? Lancet 1987; ii: 658-61.
21. Schrader J, Haddy FJ, Gerlach E. Release of adenosine, inosine and hypoxia, flow-autoregulation and reactive hyperaemia. Phlügers Arch, Eur J Physiol 1977; 369: 1-6.
22. Rubio R, Wiedmeier VT, Berne RM. Relationship between coronary flow and adenosine production and release. J Moll Cell Cardiol 1974; 6: 561-66.
23. Stafford A. Potentiation of adenosine and the adenine nucleotides by dipyridamole. Br J Pharmacol 1966; 28: 218-27.
24. Nott MW. The possible role of adenosine in the coronary dilator action of some purimidopyrimidines and pteridines. Br J Pharmacol 1970; 39: 287-95.

25. Belloni FL, Sparks HV. Dynamics of myocardial oxygen consumption and coronary vascular resistance. Am J Physiol 1977; 233: H34-H43.
26. Case RB, Greenberg H, Moskowitz R. Alterations in coronary sinus pO_2 and O_2 saturation resulting from pCO_2 changes. Cardiovasc Res 1975; 9: 167-77.
27. Case RB, Felix A, Wachter M, Kyriakidis, Castellana F. Relative effect of CO_2 on canine coronary vascular resistance. Circ Res 1978; 42: 410-8.
28. Merrill GF, Haddy FJ, Dabney JM. Adenosine, theophylline, and perfusate pH in the isolated, perfused guinea pig heart. Circ Res 1978; 42: 225-9.
29. Kline RP, Morad M. Potassium efflux in heart muscle during activity: Extracelluar accumulation and its implications. J Physiol (Lond) 1978; 280; 537-58.
30. Zuberbuhler BC, Bohr DF. Responses of coronary smooth muscle to catecholamines. Circ Res 1965; 16: 431-40.
31. Granata L, Olsson RA, Huvos A, Gregg DE. Coronary inflow and oxygen usage following cardiac sympathetic nerve stimulation in unanesthetized dogs. Circ Res 1965; 16: 114-20.
32. Gross GJ, Buck JD, Warltier DC. Transmural distribution of blood flow during activation of coronary muscarinic receptors. Am J Physiol 1981; 240: H941-6.
33. Vatner SF, McRitchie RJ. Interaction of the chemoreflex and the pulmonary inflation reflex in the regulation of coronary circulation in conscious dogs. Circ Res 1975; 37: 644-73.
34. Wharton J, Gulbenkian S. Peptides in the mammalian cardiovascular system. Experimenta 1987; 43: 821-32.
35. Svendsen JH, Sheik SP, Jørgensen J, et al. Neuropeptide Y modulates regional blood flow in canine myocardium during reactive hyperaemia. J Moll Cell Cardiol 1989; 21 (suppl. II): 105 (abstr).
36. Ezra D, Laurindo FRM, Goldstein DS, Goldstein RE, Feuerstein G. Calcitonin gene related peptide: a potent modulator of coronary flow. Eur J Pharmacol 1987; 137: 101-5.
37. Marcus ML. Humoral control of the coronary circulation. In: The coronary circulation in health and disease. New York: McGraw-Hill, 1982, 15-190.
38. Thilo-Korner DGS, Freshney RJ. The endothelial cell – a pluripotent control cell of the vessel wall. Basel: Karger, 1983.
39. Moncada S, Vane JR. Arachidonic acid metabolites and the interactions between platelets and blood-vessel walls. N Engl J Med 1979; 300: 1142-7.
40. Vanhoutte PM, Shimokawa H. Endothelium-derived relaxing factor and coronary vasospasm. Circulation 1989; 80: 1-9.
41. Yanagisawa M, Kurihara H, Kimura S, et al. A novel potent vasoconstrictor peptide produced by vascular endothelial cells. Nature 1988; 332: 411-5.
42. Lambert PR, Hess DS, Bache RJ. Effect of exercise on perfusion of collateral-dependent myocardium in dogs with chronic coronary artery occlusion. J Clin Invest 1977; 59: 1-7.
43. Brown BG, Gundel WD, Gott VL, Covell JW. Coronary collateral flow following acute coronary occlusion: a diastolic phenomenon. Cardiovasc Res 1974; 8: 621-31.
44. Russell RE, Chagrasulis RW, Downey JM. Inhibitory effect of cardiac contraction on coronary collateral blood flow. Am J Physiol 1977; 233: H541-6.
45. Schelbert HR. Myocardial ischemia and clinical applications of positron emission tomography. Am J Cardiol 1989; 64: 46E-53E.

2

The dynamic coronary artery obstruction

KLAUS RASMUSSEN

Introduction

A hundred years ago it was suggested that coronary vasoconstriction might be a pathogenetic mechanism in angina pectoris (1). This hypothesis was rejected in this century when angina pectoris and acute myocardial infarction (AMI) became related to coronary atherosclerosis by autopsy studies (2, 3). However, in 1959 Prinzmetal et al suggested that variant angina was caused by increased coronary arterial tone in a vessel with an atherosclerotic lesion (4). This theory was accepted in the 1970s (5). In 1978 Maseri et al showed that coronary arterial spasm or increased coronary tone was a pathogenetic mechanism not only in variant angina, but in a broad spectrum of patients with ischaemic heart disease (6).

In the 1980s basic experimental studies increased our understanding of the cellular and molecular mechanisms of normal and abnormal vasoconstriction, with Furchgott's discovery of endothelial derived vascular relaxant factor (EDRF) as one of the most important contributions (7).

This chapter reviews the mechanisms of coronary vasomotion and some of its clinical aspects in ischaemic heart disease. The term "dynamic coronary obstruction" is used to denote any diffuse or localized vasoconstriction of an epicardial coronary artery that is of sufficient extent to cause myocardial ischaemia. A coronary artery stenosis is denoted "fixed" if it persists after the vessel has been dilated with nitroglycerin, and "significant" if it reduces the coronary diameter by at least 50%

The mechanisms of normal coronary vasomotion

Molecular mechanisms: The vascular tone is determined by the contractile state of the vascular smooth muscles. The contractile state is determined by the intracellular calcium-ion concentration (8).

Table 1. *Some endogenous stimuli influencing the tone of the epicardial coronary arteries.*

Increased tone	Decreased tone
	A. Directly acting
Sympathetic nerves (alfa-rec)	Sympathetic nerves (beta-rec)
Adrenaline (alfa-rec)	Adrenaline (beta-rec)
Noradrenaline (alfa-rec)	Noradrenaline (beta-rec)
Acetylcholine	AMP
Angiotensin II	Adenosine
Serotonine	Histamine (H2-rec)
Thromboxane A2	Prostacyclin
Histamine (H1-rec)	
Neuropeptide Y	*B. EDRF-releasers*
Vasopressin	Acetylcholine
Endothelin	Serotonine
Alkalosis	ATP, ADP
Hypercalcaemia	Histamine (H1-rec)
Hypomagnesaemia	Bradykinin
	Thrombin
	n3PUFA
	Vasoactive intestinal peptide
	Cholecystokinin

Abbreviation: rec = receptor, n3PUFA = n3-poly-unsaturated-fatty-acid,

Neural and humoral vasoconstrictive agents (Table 1) stimulate and open the voltage- or receptor-operated calcium channels of the sarcolemma, leading to flux of calcium-ions into the muscle cell from the extracellular space, where the concentration of this ion is 10.000 times higher, together with mobilisation of calcium-ions from intracellular stores (8). Intracellularly the calcium-ions combine with a regulator protein (calmodulin) which initiates a chain of events, leading to activation of the actomyosin ATPase and the interaction between actin and myosin that constitutes the smooth muscle contraction (8, 9).

Relaxation of vascular smooth muscle is achieved either by stimulation of receptors of the cell or stimulation of the endothelium, which leads to release of EDRF (Table 1). EDRF causes intracellular production of cyclic-GMP, and beta-agonists leading to production of cyclic-AMP and both cyclic substances are supposed to cause reduction of the intracellular calcium-ion concentration by extrusion of ions across the sarcolemma together with sequestration in the intracellular stores (10).

Endothelium: EDRF was discovered by Furchgott, who showed that acetylcholine caused relaxation of isolated rabbit aorta with intact endothelium, but lack of relaxation when the endothelium had been removed (7, 11). EDRF is constantly produced by intact endothelial cells as the result of mechanical stimulation (shear stress) by erythrocytes (10, 11). In addition, many endogenous agents cause EDRF-release (Table 1). The half-life of EDRF is a few seconds, the nature of this labile substance is as yet unknown, but several observations suggest it may be nitric oxide (10). Its action is inhibited by superoxide anions and haemoglobin. Thus, although EDRF is systemically released, it acts locally.

It is noteworthy that many agents have a dual influence on the coronary tone (table 1). Catecholamines cause vasoconstriction by stimulation of alfa-receptors and vasodilation by stimulation of beta-receptors (12, 13). Acetylcholine and serotonine have dual actions due to stimulation of both the smooth muscles and the endothelial cells. Histamine appears to have a triple action (Table 1).

The endothelial cell has in itself a dual influence on arterial tone, since it also produces endothelin, a peptide with pronounced vasoconstrictive activity of slow onset and long duration. In vitro studies have shown that endothelin produces vasoconstriction in human coronary arteries (14, 15).

Exercise: The relative importance of the many tone-regulating mechanisms in different physiologic conditions is incompletely understood. During dynamic muscular exercise increased coronary flow leads to increased EDRF-release due to increased sheer stress, which tends to cause vasodilation. However, this may be counter-balanced by increased concentration of circulating catecholamines that cause vasoconstriction due to alfa-receptor stimulation. Isometric exercise produces coronary vasoconstriction probably due to alfa-receptor stimulation (16), which may only be modestly counterbalanced by increased EDRF-release, since isometric exercise causes a little increase in coronary blood flow only (17).

Thus, the tone of the epicardial coronary arteries is the result of a balance between many opposing forces. This balance may readily be upset by pathological processes.

Pathogenesis of dynamic coronary obstruction

Animal experiments: In dogs and pigs local destruction of the coronary endothelium and high-cholesterol feeding of the animals produced coronary atherosclerotic lesions that showed enhanced in vivo vasoconstriction in response to intracoronary serotonine and histamine (18, 19). Thus, it appears that atherosclerosis may change the balance between constrictive and dilative forces in favour of constriction.

Angiographic observations: These experimental studies are in accordance with numerous clinical observations in European and American patients, showing significant, fixed coronary stenoses in about 70%-90% of patients with dynamic obstructions (20), Japanese patients appear to be an exception (21). Completely normal coronary arteries at angiography were found in only a few per cent of angina patients with dynamic coronary obstruction (22). Coronary angiography performed during spontaneous or provoked coronary vasoconstriction showed the most pronounced constriction usually to occur at the site of an atherosclerotic lesion (23). Thus, the relation between dynamic coronary obstruction and coronary atherosclerosis is well established.

Influence of atherosclerosis: This influence of atherosclerosis upon coronary vasomotion may be a result of impaired EDRF production by damaged endothelial cells and reduced production of prostacyclin by the vessel wall, but also local platelet aggregation at the site of damaged endothelium with release of thromboxane-A2 and serotonine may contribute (24). In isolated human coronary arteries impaired beta-receptor mediated relaxation was demonstrated in vessels with atherosclerosis (25). Mast cells, which were demonstrated to infiltrate a dynamic coronary lesion might also play a pathogenetic role due to release of histamine, prostaglandins, and leukotrienes (26). Neovascularization of atherosclerotic lesions by vasa vasorum, which was demonstrated in human hearts, might lead to local hypercontractility due to a higher concentration of circulating vasoconstrictors in atherosclerotic than in normal wall segments (27).

Geometric factors: Some stenoses may be dynamic due to simple geometric and hydraulic mechanisms. Due to the inverse relation between stenosis resistance and the fourth power of stenosis diameter a physiologic vasomotor reduction of diameter may be enough to cause a dramatic increase in resistance of very severe fixed stenoses (80%-90% diameter reduction). It was suggested that excentric lesions might be more prone to show dynamic behaviour than concentric ones (28). Excentric lesions were found in 70% of significant coronary stenoses (29).

Generalized mechanisms: Local mechanisms may not explain all clinical observations in patients with dynamic obstructions. Several authors demonstrated angiographically generalized coronary vasoconstriction in patients with coronary spasm (22, 23, 30). *Rasmussen* found increased coronary vasoconstriction even in those coronary vessels that were ischaemia-unrelated in angina patients with dynamic obstructions, which suggested the existence of generalized hypercontractility (20). A relation between coronary spasm and migraine and Raynaud's phenomenon was found by Miller et al (31). A relation to arterial hypertension was suggested by *Freedman's* finding of arterial hypertension in 37% of 47 patients with coronary spasm (32). *Rasmussen et al* found significantly higher diastolic blood pressure and

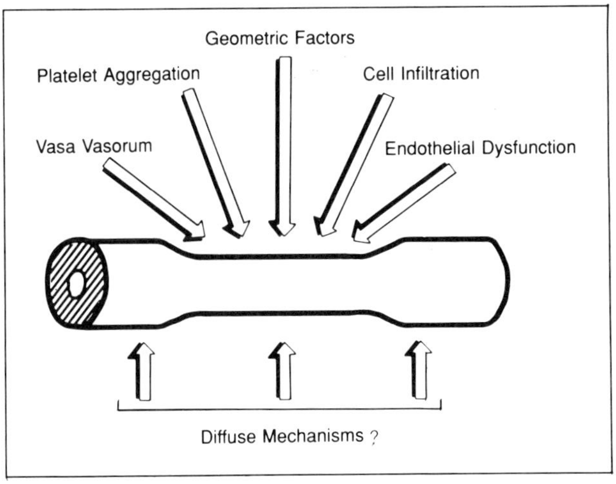

Fig. 1. *Dynamic coronary obstruction as seen as a result of an interaction between local vascular mechanisms related to atherosclerosis and diffuse, as yet hypothetical mechanisms.*

a more pronounced blood pressure increase in response to cold pressor and hyperventilation (HVT) in angina patients with dynamic coronary obstruction than in patients without (33, 34). A relation between coronary spasm and diffuse oesophageal spasms as demonstrated by oesophageal manometry also suggested the existence of generalized mechanisms (35).

Thus, dynamic coronary obstruction might be the result of an interaction between well defined, local factors related to atherosclerosis and diffuse, as yet undefined systemic factors (Fig. 1).

Clinical aspects of dynamic coronary obstruction

Dynamic coronary obstruction may be a pathophysiologic mechanism in many ischaemic heart syndromes.

Angina pectoris: Variant angina, defined by ST-elevation and chest pain at rest is the best known and most dramatic manifestation of coronary vasoconstriction, often accompanied by severe cardiac arrhythmias (6), but dynamic coronary obstruction may also be of importance in "mixed angina" and stable, exertional angina. Ambulatory ECG monitoring of angina patients has shown that many silent ischaemic episodes are not preceded by an increase in heart rate, suggesting coronary vasoconstriction to be the cause (36). The prevalence-rate of dynamic coronary obstruction in angina patients was shown in a recent review to be in the range from 15% to 35% as assessed by provocative testing (20). Dynamic coronary obstruction may cause angina after by-pass surgery due to spasm of vein grafts or native coronary vessels (37, 38). New observations suggest that coronary vasoconstriction routinely occurs after coronary angioplasty (39).

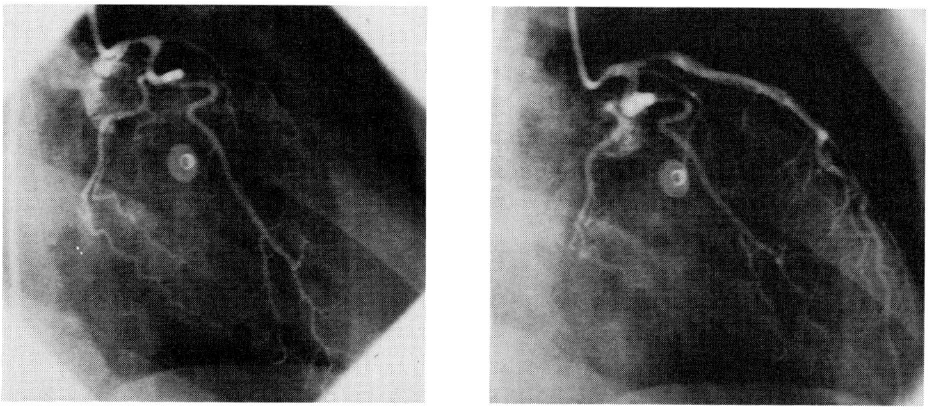

Fig. 2. *Acute coronary angiogram (projection: 30 RAO) from a young female patient, admitted with ventricular fibrillation. After resuscitation ECG showed evidence of extensive transmural anterior ischaemia, and an anterior myocardial infarction developed. Left: control, showing spasm of the main stem and occlusion of the left anterior descendant artery (LAD). Right: after intracoronary nitroglycerin spasm in the main stem and LAD is relieved. A minimal stenosis with a probable intracoronary thrombus is seen in the proximal LAD.*

Acute myocardial infarction: The role of coronary vasoconstriction in AMI is controversial. Oliva & Breckinridge found evidence of coronary spasm in 40% of patients with AMI (40). This observation has never been confirmed by others, and it is now generally accepted that occlusive coronary thrombosis is the cause of AMI. Pathoanatomic observations suggest that the chain of events, which ultimately cause coronary thrombosis may be initiated by a fissure of a coronary atherosclerotic plaque (41). During intracoronary thrombolysis in AMI Hackett et al demonstrated the existence of vasomotion in relation to thrombosis (42). This observation suggests that plaque fissuring might sometimes be initiated by coronary vasoconstriction. Coronary spasm in normal or almost normal vessels is a very rare cause of AMI (Fig. 2).

Syndrome-X: This syndrome is often defined as, angina pectoris in patients without significant fixed coronary stenosis, and without spasm of major coronary vessels. Canon et al demonstrated reduced small vessel vasodilator capacity in such patients (43). *Bortone et al* angiographically demonstrated vasoconstriction of distal coronary arteries during supine bicycle exercise in patients with Syndrome-X (44), suggesting that abnormal small vessel vasoconstriction may be one cause of this syndrome.

Provocative testing: Application of a vasoconstrictor stimulus (Table 2) with simultaneous recording of ECG and coronary angiogram has been widely used to identify patients with dynamic coronary obstructions. A test is considered "positive" if myocardial ischaemia is induced in the face of unchanged or only minimally increased myocardial metabolic demands.

Intravenous injection of ergometrine in divided doses to a dosage of 0.4 mg is the classical test, which showed a sensitivity from 57% to 98% in patients with variant angina in several studies (20). Ergometrine testing is safe in experienced hands (45), but it may cause serious complications (46). Ergometrine probably stimulates vascular alfa- or serotonergic-receptors.

Hyperventilation for 6 minutes with 30 deep respirations per minute causes respiratory alkalosis with arterial pH about 7.6-7.65, this may lead to vasoconstriction, probably because the hydrogen-ion is a calcium-ion antagonist. HVT procedure was shown to be a useful test in angina patients (34, 47). A comparative angiographic study showed ergometrine and HVT to have the same vasoconstrictive potency (48), but other studies suggested the ergometrine test might be slightly more sensitive (49). The HVT is considered safe, but complications may occur (50).

In variant angina, bicycle exercise testing may induce coronary vasoconstriction accompanied by ST-segment elevation or depression even in patients without significant fixed coronary stenoses (51). Gage et al found that bicycle exercise decreased the lumen area of stenotic coronary arterial segments in patients with classical angina (52).

Intracoronary injection of acetylcholine may be especially useful for identifying patients with endothelial dysfunction since acetylcholine dilates normal coronary arterial segments, while abnormal segments constrict. This test induced coronary vasoconstriction and ST-segment changes in 25 of 27 patients with variant angina (53).

Isometric exercise induced by hand-grip testing (16), infusion of histamine

Table 2. *Some provocative tests that are used to identify patients with dynamic coronary obstruction.*

Ergometrine, i.v. injection
Methylergometrine, i.v. injection
Hyperventilation (HVT)
HVT + Tris-buffer infusion
Acetylcholine infusion, intracoronary
Methacholine, i.v. injection
Adrenaline, i.v. injection
Histamine, i.v. injection
Bicycle exercise testing
Hand-grip testing
Cold pressor testing
Alcohol

(54), and cold pressor testing (34) may also induce myocardial ischaemia due to coronary vasoconstriction.

Therapy and prognosis: Nitroglycerin is a powerful dilator of the epicardial coronary arteries and is usually effective in terminating acute anginal attacks caused by coronary vasoconstriction. Beta-blockers may aggravate attacks in patients with variant angina (55) and should be used with caution if dynamic coronary obstruction is suspected. Calcium-blockers reduced angina frequency by 50% to 85% in patients with dynamic obstruction (56, 57). Thus, calcium-entry blockers are generally considered the best medical treatment of such patients.

PTCA can be performed with the same primary success rate in patients with dynamic coronary obstruction as in patients without, but the recurrence-rate is probably higher (58). Early mortality after by-pass surgery appears to be increased in patients with dynamic obstructions (59).

A high frequency of major cardiac complications in angina patients with dynamic coronary obstructions was reported in several studies (60-62). Harris et al followed 1241 patients with ischaemic heart disease and found that variant angina was an independent risk factor (62). In angina patients Rasmussen et al found that dynamic obstruction, as defined by a positive response to HVT, independently implied a poor prognosis (33). However, only patients with significant, fixed stenosis have a poor prognosis, while patients without significant stenosis have few complications and frequent remissions (63).

Conclusion

In contrast to what was previously thought (2), atherosclerosis may change vascular reactivity, leading to dynamic obstruction of major coronary vessels. Dynamic coronary obstruction independently influences the clinical picture and prognosis in angina patients. Its possible role in AMI as a mechanism that may initiate plaque fissuring and thus coronary thrombosis, and contribute to coronary reocclusion after thrombolysis might be a topic of future research. Provocative testing with ergometrine, HVT or acetylcholine might identify patients with coronary lesions that are unstable due to endothelial dysfunction. Mechanisms responsible for generalized hypercontractility should be identified. Further studies of the vasomotion of distal coronary arteries in syndrome-X are warranted. The possible influence of dietary factors upon coronary vasomotion deserves further consideration, since fish oil may improve endothelial dependent vasomotor function in atherosclerotic coronary arteries (64).

References

1. Huchard H. Traité des maladies du Coeur et des Vaisseaux. Paris 1889; 466-7.
2. Keefer CS, Resnik WH. A syndrome caused by anoxemia of the myocardium. Arch Int Med 1928; 41: 769-806.
3. Zoll PM, Wessler S, Blumgart HL. Angina pectoris. A clinical and pathological correlation. Am J Med 1951; 11: 331-57.
4. Prinzmetal M, Kennamer R, Merliss R, et al. Angina pectoris I. A variant form of angina pectoris. Am J Med 1959; 27: 375-88.
5. Meller J, Pichard A, Dack S. Coronary arterial spasm in Prinzmetal's angina. A proved hypothesis. Am J Cardiol 1976; 37: 938-40.
6. Maseri A, Severi S, De Nes M, et al. "Variant angina": One aspect of a continuous spectrum of vasospastic myocardial ischaemia. Am J Cardiol 1978; 42: 1019-35.
7. Furchgott RF, Zawadzki JV. The obligatory role of endothelial cells in the relaxation of arterial smooth muscle by acetylcholine.Nature 1980; 288: 373-6.
8. Webb RF, Bohr DF. Regulation of vascular tone, molecular mechanisms. Prog Cardiovasc Dis 1981; 24: 213-42.
9. Cheung WY. Ca modulin plays a pivotal role in cellular regulation. Science 1980; 207: 19-27.
10. Henderson AH. Vascular endothelium in ischemic heart disease: Possible role for endothelium-derived relaxing factor.Cardiovasc Drugs Ther 1989; 3: 241-8.
11. Furchgott RF. Role of endothelium in responces of vascular smooth muscle. Circ Res 1983; 53: 559-73.
12. Andresson R, Holmberg S, Svedmy N, et al. Adrenergic alpha- and beta-receptors in coronary vessels in man. Acta Med Scand 1972; 191: 241-4.
13. Vedernikov YP. Mechanisms of coronary spasm of isolated human epicardial coronary segments excised 3 to 5 hours after sudden death. J Am Coll Cardiol 1986; 42A-9A.
14. Hickey KA, Rubanyi G, Highsmith RF. Characterization of a coronary vasoconstrictor produced by cultured endothelial cells. Am J Physiol 1985; 248: C550-C6.
15. Chester AH, Dashwood MR, Clarke JG, et al. Influences of endothelin on human coronary arteries and localization of its binding sites.Am J Cardiol 1989; 63: 1395-8.
16. Brown BG, Lee AB, Bolson EL, et al. Reflex constriction of significant coronary stenosis as a mechanism contributing to left ventricular dysfunction during isometric exercise. Circulation 1984; 70: 18-24.
17. Brown BG, Josephson MA, Petersen RB, et al. Intravenous Dipyridamole combined with isometric handgrip for near maximal acute increase in coronary flow in patients with coronary artery disease. Am J Cardiol 1981; 48: 1077-85.
18. Kawachi Y, Tomoike H, Maruoka Y, et al. Selective hypercontraction caused by ergonovine in the canine coronary artery under conditions of induced atherosclerosis. Circulation 1984; 69: 441-50.
19. Shimokowa H, Tomoike H, Nabeyama S, et al. Coronary spasm induced in miniature swine: Angiographic evidence and relation to coronary atherosclerosis.Am Heart J 1985; 110: 300-10.
20. Rasmussen K. Clinical aspects of coronary arterial vasomotion in angina pectoris. Dan Med Bull 1989; 36: 125-41.
21. Sato I, Tomito O, O1he T, et al. Age-related changes of clinical features and prevalences of coronary risk factors in Japanese patients with vasospastic angina. Chest 1986; 89: 12-9.
22. Maseri A, Pezzola A, Marzilli M, et al. Coronary vasospasm in angina pectoris. Lancet 1977; i: 713-7.

23. McAlpin R. Relation of coronary arterial spasm to sites of organic stenosis. Am J Cardiol 1980; 46: 143-53.
24. Shephard JT, Vanhoutte PM. Mechanisms responsible for coronary vasospasm. J Am Coll Cardiol 1986; 8: 50A-4A.
25. Berkenboom B, Depierreux M, Fontaine J. The influences of atherosclerosis on the mechanical resonses of human isolated coronary arteries to substance P, isoprenaline and noradrenaline. Br J Pharmacol 1987; 92: 113-20.
26. Forman MB, Oates JA, Robertson D, et al. Increased adventitial mast cells in a patients with coronary spasm. N Eng J Med 1985; 313: 1138-41.
27. Barger AC, Beeuwkes R, Lainey LL, et al. Hypothesis: Vasa vasorum and neovascularization of human coronary arteries. N Eng J Med 1984; 310: 175-7.
28. Brown BR, Bolson EL, Dodge HT. Dynamic mechanisms in human coronary stenosis. Circulation 1984; 70: 917-22.
29. Freudenberg H, Lichtlen PR. Das nomale wandsegment bei koronarstenosen-eine postmortale studie. Z Kardiol 1981; 70: 863-9.
30. Wiener L, Kasparian H, Duca PR, et al. Spectrum of coronary arterial spasm. Clinical, angiographic and myocardial metabolic experience in 29 cases. Am J Cardiol 1976; 38: 945-55.
31. Miller D, Waters DD, Warnica W, et al. Is variant angina the coronary manifestation of a generalized vasospastic disorder? N Eng J Med 1981; 304: 763-6.
32. Freedman SB, Richmond DR, Kelly DT. Long-term follow-up of verapamil and nitrate treatment for coronary artery spasm. Am J Cardiol 1982; 50: 711-5.
33. Rasmussen K, Juul S, Bagger JP, et al. Usefulness of ST deviation induced by prolonged hyperventilation as a predictor of cardiac death in angina pectoris. Am J Cardiol 1987; 59: 763-8.
34. Rasmussen K, Bagger JP, Bøttzauw J, et al. Prevalence of vasospastic ischaemia induced by the cold pressor test or hyperventilation in patients with severe angina. Eur Heart J 1984; 5: 354-61.
35. Rasmussen K, Ravnsbaek J, Funch-Jensen P, et al. Oesophageal spasm in patients with coronary artery spasm. Lancet 1986; i: 174-6.
36. Friesinger GC. Silent myocardial ischaemia and the importance of coronary vasoconstriction. Curr Opin Cardiol 1989; 4: 492-8.
37. Baduini G, Marra S, Angelino PF. Sudden occlusion of a saphenous vein bypass graft relieved by direct injection of nitroglycerine. Cath Cardiovasc Diagn 1981; 7: 87-95.
38. Waters DD, Theroux P, Crittin J, et al. Previously undiagnosed variant angina as a cause of chest pain after coronary artery bypass surgery. Circulation 1980; 61: 1159-64.
39. Fischell TA, Derby G, Tse TM, et al. Coronary artery vasoconstriction routinely occurs after percutaneous transluminal coronary angioplasty. Circulation 1988; 78: 1323-34.
40. Oliva PB, Breckenridge JC. Arteriographic evidence of coronary arterial spasm in acute myocardial infarction. Circulation 1977; 56: 366-74.
41. Falk E. Unstable angina with fatal outcome: dynamic coronary thrombosis leading to infarction and/or sudden death. Circulation 1985; 71: 699-708.
42. Hackett D, Davies G, Chierchia S, et al. Intermittent coronary occlusion in acute myocardial infarction. N Eng J Med 1987; 317: 1055-9.
43. Canon RO, Leon MB, Watson RM, et al. Chest pain and normal coronary arteries-Role of small coronary arteries. Am J Cardiol 1985; 55: 50B-60B.
44. Bortone AS, Hess OM, Eberli FR, et al. Abnormal coronary vasomotion during exercise in patients with normal coronary arteries and reduced coronary flow reserve. Circulation 1989; 79: 516-27.
45. Bertrand ME, Lablanche JM, Tilmant PY, et al. Frequency of provoked coronary arte-

rial spasm in 1089 consecutive patients undergoing coronary arteriography. Circulation 1982; 65: 1299-306.
46. Buxton A, Goldberg S, Hirsfeld JW, et al. Refractory ergonovine-induced coronary vasospasm: Importance of intracoronary nitroglycerin. Am J Cardiol 1980; 46: 329-34.
47. Weber S, Cabanes L, Simon J-C, et al. Systemic alcalosis as a provocative test for coronary artery spasm in patients with infrequent resting chest pain. Am Heart J 1988; 115: 54-9.
48. Rasmussen K, Henningsen P. Provocative testing with prolonged hyperventilation and ergometrine in patients suspected of coronary artery spasm: A comparative study. Int J Cardiol 1987; 15: 151-63.
49. Previtali M, Ardissino D, Barberis P, et al. Hyperventilation and ergonovine tests in Prinzmetal's variant angina pectoris in men. Am J Cardiol 1989; 63: 17-20.
50. Mortensen SA, Vilhelmsen R, Sandøe E. Non-pharmacologic provocation of coronary vasospasm. Experience with prolonged hyperventilation in the coronary care unit. Eur Heart J 1983; 4: 391-7.
51. Specchia G, DeServi S, Falcone C, et al. Coronary arterial spasm as a cause of exercise-induced ST-segment elevation in patients with variant angina. Circulation 1979; 59: 948-54.
52. Gage J, Hess OM, Murakami T, et al. Vasoconstriction of stenotic coronary arteries during dynamic exercise in patients with classic angina pectoris: reversibility by nitroglyccerin. Circulation 1986; 73: 865-76.
53. Yasue H, Horio Y, Nakamura N, et al. Induction of coronary arterial spasm by acetylcholine in patients with variant angina: possible role of the parasympathetic nervous system in the pathogenesis of coronary artery spasm. Circulation 1986; 74: 955-63.
54. Ginsburg R, Bristow MR, Kantrowitz N, et al. Histamine provocation of clinical coronary artery spasm: Implications concerning pathogenesis of variant angina pectoris. Am Heart J 1981; 102: 819-22.
55. Tilmant PY, Lablanche JM, Thieuleux FA, et al. Detrimental effect of propranolol in patients with coronary arterial spasm countered by combination with diltiazem. Am J Cardiol 1983; 52: 230-3.
56. Schroeder JS, Feldman RL, Giles TD, et al. Multiclinic controlled trial of diltiazem for Prinzmetal's angina. Am J Med 1982; 72: 227-32.
57. Johnson SM, Mauritson DR, Willerson JT, et al. Comparison of verapamil and nifedipine in the treatment of variant angina pectoris: Preliminary observations on 10 patients. Am J Cardiol 1981; 47: 1295-300.
58. Bertrand ME, LaBlanche JM, Fourrier JL, et al. Percutaneous transluminal coronary angioplasty superimposed on atherosclerotic narrowings. Br Heart J 1987; 58: 469-72.
59. Bertrand JM, LaBlanche JM, Rousseau MF, et al. Surgical treatment of variant angina: Use of plexectomy with aortocoronary bypass. Circulation 1980; 61: 877-82.
60. Waters DD, Miller DD, Szlachcic J, et al. Factors influencing the long-term prognosis of treated patients with variant angina. Circulation 1983; 68: 258-65.
61. Severi S,Davies G, Maseri A, et al. Long-term prognosis of variant angina with medical treatment. Am J Cardiol 1980; 46: 226-32.
62. Harris PJ, Lee KL, Harrell FE, et al. Outcome in medically treated coronary artery disease. Circulation 1980; 62A: 718-26.
63. Freedman BS, Richmond DR, Alwyn M, et al. Late follow-up (41 to 102 months) of medically treated patients with coronary artery spasm and minor atherosclerotic coronary obstructions. Am J Cardiol 1986; 57: 1261-3.
64. Shimakowa H, Vanhoutte PM. Dietary cod-liver oil improves endothelium-dependent responses in hypercholesterolemic and atherosclerotic porcine coronary arteries. Circulation 1988; 78: 1421-30.

3

Dynamic coronary thrombosis*

ERLING FALK

Coronary lesions: progression

Slow versus rapid plaque progression: Coronary atherosclerosis usually evolves over a period of time by lipid accumulation, macrophage infiltration, and smooth muscle cell proliferation causing progressive luminal narrowing *slowly* – usually considered the atherosclerotic process proper (uncomplicated atherosclerosis). This slow plaque progression, however, may be punctuated by sudden rupture of the plaque surface which may be accompanied by haemorrhage into the plaque (also called "intraintimal" thrombus) and luminal thrombosis causing *rapid* plaque progression – a process quite different from the underlying atherosclerotic process proper (1).

Plaques "at risk": Patients with stable angina usually have a mixture of plaques, some being "hard" collagen-rich with barely detectable lipids, others being "soft" with a prominent pool of extracellular lipid (semifluid at body temperature?) separated from the arterial lumen by a cap of fibrous tissue, and many plaques are in between (2). There is no good explanation for this variety in plaque morphology often within the same artery. Uncomplicated atherosclerosis may cause luminal narrowing and consequently angina pectoris, but coronary atherosclerosis *per se* is otherwise a benign disease with which patients may live for years. Patients with "soft" plaques, however, are at increased risk of complications, because the fibrous cap of such plaques have a propensity to rupture exposing thrombogenic material to the flowing blood.

Plaque rupture +/– stenosis: Rupture of the plaque surface may cause rapid plaque progression due to haemorrhage into the plaque or luminal

* Figures illustrating the text have been published previously (1, 3, 8, 12).

Coronary thrombosis: pathogenesis

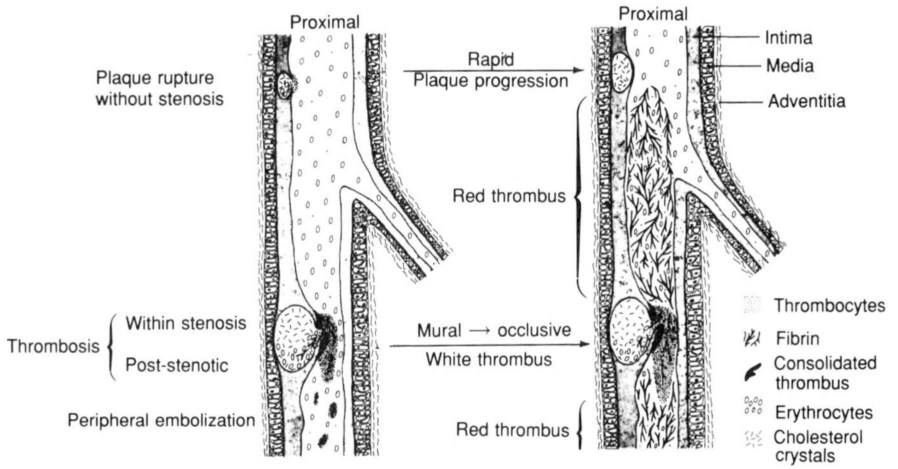

Initiation:	Plaque rupture exposing thrombogenic material
Promotion:	Stenosis causing shear-induced platelet aggregation (white thrombus)
Extension:	Post-stenotic platelet aggregation
Consolidation:	Fibrin-stabilization of the platelet thrombus
Dynamic:	Recurrent thrombosis and peripheral embolization
Propagation:	Secondary blood stagnation causing coagulation (red thrombus)

thrombosis, or both. Autopsy studies suggest that the degree of pre-existing atherosclerotic stenosis at the rupture site is decisive for the outcome: the incidence of occlusive thrombosis increases with increasing degree of pre-existing stenosis (3, 4). This patho-anatomical observation agrees with experimental studies showing that stenoses promote arterial thrombosis (5), probably via shear induced platelet aggregation (6).

Conorary thrombosis: patho-anatomy

When discussing thrombogenesis it may be helpful to separate the following "components", which are depicted in the Figure.

Initiation: If coronary thrombi are examined by serial sectioning technique a ruptured "soft" atherosclerotic plaque will be found beneath more than 80% (3, 7, 8), often with displaced atheromatous plaque material buried deeply in the thrombus, clearly indicating that rupture of the plaque surface has preceded (initiated) luminal thrombosis, and not vice versa (3, 8). Minor and more superficial intimal irregularities are generally found beneath the rest – usually in combination with a severe atherosclerotic stenosis.

Extension: Thrombus formation usually takes place *within* a stenosis with ruptured surface. It may, however, also take place or extend *post-*

stenotically (1) where flow separation, recirculation, and turbulence probably offer ideal fluid dynamic conditions for the progressive growth of the thrombus by further platelet aggregation. Such a freely floating tail of the thrombus extending downstream post-stenotically probably has a high potential to embolize.

Consolidation: In patients dying soon after the onset of an acute heart attack, platelets can usually be identified as the major component of the most recent part of the thrombus at the rupture site (early platelet thrombus), whereas older parts nearer the vessel wall are condensed and much richer in fibrin concealing the platelets in a homogeneous mass (8).

So, both platelets and fibrin play a role in the evolution of a coronary thrombus. The primary flow obstruction is usually due to platelet aggregation, but a platelet thrombus is very unstable and it can easily be swept away by the flowing blood unless fibrin secondarily enmeshes the platelets and thus stabilizes the thrombus. Such a temporal interplay between platelets and fibrin agrees with experimental studies, which also show that fresh thrombi are easier lysed than old ones (9, 10, 11).

Dynamic: More than 80% of thrombi formed within stenoses have a layered structure with thrombus material of differing age indicating an episodic growth by repeated mural deposits (12). Furthermore, episodic growth seems to alternate with thrombus fragmentation and peripheral embolization documented by the frequent finding of small fragments of thrombus material impacted in intramyocardial arteries downstream to evolving coronary thrombi, often associated with microinfarcts (12-14). Such microemboli are especially frequent in sudden ischaemic death preceded by unstable angina (13). Consequently, coronary thrombosis is usually a "dynamic" process where the thrombus waxes and wanes over a period of time, in full agreement with experimental arterial thrombosis in animals (9).

Propagation: Secondarily to the reduced flow caused by the white platelet-rich thrombus at the rupture site the blood proximal and distal to the occlusion may stagnate and coagulate giving rise to a red stagnation thrombosis consisting of erythrocytes held together by fibrin membranes like a venous thrombus formed in stagnant blood.

A stagnation thrombus may propagate *upstream* as an occlusive thrombus to the nearest side branch and even further as a non-occlusive thrombus without occluding major side branches. Consequently, re-infarction and infarct extension cannot be explained by thrombus propagation as suggested (15, 16). Downstream thrombus propagation, however, may occlude side branches, which theoretically may impede the collateral flow (and hamper access of thrombolytic agents to the thrombus?).

A stagnation thrombus may be several centimetres long (especially in the right coronary artery with its few major side branches), and if so it probably is hard to lyse being one of the mechanisms underlying failure of thrombolytic therapy for myocardial infarction.

What causes plaque rupture?

Ruptured (= "fissured") plaques are frequently found in the coronary arteries of patients dying from ischaemic heart disease (IHD) and are not infrequently found incidentally in individuals dying suddenly from non-cardiac causes. In the latter group, ruptured plaques without occlusive thrombi were present in 6 of 69 individuals without atheroma-related diseases and in 13 of 60 individuals with "atheroma-related" non-cardiac diseases (17), while 103 ruptured plaques were found in 47 patients dying from IHD, and only 40 of these ruptured plaques were associated with a major luminal thrombus – the one responsible for the final heart attack (3). So, the risk of plaque rupture increases with increasing severity of atherosclerosis, but it is probably silent clinically in the great majority of cases.

Rupture of the fibrous cap occurs most often at its junction with the adjacent more normal intima and less frequently through the centre of the cap – probably sites of high circumferential stress (7). The actual point of rupture is probably a function of the stress applied (impact) and the resistance of the cap which may exhibit local variations in mechanical strength. Local weakening could be due to foam cell infiltration which is frequenty found at the rupture site (3, 7). Focal inflammation in a thinned fibrous cap has been suggested as a marker of instability of plaques at the carotid bifurcation where rupture apparently occurs in the most stenotic region (18). In the coronary arteries, rupture occurs within the stenosis, according to Ambrose et al. (quoting M. Davies) preferentially a little bit upstream from the point of maximal stenosis where the shear forces are highest (19).

Coronary arteries are constantly exposed to a variety of stresses such as bending and twisting during each heart contraction, pulsatile flow and variations in blood pressure. In stenotic areas, high wall shear stress, wall vibration, flutter, and collapse could induce disruption of the plaque surface (18). When no more than such "daily" haemodynamic stresses may be enough to disrupt a thinned and atenuated fibrous cap, then it probably just happens – incidentally. If so, then rupture of the plaque surface may be considered a random event in the evolution and growth of the atherosclerotic lesion.

Haemodynamic and metabolic factors that may influence plaque progression and its structural integrity need further study.

Infarct-related lesion after thrombolysis

Theoretically, thrombolytic treatment might cause progressive growth of the plaque because of continuing bleeding from the lumen into the plaque through the ruptured surface. Patho-anatomical data, however, provide no support for such a theory – maybe except when thrombolysis is performed together with angioplasty (20).

Failure in recanalizing the infarct related artery with thrombolytic treatment does not indicate that the occlusion is non-thrombotic (21). The reasons for such treatment failure, however, are unknown. Based on a small autopsy series of 8 patients, it has recently been suggested, that thrombi overlying stenotic plaques with a ruptured surface may be more difficult to lyse than thrombi overlying less stenotic and uncomplicated plaques (22). This theory, however, was not substantiated in another patho-anatomical study published on the preceding pages of the same journal, where no clear morphological reason for the failures to re-open thrombosed arteries was found (21). In recanalized arteries the residual stenosis was caused by atheromas with rupture and haemorrhage usually completely without residual luminal thrombosis.

Rupture, thrombosis and spasm

An unstable (ruptured) plaque with a variable degree of haemorrhage into the plaque and luminal thrombosis could explain a possible concomitant vasospasm. Enhanced vasoreactivity locally (spasm) could be due to vasoactive substances liberated from aggregating platelets at the rupture site, or could be due to a disruptive intimal haemorrhage dissecting its way to the base of the plaque stimulating or sensitizing the adjacent smooth muscle cells of the media.

So, unstable plaques could be associated with spasm or thrombosis, or both.

Clinical correlations

Insight into disease processes derived from autopsy studies (fatal cases) may not necessarily apply to the living patient. The patho-anatomical data presented, however, are consistent with the following clinical experiences.

Plaque progression: The natural progression of coronary lesions seems to involve 2 distinct processes (23): one that is time-dependent causing non-occlusive luminal narrowing slowly suggesting a *chronic* process (atherosclerosis), and a second one that is time-independent causing sudden, usually unpredicted, and rapid vascular occlusion suggesting an *acute* event (plaque rupture, haemorrhage and thrombosis).

Natural history of plaque rupture: Acute heart attacks usually occur without any obvious precipitating cause fitting the theory, that plaque rupture is a random event in the evolution and growth of the atherosclerotic lesion. The observed circadian variation in acute coronary syndromes (24) could reflect a corresponding circadian variation in plaque rupture (increased sympatic tone and haemodynamic stresses in the morning hours?) or could be due to a similar circadian variation in platelet aggregability and response to thrombogenic stimuli from ruptured plaques.

Coronary angiographic (19) and angioscopic (25) data indicate, that unstable angina is a good clinical marker of unstable (ruptured) plaques in the coronary arteries. Sudden progression of insignificant lesions to bigger but still insignificant ones may, however, be totally silent clinically (26). The natural history of unstable angina probably mirrors that of the underlying ruptured plaque: stabilization (the rupture reseal), accentuation of symptoms (rapid plaque progression), or infarction (occlusive thrombosis).

Plaque rupture initiates thrombosis: Unstable (versus stable) *angina* is characterized angiographically by irregular and rapidly progressing coronary stenoses which during the acute phase of the disease are often associated with intraluminal filling defects within and/or distal to the stenoses – frequently accompanied by vasospasm: *A dynamic stenosis* (1). Post-mortem studies suggest that most irregular stenoses +/– filling defects represent ruptured plaques +/– thrombosis (27). Such a plaque morphology can be identified angiographically in most patients surviving myocardial infarction (28). So, plaque rupture initiates the majority of coronary thrombi – fatal as well as non-fatal.

Stenosis promotes thrombosis: This principle seems to be valid in many different clinical situations:

1. The degree of atherosclerotic stenosis seems to be a powerful predictor of the natural progression to total (=thrombotic) occlusion (23, 29, 30). Stenosis severity is also a risk marker for subsequent development of myocardial infarction (31), but it seems to be impossible on an individual basis to predict the clinical course and the location of a subsequent infarction from analysis of a previous coronary angiogram (32), partly

because thrombotic occlusion – especially in cases of pre-existing stenosis >70-90% – may occur silently without infarction (30, 33).

2. Rethrombosis after otherwise successful thrombolysis is clearly related to the severity of the residual stenosis immediately after the intervention (34).
3. The risk of thrombotic complications to coronary angioplasty seems to be related to the severity of the residual stenosis after dilatation, in addition to the extent of arterial disruption (35, 36).
4. Progression of unstable angina to infarction and/or sudden death (thrombotic complications) is related to the severity of fixed atherosclerotic changes (37).
5. In vasospastic angina increases the risk of thrombotic complications with increasing degree of underlying fixed atherosclerotic obstruction (fixed stenoses < 75%, 75-90%, and > 90% are reported to be associated with infarction risks of 2%, 5%, and 15%, respectively) (38).

Thrombus within or distal to stenosis: The pathogenesis and clinical significance of thrombi formed *within* or *distal* to stenoses may differ. The relatively small thrombus formed within the stenosis is probably the most dangerous part of the thrombus, because 1) the most severe flow-obstruction is here, 2) progression to total occlusion takes also place here, and 3) thrombus formed within stenoses may be very resistant (residual thrombus often persists here even after prolonged intracoronary streptokinase infusion (39)). On the other hand, the freely floating tail of the thrombus extending post-stenotically seems to have a much greater potential to embolize causing peripheral microvascular occlusion (39, 40).

Dynamic thrombosis: Angiography performed during acute heart attacks often reveals transient non-occlusive thrombi in unstable angina (41), mural thrombi which may progress to total occlusion in non-Q-wave infarction (42), and occlusive thrombi which may persist or lyse spontaneously in Q-wave infarction (43). The dynamic occlusion observed during the early phase of acute infarction probably results from a variable combination of thrombosis and vasoconstriction, but only thrombolysis and not vasodilators is usually effective regarding the initial opening of the totally occluded vessel (44).

Coronary thrombosis seems also to be present in the early hours of myocardial infarction with "normal coronary arteries" (45).

Determinants of thrombosis: The character of the atherosclerotic changes underlying coronary thrombi vary considerably. The pre-existing stenosis is not always severe (39,46), and a ruptured plaque surface is not universally present (28). So, in addition to the *severity of stenosis* and the *degree of intimal damage* other factors may be of importance too. Indeed, the actual *thrombotic-thrombolytic equilibrium* seems to be a very important determinant of thrombus formation documented by the beneficial effect of both anti-platelet agents and anti-coagulants in patients at risk of coronary thrombosis (47).

Clinical experience suggests that old thrombi are more stable than young ones, as indicated by a faster and more effective thrombolysis the quicker the treatment can be initiated (48,49).

Remodelling after thrombolysis: A severe stenosis due to atherosclerosis and residual thrombosis usually remains immediately after otherwise successful thrombolysis, but continuing endogeneous thrombolysis and remodelling may result in further regression of the stenosis with time (50).

Spasm and acute coronary events: Spasm and thrombosis accompany each other in many patients with an acute coronary syndrome (51). If spasm occurs, it usually does so at the site of an atherosclerotic but not necessarily stenotic lesion, and a ruptured plaque surface could explain an increased propensity for spasm as well as for thrombosis. Treatment directed against a possible vasospasm usually relieves pain during unstable angina, but the incidence of myocardial infarction or sudden death is not reduced (52). Maybe apart from some patients with non-Q-wave infarction the same is true for spasmolytic treatment during or after infarction (52).

So, from a prognostic point of view thrombosis rather than spasm is the most important.

Thrombogenesis: Summary and conclusion

Initiation: Most coronary thrombi are initiated by a sudden rupture of the plaque surface causing platelet aggregation where thrombogenic subendothelial tissue has been exposed.

The pathogenesis of plaque rupture is unknown.

Promotion: 1) The severity of pre-existing atherosclerotic stenosis at the rupture site seems to be decisive for whether the platelet nidus remains mural and limited (just sealing the rupture) or evolves into an occlusive thrombosis. Other major determinants for *occlusive* thrombosis seem to be 2) the character and degree of intimal damage, and 3) the actual thrombotic-thrombolytic equilibrium.

Extension: Platelet aggregation and thrombus formation may take place *within* the stenosis where the flow velocity and shear forces are highest, or it may take place or extend *post-stenotically* where recirculation, turbulence, and vortex formation probably offer ideal fluid dynamic conditions for progressive thrombus formation by platelet aggregation.

Dynamic: Coronary thrombus formation is usually a dynamic process where recurrent mural thrombosis alternates with thrombus fragmentation and peripheral embolization.

Propagation: A red stagnation thrombosis (rich in erythrocytes) may form *secondarily* to the reduced flow caused by the *primary* platelet-rich thrombus at the rupture site. This stagnation thrombosis may propagate upstream without occluding major side branches while downstream thrombus propagation may cause side branch occlusion.

The clinical significance, if any, of downstream side branch occlusion is unknown.

Composition: Displaced atheromatous plaque material is often found buried deeply in the luminal thrombus at the rupture site clearly indicating that rupture of the plaque surface has occurred just before thrombus formation, and not vice versa. Fatty plaque material extruded through the ruptured surface may in exceptional cases occlude the lumen locally but otherwise platelet aggregation seems to be responsible for the primary flow obstruction while fibrinogen/fibrin subsequently infiltrate and stabilize the early platelet-rich thrombus. Fibrin is also found in the secondarily formed erythrocyte-rich red stagnation thrombosis.

So, both platelets and the coagulation system are involved in the evolution of a coronary thrombus.

References

1. Falk E. Morphologic features of unstable atherothrombotic plaques underlying acute coronary syndromes. Am J Cardiol 1989; 63: 114E-20E.
2. Hangartner JRW, Charleston AJ, Davies MJ, Thomas AC. Morphological characteristics of clinically significant coronary artery stenosis in stable angina. Br Heart J 1986; 56: 501-8.
3. Falk E. Plaque rupture with severe pre-existing stenosis precipitating coronary thrombosis. Characteristics of coronary atherosclerotic plaques underlying fatal occlusive thrombi. Br Heart J 1983; 50: 127-34.
4. El Fawal MA, Berg GA, Wheatley DJ, Harland WA. Sudden coronary death in Glasgow: nature and frequency of acute coronary lesions. Br Heart J 1987; 57: 329-35.
5. Willerson JT, Golind P, Eudt J, Campbell WB, Buja LM. Specific platelet mediators and unstable coronary artery lesions. Experimental evidence and potential clinical implications. Circulation 1989; 80: 198-205.
6. Badimon L, Badimon JJ, Turitto VT, Vallabhajosula S, Fuster V. Platelet thrombus formation on collagen type I. A model of deep vessel injury. Influence of blood rheology, von Willebrand factor, and blood coagulation. Circulation 1988; 78: 1431-42.

7. Richardson PD, Davies MJ, Born GVR. Influence of plaque configuration and stress distribution on fissuring of coronary atherosclerotic plaques. Lancet 1989; ii: 941-4.
8. Falk E. Thrombosis in unstable angina: Pathologic aspects. In: Mehta JL, Conti CR, eds. Thrombosis and platelets in myocardial ischemia. Cardiovascular Clinics, Philadelphia: F. A. Davis, 1987, 18/1: Chapter 9.
9. Jørgensen L. Experimental platelet and coagulation thrombi. A histological study of arterial and venous thrombi of varying age in untreated and heparinized rabbits. Acta Path Microbiol Scand 1964; 62: 189-223.
10. Jørgensen L, Rowsell HC, Hovig T, Mustard JF. Resolution and organization of platelet-rich mural thrombi in carotid arteries of swine. Acta Path Microbiol Scand 1967; 51: 681-719.
11. Cercek B, Hod H, Lew AS. 4-hr old arterial thrombi are bigger and more resistant to lysis than 1-hr old thrombi (abstract). Clin Res 1986; 34: 5A.
12. Falk E. Unstable angina with fatal outcome: dynamic coronary thrombosis leading to infarction and/or sudden death. Autopsy evidence of recurrent mural thrombosis with peripheral embolization culminating in total vascular occlusion. Circulation 1985; 71: 699-708.
13. Davies MJ, Thomas AC, Knapman PA, Hangartner JR. Intramyocardial platelet aggregation in patients with unstable angina suffering sudden ischemic cardiac death. Circulation 1986; 73: 418-27.
14. Frink RJ, Rooney PA, Trowbridge JO, Rose JP. Coronary thrombosis and platelet/fibrin microemboli in death associated with acute myocardial infarction. Br Heart J 1988; 59: 196-200.
15. Swan HJC, Shah PK, Rubin S. Role of vasodilators in the changing phases of acute myocardial infarction. Am Heart J 1982; 103: 707-15.
16. Chamberlain DA. Unanswered Questions in Thrombolysis. Am J Cardiol 1989; 63: 34A-40A.
17. Davies MJ, Bland JM, Hangartner, Angelini A, Thomas AC. Factors influencing the presence or absence of acute coronary artery thrombi in sudden ischaemic death. Eur Heart J 1989; 10: 203-8.
18. Bassinouny HS, Davis H, Massawa N, Gewertz BL, Glagov S, Zarins CK: Critical carotid stenoses: Morphologic and chemical similarity between symptomatic and asymptomatic plaques. J Vasc Surg 1989; 9: 202-12.
19. Ambrose JA, Hjemdal-Monsen CE. Arteriographic anatomy and mechanisms of myocardial ischemia in unstable angina. J Am Coll Cardiol 1987; 9: 1397-402.
20. Waller BF, Rothbaum DA, Pinkerton CA. Status of the myocardium and infarct-related coronary artery in 19 necropsy patients with acute recanalization using pharmacologic (streptokinase, r-tissue plasminogen activator), mechanical (percutaneous transluminal coronary angioplasty) or combined types of reperfusion therapy. J Am Coll Cardiol 1987; 9:785-801.
21. Onodera T, Fujiwara H, Tanaka M. Cineangiographic and pathological features of the infarct related vessel in successful and unsuccesful thrombolysis. Br Heart J 1989; 61: 385-9.
22. Richardson SG, Callen D, Morton P, Murtagh JG, Scott ME, O'Keeffe DB. Pathological changes after intravenous streptokinase treatment in eight patients with acute myocardial infarction. Br Heart J 1989; 61: 390-5.
23. Kramer JR, Kitazume H, Proudfit WL. Segmental analysis of the rate of progression in patients with progressive coronary atherosclerosis. Am Heart J 1983; 106: 1427-31.
24. Muller JE, Toffler GH, Stone PH. Circadian variation and triggers of onset of acute cardiovascular disease. Circulation 1989; 79: 733-43.

25. Forrester JS, Litvack F, Grundfest W, Hickey A. A perspective of coronary disease seen through the arteries of living man. Circulation 1987; 75: 505-13.
26. Singh RN. Progression of coronary atherosclerosis. Clues to pathogenesis from serial coronary arteriography. Br Heart J 1984; 52: 451-61.
27. Levin DC, Gardiner GA. Complex and simple coronary artery stenoses: A new way to interpret coronary angiograms based on morphologic features of lesions. Radiology 1987; 164: 675-80.
28. Nakagawa S, Hanada Y, Koiwaya Y, Tanaka K. Angiographic features in the infarct-related artery after intracoronary urokinase followed by prolonged anticoagulation. Role of ruptured atheromatous plaque and adherent thrombus in acute myocardial infarction in vivo. Circulation 1988; 78: 1335-44.
29. Moise A, Lesoérance J, Théroux P, Taeymans Y, Goulet C, Bourassa MG. Clinical and angiographic predictors of new total coronary occlusion in coronary artery disease: analysis of 313 nonoperated patients. Am J Cardiol 1984; 54: 1176-81.
30. Danchin N, Osvald T, Voiriot P, Juillière Y, Cherrier F. Significance of spontaneous obstruction of high degree coronary artery stenoses between diagnostic angiography and later percutaneous transluminal coronary angioplasty. Am J Cardiol 1989; 63: 660-2. 660-2.
31. Ellis S, Alderman E, Cain K. Prediction of risk of anterior myocardial infarction by lesion severity and measurement method of stenoses in the left anterior descending coronary distribution: A CASS registry study. J Am Coll Cardiol 1988; 11: 908-16.
32. Little WC, Constantinescu M, Applegate RJ. Can coronary angiography predict the site of a subsequent myocardial infarction in patients with mild-to-moderate coronary artery disease? Circulation 1988; 78: 1157-66.
33. Ambrose JA, Tannembaum MA, Alexopoulos D. Angiographic progression of coronary artery disease and the development of myocardial infarction. J Am Coll Cardiol 1988; 12: 56-62.
34. Harrison DG, Ferguson DW, Collins SM. Rethrombosis after reperfusion with streptokinase: importance of geometry of residual lesions. Circulation 1984; 69: 991-9.
35. Ellis SG, Roubin GS, King SB. Angiographic and clinical predictors of acute closure after native vessel coronary angioplasty. Circulation 1988; 77: 372-9.
36. Black AJR, Namay DL, Niederman AL: Tear or dissection after coronary angioplasty. Morphologic correlates of an ischemic complication. Circulation 1989; 79: 1035-42.
37. Alison HW, Rusell RO, Mantle JA, Kouchoukos NT, Moraski RE, Rackley CE. Coronary anatomy and arteriography in patients with unstable angina pectoris. Am J Cardiol 1978; 41: 204-9.
38. Nakamura M, Takeshita A, Nose Y. Clinical characteristics associated with myocardial infarction, arrhythmias, and sudden death in patients with vasospastic angina. Circulation 1987; 75: 1110-16.
39. Brown BG, Gallery CA, Badger RS. Incomplete lysis of thrombus in the moderate underlying atherosclerotic lesion during intracoronary infusion of streptokinase for acute myocardial infarction: quantitative angiographic observations. Circulation 1986; 73: 653-61.
40. Terrosi P, Ibba GV, Contini GM, Franceschino V. Angiographic features of the coronary arteries during intracoronary thrombolysis. Br Heart J 1984; 52: 154-63.
41. Capone G, Wolf NM, Meyer B, Meister SG. Frequency of intracoronary filling defects by angiography in angina pectoris at rest. Am J Cardiol 1985; 56: 403-6.
42. DeWood MA, Stifter WF, Simpson CS. Coronary arteriographic findings soon after non-Q-wave myocardial infarction. N Engl J Med 1986; 315: 417-23.
43. DeWood MA, Spores J, Notske R, et al. Prevalence of total coronary occlusion during

the early hours of transmural myocardial infarction. N Engl J Med 1980; 303: 897-902.
44. Hackett D, Davies G, Chierchia S, Maseri A. Intermittent coronary occlusion in acute myocardial infarction. Value of combined thrombolytic and vasodilator therapy. N Engl J Med 1987; 317: 1055-9.
45. Rapold HJ, Haeberli A, Kuemmerli H, Weiss M, Baur HR, Straub WP. Fibrin formation and platelet activation in patients with myocardial infarction and normal coronary arteries. Eur Heart J 1989; 10: 323-33.
46. Hackett D, Davies G, Maseri A. Pre-existing coronary stenoses in patients with first myocardial infarction are not necessarily severe. Eur Heart J 1988; 9: 1317-23.
47. Stein B, Fuster V, Israel DH. Platelet inhibitor agents in cardiovascular disease: An update. J Am Coll Cardiol 1989; 14: 813-36.
48. Lew AS, Larae P, Cercek B, Rodriguez L, Shah PK, Ganz W. The effects of the rate of intravenous infusion of streptokinase and the duration of symptoms on the time interval to reperfusion in patients with acute myocardial infarction. Circulation 1985; 72: 1053-8.
49. Topol EJ, Bates ER, Walton JA. Community hospital administration of intraveneous tissue plasminogen activator in acute myocardial infarction: Improved timing, thrombolytic efficacy and ventricular function. J Am Coll Cardiol 1987; 10: 1173-7.
50. Schmidt WG, Uebis R, v.Essen R. Residual coronary stenosis after thrombolysis with rt-PA or streptokinase: acute results and 3 weeks follow-up. Eur Heart J 1987; 8: 1182-8.
51. Bertrand ME, Lablanche JM, Tilmant PY, Thieuleux FA. Frequency of provoked coronary arterial spasm in 1089 consecutive patients undergoing coronary arteriography. Circulation 1982; 65: 1299-306.
52. Held PH, Yusuf S, Furberg CD. Calcium channel blockers in acute myocardial infarction and unstable angina: an overview. Br Med J 1989; 299: 1187-92.

4

Thrombocyte aggregation and coronary artery disease

ERIK THAULOW,
JAN ERIKSSEN,
GUNNAR ERIKSSEN

Introduction

Blood platelets may play a role in the development, the course of, as well as the symptoms of coronary artery disease (CAD).

Atherogenesis

Experimental studies suggest blood platelet involvement in atherogenesis. Possibly, the initial step in the formation of an atherosclerotic lesion is damage of the intima followed by platelet adhesion and aggregation to endothelial cells and release of platelet smooth muscle growth stimulating factor, which induces cell proliferation in the media. Increased platelet responsiveness may be important for the development of CAD, since abnormal platelet functions are common in subjects with hypertension (1), hyperlipaemia (2) and in smokers (3) as well as in familial CAD (4).

In a prospective study the prevalence of coronary heart disease (CHD) was examined in 2014 apparently healthy middle aged men, who underwent a comprehensive examination including clinical examination, questionnaire, x-ray of the chest, blood tests, ECG and a submaximal bicycle exercise ECG-test (5). Blood platelet counts (n=487) and blood platelet aggregation tests (n=150) were included in a random sub-sample. Platelet aggregability was assessed by lag time and by maximal rate (6). Annual total- and CHD-mortality has been monitored continuously (7), and the incidence of non-fatal CHD has been determined by follow-up examinations 7½ years (completed) and 15 years (on-going) after the baseline study-programme. Blood platelet count was unrelated to markers of increasing coronary atherosclerosis i.e angina pectoris (AP) / positive-exercise ECG de novo (Pos-ECG)

Table 1. *Annual incidence of angina pectoris (AP), positive exercise ECG response de novo (Pos-ECG) (both 7 years follow-up) and death (total- and CHD-death) (13 1/2 years follow up) in 487 apparently healthy middle aged men. Material divided into four quartiles according to platelet counts.*

Quartiles:	I	II	III	IV
AP	1.7%	2.3%	2.0%	2.1%
Pos-ECG	3.5%	2.7%	3.8%	3.4%
Total-death	0.7%	0.9%	0.9%	1.5%
CHD-death	0.4%	0.4%	0.4%	1.0%

(table 1), and there were no differences in signs of CAD (AP/pos-ECG) in the 50% with the most pronounced aggregation response compared with the others (8). These data from the Oslo-ischaemia study do not support the hypothesis, derived from animal experiments suggesting that blood platelets are related to the atherosclerotic process itself. No other prospective data are available relating platelet aggregability to the development of ischaemic heart disease in man.

Complications to coronary artery disease

Platelets have been assumed to precipitate thrombotic CAD-complications, since occlusion of stenotic arteries is most often caused by a thrombus mainly consisting of platelets (9). Coronary angiography has documented a dynamic build-up of coronary artery thrombotic masses (10) and thus involvement of platelet aggregates in unstable ischaemic heart disease, especially in unstable AP. Elevated thromboxane plasma levels have further documented the involvement of blood platelets in unstable angina (11). Several studies therefore suggest enhanced platelet responsiveness to be part of the acute ischaemic syndromes. Reduced death and reinfarction in subjects treated with acetylsalicylic acid (ASA) in conjunction with acute myocardial infarction (12) strongly indicate that platelets play a primary role. This is substantiated by reports of improved prognosis in patients with unstable AP treated with ASA (13-15). The Oslo-ischaemia-study confirmed the impact of blood platelet counts and aggregability on cardiovascular death. Annual total mortality was significantly higher in the quartile with the highest platelet count (Table I). The mortality was especially increased in the 10 per cent with the highest platelet concentration. Of these, 6 men had platelet counts above 400.000 pr ml, but among them only one man died, therefore the high death-rate is not related to *pathologically* elevated platelet counts. The increased annual mortality was solely due to increased cardiovascular death, since non-cardiovascular deaths were distributed equally in the four quartiles (8). These data are the first to demonstrate a link between blood platelet count and risk of fatal coronary artery thrombotic complications. It was evident using a proportional hazard model that the CHD death-rate was 2.6 times higher in the fourth than in the other three quartiles, after adjusting the data for age, smoking, cholesterol and blood pressure. Thus, blood platelet count was identified to be a strong, independent CHD-death risk factor in apparently healthy middle aged men.

In the 50 per cent with the most pronounced platelet aggregability annual total mortality was significantly increased as compared to the others due to a fourfold increase in CHD-mortality. Thus, blood platelets are linked to fatal CAD-complications, but the mechanisms (thrombus/micro-aggregates/vasospasm) involved are unsettled.

Platelet aggregates are more often found in epicardial vessels in patients with asymptomatic CAD who died suddenly than in patients who died from symptomatic CAD (16). Platelet aggregates may have occluded small coronary vessels and induced focal ischaemic lesions in which lethal arrhythmias have been triggered. Infusion of glass beads into coronary arteries of dogs induced formation of small platelet aggregates and subsequently lethal arrhythmias, which were effectively prevented by platelet depressing drugs (17). Animal studies have further revealed that platelet aggregates formed at non-obstructing stenotic lesions are shed into the blood stream like emboli and may impair myocardial perfusion (18). However, thromboxane synthetase inhibition had no effect on the induction of ventricular tachycardia or fibrillation in dogs which had been subjected to myocardial infarction (19). In 72 patients examined one month after the onset of myocardial infarction, patients who displayed complex arrhythmias had higher platelet aggregability than subjects with stable rhythm (20). We found no relationship between ventricular arrhythmias and platelet aggregability in patients examined in a stable phase several months after acute myocardial infarction (21).

Twentyfour hours ECG monitoring has revealed a circadian distribution of ischaemic episodes with a peak in the early morning hours and in the afternoon. Platelet aggregability is increased at the same times, as is also sudden death and non-fatal myocardial infarction, suggesting that myocardial ischaemia, platelet aggregability and coronary artery occlusions are linked (22, 23).

Blood platelets may not only induce but also aggravate myocardial ischaemia either by mechanical obstruction of small vessels or by release of vasoconstricting thromboxane. In order to study the interplay between blood platelets and myocardial ischaemia, blood was sampled from the coronary sinus and from a reference point (aorta or superior caval vein) (6). Alterations in platelet function induced in the coronary circulation could be examined at rest and during angina induced by atrial pacing. Blood platelets or their products are thought to be of importance for myocardial perfusion, especially in unstable angina and in non-exertional ischaemia. Since 24-hour ECG-monitoring has documented a significant incidence of asymptomatic and non-exertional ischaemia in patients with stable AP also, platelet involvement may differ quantitatively rather than qualitatively in stable and unstable phases of CAD. Studies during pacing-induced AP may therefore have general relevance.There are several methodological concerns using the model described. Blood-sampling through 100 cm long catheters affects blood function (24), but as long as only relative differences between parallell samples are studied, and lactate measurements are used to verify that coronary sinus-blood is sampled from predominantly ischaemic myocardium (net lactate production), relevant information can be obtained.

Our studies showed that blood platelet aggregability was reduced in blood passing the coronary circulation when the patients were at rest (25). The mechanisms responsible for the depressed responsiveness are unknown, but the reduced aggregability hardly represents a refractory state after intracoronary stimulation, since there was no evidence from beta-thromboglobulin (BTG) or thromboxane measurements that blood platelets had been stimulated. Furthermore, release of platelet inhibiting prostacyclin does not explain the reduced platelet function, since ASA failed to normalize the depressed response (25).

In 50 patients with angiographically verified CAD, heart rate was increased gradually by atrial pacing until AP. In 27 patients lactate measurements verified that coronary sinus-blood was sampled from ischaemic myocardium and in 23 patients that blood was sampled from predominantly non-ischaemic myocardium. In blood from ischaemic myocardium, ADP-induced and collagen-induced aggregation, platelet retention and plasma-BTG-levels remained unchanged. Platelet activation was evident in blood from non-ischaemic myocardium (26), a finding in agreement with others (27), but in conflict with some (28) who found platelet activation in coronary sinus-blood during angina not including lactate measurements. Our data suggest that factors other than ischaemia activate platelets in the coronary circulation during tachycardia stress. It is possible that endogenous catecholamines are involved since a non-selective beta adrenoceptor blocking drug (timolol) abolished the induced platelet activation (29).

The model was furthermore used to study the effect of platelet inhibition on myocardial ischaemia. In patients with CAD two identical atrial pacing stress tests were performed before and after ASA (n=10) or thromboxane synthetase inhibition (dazoxiben)(n=15)(30). The ischaemic response, quantified by coronary sinus lactate levels and with ST-depressions, was significantly reduced after dazoxiben, but not after ASA. Both drugs reduced thromboxane formation equally, therefore improved blood flow to ischaemic regions because of enhanced prostacyclin synthesis may explain the beneficial effect of dazoxiben. In another model selective thromboxane synthetase inhibiton reduced experimental infarct size (31), as did prostacyclin (32). Thromboxane synthetase inhibition had no effect on effort AP in another study (33). A low dose of ASA had no effect on variant AP (34), while 4 gm of ASA reduced exercise tolerance in patients with unstable AP (35).

Conclusion

Blood platelets are linked to complicating events in ischaemic heart disease, verified by increased mortality in subjects with a high platelet count or enhanced platelet aggregability. Platelets are not activated in ischaemic myocardium, but in non-ischaemic regions during tachycardia stress, possibly secondary to endogenous catecholamine release. Myocardial perfusion to ischaemic myocardium can be improved by interventions that enhance prostacyclin formation, while thromboxane seems to have little impact on myocardial blood flow in pacing-induced angina. Blood platelet inhibition is especially beneficial in unstable ischaemic heart disease, suggesting that blood platelets play an important role in this phase of CAD.

References

1. Mehta J, Mehta P. Platelet function in hypertension and effects of therapy. Am J Cardiol 1981; 47: 331-4.
2. Carvalho ACA, Colman RW, Lees RS. Platelet function in hyper-lipoproteinemia. N Engl J Med 1974; 290: 434-8.
3. Davis JW, Davis RF. Prevention of sigarette smoking-induced platelet aggregate formation by aspirin. Arch Intern Med 1981; 141: 206-7.
4. Hampton JR, Gorlin R. Platelet studies in patients with coronary artery disease and in their relatives. Br Heart J 1972; 34: 465-71.
5. Erikssen J, Rasmussen K, Forfang K, Storstein O. Exercise ECG and case history in the diagnosis of latent coronary heart disease among presumably healthy middle-aged men. Eur J Cardiol 1977; 5/6: 463-76.
6. Thaulow E, Dale J, Kjekshus J, Simonsen S, Hovig T, Solum N-O. Pacing induced angina and platelet reactivity. Scan J Clin Lab Invest 1982; 42: 607-11.

7. Erikssen J, Mundal R. The non-infarct patient with coronary artery disease: Can a high risk group be identified. Ann NY Acad Sci 1981; 382: 438-51.
8. Thaulow E, Erikssen J, Sandvik L, Cohn PF. Blood platelet count is related to cardiovascular death in apparently healthy men (abstr). Circulation 1989; 80: II-299.
9. Moore S. Platelet aggregation secondary to coronary obstruction. Circulation 1976; 53: 166-72.
10. Holmes DR Jr., Hartzler GO, Smith HC, Fuster V. Coronary artery thrombosis in patients with unstable angina. Br Heart J 1981; 45: 411-6.
11. NeriSerneri GG, Gensini GF, Abbate R, et al. Abnormal cardiocoronary thromboxane A2 production in patients with unstable angina. Am Heart J 1985; 109: 732-8.
12. ISIS-2 Collaborative group. Randomised trial of intravenous streptokinase, oral aspirin, both or neither among 17 187 cases of suspected acute myocardial infarction: ISIS 2. Lancet 1988; II:349-60.
13. Lewis DH Jr., Davis JW, Archibald DG, et al. Protective effects of aspirin against acute myocardial infarction and death in men with unstable angina. N Engl J Med 1983; 309: 396-403.
14. Cairns JA, Gent M, Singer J, et al. Aspirin, sulfinpyrazone, or both in unstable angina. N Engl J Med 1985; 313: 1369-75.
15. Theroux P, Ouimet H, McCans J, et al. Aspirin, heparin, or both to treat acute unstable angina. N Engl J Med 1988; 319: 1105-11.
16. Hærem JW. Platelet aggregates in intramyocardial vessels of patients dying suddenly and unexpectedly of coronary artery disease. Atherosclerosis 1972; 15: 199-213.
17. Franciosa JA, Heckel R. Significance of hypotension preceding ventricular tachyarrhythmias in post coronary obstruction sudden death. Am Heart J 1981; 101: 421-7.
18. Folts JD, Crowell EB, Rowe GG. Platelet aggregation in partially obstructed vessels and its elimination with aspirin. Circulation 1976; 54: 365-70.
19. Kitzen JM, Lynch JJ, Uprichard AC, Venkatesh N, Lucchesi BR. Failure of thromboxane synthetase inhibition to protect the postinfarcted heart against the induction of ventricular tachycardia and ventricular fibrillation in a conscious canine model of sudden coronary death. Pharmacology 1988; 37: 171-86.
20. Geblaska J, Dluzniewski M, Cermuzynski L. Platelet aggregation and arrhythmias after myocardial infarction. Int J Cardiol 1989; 23: 137-8.
21. Thaulow E, Kjekshus J, Erikssen J. The effects of timolol on platelet aggregation. Acta Med Scand 1981; 210 (suppl): 101-9.
22. Tofler GH, Brezinski D, Schafer AI, et al. Concurrernt morning increase in platelet aggregability and the risk of myocardial infarction and sudden cardiac death. N Engl J Med 1987; 316: 1514-8.
23. Mulcahy D, Keegan J, Crean P. Silent myocardial ischemia in chronic stable angina: a study of its frequency and characteristics in 150 patients. Br Heart J 1988; 60: 417-23.
24. Thaulow E. Platelet function in blood sampled through heart catheters. Acta Med Scand 1984; 216: 187-92.
25. Thaulow E. Platelet function in blood from the coronary sinus in patients with arteriosclerotic heart disease. Thromb Haemost 1983; 50: 629-32.
26. Thaulow E. Effects induced on blood platelets in ischemic and nonischemic myocardium. Am J Cardiol 1983; 52: 466-9.
27. Remme WJ, Zijlstra FJ, van de Berg R, Look MP. Myocardial ischemia activates catecholamines and thromboxane. Evidence for cardiac uptake, not release. Circulation (abstr) 1989; 80: II-234.
28. Mehta J, Mehta P, Pepine CJ. Platelet aggregation in aortic and coronary venous blood in patients with and without coronary disease. III. Role of tachycardia stress and propranolol. Circulation 1978; 58: 881-6.

29. Thaulow E, Dale J. Effects of timolol on platelets in coronary sinus blood and on myocardial ischemia during pacing-induced angina. Acta Med Scand 1984; 216: 193-8.
30. Thaulow, E, Dale J, Myhre E. Effects of a selective thromboxane synthetase inhibitor, dixazosin, and of acetylsalicylic acid on myocardial ischemia in patients with coronary artery disease. Am J Cardiol 1984; 53: 1255-8.
31. Burke SE, Lefer AM, Smith GM, Smith JB. Prevention of extension of ischemic damage following acute myocardial ischemia by Doxiben, a new thromboxane synthetase inhibitor. Br J Clin Pharmacol 1983; 15: 97S-101S.
32. Araki H, Lefer AM. Role of prostacyclin in the preservation of ischemic myocardial tissue in the perfused cat heart. Circ Res 1980; 47: 757-63.
33. Reuben SR, Kuan P, Cairns J, Gyde OH. Effects of Doxiben on exercise performance in chronic stable angina. Br J Clin Pharmacol 1983; 15: 83S-6S.
34. Chierchia S, DeCatharina R, Crea F, Patrono C, Maseri A. Failure of thromboxane A2 blockade to prevent attacks of vasospastic angina. Circulation 1982; 66: 702-5.
35. Miwa K, Kambara H, Kawai C. Exercise-induced angina provoked by aspirin administration in patients with variant angina. Am J Cardiol 1981; 47: 1210-4.

Myocardial metabolism and tissue injury

5

Myocardial metabolism

ANNE RAHBEK THOMASSEN,
TORSTEN TOFTEGAARD NIELSEN,
JENS PEDER BAGGER

Myocardial lipid and carbohydrate metabolism

Phasic mechanical activity of the heart neccessitates a continuous supply of nutrients and oxygen for energy production. The regulation of myocardial energy metabolism has been excellently reviewed (1, 2). A brief synopsis of cardiac lipid and carbohydrate metabolism is given here that bears relationships to metabolic diagnosis and treatment of myocardial ischaemia in clinical settings.

The normal heart possesses a remarkable ability to choose between and to oxidize a number of circulating substrates (3). However, under physiological conditions, the only fuels of quantitative importance are free fatty acids *(FFA)*, glucose and lactate that act as competitive substrates (1-3). In the fasting state, with high circulating levels of FFA and low glucose levels, FFA are the preferred fuel, accounting for 60-80% of myocardial energy production (3, 4). Cardiac uptake and oxidation of FFA are linearly related to plasma fatty acid content (1, 2, 4-6) and are decisive for the maintenance of normal cellular function (7). After a carrier mediated influx into the cell (6), FFA are transformed succesively to acyl-coenzyme A and acyl-carnitine and inside the mitochondria again to acyl-coenzyme A that undergoes beta-oxidation to form acetyl-coenzyme A which finally enters the Krebs-cycle (1, 2). Oxygenation of FFA restricts breakdown of glucose and lactate due to inhibition of glycolytic key enzymes (see below) (1,2). Arterial FFA concentration thus becomes a main determinant of myocardial substrate selection being related positively to myocardial uptake of FFA and negatively to the uptake of both glucose and lactate (4, 8).

The normal rates of glucose utilization are low accounting for only 30% of cardiac energy requirements (1, 3). In the presence of insulin, the glycolytic pathway exhibits 2 major control points: phosphofructokinase and glyceraldehyde 3-P dehydrogenase (1, 2). Under most physiologic conditions, phosphofructokinase is the rate-controlling step of glycolysis. Its activity is strongly inhibited by citrate that accumulates during FFA oxidation and is considered to be a main mediator of fatty acid-induced inhibition of glucose breakdown (1, 2, 4, 9). When glycolysis is accelerated due to stimulation of phosphofructokinase, flux through the other control step glyceraldehyde 3-P dehydrogenase becomes rate-limiting due to inhibition by its product NADH (7). Inability of cardiac cells to rapidly remove cytosolic NADH is the reason why neither glucose nor lactate, are solely capable of supplying adequate amounts of acetyl-coenzyme A for oxidative metabolism, whereas pyruvate, the next product in glycolysis, is oxidized readily (7). In the aerobic heart, disposal and reoxidation of cytosolic NADH occurs indirectly by way of the malate-aspartate cycle. Flux through this shuttle is partly regulated by cytosolic glutamate concentration and requires import of glutamate (10). In man, myocardial glutamate uptake is positively related to the uptake of glucose and lactate, suggesting that exogenous glutamate may be of importance for carbohydrate breakdown (4).

Acute myocardial ischaemia (AMI) is associated with dramatic changes in substrate utilization due to alterations of the key regulatory steps in FFA and glucose metabolism. Beta-oxidation of FFA is immediately depressed, because of a rise in mitochondrial NADH (1, 2). Consequently, acyl coenzyme A and acylcarnitine accumulate (11), uptake of FFA decreases (4-6) and a greater fraction of extracted FFA is build into tissue triglycerides, or back-diffuses to the circulation without having undergone metabolic alteration (5). The FFA intermediates may, due to uncoupling and detergent effects, contribute to ischaemic cellular damage (11).

Oxygen deficiency is a strong stimulus for increased glycolysis due to activation of phosphofructokinase by the decreased cellular energy charge (1, 2, 12). The utilization rates of both exogenous glucose and tissue glycogen are accelerated (1, 2, 4, 12). Anaerobic glycolysis with transformation of pyruvate to lactate is compulsory, but despite a pronounced decrease in overall oxidative metabolism, aerobic glycolysis remains the predominant source (90%) of ATP production. In cases of severe ischaemia the initial augmentation of glycolytic flux is short lived. Accumulating lactate, NADH and hydrogen ions depress the activity of rate-limiting glycolytic enzymes (1, 2, 7, 12). Washout of the interstitial space by residual coronary flow assists the efflux of toxic metabolites from the cell and is an important factor in maintaining an accelerated glycolysis (1).

The heart responds to ischaemia by increasing its uptake of glutamate (4, 13) and tissue glutamate is depleted (14). Glutamate may act not only

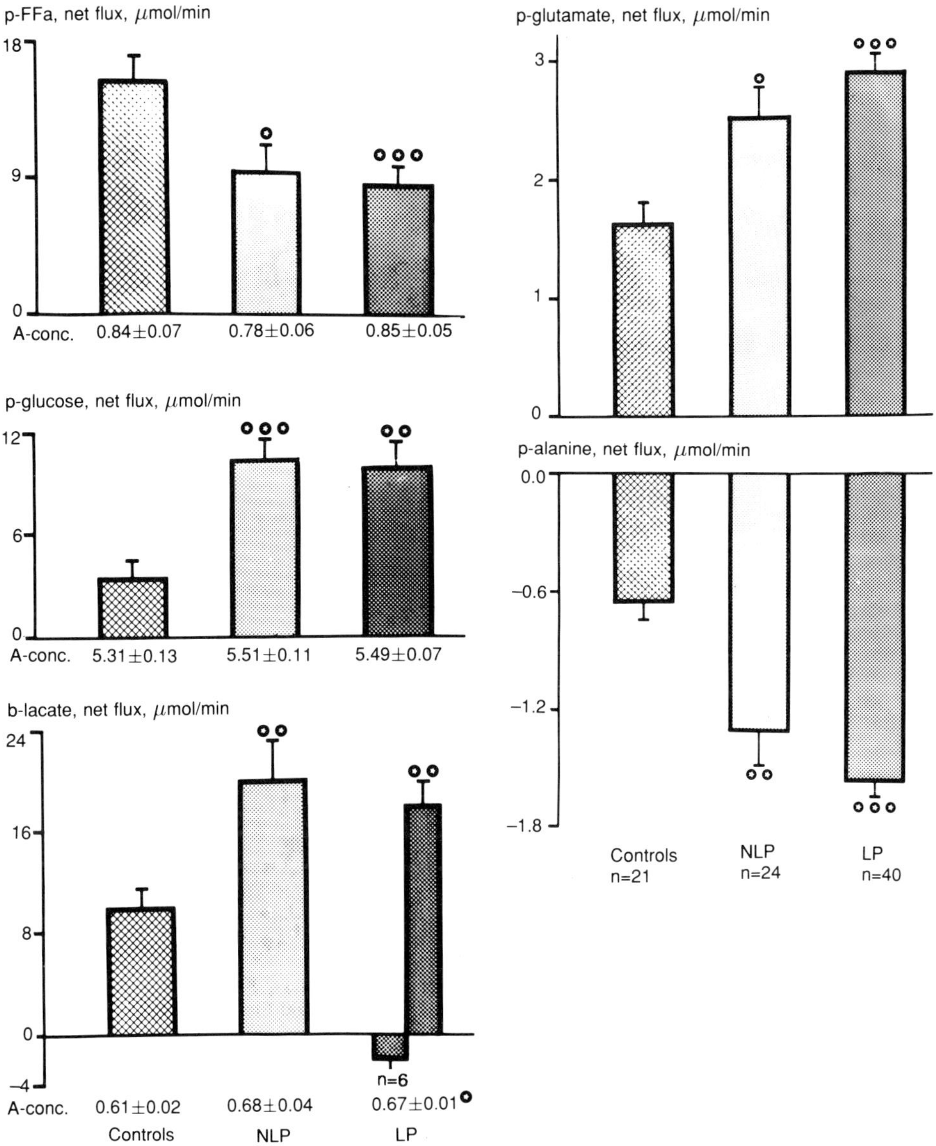

Fig. 1. *Net uptake/release of free fatty acids (FFA), glucose, lactate (left), glutamate and alanine (right) across the non-stressed heart in control patients with normal coronary anatomy and no evidence of heart disease, and in patients with stable effort angina and fixed coronary artery disease. The latter were classified as nonlactate producers (NLP) or lactate producers (LP), depending on whether atrial pacing did or did not induce myocardial lactate release. On average LP were more severe coronary diseased than NLP, and 6 patients showed myocardial lactate release in unstressed state. Data are mean+SEM. A.-conc.= arterial concentration. Difference from controls:* ∘ $P<0.05$, ∘∘ $P<0.01$, ∘∘∘ $P<0.001$. *From (4).*

as aerobic but also as anaerobic fuel via conversion to succinate (15). By transamination, glutamate may transform glycolytic pyruvate to alanine instead of lactate and thereby diminish lactate intoxication (4).

Although energy expenditures are diminished by disruption of mechanical performance, a gross imbalance between ATP supply and demand persists during severe ischaemia. This leads to an accelerated adenine nucleotide degradation along the following pathway: ATP – ADP – AMP – adenosine – inosine – hypoxanthine. Adenosine is lost by penetration of the cell membrane and accounts for a net decrease of the total adenine nucleotide pool and failure to restore ATP levels with reoxygenation (16). Irreversible myocardial damage may result when ATP levels are too low to support critical cellular function.

Recovery occurs quickly after a short attack of ischaemia and is accompanied by an early washout of lactate and an increase in glucose uptake for glycogen replenishment (4). A severe transient ischaemic insult without necrosis may be followed by prolonged depression of myocardial contractile function, the socalled *stunning* (17). The exact mechanism of stunning is controversial, but it is associated with prolonged abnormalities of myocardial energy and substrate metabolism. These include failure to restore ATP levels (16), decreased FFA oxidation and increased glucose utilization (18, 19). Anaerobic glycolysis may persist for up to 24 hours (20). Restoration of metabolic function occurs slowly and parallels functional recovery (19).

Chronic ischaemia. Metabolic investigations in patients with severe coronary artery disease in a resting asymptomatic state and without electrocardiographic evidence of acute ischaemia, have revealed "persistent" changes in regional (18) and global (4) substrate preference. Utilization of FFA is decreased while the consumption of glucose is augmented, regardless of arterial levels (4, 18, 20). Even production of lactate occurs (4, 21). Furthermore, as seen in Figure 1, increased amounts of glutamate are taken up and are released by the heart via alanine (4). The disturbancies in substrate metabolism are related to severity of the disease (4, 21). It remains to be established whether these metabolic changes represent an adaptation to a persistent reduction in myocardial perfusion i.e. chronic ischaemic or hibernating myocardium (22) or whether they are caused by repeated episodes of acute ischaemia followed by periods of incomplete recovery (stunning) that may last until renewed ischaemic insults (20).

Clinical methods of estimating myocardial energy metabolism

Coronary sinus catheterization. The coronary sinus collects cardiac venous efflux, mainly from the left coronary artery tree. Since the discovery by Bing (3) that the coronary sinus can be catheterized from the right atrium, measurements of aorto-coronary sinus substrate differences have been widely used for studying myocardial metabolism in man. Blood flow in the coronary sinus can be estimated by the thermodilution technique (23). Rapid atrial pacing is to be preferred for stressing the heart, because pressure work is neglible and ischaemia is provoked by shortening of the diastolic perfusion time only. We have performed more than 500 pacing studies without serious events. In contrast to exercise or stimulation with adrenergic drugs, heart rate returns to basal level within seconds after pacing is stopped and arterial metabolite concentrations remain unchanged, which is of critical importance for evaluating cardiac substrate exchanges. Atrial pacing can be performed in a haemodynamic and metabolic reproducible manner and thus allows intervention studies with the single patient being his own control. Several metabolites can be measured simultaneously and minute-to-minute changes can be monitored. However, chemically determined aorto-coronary sinus differences represent the net sum of oxidation, storage and possible release of metabolites. This problem may be overcome, to some extent, by using tracer metabolites (21). Interpretations of arterio-venous substrate differences may further be hampered by small absolute values near the analytical precision (glucose, citrate). Despite these limitations, we have defined a useful diagnostic metabolic profile of pacing-induced ischaemia by measurements of several metabolites before, during and after pacing (4). The ischaemic response, which is related to the severity of the disease, includes decreased FFA uptake and increased lactate release during pacing, increased glucose uptake and citrate release within the first minutes of recovery and increased glutamate uptake and alanine release throughout the study (4).

While evaluation of myocardial metabolism by the coronary sinus catheterization technique is easy to perform, safe, reproducible and inexpensive, it permits an estimate of global metabolic disturbancies only. By nature, flow and metabolic disturbancies in ischaemic heart disease are regional. Dilution of effluents from ischaemic zones with flow from normal areas decreases the diagnostic sensitivity.

Positron emmission tomography (PET). With the development of PET it has become possible noninvasively to study regional metabolism of the human heart (20). By tagging short-lived (half-life: 2-112 min) positron emitting tracers of oxygen, nitrogen, carbon and fluorine to natural substrates without affecting their biochemical properties, PET permits evaluation of regional myocardial blood flow (^{82}Ru, ^{13}N-ammonia), glucose utilization (^{18}F-2-deoxyglucose), FFA oxidation (^{11}C-palmitate), amino acid metabolism

(^{13}N-glutamate) and oxygen consumption (^{11}C-acetate) (5, 6, 12, 18, 20). Considerable insight into the regional utilization rates and fate of substrates in coronary artery disease, and thereby in the nature of the disease, have been gained from PET. In fact, the idea of a chronic ischaemic state and the hibernating myocardium with reduced blood flow but maintained residual metabolism (flow-metabolism mismatch) have been conceived on the basis of PET studies. PET is able to differentiate between normal, viable but ischaemic tissue and myocardial necrosis by quantification of regional disturbancies in blood flow and glucose utilization. This may be of considerable clinical relevance with regard to the selection of patients for medical or surgical interventional treatment (20).

Although PET is unique for imaging moment to moment regional changes in myocardial metabolism and perfusion, its research as well as clinical application will probably be limited by the high costs. A full operating PET centre necessitates an in-house cyclotron, due to the short half-life of tracers and radiochemicals.

Endomyocardial biopsy. Biochemical evaluation of myocardial biopsies (measurements of enzyme activities, content of essential cofactors, lipid and glycogen stores, and energy rich phoshate compounds) may prove to be of value in the future, especially for the classification of cardiomyopathies. The main methodological problems are those of sampling error and contamination with blood and connective tissue. Biochemical analysis of biopsy tissue may be representative and informative only in patients with homogenous heart diseases. Metabolite measurements have been related to the content of intracellular heart cell markers (creatine) in order to overcome blood and tissue contamination (24). So far, only scattered reports have appeared. A decreased ATP content in endomyocardial biopsies has been reported in congestive cardiomyopathy related to the increase in right and left ventricular end diastolic pressure (24), and low levels of coenzyme Q-10 (25).

Metabolic intervention

Knowledge of specific myocardial metabolic changes in response to ischaemia forms the basis of and inspires to more effective treatment. Thus, it is logical to propose limitation of fatty acid metabolism and promotion of glycolysis as a means of improving cardiac performance during and after ischaemia. In man, metabolic support with glucose-insulin-potassium infusion or glucose alone has been demonstrated to increase the tolerance to pacing-induced ischaemia (26), to enhance myocardial preservation during aortic cross-clamping (27) and to improve the outcome of AMI both when the infusion is given alone (28) or in combination with streptokinase (29). Augmented provision of insulin and glucose increases tissue glycogen (12, 27) and may accelerate glycolysis during moderate ischaemia but cannot be expected to surmount the intracellular block of glycolysis that characterizes severe ischaemia (12). Several promising studies have been performed in attempts to avoid the limiting steps of glycolysis, using short-carbon derivatives that can enter the mitochondria or even the Krebs cycle directly. They include pyruvate (30), acetate (31), aspartate and glutamate (32) all of which provide protection in ischaemic animal heart preparations. In patients with stable angina pectoris, exercise tolerance is increased after pretreatment with glutamate orally or intravenously (33). Intravenous infusion of glutamate (34) and application of glutamate-enriched cardioplegia (35) to patients with cardiac failure is associated with improved left ventricular function and preserved tissue ATP stores (14). *Allen et al* (36) noted remarkable improvement in regional wall motion score after operative revascularization as long as 8 hours after AMI in a small clinical series in which they applied glutamate and aspartate enhanced cardioplegia during the operative procedure. Recently in our own laboratory, we found that systemic administration of glutamate in man, not only increases cardiac utilization of glutamate, but also stimulates endogenous insulin secretion, augments arterial levels and cardiac consumption of glucose, while circulating levels and cardiac uptake of free fatty acids are diminished (37). Further, investigations of the effects of systemic glutamate are needed before it can be advocated for the treatment of acute ischaemia in man.

Despite the positive reports, clinical application of metabolic intervention has not yet gained widespread acceptance as has the use of drugs, especially beta-adrenergic blockers, for protection of the heart in acute ischaemic syndromes. However, the well-known beneficial effects of beta-blockers are not entirely caused by a haemodynamic reduction in myocardial oxygen demand but are also associated with an increased uptake of glucose and glutamate in the ischaemic heart on one side and a decreased fatty acid load and extraction on the other (38).

Summary

The normal, well-oxygenated heart prefers free fatty acids *(FFA)* as fuel. During acute ischaemia, oxidation and uptake of FFA is depressed and the heart becomes dependent upon increased aerobic and anaerobic breakdown of glucose and glycogen. Lactate accumulates and may secondarily inhibit glycolysis. Glutamate is an alternative anaerobic substrate that is converted to alanine and succinate. Metabolic diagnosis of ischaemia in man is possible by coronary sinus catheterization or positron emmision tomography *(PET)* showing decreased extraction of FFA, increased utilization of glucose and glutamate and cardiac release of lactate and alanine. PET may differentiate between myocardial necrosis and chronically jeopardized tissue, the latter being characterized by reduced blood flow but maintained glucose metabolism. Biochemical evaluation of endomyocardial biopsies may become of clinical importance in the characterization of cardiomyopathies in the future. Knowledge of the metabolic response to ischaemia has inspired several promising studies that show improved protection against ischaemic damage during metabolic support with glucose-insulin-potassium, pyruvate, acetate, aspartate and glutamate.

References

1. Neely JR, Morgan HE. Relationship between carbohydrate and lipid metabolism and the energy balance of the heart muscle. Annu Rev Physiol 1974; 36: 413-59.
2. Randle PJ, Tubbs PK. Carbohydrate and fatty acid metabolism. In: Berne RM, Speralakis N, Geiger SR, eds. Handbook of physiology. The cardiovascular system. Vol I. The heart. Bethesda, Am Physiol Soc, 1979: 805-44.
3. Bing RJ. The metabolism of the heart. Harvey Lecture series. New York, Academic Press, Inc., 1954-1955: 27-70.
4. Thomassen A, Bagger JP, Nielsen TT, Henningsen P. Altered global myocardial substrate preference at rest and during pacing in coronary artery disease with stable angina pectoris. Am J Cardiol 1988; 62: 686-93.
5. Fox KAA, Abendschein DR, Ambos HD, Sobel BE, Bergmann SR. Efflux of metabolized and nonmetabolized fatty acid from canine myocardium. Implication for quantifying myocardial metabolism tomographically. Circ Res 1985; 57: 232-43.
6. Vyska K, Machulla HJ, Stremmel W, et al. Regional myocardial free fatty acid extraction in normal and ischaemic myocardium. Circulation 1988; 78: 1218-33.
7. Kobayashi K, Neely JR. Control of maximum rates of glycolysis in rat cardiac muscle. Circ Res 1979; 44: 166-75.
8. Lassers BW, Wahlquist ML, Kaijser L, Carlson LA. Relationship in man between plasma free fatty acids and myocardial metabolism of carbohydrate substrates. Lancet 1971; II: 448-50.
9. Nielsen TT. Plasma citrate in relation to glucose and free fatty acid metabolism in man. Thesis. Dan Med Bull 1983; 30: 357-78.
10. Digerness SB, Reddy WJ. The malate-aspartate shuttle in heart mitochondria. J Mol Cell Cardiol 1976; 8: 779-85.
11. Liedtke AJ, Nellis S, Neely JR. Effects of excess free fatty acids on mechanical and metabolic function in normal and ischaemic myocardium in swine. Circ Res 1978; 43: 652-61.
12. Opie LH. Effects of regional ischaemia on metabolism of glucose and fatty acids. Circ Res 1976; 38 (suppl 1): 152-68.
13. Zimmermann R, Tillmanns H, Knapp WH, et al. Regional myocardial nitrogen-13 glutamate uptake in patients with coronary artery disease: Inverse post-stress relation to thallium-201 uptake in ischaemia. J Am Coll Cardiol 1988; 11: 549-56.

14. Pisarenko OI, Portney VF, Studneva IM, Arapov AD, Korostylev AN. Glutamate-blood cardioplegia improves ATP preservation in human myocardium. Biomed Biochim Acta 1987; 46: 499-504.
15. Sanborn T, Gavin W, Berkowitz S, Perille T, Lesch M. Augmented conversion of aspartate and glutamate to succinate during anoxia in rabbit heart. Am J Physiol 1979; 237: H535-41.
16. Reibel DK, Rovetto MJ. Myocardial adenosine salvage rates and restoration of ATP content following ischaemia. Am J Physiol 1979; 237: H247-52.
17. Braunwald E, Kloner RA. The stunned myocardium: prolonged post-ischaemic ventricular dysfunction. Circulation 1982; 66: 1146-9.
18. Marshall RC, Tillisch JH, Phelps ME, et al. Identification and differentiation of resting myocardial ischaemia and infarction in man with positron computed tomography, 18F-labeled fluorodeoxyglucose and N13 ammonia. Circulation 1983; 67: 766-78.
19. Schwalger M, Schelbert HR, Ellison D, et al. Sustained regional abnormalities in cardiac metabolism after transient ischaemia in the chronic dog model. J Am Coll Cardiol 1985; 6: 336-47.
20. Schelbert HR, Buxton DB. Insights into coronary artery disease gained from metabolic imaging. Circulation 1988; 78: 496-505.
21. Gertz EW, Wisneski JA, Neese R, Bristow JP, Searle GL, Hanlon JT. Myocardial lactate metabolism: Evidence of lactate release during net chemical extraction in man. Circulation 1981; 63: 1273-1279.
22. Braunwald E, Rutherford JD. Reversible ischaemic left ventricular dysfunction: Evidence for the "Hibernating Myocardium". J Am Coll Cardiol 1986; 8: 1467-70.
23. Ganz W, Tamura K, Marcus HS, Donoso R, Yoshida S, Swan HJC. Measurement of coronary sinus blood flow by continuous thernodilution in man. Circulation 1971; 44: 181-95.
24. Unverfeth DV, Fertal RH, Altschuld R, Magorien RD, Lewis RP, Leier CV. Biochemical measurements of endomyocardial biopsies. Cath Cardiovasc Diagn 1981; 7: 55-64.
25. Mortensen SA. Endomyocardial biopsy. Thesis. Copenhagen, Lægeforeningens Forlag, 1989.
26. Thomassen A, Nielsen TT, Bagger JP, Henningsen P. Antianginal and cardiac metabolic effects of low dose glucose infusion during pacing in patients with and without coronary artery disease. Am Heart J 1989; 118: 25-32.
27. Berggren H, Ekroth R, Herlitz J, et al. Improved myocardial protection during cold cardioplegia by means of increased myocardial glycogen stores. Thorac cardiovasc Surgeon 1982; 30: 389-92.
28. Whitlow PL, Rogers WJ, Smith LR, et al. Enhancement of left ventricular function by glucose-insulin-potassium infusion in acute myocardial infarction. Am J Cardiol 1983; 49: 811-20.
29. Satler LF, Green CE, Kent KM, Pallas RS, Pearle DL, Rackley CE. Metabolic support during coronary reperfusion. Am Heart J 1987; 114: 54-8.
30. Regitz V, Azumi T, Stephan H, Naujocks S, Schaper W. Biochemical mechanism of infarct size reduction by pyruvate. Cardiovasc Res 1981; 15: 652-8.
31. Vary TC, Angelakos ET, Schaffer SW. Relationship between adenine nucleotide metabolism and irreversible ischaemic tissue damage in isolated perfused rat heart. Circ Res 1979; 45: 218-25.
32. Rau EE, Shine KI, Gervais A, Douglas AM, Amos EC. Enhanced mechanical recovery of anoxic and ischaemic myocardium by amino acid perfusion. Am J Physiol 1979; 236: H873-9.
33. Thomassen A, Bøtker HE, Nielsen TT, Thygesen K, Henningsen P. Effects of glutamate

on exercise tolerance and circulating substrate levels in stable angina pectoris. Am J Cardiol 1990; 65: 173-8.

34. Pisarenko OI, Lepilin MG, Ivanov VE. Cardiac metabolism and performance during L-glutamic acid infusion in postoperative failure. Clin Sci 1986; 70: 7-12.
35. Rosenkranz ER, Buckberg GD, Laks H, Mulder DG. Warm induction of cardioplegia with glutamate-enriched blood in coronary patients with cardiogenic shock who are dependent on inotropic drugs and intra-aortic balloon support. J Thorac Cardiovasc Surg 1983; 86: 507-18.
36. Allen BS, Buckberg GD, Schwaiger M, et al. Studies of controlled reperfusion after ischaemia XVI. Early recovery of regional wall motion in patients following surgical revascularization after eight hours of acute coronary occlusion. J Thorac Cardiovasc Surg 1986; 92: 636-48.
37. Thomassen A, Nielsen TT, Bagger JP, Henningsen P. Systemic and cardiac metabolism and hemodynamic effects of intravenous glutamate in man. Metabolism 1990 (submitted).
38. Nielsen TT, Bagger JP, Thomassen A. Improved myocardial lactate extraction after propranolol in coronary artery disease: effected by peripheral glutamate and free fatty acid metabolism. Br Heart J 1986; 55: 140-7.

6

Lipid accumulation in the myocardium during ischaemia

HARALD JODALEN,
GOTFRIED GREVE,
SVEIN ROTEVATN

Fatty change is observed in a number of diseases in various organ systems like the liver, kidney, and heart. In the heart, neutral fat may accumulate in diabetes, starvation, myocarditis, heart failure, poisoning (e.g. ethanol, phosphorus), and ischaemia (1). This morphological manifestation of an altered lipid metabolism, was earlier described by pathologists as fatty degeneration or fatty infiltration (2, 3). These terms have today been replaced by the more descriptive term fatty change.

Lipid metabolism

Cardiac energy production is regulated by the needs of the myocardium (4, 5), and a number of substrates are utilized. Glucose and fatty acids are the major oxidative substrates, but lactate, pyruvate, ketone bodies, and amino acids can all contribute. Their relative contribution depends on the supply from the circulation, availability of alternative substrates, oxygen supply, rate of oxidative respiration, and mechanical activity (6-8).

In a majority of metabolic situations, oxidative phosphorylation supplies the myocardium with more than 90% of the total ATP supply and, thus, is the most important source of ATP (9). Fatty acids are the preferred fuel for the aerobic myocardium. In a fasting condition, 60-90% of the total oxygen consumption may be ascribed to the β-oxidation of fatty acids (4, 6, 10), while in the presence of exogenous glucose, it may account for 35-70% (11). The energy reserves in the heart are limited. As much as 5% of the ATP and creatine phosphate stored, may be consumed per beat. The triacylglycerol (triglyceride) reserves in the heart thus provide enough energy to maintain a high ventricular function for no more than 12 minutes (12). A continuous supply of substrates and oxygen is crucial for proper function of the heart.

The heart contributes only about 0.1% of the total fatty acid production in the body. For all practical purposes fatty acids stem from extracardiac sources (13). Fatty acids are supplied by the blood either in the form of non-esterified fatty acids bound to albumin or as elements of triacylglycerols in lipoproteins and chylomicrons (14). Fatty acids from circulating phospholipids are not taken up by the heart (15). Experiments in perfused isolated rat hearts have shown a significant uptake of fatty acids from triacylglycerols (15). It is technically difficult to detect similar mechanisms *in vivo*, as a 1-2% arterio-venous difference in the concentration of triacylglycerols may represent 15% of the total myocardial energy consumption (16). Uptake and utilization of fatty acids are limited by the fatty acid to albumin ratio in plasma and by the metabolic state of the cardiac myocytes (4, 17, 18). Because the plasma albumin levels tend to be fairly constant, the supply of fatty acids is mainly determined by their concentrations in the plasma (19). Fatty acids, released from adipose tissues by hormone sensitive lipolysis, are the main source of the albumin bound fatty acids. In the plasma 5-10% of the total content of fatty acids is in the form of non-esterified fatty acids, and the half-life of this pool is 2-3 minutes (20).

Approximately 10% of the non-esterified fatty acids in the plasma is taken up by the heart (21). In the rat, there is a strong concentration gradient for non-esterified fatty acids from arterial blood (310 μM) to the cytoplasm (21 μM)(22). Non-esterified fatty acids are taken up from the circulation by the capillary endothelium and transported to the myocytes (Fig. 1). Fatty acids bound in triacylglycerols, can only pass the capillary endothelium after hydrolysis from glycerol (23). Only non-esterified fatty acids are taken up by the capillary endothelium lower case from the circulation, and not the glycerol component of the triacylglycerols (24, 25). Catecholamine stimulated lipoprotein lipases in the capillary endothelium mediate hydrolysis of triacylglycerols in chylomicrons, very-low-density lipoproteins, and low-density lipoproteins (26, 27). There are specific albumin receptors on the luminal surface of the endothelial cells which may account for the transcapillary transfer (28). There are also reports suggesting an albumin receptor on the sarcolemma (29). The transport of fatty acids over the sarcolemma may be mediated by specific fatty acid-binding proteins in the membrane (30). Another fatty acid-binding protein has been isolated in the cytoplasm, which may represent an intracellular transport mechanism (31).

In the cytoplasm, fatty acids are activated by ATP-dependent esterification to coenzyme A by the enzyme acyl-CoA synthetase (32). Cytoplasmic fatty acyl-CoA may be utilized for energy production in the mitochondria,

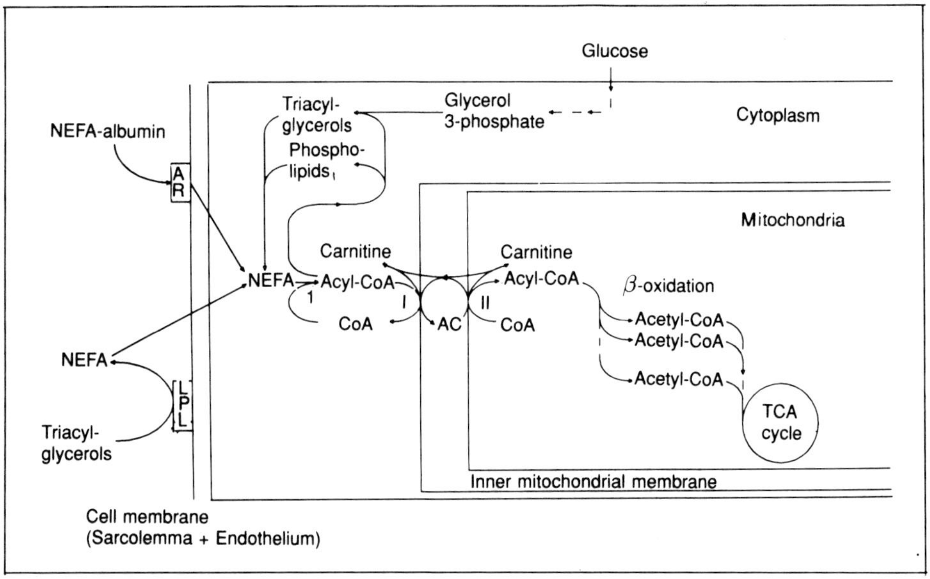

Fig. 1. *Uptake, transport, and metabolism of non-esterified fatty acid in cardiac muscle cells. NEFA = non-esterified fatty acids. AR = albumin receptor. LPL = lipoprotein lipase. AC = acyl carnitine. I = carnitine acyltransferase I. II = carnitine acyltransferase II. 1 = acyl-CoA synthetase. TCA cycle = tricarboxylic acid cycle.*

or be utilized for synthesis of complex lipids such as triacylglycerols and phospholipids (Fig. 1).

Fatty acyl-CoA cannot cross the inner mitochondrial membrane, and the acyl component is transferred to carnitine by carnitine acyltransferase I to be shuttled as acyl carnitine into the mitochondria by an acyl carnitine carrier. Reconversion of the acyl group to acyl-CoA inside the mitochondria is catalysed by carnitine acyltransferase II (Fig. 1). As much as 95% of the total cellular content of carnitine is found in the cytoplasm, whereas 95% of the total cellular content of coenzyme A is mitochondrial (14).

Ischaemia

The supply of fatty acids from the circulation, from albumin bound non-esterified fatty acids and triacylglycerols, increases during ischaemia. Increased catecholamine release mobilizes fatty acids from the lipid stores in the body by stimulating the lipase activity in lipocytes and, thus, increases the level of fatty acids in the circulation. There is also some support for an increased lipoprotein lipase activity in the capillary endothelium during ischaemia due to catecholamine stimulation (33). Fatty acids are, thereby, released from the triacylglycerols of circulating lipoproteins.

Coronary artery occlusion induces an abrupt fall in the supply of oxygen and substrates necessary for energy production. Simultaneously, metabolites from the ischaemic myocardium accumulate as their transport from the heart ceases. The rate limiting step in the utilization of fatty acids shifts from transport of fatty acids into the cell, to mitochondrial oxidation (34, 35). Initially there is stimulation of the glycogenolysis and glycolysis, and, hence, the energy supply shifts from mainly β-oxidation of fatty acids to anaerobic glycolysis. Due to the high demand for ATP, to maintain contractile activity and ion gradients, there is a rapid fall in creatine phosphate and ATP during the first minutes of myocardial ischaemia (36-38). As a consequence of the increased glycolysis, lactate accumulates in the myocardium, and the resulting acidification impairs a number of cellular processes. At later stages of ischaemia, the glycolysis is inhibited due to accumulation of lactate, H^+, and other metabolites (4, 39, 40). Because of the inadequate supply of oxygen, and resulting depression of β-oxidation, there is an accumulation of fatty acid intermediates; acyl carnitine in the cytosol and acyl-CoA in the mitochondria (41, 42). In addition, glyceraldehyde 3-phosphate dehydrogenase is impaired by ischaemia and adrenergic agents, resulting in accumulation of glycerol 3-phosphate which is a substrate for triacylglycerol formation (43).

The transport of fatty acyl derivatives into the mitochondria for β-oxidation is dependent on the acyl carnitine carrier system which may be impaired by lactate, an inhibitor of carnitine acyltransferase (44). Lactate from the ischaemic tissue may, thus, induce accumulation of substrates for esterification of fatty acids to triacylglycerols in the cytoplasm of cells both in the central ischaemic area and its periphery, the border zone.

Accumulation of fatty acids and other amphipathic metabolites within the myocardium has been reported to be associated with arrhythmia (45), increased myocardial oxygen demand, and depressed left ventricular function (46-48).

In addition to the increased supply from external sources, there is a potential for mobilizing fatty acids from cell membranes due to increased phospholipase activity. Thus, there are concentrations of intracellular metabolites of fatty acids, acyl-CoA, and acyl carnitine, which have been suggested to exert detergent effects on cell membranes (49). Esterification of the lipid metabolites to triacylglycerols may represent a protective mechanism against their detergent effect.

Morphological consequences

Morphological manifestation of lipid accumulation is found in the form of

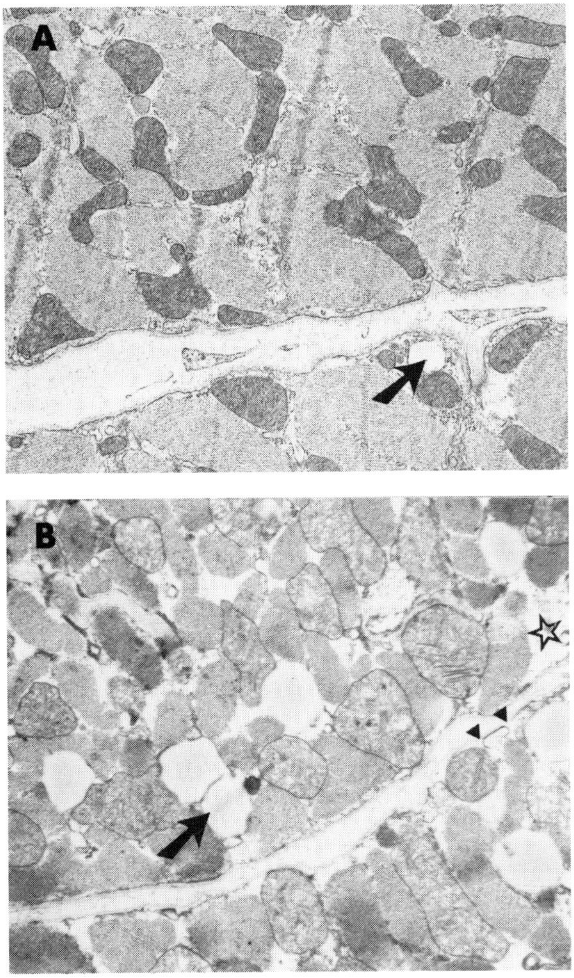

Fig. 2. *Micrographs from left ventricular myocardium of a sham operated cat (A), and from the border zone of a heart after three hours occlusion of the left anterior descending coronary artery (B), showing severe injury. Arrows indicate lipid droplets, arrowheads sarcolemmal disruption, and asterisks cytoplasmic oedema. Sections stained by uranyl acetate and lead citrate. Magnification X 9600.*

spherical non-membrane bound structures (Fig. 2). These vaguely opaque lipid droplets are often observed in close proximity to the mitochondria which are arranged in rows between the myofibrils. They are believed to represent triacylglycerols (50) and can, hence, be used to obtain metabolic information by morphological analysis. This can be performed in samples consisting of only a few cells or even single cells if serial sections are studied.

There is some evidence from morphological studies of increased fragility of the cell membrane in the early stages of ischaemia as well as in cells otherwise appearing structurally intact in the border zone (51, 52). There is, however, a coincidence of membrane fragility and accumulation of lipid droplets which is consistent with the hypothesis of a contribution of lipids from the cell membranes to the lipid droplets (Fig. 3) (51).

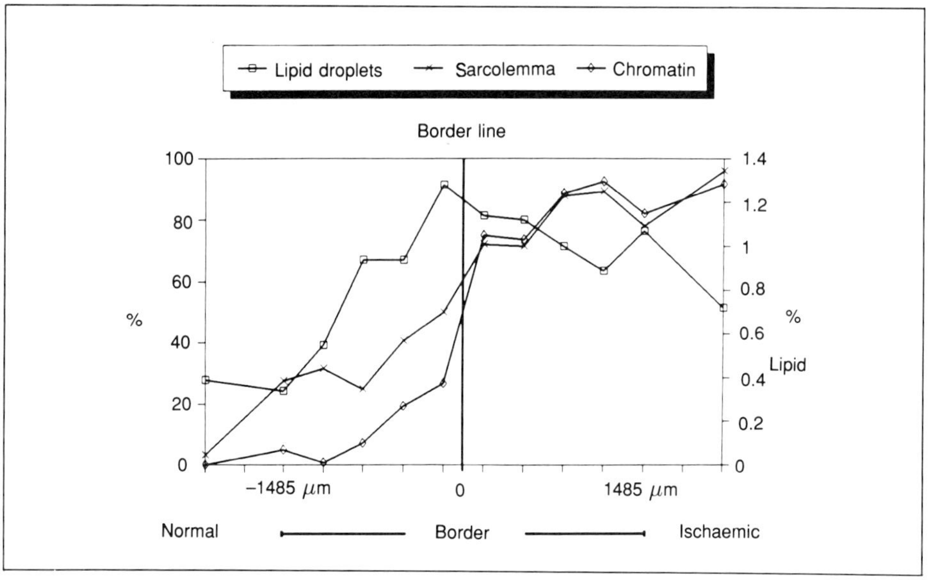

Fig. 3. *Level of cell injury in the central ischaemic and border zones of cat hearts three hours after occlusion of the left anterior descending coronary artery. Shown are the percentages of myocytes with sarcolemmal disruption (X) and chromatin clumping or margination (dimonds) obtained after assessing 480 myocytes in the normal and central ischaemic zones, and 4800 myocytes in twenty subsequent areas of the border zone. The areas were located 165 μm apart. The border line is defined by the abrupt increase in these variables, which are closely correlated. The diagram also shows the corresponding fractional volumes of lipid droplets (squares) measured in the same sections. Towards the normally perfused side of the border line, one can observe areas with considerable lipid accumulation.*

In healthy hearts and in the normally perfused part of hearts with regional ischaemia, there are only a few lipid droplets. During myocardial ischaemia they become more numerous, especially in the border zone surrounding the infarct (Figs. 2 and 3) (50). Across this zone there is also a marked increase in the number of cells showing sarcolemmal damage and chromatin clumping (referred to as *border line*). Quantitative analyses from hearts with regional ischaemia have shown a distinct pattern in the fractional volume of lipid droplets in respect of the sarcolemmal and nuclear changes (50, 51). On the normal side of this border line there is a zone characterized by lipid droplet accumulation, mitochondrial oedema, and sarcolemmal fragility (Fig. 3). The cells in this zone also have a mild cytoplasmic oedema (50, 51). Similar alterations, except a less prominent mitochondrial swelling, can be observed in early stages of ischaemic cell injury in the central parts of the ischaemic zone (Fig. 4) (52). The lipid droplet accumulation observed in the border zone, may be explained by a larger delivery of fatty acids to the myocardium here. Coronary occlusion induces mobilization of fatty acids from peripheral depots and, thereby, increases the plasma content (50). Accordingly, an increased supply of fatty acids may well represent the major determinant of lipid accumulation in the border zone, whereas a reduced capacity to utilize fatty acids represents the limiting factor in the central ischaemic zone. As in low flow ischaemia, the collateral blood supply to the border zone, may supply sufficient oxygen for oxidation of some lactate and fatty acids. Thus, the cell may function by a mixture of aerobic and anaerobic metabolism (53, 54).

Pharmacological intervention

Drugs commonly used in the treatment of patients with myocardial ischaemia interact with lipid metabolism. The conventional analgetic treatment with morphine in acute myocardial infarction is likely to reduce catecholamine release and, thus, the supply of fatty acids. The synthetic catecholamine isoproterenol has been found to induce marked accumulation of

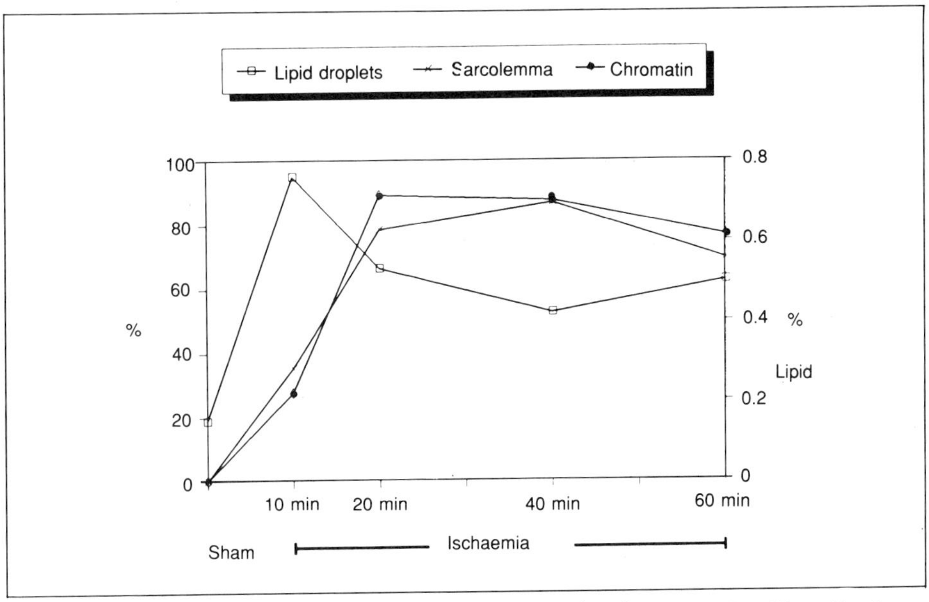

Fig. 4. *Level of cell injury in the central ischaemic zone of cat hearts 10, 20, 40 or 60 minutes after occlusion of the left anterior descending coronary artery. Shown are the percentages of myocytes with sarcolemmal disruption (X) and chromatin clumping or margination (dimonds) obtained after assessing a total number of 2400 myocytes in the central ischaemic zone and in sham operated cats. The figure also shows the corresponding fractional volumes of lipid droplets (squares) measured in the same sections. Sarcolemmal damage and nuclear alterations are closely correlated, and are preceded by peak values of lipid droplet accumulation after 10 minutes.*

lipid droplets (55). This is interpreted as resulting from an increased supply of non-esterified fatty acids, both from mobilization in lipocytes, and activation of the lipoprotein lipase in coronary capillaries. Cathecholamine stimulation of the mechanical activity and β-oxidation is not sufficient to consume the increased supply. The β-blocker, propranolol, does also induce lipid accumulation, probably because it impairs the β-oxidation without reducing the supply of fatty acids. In hearts with regional ischaemia, the β-blocker timolol, reduces the lipid accumulation in the border zone, but not in the central ischaemic zone (56). Timolol inhibits the increase in plasma fatty acids otherwise seen in ischaemia. Calcium channel blockade by verapamil increases lipid accumulation in the central ischaemic area, but not in the border zone (57). Verapamil induces an increased supply of fatty acids in ischaemia, and it has also been speculated that verapamil may improve the ability of the myocytes to esterify fatty acid intermediates.

Conclusion

Lipid droplets accumulate as a result of two major factors, increased supply of fatty acids from plasma non-esterified fatty acids and lipoproteins, and from reduced β-oxidation. Lipid droplet accumulation is reversible (58, 59) and is not directly related to cell damage. It can, therefore, not be used as an indicator of cell injury. Rather, it is an indicator of the metabolic state, to be interpreted in context with other variables. Advanced technology like positron emission tomography has been applied to non-invasively assess lipid accumulation in the heart (60). Thus, the myocardial fatty change associated with ischaemia, as described by the early masters of pathology (2, 3), makes possible a method of metabolic imaging which contributes to the detection and localization of myocardial ischaemia.

References

1. Alavaikko M, Hirvonen J, Räsänen O. Fatty change in papillary heart muscle and its arterioles. Acta Path Microbil Immunol Scand Sect A 1970; 78: 458-72.
2. Virchow R. Cellular pathology as based upon physiological and pathological histology. Philadelphia: P Blakiston Son & Co, 1860.
3. Rokitansky C. A manual of pathological anatomy. London: Sydenham Society, Vol 4, 1854.
4. Neely JR, Morgan HE. Relationship between carbohydrate and lipid metabolism and energy balance of heart muscle. Ann Rev Physiol 1974; 36: 413-59.
5. Randle PJ, Tubbs PK. Carbohydrate and fatty acid metabolism. In: Berne RM, ed. Handbook of physiology. Bethesda: American Physiological Society, 1979: 805.

6. Opie LH. Metabolism in the heart in health and disease. Part II. Am Heart J 1969; 77: 100-22.
7. Neely JR, Rovetto MJ, Oram JF. Myocardial utilization of carbohydrate and lipids. Prog Cardiovasc Dis 1972; 15: 289-327.
8. Mjøs OD. Effect of free fatty acids on myocardial function and oxygen consumption in intact dogs. J Clin Invest 1971; 50: 1386-9.
9. Kobayashi K, Neely JR. Control of maximum rates of glycolysis in rat cardiac muscle. Circ Res 1979; 44: 166-75 .
10. Lassers BW, Carlson LA, Kaijser L, Wahlquist M. The nature and control of myocardial substrate metabolism in healthy man. In: Oliver MF, Julian DG, Donald KW, eds. Effects of acute ischemia on myocardial function. London: Churchill Livingstone, 1972: 200-12.
11. Crass III MF, Shipp JC. Metabolism of exogenous and endogenous fatty acids in the heart. In: Bajusz E, Rona G, eds. Recent advances in studies on cardiac structure and metabolism. Baltimore: University Park Press, 1970: 115-25.
12. Morgan HE, Neely JR. Metabolic regulation and myocardial function. In: Hurst JW, ed. The heart. New York: McGraw-Hill, 1985: 85-100.
13. Gandemer GG, Durand G, Pascal G. Relative contribution of the main tissues and organs to fatty acid synthesis in the rat. Lipids 1983; 18: 223-8.
14. Idell-Wenger JA, Neely JR. Regulation of uptake and metabolism of fatty acids by muscle. In: Dietschy JM, Gotto AM, Ontko JA, eds. Disturbances in lipid and lipoprotein metabolism. Bethesda: American Physiological Society, 1978: 269-84.
15. Delcher HK, Fried M, Shipp JC. Metabolism of lipoprotein lipid in the isolated perfused rat heart. Biochim Biophys Acta 1965; 106: 10-8.
16. Willebrands AF. Myocardial extraction of individual non-esterified fatty acids, esterified fatty acids and aceto-acetate in the fasting human. Clin Chim Acta 1964; 10: 435-46.
17. Oram JF, Bennetsch SL, Neely JR. Regulation of fatty acid utilization in isolated perfused rat hearts. J Biol Chem 1973; 248: 5299-309.
18. Miller NE, Mjøs OD, Oliver MF. Relationship of epicardial ST-segment elevation to the plasma free fatty acid/albumin ratio during coronary occlusion in dogs. Clin Sci Mol Med 1976; 51: 209-13.
19. Carlsten A, Hallgren B, Jagenburg R, Svanborg A, Werkø L. Myocardial metabolism of glucose, lactic acid, amino acids and fatty acids in healthy human individuals at rest and at different work loads. Scand J Clin Lab Invest 1961; 13: 418-25.
20. Spector AA. The transport and utilization of free fatty acids. Ann NY Acad Sci 1968; 149: 768-83.
21. Miller HI, Yum KY, Durham BC. Myocardial free fatty acid in unanaesthetized dogs at rest and during exercise. Am J Physiol 1971; 220: 589-96.
22. Van der Vusse GJ, Roemen THM, Flameng W, Reneman RS. Serum-myocardium gradients of non-esterified fatty acids in dog, rat and man. Biochim Biophys Acta 1983; 752: 361-70.
23. Stam H, Huelsmann WC. Regulation of lipases involved in the supply of substance fatty acids for the heart. Eur Heart J 1985; 6: 158-67.
24. Scheuer J, Olson RE. Metabolism of exogenous triglyceride by the isolated perfused rat heart. Am J Physiol 1967; 212: 301-7.
25. Tamboli A, O'Looney P, van der Maten M, Vahouny GV. Metabolism of fatty acids, glycerol and a monoglyceride analogue by cardiac myocytes and perfused hearts. Lipids 1983; 18: 808-13.
26. Kreisberg RA. Effect of epinephrine on myocardial triglyceride and free fatty acid utilization. Am J Physiol 1966; 210: 385-9.

27. Pedersen ME, Cohen M, Schotz MC. Immunocytochemical localization of the functional fraction of lipoprotein lipase in the perfused heart. J Lipid Res 1983; 24: 512-21.
28. Ghitescu L, Fixman A, Simionescu M, Simionescu N. Spesific binding sites for albumin restricted to plasmalemmal vesicles of continuous capillary endothelium: Receptor-mediated transcytosis. J Cell Biol 1986; 102: 1304-11.
29. Hutter JF, Piper HM, Spieckermann PG. Kinetic analysis of myocardial fatty acid oxidation suggesting an albumin receptor mediated uptake process. J Mol Cell Cardiol 1984; 16: 219-26.
30. Stremmel W, Strohmeyer G, Borchard F, Kochwa S, Berk PD. Isolation and partial characterization of a fatty acid binding protein in rat liver plasma membrane. Proc Nat Acad Sci USA 1985; 82: 4-8.
31. Fournier N, Rahim M. Control of energy production in the heart. A new function for fatty acid binding protein. Biochemistry 1985; 24: 2387-96.
32. Groot PHE, Scholte HR, Huelsmann WC. Fatty acid activation: specificity, localization and function. Adv Lip Res 1976; 14: 75-126.
33. Franson RC, Pang DC, Weglicki WB. Modulation of lipolytic activity in isolated canine cardiac sarcolemma by isoproterenol and propranolol. Biochem Biophys Res Commun 1979; 90: 956-62.
34. Liedtke AJ, Orie JE, Toggart EJ. Carbohyderate and lipid metabolism in ischemia. In: Stone HL, Weglicki WB, eds. Pathobiology of cardiovascular injury. Boston: Martinus Nijhoff Publishing, 1985: 190-201.
35. Ward BJ, Harris P. Incorporatin and distribution of 3H oleic acid in the isolated, perfused guinea-pig heart made hypoxic. J Mol Cell Cardiol 1984; 16: 765-70.
36. Christian DR, Kilsheimer GS, Petlett G, Paradise R, Ashmore J. Regulation of lipolysis in cardiac muscle: A system similar to hormone-sensitive lipase of adipose tissue. Adv Enzym Regul 1969; 7: 71-82.
37. Kubler W, Spieckermann PG. Changes in glycolysis and in high energy phosphates during myocardial ischemia with intermittent coronary perfusion. Cardiology 1971; 56: 100-7.
38. Neely JR, Rovetto MJ, Whitmer JT, Morgan HE. Effects of ischemia on ventricular function and metabolism in isolated working rat heart. Am J Physiol 1973; 225: 651-8.
39. Rovetto MJ, Whitmer JT, Neely JR. Comparison of effects of anoxia and whole heart ischemia on carbohydrate utilization in isolated working rat hearts. Circ Res 1973; 32: 699-711.
40. Whitmer JT, Idell-Wenger JA, Rovetto MJ, Neely JR. Control of fatty acid metabolism in ischemic and hypoxic hearts. J Biol Chem 1978; 253: 4305-9.
41. Shug AL, Thomsen JH, Folts JD, et al. Changes in tissue levels of carnitine and other metabolites during myocardial ischemia and anoxia. Arch Biochem Biophys 1978; 187: 25-33.
42. Neely JR, Garber D, McDonough K, Idell-Wenger J. Relationship between ventricular function and intermediates of fatty acid metabolism during myocardial ischemia: Effects of carnitine. In: Winbury MM, Abiko Y, eds. Perspectives in cardiovascular research. 3. Ischemic myocardium and antianginal drugs. New York: Raven Press, 1979: 225-39.
43. Heathers GP, Al-Muhtaseb N, Brunt RV. The effect of adrenergic agents on the activities of glycerol 3-phosphate acyltransferase and triglycerid lipase in the isolated perfused rat heart. J Mol Cell Cardiol 1985; 17: 785-96.
44. Bielefeld DR, Vary CT, Neely JR. Inhibition of carnitine palmitoyl-CoA transferase activity and fatty acid oxydation by lactate and oxfenicine in cardiac muscle. J Mol Cell Cardiol 1985; 17: 619-25.
45. Corr PB, Gross RW, Sobel BE. Amphipathic metabolites and membrane dysfunction in ischaemic myocardium. Circ Res 1984; 55: 135-54.
46. Smiseth OA, Mjøs OD. Haemodynamic and metabolic consequences of elevated plasma

free fatty acids during acute ischaemic left ventricular failure in dogs. Scand J Clin Lab Invest 1985; 45: 15-520.
47. Simonsen S, Kjekshus JK. The effect of free fatty acids on myocardial oxygen consumption during atrial pacing and cathecholamine infusion in man. Circulation 1978; 58: 484-91.
48. Vik-Mo H, Mjøs OD. Influence of free fatty acids on myocardial oxygen consumption on ischemic injury. Am J Cardiol 1981; 48: 361-5.
49. Katz AM, Messineo FC. Lipid-membrane interactions and the pathogenesis of ischemic damage in the myocardium. Circ Res 1981; 48: 1-16.
50. Jodalen H, Stangeland L, Grong K, Vik-Mo H, Lekven J. Lipid accumulation in the myocardium during acute regional ischaemia in cats. J Mol Cell Cardiol 1985; 17: 973-80.
51. Greve G, Rotevatn S, Stangeland L. Morphological alterations across the border zone of cat hearts subjected to regional ischemia. Virchows Arch A (Pathol Anat) 1989; 415 (2): 323-33.
52. Greve G, Rotevatn S, Svendby K, Grong K. Early morphological changes in cat heart muscle cells following acute coronary artery occlusion. Am J Pathol 1990; 136: 273-83.
53. Janse MJ, Cinca J, Moréna H, et al. The "border zone" in myocardial ischemia. A electrophysiological, metabolic, and histochemical correlation in the pig heart. Circ Res 1979; 44: 576-88.
54. Jennings RB, Ganote CE. Mitochondrial structure and function in acute myocardial ischemic injury. Circ Res 1976; 5 (suppl.1): I-80-I-91.
55. Jodalen H, Lie R, Rotevatn S. Effect of isoproterenol on lipid accumulation in myocardial cells. Res Exp Med 1982; 181: 239-44.
56. Grong K, Jodalen H, Stangeland L, Vik-Mo H, Lekven J. Cellular lipid accumulation in different regions of myocardial infarcts in cats during beta-adrenergic blockade with timolol. Cardiovasc Res 1986; 20: 248-55.
57. Jodalen H, Rotevatn S, Stangeland L, Grong K, Vik-Mo H. Effects of verapamil on intracellular lipid accumulation in cat hearts with 3 h of regional-ischaemia. Scand J Clin Lab Invest 1989; 49: 55-61.
58. Ursell PC, Gardner PI, Albala A, Fenoglio Jr JJ, Wit AL. Structural and electrophysiological changes in the epicardial border zone of canine myocardial infarcts during infarct healing. Circ Res 1985; 56: 436-51.
59. Lindal S, Smiseth OA, Mjøs OD, Myklebust R, Jørgensen L. Reversible and irreversible changes in the dog heart during acute left ventricular failure due to experimental multifocal ischemia. Acta Path Microbil Immunol Scand Sect A 1986; 94: 177-86.
60. Schwaiger M, Fishbein MC, Block M, et al. Metabolic and ultrastructural abnormalities during ischemia in canine myocardium: Noninvasive assessment by positron emission tomography. J Mol Cell Cardiol 1987; 19: 259-69.

7

Reperfusion damage of the myocardium

JARLE VAAGE

Does reperfusion injury really exist?

In order to salvage ischaemic myocardium and to resume normal function, the restoration of blood flow is a *conditio sine qua non.* However, sudden reperfusion and reoxygenation may be associated with acceleration or even extension of irreversible myocardial cell injury (1). Reperfusion injury is of increasing importance due to new techniques of restoring blood flow to acutely ischaemic areas by means of thrombolysis, angioplasty, or acute coronary artery bypass surgery. With the evolvement of open-heart surgery with cardioplegic arrest reperfusion is an everyday procedure.

A major controversy exists as to whether reperfusion injury merely represents an acceleration of ischaemic damage, or whether reperfusion causes a specific additional injury. In order to assess any damage by reperfusion, it is important to distinguish those cells that are irreversibly damaged by ischaemia from those that are potentially viable, but become lethally damaged during reperfusion. There are intrinsic difficulties in differentiating between these two possibilities, since it is not possible to have a model of myocardial reperfusion without preceding ischaemia. The definition of reperfusion injury is crucial. *Jennings et al* (2) argue that "reperfusion injury should be restricted to mean cell death caused by reperfusion". Others have referred to reperfusion injury as a series of reperfusion-related phenomena (3, 4). The strongest support for reperfusion injury as a particular entity comes from studies demonstrating that the ischaemic injury may be attenuated and modified at the time of reperfusion (5-10).

Ischaemia-reperfusion and coronary vascular tone. The no-reflow phenomenon

The mechanism of reactive hyperaemia in the coronary circulation is complex. Potassium, acetate, adenosine, kinins and a number of metabolites are possible mediators, as well as the direct effects of hypoxia itself. Hypoxia activates arachidonic acid metabolism in coronary endothelial cells. The predominant metabolite is prostaglandin I_2 (PGI_2), which may be a mediator of hypoxia-induced coronary vasodilation (11). The endothelium is also the source of other vasodilators such as Endothelium – derived Relaxing Factor (EDRF) (12).

Coronary blood flow is not completely restored by reperfusion after a moderate to longer period of ischaemia (13, 14). Particular emphasis has been on the possible role of capillary obstruction by leukocytes (6). During reperfusion, accumulation of neutrophil granulocytes occurs due to locally active chemotactic factors and changes in leukocyte-endothelium interaction. The no-reflow phenomenon is inhibited when reperfusion is carried out using leukocyte-depleted blood (6). Activated granulocytes increase coronary vascular resistance, probably due to some vasoconstrictor effect(s) rather than by mechanical obstruction (15).

Longer lasting ischaemia alters arachidonic acid metabolism away from PGI_2 towards the vasoconstrictive thromboxane A_2 (TxA_2) and leukotrienes (LTs) (9). These changes in arachidonic acid metabolism are associated with endothelial damage and enhanced accumulation of leukocytes and platelets. LTs and TxA_2 may well be derived from these blood cells (9). Concomitantly, endothelial dysfunction decreases production of PGI_2, reducing coronary vasodilation and endothelial platelet inhibition. The endothelial injury of ischaemia and reperfusion might also reduce EDRF production and trigger the release of endothelium-derived constricting factors (12, 16, 17). Toxic oxygen metabolites (TOM), which are probable mediators of reperfusion injury (see later), may destroy EDRF and are cytotoxic against endothelial cells. Consequently, in situations with endothelial dysfunction a variety of agents and/or situations, which normally induce coronary vasodilation, may cause a vasoconstrictor response (12, 16, 17).

Reperfusion arrhythmias

Arrhythmias appear to be specific reperfusion-related events (18). Ventricular fibrillation occurs abruptly without warning following reperfusion, but is much less common in patients than in animal experiments (19). Chemical and electrical gradients caused by rapid intramyocardial changes of metabolites and electrolytes, such as potassium, calcium, hydrogen and catecholamines, may be responsible for reperfusion arrhythmias. Particular interest has focussed on abnormal control of calcium movements (18).

However, the evidence that calcium blockers reduce reperfusion arrhythmias remains inconclusive, probably due to the existence of different calcium channels.

Toxic oxygen metabolites have been suggested as potential mediators of reperfusion arrhythmias (20). TOM may interact with calcium haemeostasis to trigger arrhythmias (21), or act through lipid peroxidation (22). Changes in membrane phospholipids, plasmalogens, lysophospholipids, and free fatty acids may also mediate reperfusion arrhythmias (23, 24).

The "stunned" myocardium

Reperfusion after a brief episode of myocardial ischaemia induces a prolonged, but reversible myocardial dysfunction known as "myocardial stunning" (25). Implicit in the definition of "stunning" is that the postischaemic dysfunction, no matter how prolonged, is reversible. The return of contractility in myocardium salvaged by reperfusion is delayed for hours, days, or even weeks (3, 25-27). Both moderate and severe post-cardioplegic "stunning" of the myocardium with delayed recovery have been reported in patients after cardiac surgery (28,29). "Stunning" is associated not only with impaired contractile power, but also with prolonged abnormalities of relaxation; thus involving both systolic and diastolic function (30).

The primary determinant of myocardial "stunning" is the severity or duration of ischaemia (27). Even small differences in ischaemic perfusion during regional coronary occlusion are associated with large differences in postischaemic recovery. In such a setting, collateral blood flow becomes very important. The speed of reperfusion may be a determinant of myocardial "stunning". There are investigators claiming that a more gradual reperfusion might be beneficial (10). Others claim that reactive hyperaemia is important for functional recovery (31), or that the mode of reperfusion does not influence postischaemic damage (32).

The cause of "stunning" has been related to loss and impaired synthesis of ATP (25). But despite reduced ATP in the "stunned" myocardium, inotropic stimulation elicits a substantial increase in mechanical activity and enhances contractile function (33). Thus, considerable evidence refutes the theory that lack of and/or inability to synthesize high energy phosphates is the main cause of postischaemic myocardial dysfunction. At present intracellular Ca-accumulation with disturbed excitation-contraction coupling is suggested as the most likely mechanism (34). However, the evidence that calcium blockers are cardio-protective is far from conclusive.

Mode and speed of reperfusion: The speed of reperfusion may be of importance for postischaemic myocardial dysfunction (see above). Gentle reperfusion has also been suggested to be beneficial for energy preservation of the myocardium (35), and to ameliorate ultrastructural reperfusion damage in isolated rat hearts (36). Other studies have shown that asanguineous reperfusion of the globally ischaemic heart reduces reperfusion-induced ultrastructural damage and attenuates deterioriation of left ventricular diastolic compliance (37).

Calcium: Defective regulation of calcium homaeostasis in postischaemic cells may contribute to reperfusion injury (see above) (34, 38, 39). Calcium overload as a cell-toxic event is clearly demonstrated in the so-called calcium-paradox (1). However, whether calcium has deleterious effects on injured, but still viable cells in vivo is not verified. It has been suggested that ischaemia induces susceptibility to calcium-damage which may involve enhanced membrane fragility. Reperfusion is then accompanied by cellular accumulation of calcium. Calcium probably enters the cell via several routes. Why cellular calcium overload causes injury is not clear, but may trigger a turbulent cascade of events such as activation of phospholipases and/or production of oxygen free radicals.

Toxic oxygen metabolites (TOM): An abundant litterature exists regarding a possible role of TOM in reperfusion injury (see reviews: 5, 7, 8, 40). The data are somewhat conflicting, but suggest an important role of TOM in myocardial ischaemia-reperfusion injury. TOM have been demonstrated in the coronary venous blood during reperfusion of globally or regionally ischaemic myocardium (40). However, due to major technical difficulties in directly detecting TOM, most of the data is derived from studies using scavengers of oxygen-derived free radicals (see reviews). During ischaemia-reperfusion TOM are produced in mitochondria via univalent reduction of oxygen in the electron transport chain. In addition, endothelial cells contain the enzyme xanthine dehydrogenase, which is rapidly converted to xanthine oxidase during ischaemia. During reoxygenation a burst of TOM is generated by xanthine oxidase. However, the amount of xanthine oxidase is species-dependent, and appears undetectable in the human heart. Finally TOM are also produced by activated neutrophils (see later).

Intracellular scavengers (superoxide dismutase (SOD), catalase, and glutathione peroxidase) normally rapidly break down TOM. These defense mechanisms may be overwhelmed in situations with increased production of TOM. Several studies have presented substantial evidence of antioxidant depletion during ischaemia, hypoxia and reperfusion. Experimentally generated TOM are shown to deplete the isolated, perfused rat heart of SOD, reduced glutathione, and the antioxidant vitamin E, indicating that TOM themselves deplete the myocardium of its antioxidants (41).

Clinical data are lacking regarding a possible role of TOM in ischaemia-reperfusion, partly because the ideal scavenger/antioxidant has not been found. The usefulness of exogenous SOD and catalase is limited by their large molecular weight inhibiting extravascular and intracellular penetration. Other scavengers and antioxidants may potentially have therapeutic use.

Neutrophil granulocytes: Neutrophil infiltration of the myocardium starts within one hour of ischaemia and is markedly accelerated by reperfusion (6). In cardiac surgery, leukocytes are trapped across the coronary circulation during reperfusion after cold, cardioplegic arrest (42). Neutrophil depletion reduces infarct size after coronary occlusion followed by reperfusion (5, 6, 9, 43). Apparently, the injurious effects of neutrophil granulocytes are closely connected to production of TOM and eicosanoids. The role of neutrophils as a cause of myocyte injury is, however, controversial (44). Postischaemic contractile dysfunction may be attenuated by neutrophil depletion (45). Others have concluded that neutrophil depletion does not enhance contractile performance of stunned myocardium (46). Activated leukocytes have been found to impair contractile power and reduce coronary flow in isolated rat hearts. These effects were blocked by scavengers of TOM (15) and by lipoxygenase inhibitors (47).

Arachidonic acid metabolites: The myocytes have a certain production of lipoxygenase (LO) products, whereas the formation of cyclooxygenase (CO) products is negligible (9). The major source of CO products in the heart is the vascular wall, in particular the endothelium. The major prostanoid released into the effluent of isolated, perfused hearts is PGI_2. With blood perfusion two important additional sources of eicosanoids are the circulating leukocytes and platelets. Platelet aggregation and activation induces formation of TxA_2, which is vasospastic, augments platelet aggregation, and may precipitate ventricular arrhythmias and fibrillation (19). Cardiac release of PGI_2 and TxA_2 has been detected during the early reperfusion period in cardiac surgery (42, 48). Their role in reperfusion injury is not clarified, and PGI_2 has been reported to be cardio-protective (49).

The neutrophil granulocytes are a major source of eicosanoids. These include LO products that influence coronary vascular tone, contractility, and are potentially important for reperfusion injury (9). Apparently, the enhanced formation of 12-LO products in myocardial ischaemia-reperfusion is due to granulocytes (9). The role of this pathway in myocardial ischaemia-reperfusion is highly controversial. In recent years products of the 5-LO enzyme such as LTA_4, LTB_4, LTC_4, and LTD_4, have received most attention. 5-LO-inhibitors are able to reduce experimental reperfusion injury and infarct size (9). Such findings infer that the formation of LO-products are important mediators. However, the benefits of LO inhibitors are related to suppression of neutrophil accumulation. Obviously, there is a close relationship between leukotrienes and granulocytes in myocardial injury (9). In isolated, perfused rat hearts the detrimental effects of activated granulocytes are inhibited by LO-inhibitors (47). During myocardial reperfusion in cardiac surgery LTB_4 is released concomitanttly with granulocyte trapping in the coronary circulation (42).

Platelets: Platelets accumulate in reperfused myocardium (50), and they are able to cause coronary vascular injury (51). Experimentally induced platelet activation induces cardiac ischaemia, most likely due to generation of CO products (52). Platelet-derived TxA_2 may have a role in the pathophysiology of myocardial reperfusion injury (9). However, platelet depletion did not reduce infarct size in a canine ischaemia-reperfusion model (53).

Complement: The ischaemic and reperfused myocardium activates complement and traps complement factors and their activation products (34). Complement activation has been demonstrated in patients with acute myocardial infarction (55). Complement split products may have direct detrimental effects on cardiac function (56), or they may act through leukocyte attraction and activation. During myocardial ischaemia, chemotactic activity has been found in the coronary sinus (57). Chemotactic and neutrophil-stimulating activity, partly derived from the complement system, has been obtained from cardiac lymph during reperfusion of ischaemic myocardium (58).

Miscellaneous: Evidence suggests that intramyocardial fatty acids, phospholipids, lysophospholipids, fatty acid esters and a variety of lipid derivates may have important functions in ischaemia-reperfusion injury (23, 59, 60). Possibly due to its interference with triglyceride and fatty acid metabolism, increased levels of free carnitine may benefit the ischaemic, reperfused heart (59). A particular phospholipid being synthesized by various inflammatory cells is platelet activating factor (PAF). PAF has been implicated as a potential mediator of ischaemia-reperfusion injury (61).

Adenosine has been shown to reduce experimental infarct size after reperfusion, reduce neutrophil accumulation, improve ventricular function, reduce ultrastructural and functional abnormalities of the coronary microvasculature, and decrease ATP degradation (62, 63). Adenosine may be an anti-inflammatory autacoid preventing reperfusion injury by inhibition of granulocyte adherence, microvascular obstruction and superoxide anion formation.

Conclusion

There is good evidence favouring the view that reperfusion injury exists, and that ischaemic injury may be influenced by the mode of reperfusion. The complex group of phenomena associated with reperfusion include: No-reflow, arrhythmias, impaired contractile power and abnormalities of relaxation. The causal factors of reperfusion injury are not clarified, but include calcium and various inflammatory mediators.

References

1. Hearse DJ. Reperfusion of the ischaemic myocardium. J Mol Cell Cardiol 1977; 9: 605-16.
2. Jennings RB, Reiner KA, Steenbergen C. Myocardial ischaemia revisited: The osmolar load, membrane damage, and reperfusion. J Mol Cell Cardiol 1986; 18: 769-80.
3. Braunwald E, Kloner RA. Myocardial reperfusion: A double-edged sword? J Clin Invest 1985; 76: 1713-9.
4. Nayler WG, Elz JS. Reperfusion injury: Laboratory artifact or clinical dilemma? Circulation 1986; 74: 215-21.
5. Simpson PJ, Lucchesi BR. Free radicals and myocardial ischaemia and reperfusion injury. J Lab Clin Med 1987; 110: 13-30.
6. Schmid-Schönbein GW, Engler RL. Granulocytes as active participants in acute myocardial ischaemia and infarct. Am J Cardiovasc Pathol 1986; 1: 15-30.
7. Kloner RA, Przyklenk K, Wittaker P. Deleterious effects of oxygen radicals in ischaemia/reperfusion. Resolved and unresolved issues. Circulation 1989; 80: 1115-27.
8. Maza SR, Frishman WH. Therapeutic options to minimize free radical damage and thrombogenicity in ischaemic/reperfused myocardium. Am Heart J 1987; 114: 1206-15.
9. Mullane KM. Eicosanoids in myocardial ischaemia reperfusion injury. In: Lewis A, ed. Advances in inflammation research. New York: Raven Press, Ltd., 1988: 191-214.
10. Peng CF, Murphy ML, Colwell K, Straub KD. Controlled versus hyperemic flow during reperfusion of jeopardized ischaemic myocardium. Am Heart J 1989; 117: 515-22.
11. Busse R, Forstermann, Matsunda H, Pohl U. The role of prostaglandins in the endothelium - mediated vasodilatory response to hypoxia. Pflügers Arch 1984; 401: 77-83.
12. Vanhoutte PM, Shimokawa H. Endothelium - derived relaxing factor and coronary vasospasm. Circulation 1989; 80: 1-9.
13. Kloner RA, Grandte CE, Jennings RB. The "no-reflow" phenomenon after temporary coronary occlusion in the dog. J Clin Invest 1974; 54: 1496-1508.
14. Schofer J, Montz R, Mathey DG. Scintigraphic evidence of the "no reflow" phenomenon in human beings after coronary thrombolysis. J Am Coll Cardiol 1985; 5: 593-8.
15. Semb AG, Ytrehus K, Vaage J, Myklebust R, Mjøs OD. Functional impairment in isolated rat hearts induced by activated leukocytes: Protective effect of oxygen free radical scavengers. J Mol Cell Cardiol 1989; 21: 877-87.

16. Lüscher TF. Endothelium – derived relaxing factors: potential role in coronary artery disease. Eur Heart J 1989; 10: 847-57.
17. Forman MB, Puett DW, Virmani R. Endothelial and myocardial injury during ischaemia and reperfusion: Pathogenesis and therapeutic implications. J Am Coll Cardiol 1989; 13: 450-9.
18. Opie LH, Coetze WA, Dennis SC, et al. A potential role of calcium ions in early ishemic and reperfusion arrhythmias. Ann NY Acad Sci 1988; 522: 446-77.
19. Maras P, Della Grazia E, Klugmann S, et al. Reperfusion ventricular arrhythmias during intracoronary thrombolysis. Eur Heart J 1986; 7 (suppl A): 23-30.
20. Manning AS. Reperfusion-induced arrhythmias: Do free radicals play a critical role? Free Radical Biol Med 1988; 4: 305-16.
21. Hearse DJ, Tosaki A. Free radicals and calcium: Simultaneously acting triggers as determinants of vulnerability to reperfusion-induced arrhythmias in the rat heart. J Mol Cell Cardiol 1988; 20: 213-23.
22. Merson FZ, Belkina LM, Sazontova TG, Saltykova VA, Arhgipenko YV. The role of lipid peroxidation in pathogenesis of arrhythmias and prevention of cardiac fibrillation with antioxidants. Basic Res Cardiol 1987; 82: 123-37.
23. Kako KJ. Membrane phospholipids and plasmalogens in the ischaemic myocardium. Can J Cardiol 1986; 2: 184-94.
24. Sugiyama S, Osawa T. Biochemical basis for reperfusion arrhythmias. J Mol Cell Cardiol 1987; 19 (suppl V): 67-75.
25. Braunwald E, Kloner RA. The stunned myocardium: Prolonged postischaemic ventricular dysfunction. Circulation 1982; 66: 1146-9.
26. Matsizaki M, Gallagher KP, Kemper WS, White F, Ross J jr. Sustained regional dysfunction produced by prolonged coronary stenosis: gradual recovery after reperfusion. Circulation 1983; 68: 170-2.
27. Bolli R, Zhu WX, Thornby JI, O'Neill PG, Roberts R. Time-course and determinants of recovery of function after reversible ischaemia in conscious dogs. Am J Physiol 1988; 254: H 102-14.
28. Reduto LA, Lawrie GM, Reid JW, et al. Sequential postoperative assessment of left ventricular performance with gated cardiac blood pool imaging following aortocoronary bypass surgery. Am Heart J 1981; 101: 59-66.
29. Ballantyne CM, Verani MS, Short D, Hyatt C, Noon GP. Delayed recovery of severely "stunned" myocardium with the support of a left ventricular assist device after coronary artery bypass surgery. J Am Coll Cardiol 1987; 10: 710-2.
30. Verani MS, Bolli R, Tadros S, et al. Dissociation between global and regional systolic and diastolic ventricular function during coronary occlusion and reperfusion. Am Heart J 1987; 114: 687-95.
31. Farber NE, Pieper GM, Gross GJ. Postischemic recovery in the stunned myocardium after reperfusion in the presence or absence of a flow-limiting coronary artery stenosis. Am Heart J 1988; 116: 407-20.
32. Granato JE, Watson DD, Flanagan TL, Beller GA. Myocardial thallium-201 kinetics and regional flow alterations with 3 hours of coronary occlusion and either rapid reperfusion through a totally patent vessel or slow reperfusion through a critical stenosis. J Am Coll Cardiol 1987; 9: 109-18.
33. Ambrosio G, Jacobus WE, Bergman CA. Preserved high energy phosphate metabolic reserve in globally "stunned" hearts despite reduction of basal ATP content and contractility. J Mol Cell Cardiol 1987; 19: 953-64.
34. Kusuoka H, Porterfield JK, Weisman HF, Weisfeldt, Marban E. Pathophysiology and pathogenesis of stunned myocardium. Depressed Ca^{2+} activation of contraction as a

consequence of reperfusion induced cellular calcium overload in ferret hearts. J Clin Invest 1987; 89: 950-61.
35. Gunnes S, Ytrehus K, Sørlie D, Helgesen KG, Mjøs OD. Improved energy preservation following gentle reperfusion after hypothermic, ischaemic cardioplegia in infarcted rat hearts. Eur J Cardio-thorac Surg 1987; 1: 139-47.
36. Lindal S, Gunnes S, Ytrehus K, Straume BK, Jørgensen L, Sørlie D. Amelioration of reperfusion injury following hypothermic, ischaemic cardioplegia in isolated infarcted rat hearts. Eur J Cardio-thorac Surg 1990; 4: in press.
37. Rebeyka I, Wilson GJ, Axford-Gatley RA, Romaschin AD, Mickle DAG. Asangineous reperfusion in a canine model of cardiopulmonary bypass and controlled postischaemic work. Ann Thorac Surg 1989; 48: 397-403.
38. Cheung JY, Bonventre JV, Malis CD, Leaf A. Calcium and ischaemic injury. N Engl J Med 1986; 314: 1670-6.
39. Nayler WG, Panagiotopoulos S, Elz JS, Daly MJ. Calcium-mediated damage during post-ischaemic reperfusion. J Mol Cell Cardiol 1988; 20 (suppl II): II 41-54.
40. Bolli R. Oxygen-derived free radicals and postischaemic myocardial dysfunction. J Am Coll Cardiol 1988; 12: 239-49.
41. Vaage J, Semb AG. Myocardial reperfusion injury: An inflammatory reaction? Biomed Biochim Acta 1989, 48, 63-8.
42. Semb AG, Forsdahl K, Vaage J. Granulocyte and eicosanoid gradients across the coronary circulation during myocardial reperfusion in cardiac surgery. Eur J Cardio-thorac Surg 1990; in press.
43. Werns SW, Lucchesi BR. Leukocytes, oxygen radicals and myocardial injury due to ischaemia and reperfusion. Free Radical Biol Med 1988; 4: 31-7.
44. Chatelain P, Latour JG, Tran D, et al. Neutrophil accumulation in experimental myocardial infarcts: Relation with extent of injury and effect of reperfusion. Circulation 1987; 75: 1083-90.
45. Engler RE, Covell JW. Granulocytes cause reperfusion ventricular dysfunction after 15 min of ischaemia in the dog. Circ Res 1987; 61: 20-8.
46. O'Neill PG, Charlat ML, Michael LH, Roberts R, Bolli R. Influence of neutrophil depletion on myocardial function and flow after reversible ischaemia. Am J Physiol 1989; 256: H 341-51.
47. Semb AG, Vaage J, Mjøs OD. Oxygen free radical producing leukocytes cause functional depression of isolated rat hearts: Role of leukotrienes. J Mol Cell Cardiol 1990, in press.
48. Teoh KH, Fremes SE, Weisel RD, et al. Cardiac release of prostacyclin and thromboxane A_2 during coronary revascularization. J Thorac Cardiovasc Surg 1987; 93: 120-6.
49. Araki H, Lefer AM. Role of prostacyclin in the preservation of ischemic myocardial tissue in the perfused cat heart. Circ Res 1980; 47: 757-63.
50. Feinberg H, Rosenbaum DS, Levitsky S, Silverman NA, Kohler J, Lebreton G. Platelet deposition after surgically induced myocardial ischaemia. J Thorac Cardiovasc Surg 1982; 84: 815-22.
51. Jørgensen L, Hovig T, Rowsell HC, Mustard JF. Adenosine disphosphate-induced platelet aggregation and vascular injury in swine and rabbits. Am J Pathol 1970; 61: 161-70.
52. Addonizio VP, Wetstein L, Fisher CA, Feldman P, Strauss JF, Harken AH. Mediation of cardiac ischaemia by thromboxanes released from human platelets. Surgery 1982; 92: 292-8.
53. Jolly SR, Schumaker WA, Kunkel SL, Abrams GD, Liddicoat J, Lucchesi BR. Platelet depletion in experimental myocardial infarction. Basic Res Cardiol 1985; 80: 269-9.
54. Pinchard RN, O'Rourke RA, Crawford MH, et al. Complement localization and mediation of ischemic injury in baboon myocardium. J Clin Invest 1980; 66: 1050-6.

55. Earis JE, Marcuson EC, Bernstein A. Complement activation after myocardial infarction. Chest 1985; 87: 186-90.
56. Del Balzo HM, Levi R, Polley MJ. Cardiac dysfunction caused by purified C3a anaphylatoxin. Proc Nat Acad Sci USA 1985; 82: 886-90.
57. Hartmann JR, Robinson JA, Gunnar RM. Chemotactic activity in the coronary sinus after experimental myocardial infarction: Effects of pharmacological interventions on ischaemic injury. Am J Cardiol 1977; 40: 550-5.
58. Dreyer WJ, Smith CW, Michael LH, et al. Canine neutrophil activation by cardiac lymph obtained during reperfusion of ischemic myocardium. Circ Res 1989; 65: 1751-62.
59. Corr PB, Gross RW, Sobel BE. Amphipathic metabolites and membrane dysfunction in ischemic myocardium. Circ Res 1984; 55: 135-54.
60. Das DK, Engelmann RM, Rousou JA, Breyer RH, Otani H, Lemeshow S. Role of membrane phospholipids in myocardial injury induced by ischemia and reperfusion. Am J Physiol 1986; 251: H71-9.
61. Koltai M, Tosaki A, Guillon JM, Hosford D, Braquet P. PAF antagonists as potential therapeutic agents in cardiac anaphylaxis and myocardial ischaemia. Cardiovasc Drug Rev 1989; 7: 177-98.
62. Olafsson B, Forman MB, Puett DW, et al. Reduction of reperfusion injury in the canine preparation bye intracoronary adenosine: importance of the endothelium and the no-reflow phenomenon. Circulation 1987; 76: 1135-45.
63. Babitt DG, Virmani R, Forman MB: Intracoronary adenosine administered after reperfusion limits vascular injury after prolonged ischemia in the canine model. Circulation 1989; 80: 1388-99.

8

Free oxygen radicals during acute myocardial infarction

KIRSTI YTREHUS

INTRODUCTION

The use of oxygen as an acceptor of reducing equivalents in cellular energy metabolism has probably made the evolution of multicellular species possible. In human life the danger of oxygen deprivation is illustrated above all by the serious consequences of myocardial injury due to coronary ischaemia. However, the question of a paradoxical toxicity of oxygen in heart patients suffering from severe lack of oxygen has been raised (1, 2). Experimental research performed in the late seventies/early eighties supports this view by proving free oxygen radicals to be possible mediators of ischaemic tissue damage (3-6). The present chapter deals with this question.

Free oxygen radicals

In 1931 the chemists *Haber* and *Willstatter* discovered that univalent reduction of molecular oxygen resulted in an oxygen radical, the superoxide anion (7). The biological importance of this discovery became apparent when *McCord* and *Fridovich* in 1969 identified the superoxide removing enzyme superoxide dismutase (SOD), and the toxicity of reduced oxygen intermediates was gradually established (8-14). These intermediates are superoxide anion, hydrogen peroxide and hydroxyl radical (Fig. 1). Hydrogen peroxide is not a free radical but an important product during the reduction of oxygen. Hydrogen peroxide is non-polar and able to diffuse through membranes. The hydroxyl radical is easily produced when hydrogen peroxide comes into contact with iron (Fe^{2+}) or copper (Cu^{2+}) ions. The hydroxyl radical has a high but indiscriminate reactivity. The derivates of polyunsaturated fatty acids, sulfhydryl compounds and quinone-like compounds are other possible radicals of major importance in biological systems.

Free radicals are by definition atomic or molecular species that contain in one or more orbitals (valence shells) an unpaired electron. Radicals have a net magnetic moment which can be detected by electron spin resonance spectroscopy (12, 15-17). A substance may become a radical either by gaining or loosing electrons in a reduction/oxidation reaction. Radicals are often unstable, and they generally demonstrate high chemical reactivity and chain-reaction induction, participating in hydrogen abstraction, radical addition, bond scission and annihilation reactions.

Tissue sources of free oxygen radicals: Free oxygen radicals are part of the normal cell metabolism (9, 10, 14). Organelles such as mitochondria, microsomes and nuclei have been shown to produce free oxygen radicals. Some of this oxygen radical production has been suggested as being due to auto-oxidation of reduced components of electron transport assemblies. The killing of bacteria by polymorphonuclear leucocytes is accompanied by a sudden and massive uptake of oxygen and release of oxygen radicals at the cell surface and into phagocytic vesicles (11). This is due to an oxygen radical producing enzyme system named NADPH oxidase, located in the cell membrane. Several other mammalian enzymes also produce oxygen radicals; examples are xanthine oxidase and cytochrome P450.

Defence: Defence systems against oxygen radicals seem to exist in all aerobic cells (Fig. 2). In addition to the previously mentioned enzyme SOD, there are other enzymes responsible for peroxide removal. Catalase, mainly a peroxisomal enzyme, catalyzes the conversion of hydrogen peroxide into

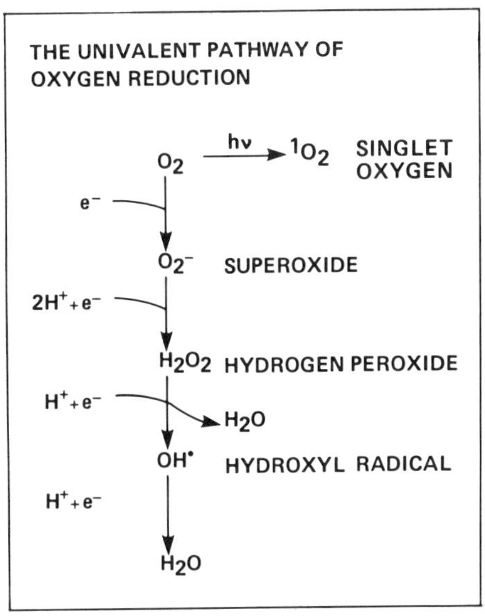

Fig. 1. *The univalent reduction of oxygen: different species of reduced oxygen are shown in protonated or nonprotonated form depending on the dominating form at pH 7.4.*

$$O_2^- + O_2^- \xrightarrow[2H^+]{SOD} H_2O_2 + O_2$$

$$2H_2O_2 \xrightarrow{catalase} O_2 + 2H_2O$$

$$H_2O_2 + 2GSH \xrightarrow{GSH\text{-}peroxidase} 2H_2O + GSSG$$

$$ROOH + 2GSH \xrightarrow{GSH\text{-}peroxidase} ROH + H_2O + GSSG$$

$$GSSG + NADPH \xrightarrow{GSSG\text{-}reductase} 2GSH + NADP^+$$

Fig. 2. *Enzymatic reactions protecting cells against superoxide, hydrogen peroxide and lipid peroxides. SOD: superoxide dismutase, GSH: reduced glutathione, GSSG: oxidized glutathione, NADPH: nicotine adenine dinucleotide phosphate.*

water and oxygen (9). The cytoplasmatic and mitochondrial enzyme glutathione peroxidase reduces both lipid peroxides and hydrogen peroxide. The function of vitamin E as a lipid-soluble antioxidant has been studied for several years. Other endogenous or exogenous substances able to act as antioxidants or oxygen scavengers are glutathione, methionine, vitamin C, urea, dimethylsulphoxide, mannitol, sodium selenite and various phenols. However, chemical antioxidant defence can be a double-edged sword. When a reducing agent scavenges a radical, its own radical is formed, and unless this radical is extremely stable a radical chain reaction continues. This is supposed to be a problem with ascorbate and urea, but not with vitamin E.

Biochemical tissue change: From a biochemical point of view toxicity of oxygen radicals is probably due to peroxidation of poly-unsaturated lipids and attacks on proteins containing sulfhydryl groups (Fig. 3). These compounds are known to react easily with oxygen radicals through hydrogen abstraction. This makes membrane structures highly vulnerable to oxygen radicals. Lipid peroxides are removed from the membranes by phospholipases (18). Oxygen radicals may also damage DNA, depolymerize hyaluronic acid, and modulate nucleotide cyclase activities as well as synthesis and action of prostaglandins and lipoxygenase products (19). The presence of bound metal promoters in compounds may favour hydroxyl radical formation and determine the vulnerability of a compound (14).

Free oxygen radicals in disease: Increased generation or decreased defence may both lead to an increased level of oxygen radicals which promote disease (Fig. 3). There are several pathological processes in which oxygen radicals may be involved (10, 12-14). With regard to the heart the following conditions will be mentioned. Cardiomyopathy after adriamycin treatment is an example of drug toxicity possibly mediated by free radicals through redox cycling of the drug (20). Selenium is an essential prostetic group for the enzyme glutathione peroxidase. Deficiency in selenium has been identified by Chinese investigators as a risk factor for the development of cardiomyopathy (21, 22). The mechanism behind may be decreased cellular defence against hydroperoxides and hydrogen peroxide. There has also been research suggesting that catecholamine-induced cardiomyopathy is related to oxidative damage (23).

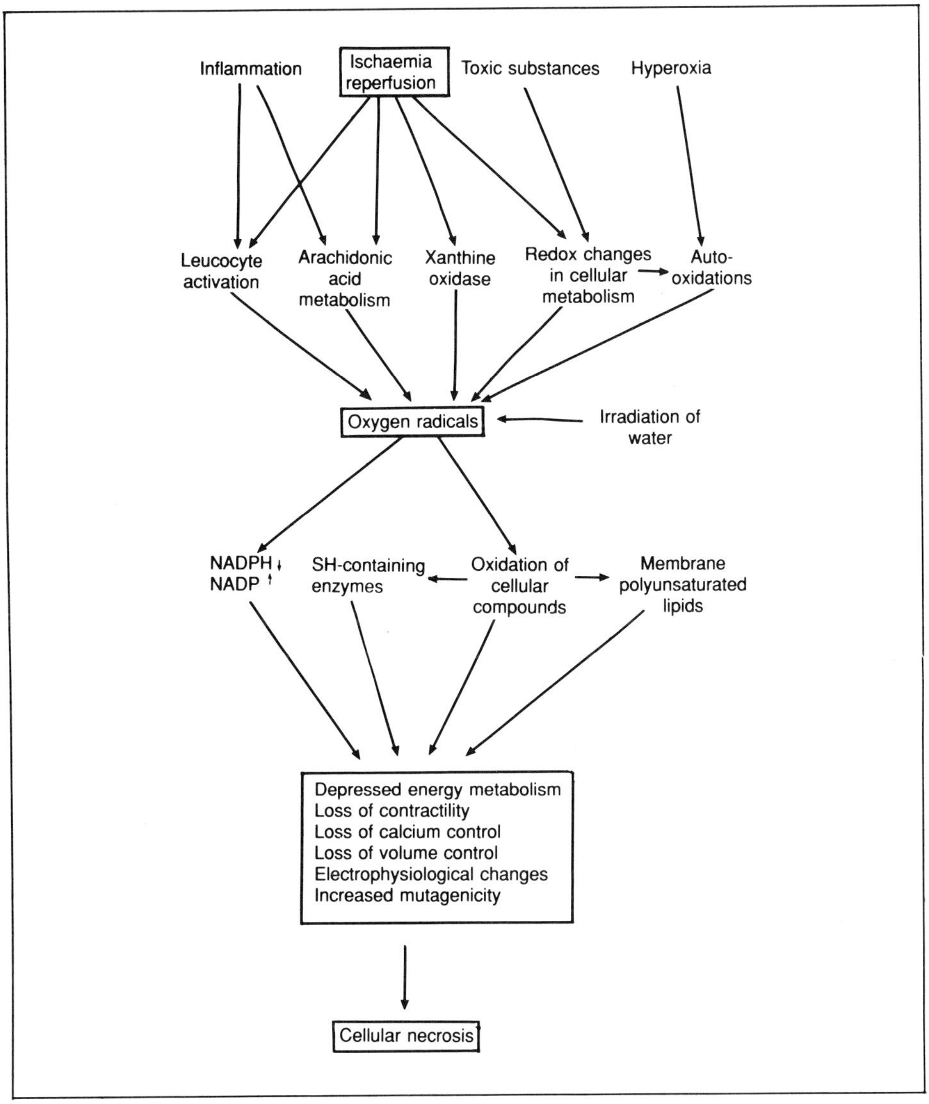

Fig. 3. *Pathophysiological conditions suggested as leading to increased free oxygen radical levels in the tissue.*

Myocardial ischaemia

Involvement of peroxidation in heart injury during reoxygenation after prolonged hypoxia was already suggested by *Hearse et al* in 1973 (24). This possibility was excluded, based on the inability of ascorbate (Vit C) to protect isolated perfused hearts against reoxygenation damage. Later, *Guarnieri et al* addressed the problem and were able to demonstrate protection by α-tocopherol and sodium-selenite (3).

The use of SOD as a protective agent in ischaemia was suggested by *Granger et al* (5). They were able to demonstrate that the increased capillary permeability seen after intestinal ischaemia was attenuated by SOD. *Shlafer et al* published two papers in 1982 describing the use of SOD and catalase in cardioplegic solutions (6, 25). These enzymes are not inotropic or cardioplegic, and thus beneficial effects are believed to be due to a reduction of oxygen radical level in the tissue. Hearts reperfused after hypothermic cardioplegic ischaemia or hearts reperfused after a brief period of ischaemia often demonstrate depressed contractility and reduced high energy phosphate content despite sparce cell damage (26, 27). This is often called "stunned myocardium" and may be explained by postischaemic dysfunction in high energy phosphate metabolism or in cellular calcium handling. Improvement of stunning by treatment with SOD and catalase or SOD alone has been demonstrated repetedly in experimental work (Fig. 4) (26-34).

It has been possible to demonstrate a reduction of infarct size in dogs after pre- plus postischaemic intravascular administration of SOD (35-39). Other investigated parameters related to ischaemic tissue damage are creatine kinase release, cell oedema and mitochondrial alterations and sarcoplasmatic reticulum dysfunction. Some studies have failed to demonstrate infarct limi-

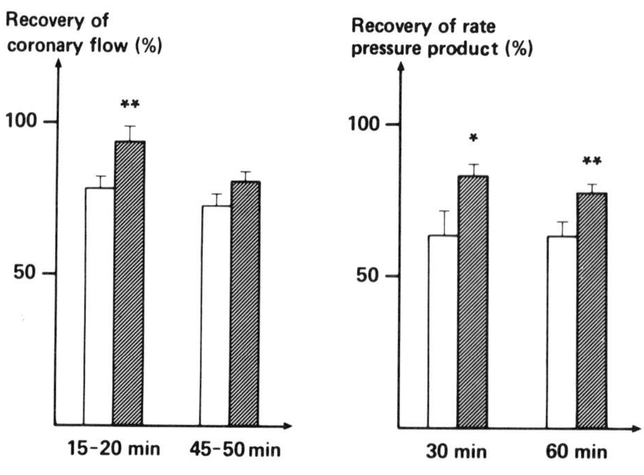

Fig. 4. *Recovery of function in isolated perfused rat hearts after prolonged ischaemia. Hearts were arrested with a cardioplegic solution and kept hypothermic during ischaemia. SOD and catalase were added to the cardioplegic solution and during initial reperfusion in one group. A significant improvement in recovery is achieved compared with a control group.* * $p<0.05$, ** $p<0.01$.

tation (40, 41). *Przyklenk & Kloner* were able to find only a delay in infarct development with SOD and catalase supplement (42). The strong model dependence of infarct size studies due to species differences in collateral flow and the use of different methods to measure infarct size make conclusions valid in human medicine, difficult at present (43, 44).

Oxygen radical scavengers, other than SOD, have also been used with success; examples are dimethylsulphoxide, mannitol, dimethylthiourea and N-2-mercaptoproprionyl glycine (45-48).

Intravascularly administrated SOD has a limited distribution volume and is rapidly metabolized. Large protein molecules as SOD probably reach the interstitial space through intercellular gap junctions. It is unlikely to reach the interior of the cells unless there are active transport mechanisms, but cell membranes of both endothelial and myocardial cells are protected against increased extracellular levels of oxygen radicals. SOD seems to improve recovery of post ischaemic coronary flow after ischaemia (Fig. 4) (6, 25, 26, 28, 32, 34, 49). This could be due to improved myocardial cell function, but also to a beneficial influence on the vessel wall. SOD preserves the endothelium derived realaxing factor (EDRF) in isolated arterial segments (50, 51). Diminished coronary vasodilatator reserve is present after temporary ischaemia. It is thus possible that SOD supports endogenous vasodilatation either by preserving the endothelium derived relaxing factor or by other mechanisms (52). A primary protection against flow perturbation due to vascular damage may secondarily improve oxygenation of myocardial cells and lead to the improved functional recovery.

Lipid peroxides and peroxidation products have been detected during reperfusion (49, 53). There is strong evidence suggesting myocardial reperfusion being a much stronger trigger for free oxygen radical production than ischaemia (34, 43, 54). Reperfusion arrhythmias have been related to free oxygen radicals. Superoxide dismutase, catalase, some oxygen radical scavengers and the xanthine oxidase inhibitor allopurinol have all been shown to reduce the incidence of reperfusion arrhythmias in rat hearts (55-57). The use of scavengers gives only indirect proof of oxygen radicals being involved in tissue damage due to ischaemia and reperfusion. Direct demonstration of the presence of oxygen radicals has been tried using electron spin resonance technique with spin trappers, and these measurements are centred around the early minutes of reperfusion (16, 17).

Free oxygen radical toxicity in the heart

Hydrogen peroxide and peroxides induce a dose-dependent decrease in con-

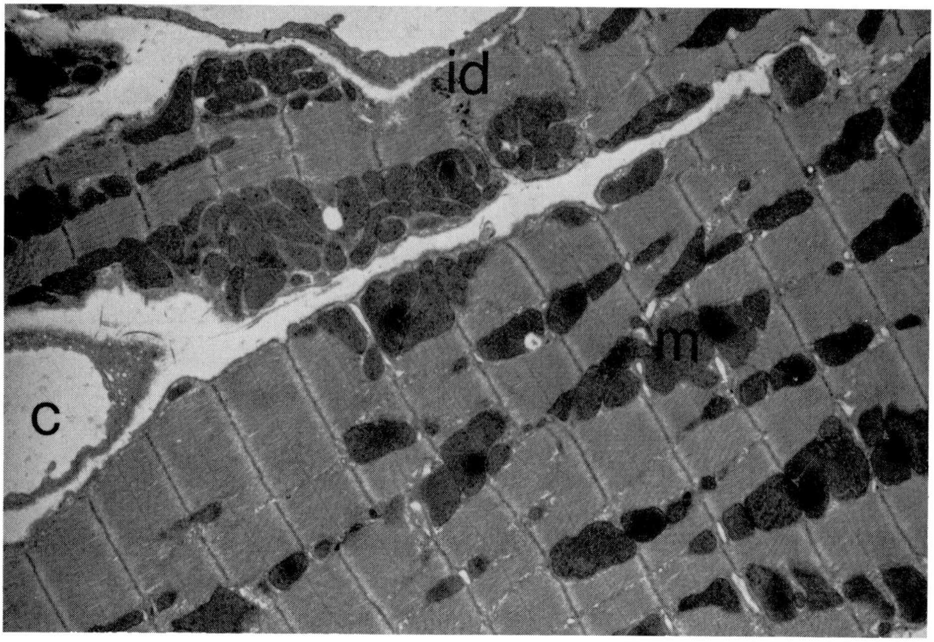

Fig. 5a. *The ultrastructure of normal myocardium (rat). id: intercalated disc, m: mitochondria, c: capillary, barr: 1μm.*

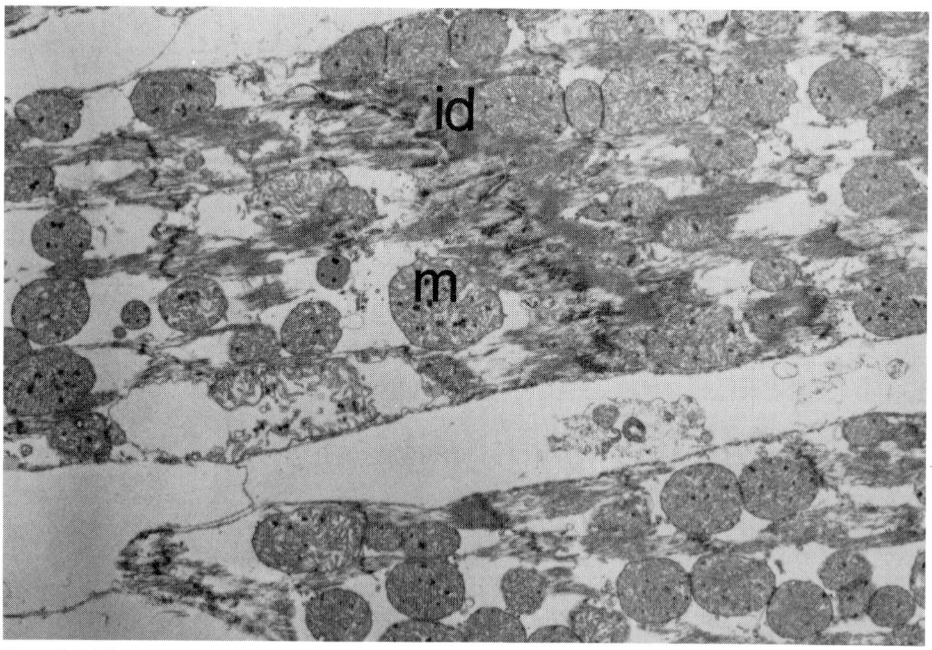

Fig. 5b. *Ultrastructural damage induced by free oxygen radicals: Swollen mitochondria with loss of contrast, intracellular oedema, filamental disruption, cell membrane disattachment. id: intercalated disc, m: mitochondria, barr: 1μm*

tractility in the isolated perfused rat heart (58-60). Initially, this is reversible, but finally the result is irreversible loss of contractility and contracture. A decrease in tissue content of high energy phosphate, adenosine triphosphate (ATP) and creatine phosphate (CP), has also been detected and seems to be a consequence of impaired mitochondrial respiration (61-63).

The myocardial cell structure gradually changes towards the characteristics of irreversibly damaged cells during perfusion with oxygen radicals, and total loss of cell organization or gross disruption of the sarcolemma has been observed (Fig. 5a and b) (64). The affected single myocardial cell seems to go through a graded process ranging from slight clearing and rounding of the mitochondria to the development of intracellular oedema and cell swelling. Similar changes have been observed in ischaemic myocardium. The early appearance of structural changes when hydrogen peroxide or other peroxides are involved is a major difference when comparing free oxygen radical-induced and ischaemia-induced changes in ultrastructure. This is an interesting observation, and the abrupt development of major ultrastructural changes effected by oxygen radicals has striking similarities with the rapid acceleration of damage in the early minutes of reperfusion.

Ischaemia, reperfusion and free oxygen radical damage have been associated with sarcolemma damage (65). ATP-dependent membrane-bound enzymes are vulnerable to ischaemia. This is only partly due to loss of high energy phosphate; a toxic influence of free oxygen radicals may also contribute (66). Cardiac sarcolemmal $Na^{+}K^{+}$ATPase, Ca^{++}-ATPase of both sarcoplasmatic reticulum and myofibrillar preparations show reduced activity during exposure to oxygen radicals (20, 67, 68). The consequences are impaired cellular volume regulation (cellular swelling) and impaired calcium handling.

The influence of free oxygen radicals is not restricted to myocardial cells. Both isolated arterial segments and intact hearts demonstrate vasodilatation upon exposure to free oxygen radicals and peroxides (69, 70). This could be a direct effect on smooth muscle or mediated through changes in other components in the vessel wall.

Source of free oxygen radicals in acute ischaemia

Endothelium, platelets and leucocytes are the most likely sources of free oxygen radicals.

The enzymatic metabolization of arachidonic acid occurring in the endothelial cells and in blood-born cells (leucocytes, platelets) may result in free oxygen radical generation (71, 72). Arachidonic acid is released from ischaemic myocardial cells and serves as a substrate (73).

In addition, endothelial cells are rich in xanthine oxidase (74, 75). Hypoxanthine and xanthine released from ischaemic myocardial cells during ATP break-down are substrates for this enzyme. Conversion of the enzyme to an oxygen radical producing form occurs rapidly in ischaemia (76), probably due to proteolytic activity in ischaemic tissue. Xanthine oxidase is able to induce detrimental effects when producing free oxygen radicals both in coronary vessels and in myocardial cells. The xanthine oxidase inhibitor allopurinol has been reported to reduce reperfusion arrhythmias in the rat, and to limit infarct development in the dog (55, 76). Whether the endothelium of the human heart contains significant amounts of xanthine oxidase is at present uncertain (74).

Leucocytes have important functions in tissue repair, but an early participation of leucocytes in ischaemia may lead to detrimental effects due to the release of free oxygen radicals, proteolytic enzymes, prostaglandins and leucotrienes. A change in leucocyte behaviour is observed within an hour in the border zone of an ischaemic area and in reperfused tissue. Increased margination and infiltration of leucocytes along blood vessels are primer events (77). The relationship between inflammatory mechanisms and oxygen radicals in myocardial ischaemia and shock was addressed by *Lefer et al* in 1981, using a combination of a free radical scavenger and an anti-inflammatory agent (4). Neutrophil depletion reduces the size of experimental infarcts in dogs. Some anti-inflammatory agents, lipoxygenase inhibitors and the cyclooxygenase inhibitor, ibuprofen, also demonstrate reduced infarct development and reduce the infarcted area in per cent of area at risk (78-82). The problem with anti-inflammatory agents in human medicine is the possibility of infarct scar thinning (83).

It is thought that during reoxygenation free oxygen radicals may be produced by mitochondria in increased quantities. Superoxide production by mitochondria is greatest when respiratory chain carriers located in the inner mitochondrial membrane are highly reduced. This is the situation when there is a limitation in oxygen supply. In situations with cell lysis and release of organelles to the extracellular space components of mitochondria, peroxisomes or microsomes may autooxidate and generate free oxygen radicals (84).

Conclusion

Our knowledge about free oxygen radicals in acute ischaemia relies mainly on animal experiments. In ischaemia and reperfusion protection against increased levels of free oxygen radicals in the interstitial space seems to improve function and delay infarct development. It is important to be aware of how free oxygen radicals disturb the interaction between blood-born cells and endothelium and between endothelium and smooth muscle in the vessel wall. The experimental findings are promising with regard to future therapeutic use of agents removing oxygen radicals, especially in clinical conditions involving reperfusion (cardioplegia, fibrinolytic therapy, transcutaneous angioplasty).

References

1. Braunwald E, Kloner RA. Myocardial reperfusion: a doubleedged sword. J Clin Invest 1985; 76: 1713-9.
2. Nayler WG, Elz JS. Reperfusion injury: laboratory artifact or clinical dilemma? Circulation 1986; 74: 215-21
3. Guarnieri C, Ferrari R, Visioli O, Caldarera CM, Nayler WG. Effect of α -tocopherol on hypoxic-perfused and reoxygenated rabbit heart muscle. J Mol Cell Cardiol 1978; 10: 893-906
4. Lefer AM, Araki H, Okamatsu S. Beneficial actions of a free radical scavenger in traumatic shock and myocardial ischemia. Circ Shock 1981; 8: 273-82
5. Granger DN, Rutili G, McCord JM. Superoxide radicals in feline intestinal ischemia. Gastroenterology 1981; 81: 22-9.
6. Shlafer M, Kane PF, Kirsh MM. Superoxide dismutase plus catalase enhances the efficiency of hypothermic cardioplegia to protect the globally ischemic, reperfused heart. Thorac Cardiovasc Surg 1982; 83: 830-9.
7. Green MJ, Hill HAO. Chemistry of dioxygen. In: Packer L, ed. Methods of enzymology. Orlando: Academic Press, 1984: 3-22.
8. McCord JM, Fridovich I. Superoxide dismutase. An enzymatic function for erythrocuprein (Hemocuprein). J Biol Chem 1969; 244: 6049-55.
9. Chance B, Sies H, Boveris A. Hydroperoxide metabolism in mammalian organs. Physiol Rev 1979; 59: 527-605.
10. Freeman BA, Crapo JD. Biology of disease. Free radicals and tissue injury. J Lab Invest 1982a; 47: 412-26.
11. Fantone JC, Ward PA. Role of oxygen-derived free radicals and metabolites in leucocyte-dependent inflammatory reactions. Am J Pathol 1982; 107: 397-418.
12. Slater TF. Free-radical mechanisms in tissue injury. Biochem J 1984; 222: 1-15.
13. Proctor PH, Reynolds ES. Free radicals and disease in man. Physiol Chem Phys Med NMR 1984; 16: 175-95.
14. Halliwell B, Gutteridge JMC. Oxygen free radicals and iron in relation to biology and medicine: some problems and concepts. Arch Biochem Biophys 1986; 246: 501-14.
15. Rao PS, Cohen MV, Muellier HS. Production of free radicals and lipid peroxides in early experimental myocardial ischemia. J Mol Cell Cardiol 1983; 15: 713-6.
16. Blasig IE, Ebert B, Löve H. Identification of free radicals trapped during myocardial ischemia in vitro by ESR. Studia Biophysica 1986; 116: 35-42.
17. Garlick PB, Davies MJ, Hearse DJ, Slater TF. Direct detection of free radicals in the reperfused rat heart using electron spin resonance spectroscopy. Circ Res 1987; 61: 757-60.

18. Sevanian A, Muakkassah-Kelly SF, Montestruque S. The influence of phospholipase A_2 and glutathione peroxidase on the elimination of membrane lipid peroxides. Arch Biochem Biophys 1983; 223: 441-52.
19. Del Maestro RF, Thaw HH, Björk J, Planker M, Arfors K-E. Free radicals as mediators of tissue injury. Acta Physiol Scand 1980; (suppl 492): 43-57.
20. Harris RN, Doroshow JH. Effect of doxorubicin-enhanced hydrogen peroxide and hydroxyl radical formation on calcium sequestration by cardiac sarcoplasmic reticulum. Biochem Biophys Res Comm 1985; 130: 739-45.
21. Yang G, Chen J, Wen Z, Ge K, Zhu L, Chen X. The role of selenium in keshan disease. Adv Nutr Res 1984; 6: 201-31.
22. Ytrehus K, Ringstad J, Myklebust R, Norheim G, Mjøs OD. The selenium-deficient rat heart with special reference to tolerance against enzymatically generated oxygen radicals. Scand J Clin Lab Invest 1988; 48: 289-95.
23. Singal PK, Kapur N, Dhillon KS, Beamish RE, Dhalla NS. Role of free radicals in catecholamine-induced cardiomyopathy. Can J Physiol Pharmacol 1982; 60: 1390-7.
24. Hearse DJ, Humphrey SM, Chain EB. Abrupt reoxygenation of the anoxic potassium-arrested perfused rat heart: a study of myocardial enzyme release. J Mol Cell Cardiol 1973; 5: 395-407.
25. Shlafer M, Kane PF, Wiggins BS, Kirsh MM. Possible role for cytotoxic oxygen metabolites in the pathogenesis of cardiac ischemic injury. Circulation 1982; 66 (suppl I): 85-92.
26. Ytrehus K, Gunnes S, Myklebust R, Mjøs OD: Protection by superoxide dismutase and catalase in the isolated rat heart reperfused after prolonged cardioplegia: a combined study of metabolic, functional, and morphometric ultrastructural variables. Cardiovasc Res 1987; 21: 492-9.
27. Lee RB, Stewart JR, Merrill WH, Frist WH, Hammon JW, Bender HV Pharmacokinetics of superoxide dismutase during hypothermic cardiopulmonary bypass. Circulation 1989; 80 (suppl III): III-25-9.
28. Gauduel Y, Duvelleroy MA. Role of oxygen radicals in cardiac injury due to reoxygenation. J Mol Cell Cardiol 1984; 16: 459-70.
30. Myers ML, Bolli R, Lekich R, Hartley CJ, Roberts R. Enhancement of recovery of myocardial function by oxygen freeradical scavengers after reversible regional ischemia. Circulation 1985; 72: 915-21.
29. Menasche P, Grousset C, Gauduel Y, Piwnica A. A comparative study of free radical scavengers in cardioplegic solutions. J Thorac Cardiovasc Surg 1986; 92: 264-71.
31. Gross GJ, Farber NE, Hardman HF, Warltier DC. Beneficial actions of superoxide dismutase and catalase in stunned myocardium of dogs. Am J Physiol 1986; 250: H372-7.
32. Myers CL, Weiss SJ, Kirsh MM, Shepard BM, Shlafer M. Effects of supplementing hypothermic crystalloid cardioplegic solution with catalase, superoxide dismutase, allopurinol, or deferoxamine on functional recovery of globally ischemic and reperfused isolated hearts. J Thorac Cardiovasc Surg 1986; 91: 281-9.
33. Przyklenk K, Kloner RA. Superoxide dismutase plus catalase improve contractile function in the canine model of the "stunned myocardium". Circ Res 1986; 58: 148-56.
34. Ambrosio G, Weisfeldt ML, Jacobus WE, Flaherty JT. Evidence for a reversible oxygen radical-mediated component of reperfusion injury: reduction by recombinant human superoxide dismutase administered at the time of reflow. Circulation 1987; 75: 282-91.
35. Jolly SR, Kane WJ, Bailie MB, Abrams GD, Lucchesi BR. Canine myocardial reperfusion injury: its reduction by the combined administration of superoxide dismutase and catalase. Circ Res 1984; 54: 277-85.
36. Ambrosio G, Becker LC, Hutchins GM, Weisman HF, Weisfeldt ML. Reduction in experimental infarct size by recombinant human superoxide dismutase: Insights into the pathophysiology of reperfusion injury. Circulation 1986; 74: 1424-33.

37. Näslund U, Häggmark S, Johanson G, Marklund SL, Reiz S, Oberg A. Superoxide dismutase and catalase reduce infarct size in a porcine myocardial occlusion-reperfusion model. J Mol Cell Cardiol 1986; 18: 1077-84.
38. Chi L, Tamura Y, Hoff PT, et al. Effect of superoxide dismutase on myocardial infarct size in the canine heart after 6 hours of regional ischemia and reperfusion: a demonstration of myocardial salvage. Circ Res 1989; 64: 665-75.
39. Przyklenk K, Kloner R. "Reperfusion Injury" by oxygen-derived free radicals? Effect of superoxide dismutase plus catalase, given at the time of reperfusion, on myocardial infarct size, contractile function, coronary microvasculature, and regional myocardial blood flow. Circ Res 1989; 64: 86-96.
40. Gallangher KP, Buda AJ, Pace D, Gerren RA, Shlafer M. Failure of superoxide dismutase and catalase to alter size of infarction in conscious dogs after 3 hours of occlusion followed by reperfusion. Circulation 1986; 73: 1065-76.
41. Uraizee A, Reimer KA, Murry CE, Jennings RB. Failure of superoxide dismutase to limit size of myocardial infarction after 40 minutes of ischemia and 4 days of reperfusion in dogs. Circulation 1987; 75: 1237-48.
42. Przyklenk K, Kloner RA. Effect of oxygen-derived free radical scavengers on infarct size following six hours of permanent coronary artery occlusion: salvage or delay of myocyte necrosis. Basic Res Cardiol 1987; 82: 146-58.
43. Opie LH. Reperfusion injury and its pharmacologic modification. Circulation 1989; 80: 1049-62.
44. Shirato C, Miura T, Ooiwa H, Toyofuku T, Wilborn WH, Downey JM. Tetrazolium artifactually indicates superoxide dismutase induced salvage in reperfused rabbit heart. J Mol Cell Cardiol 1989; 21: 1187-93.
45. Ganote CE, Sims M, Safavi S. Effects of dimethylsulfoxide (DMSO) on the oxygen paradox in perfused rat hearts. Am J Pathol 1982; 109: 207-76.
46. Magovern GJ, Bolling SF, Casale AS, Bulkley BH, Gardner TJ. The mechanism of mannitol in reducing ischemic injury: hyperosmolarity or hydroxyl scavenger? Circulation 1984; 70 (suppl 1): 91-5.
47. Mitsos SE, Fantone JC, Gallagher KP, et al. Canine myocardial reperfusion injury: Protection by a free radical scavenger, N-2-mercaptoproprionyl glycine. J Cardiovasc Pharmacol 1986; 8: 978-89.
48. Bolli R, Zhu WX, Hartley CJ, et al. Attenuation of dysfunction in the postischemic "stunned" myocardium by dimethylthiourea. Circulation 1987; 76: 458-68.
49. Otani H, Engelman RM, Rousou JA, Breyer RH, Lemeshow S, Das DK. Cardiac performance during reperfusion improved by pretreatment with oxygen free-radical scavengers. J Thorac Cardiovasc Surg 1986; 91: 290-5.
50. Rubanyi GM, Vanhoutte PM. Superoxide anions and hyperoxia inactivate endothelium-derived relaxing factor. Am J Physiol 1986b; 250: H822-7.
51. Hartmann A, Saeed M, Bing RJ. Release of endothelium-derived relaxing factor from freshly harvested porcine endothelial cells. Circ Res 1987; 61: 548-54.
52. Mehta JL, Nicols WW, Donnelly WH, et al. Protection by superoxide dismutase from myocardial dysfunction and attenuation of vasodilatator reserve after coronary occlusion and reperfusion in dogs. Circ Res 1989; 65: 1283-95.
53. Romaschin AD, Rebeyka I, Wilson GJ, Mickle DAG. Conjugated dienes in ischemic and reperfused myocardium: an in vivo chemical signature of oxygen free radical mediated injury. J Mol Cell Cardiol 1987; 19: 289-302.
54. Bolli R, Patel BS, Jeroudi MO, Lai EK, McCay PB. Demonstration of free radical generation in 'stunned' myocardium of intact dogs with the use of the spin trap α-phenyl N-tert-butyl nitrone. J Clin Invest 1988; 82: 476-85.

55. Bernier M, Hearse DJ, Manning AS. Reperfusion-induced arrhythmias and oxygen-derived free radicals. Circ Res 1986; 58: 331-40.
56. Manning AS, Coltart DJ, Hearse DJ. Ischemia and reperfusion-induced arrhythmias in the rat. Effects of xanthine oxidase inhibition with allopurinol. Circ Res 1984; 55: 545-8.
57. Woodward B, Zakaria MNM. Effect of some free radical scavengers on reperfusion induced arrhythmias in the isolated rat heart. J Mol Cell Cardiol 1985; 17: 485-93.
58. Koster JF, Slee RG, Essed CE, Stam H. Studies on cumene hydroperoxide-induced lipid peroxidation in the isolated perfused rat heart. J Mol Cell Cardiol 1985; 17: 701-8.
59. Ytrehus K, Myklebust R, Mjøs OD. Influence of oxygen radicals generated by xanthine oxidase in the isolated perfused rat heart. Cardiovasc Res 1986; 20: 597-603.
60. Miki S, Asraf M, Salka S, Sperelakis N. Myocardial dysfunction and ultrastructural alterations mediated by oxygen metabolites. J Mol Cell Cardiol 1988; 20: 1009-24.
61. Harris EJ, Booth R, Cooper MB. The effect of superoxide generation on the ability of mitochondria to take up and retain Ca^{++}. FEBS lett 1982; 46: 267-72.
62. Guarnieri C, Muscari C, Ceconi C, Flamigni F, Caldarera CM. Effect of superoxide generation on rat heart mitochondrial pyruvate utilization. J Mol Cell Cardiol 1983; 15: 859-62.
63. Hillered L, Ernster L. Respiratory activity of isolated rat brain mitochondria following in vitro exposure to oxygen radicals. J Cerebr Blood Flow Metabol 1983; 3: 207-14.
64. Ytrehus K, Myklebust R, Olsen R, Mjøs OD. Ultrastructural changes induced in the isolated rat heart by enzymatically generated oxygen radicals. J Mol Cell Cardiol 1987; 19: 389-97.
65. Jennings RB, Reimer KA, Steenbergen C. Myocardial ischemia revisited. The osmolar load, membrane damage, and reperfusion. J Mol Cell Cardiol 1986; 18: 769-80.
66. Kim M-S, Akera T. O_2 free radicals: cause of ischemia-reperfusion injury to cardiac Na^+K^+-ATPase. Am J Physiol 1987; 252: 252-7.
67. Kramer JH, Tong Mak I, Weglicki WB. Differential sensitivity of canine cardiac sarcolemmal and microsomal enzymes to inhibition by free radical-induced lipid peroxidation. Circ Res 1984: 55: 120-4.
68. Scherer NM, Deamer DW. Oxidative stress impairs the function of sarcoplasmic reticulim by oxidation of sulfhydryl groups in the Ca^{++}-ATPase. Arch Biochem Biophys 1986; 246: 589-601.
69. Rubanyi GM, Vanhoutte PM. Oxygen-derived free radicals, endothelium, and responsiveness of vascular smooth muscle. Am J Physiol 1986; 250: H815-21.
70. Greenberg B, Rhoden K, Barnes PJ. Activated oxygen molecules generated by electrical stimulation affect vascular smooth muscle. J Mol Cell Cardiol 1986; 18: 975-81.
71. Marcus AJ, Silk ST, Safier LB, Ullman HL. Superoxide production and reducing activity in human platelets. J Clin Invest 1977; 59: 149-58.
72. Kukreja RC, Kontos HA, Hess ML, Ellis EF. PGH synthase and lipoxygenase generate superoxide in the presence of NADH or NADPH. Circ Res 1986; 59: 612-9.
73. Otani H, Engelman RM, Rousou JA, Breyer RH, Das DK. Enhanced prostaglandin synthesis due to phospholipid breakdown in ischemic-reperfused myocardium. J Mol Cell Cardiol 1986; 18: 953-61.
74. Schoutsen B, de Jong JW. Age-dependent increase in xanthine oxidoreductase differs in various heart cell types. Circ Res 1987; 61: 604-7.
75. Jarasch E-D, Grund C, Bruder G, Heid HW, Keenan TW, Franker WW. Localization of xanthine oxidase in mammary-gland epithelium and capillary endothelium. Cell 1981; 25: 67-82.
76. Chambers DE, Parks DA, Patterson G, et al. Xanthine oxidase as a source of free radical damage in myocardial ischemia. J Mol Cell Cardiol 1985; 17: 145-52.

77. Engler RL, Dahlgren MD, Morris DD, Peterson MA, Schmid-Schönbein GW. Role of leucocytes in response to acute myocardial ischemia and reflow in dogs. Am J Physiol 1986; 251: H314-22.
78. Chambers DE, Yellon DM, Hearse DJ, Downey JM. Effects of flurbiprofen in altering the size of myocardial infarcts in dogs: reduction or delay? Am J Cardiol 1983; 51: 884-90.
79. Lucchesi BR, Romson JL, Jolly SR. Do leukocytes influence infarct size? In: Hearse DJ, Yellon DM, eds. Therapeutic approaches to myocardial infarct size limitation. Raven Press, 1984: 219-48.
80. Mullane KM, Read N, Salmon JA, Moncada S. Role of leucocytes in acute myocardial infarction in anesthetized dogs: relationship to myocardial salvage by anti-inflammatory drugs. J Pharmacol Exp Ther 1984; 228: 510-22.
81. Allan G, Bhattacherjee P, Brook CD, Read NG, Parke AJ. Myeloperoxidase activity as a quantitative marker of polymorphonuclear leucocyte accumulation into an experimental myocardial infarct – the effect of ibuprofen on infarct size and polymorphonuclear leucocyte accumulation. Cardiovasc Pharmacol 1985; 7: 1154-60.
82. Minta JO, Williams MD. Some nonsteroidal antiinflammatory drugs inhibit the generation of superoxide anions by activated polymorphs by blocking ligand-receptor interactions. J Rheumatol 1985; 12: 751-7.
83. Werns SW, Shea MJ, Vaporciyan A, et al. Superoxide dismutase does not cause scar thinning after myocardial infarction. J Am Coll Cardiol 1987; 9: 898-902.
84. Turrens JF, Boveris A. Generation of superoxide anion by the NADH dehydrogenase of bovine heart mitochondria. Biochem J 1980; 191: 421-7.

9

Magnesium in cardiology: Both a nutrient and a drug

PETTER C. BORCHGREVINK,
PER JYNGE

Since 1935, when successful magnesium (Mg) therapy of digitalis-induced arrhythmias was first reported (1), it has been known that Mg influences the heart. Today, Mg supplementation has some clinical use as a protective agent during open heart surgery. The two main questions concerning Mg and cardiology are whether special precautions should be taken to keep cardiac patients in optimal Mg status and whether Mg should be given during acute myocardial infarction (AMI). In an attempt to answer these questions, the present review will mainly concentrate on these subjects:

- Basic information about Mg in biology and medicine (I).
- Mg: nutrient and drug in cardiovascular diseases (II).
- Experimental data on Mg in myocardial ischaemia and reperfusion (III).

I. Basic information on Mg

Because of its small ion and its divalence, Mg forms complex ions to a special degree, combinding not only with other ions but also with many molecules of dipolar nature (2). Mg is bound to ATP and is a cofactor for about 300 enzymes, among others enzyme systems using ATP as a substrate. Thus, Mg is important in several basic physiological energy demanding and producing processes, such as muscle contraction, oxydative phosphorylation, mitochondrial function, cell membrane permeability and neuromuscular excitability (3).

Content of Mg in different body compartments

Mg has been called the neglected cation. Although the concentration in serum is only 0,70-0.95 mmol/l (4), the normal human body contains 21-

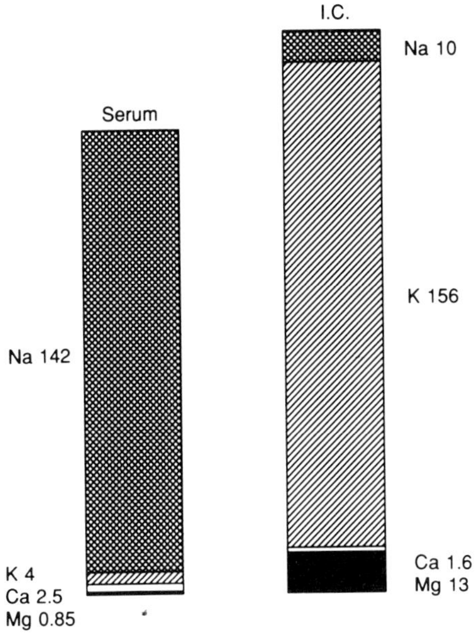

Fig. 1. *The distribution of Mg and other cations in serum and in i.c. space expressed in mmol/l (serum and cell water).*

28 grams of Mg (3), and Mg is the second most abundant cation (see Fig. 1). About 1% of Mg in the body is located in plasma, of which 55% of Mg is "free", i.e. in the ionized form. Thirtytwo per cent is protein-bound while the remainder is complexed to phosphate, citrate or other agents (5, 6). Approximately 60% of Mg in the body is located in bone.

The intracellular (i.c.) space accounts for about 40%, almost half of this being in skeletal muscle. The cell contains from 11 to 17 mmol Mg per litre cell water (7). Almost all are bound to i.c. structures. In the heart 12% of Mg was estimated to be in the mitochondria and 2-3% in the myofibrils (7). The new finding of a concentration of free i.c. Mg of 0.5 mM has been confirmed by NMR (8, 9) and dye studies (9, 10). This concentration, close to what is found extracellularly is rather low compared to what has formerly been accepted (2.5 mM) (5, 11).

Mg and ionic homeostasis

Experimental studies have shown that Mg deficiency causes increased i.c. sodium (Na) and calcium (Ca) and reduced i.c. potassium (K) and Mg levels (12, 13). A number of possible mechanisms for these interionic relationships exist. Mg deficiency may increase membrane fluidity, resulting in leaky membranes (14), and Mg has been established as an absolute requirement for Na-K-ATPase (15).

Both experimental and clinical investigations (16, 17) indicate an important role for Mg in K homeostasis as follows: 1. Mg deficiency results in decreased cell K. 2.Combined Mg and K deficiencies result in greater loss in cell K than occur in simple K deficiency. 3.Uncorrected co-exisiting Mg deficiency impairs repletion of cell K.

Mg is named nature's physiologic Ca blocker (18). In vitro studies (19) suggest that specific membrane Mg sites in vascular muscle can act physiologically to control and regulate the entry and exit of Ca. In cardiac muscle, Mg modulates the force development by its interaction with Ca (18).

Mg and cardiac contractility

High levels of Mg depress myocardial contractility through its interaction with K, Na and especially Ca (20). In rat ventricular septa there was a decline in tension development by an increasing extracellular (e.c.) Mg concentration, and Mg was found to reduce the movement of e.c. Ca into the rat myocardial cell by a competitive process localized at the sarcolemmal membrane (21).

Within the muscle cell, Mg appears to: 1. Inhibit release of Ca from sarcoplasmatic reticulum in response to a sudden influx of e.c. Ca which normally "triggers" this release. 2. Actually drive Ca into sarcoplasmatic reticulum by stimulation of Ca-ATPase enzyme activity. 3. Compete with Ca at certain binding sites on troponin-C and myosin. 4. Inhibit the ability of Ca to stimulate myocardial tension (18).

Mg and cardiac electrophysiology

Infusion of Mg produces decreased atrioventricular conduction, decreased intra-ventricular conductance and suppresion of sinus node function (20). The duration of the vulnerable period in the heart cycle is diminished (22). It has also been demonstrated that Mg elevates the ventricular threshold of premature contraction and fibrillation (23). These conditions are thought to be reversed during Mg deficiency with an increase in the discharge rate of the sinus node and a tendency to abnormal impulse formation (22).

II. Mg: Nutrient and drug in cardiovascular diseases

Several epidemiological studies from different parts of the world have reported that the regional death-rates from ischaemic heart disease including sudden death from this disease, are inversely correlated to the water hardness and the Mg content of the drinking water and to the content of the exchangeable Mg in the soil (24-27). Another argument for a connection between Mg deficiency and ischaemic heart disease has been that patients dying of cardiac conditions tend to have lower myocardial Mg in non-ischaemic areas than those dying of other causes (25, 28). These findings may, however, be a consequence of various hormonal and metabolic reactions that occur during MI, since catecholamines produce a cardiospesific loss of Mg (28).

Since Mg treatment has been useful both in Mg deficiency states and when Mg status is normal, the ion may be regarded as both an essential nutrient and a drug. In the following pages some indications of the importance of Mg in cardiovascular disease and the possible mechanisms of actions will be reviewed. We will discuss studies indicating that Mg-deficiency may predispose to, and that Mg treatment may be effective against, various types of cardiovascular diseases.

Mg and arrhythmias

Although, experimentally, it is difficult to demonstrate that Mg deficiency will lead to cardiac arrhythmias, clinically, there is some evidence that Mg deficiency may be one among other responsible factors in the development of various tachyarrhythmias (30, 31). Much of the evidence is provided by documentation that rapid replacement of Mg will convert these rhythms into a sinus mechanism, especially when conventional methods fail (32).

Different cardiac dysrhythmias may respond to $MgSO_4$, including: ventricular tachycardia (VT) and fibrillation (VF) due to massive digitalis intoxication; intractable VF; "torsades de pointes" tachycardia; hypomagnesaemic atrial tachycardia, flutter and fibrillation; and multifocal atrial tachycardia (32). The positive influence of Mg on cardiac arrhythmias may be mediated through a direct action, through interaction with K or by interfering with Ca and Na (22). See later regarding Mg and arrhythmias during AMI.

An increased sensitivity to digitalis-induced arrhythmias in hypomagnesaemia has been demonstrated both in experimental settings (33) and in clinical studies (34). Both digitalis administration and Mg deficiency reduce i.c. K (34). While a former study did not find any evidence of a change in the activity of Na-K-ATPase following alteration of e.c. Mg (35), a recent study demonstrated that the level of e.c. Mg is important for total K transport and digitalis-sensitive K transport (36).

Mg and vascular tone

Acute hypomagnesaemia in animals and man is often associated with rises in blood pressure and elevations in peripheral vascular resistance in several regional circulations (37). Reduction of e.c. Mg concentration during perfusion of isolated canine and human vessels produces vasoconstriction and potentiates the pressor effects of angiotensin II and norepinephrine (19).

The vasodilator properties of Mg have been known for many years (38). Increasing the e.c. level of Mg relaxes vascular smooth muscle and reduces pressor responses (39). Mg depletion in rats not only increases blood pressure but also reduces microcirculatory blood flow (40), while in humans Mg supplementation augments the reduction in blood pressure induced by diuretics (41). The prompt termination of Prinzmetal's angina attacks (due to coronary artery spasm) by i.v. bolus of $MgSO_4$ has been documented (42).

The mechanism of Mg-induced vasodilation is not completely understood. Evidence in vitro indicates that Mg may compete with Ca for e.c. binding sites in vascular tissue, thereby preventing Ca-induced vasoconstriction (19). In addition to Ca flux, recent results (37) suggest that prostacyclin release plays a role in mediating the vascular action of Mg in humans.

Mg and atherosclerosis

Sudden death victims in hard water areas have less atheromas than those in soft water areas (43). Experimental Mg deficiency produces vascular lesions with calcifications, while increasing the dietary intake of Mg has been shown to prevent atheroma and thrombotic complications (44). Experimental evidence suggests that Mg deficiency may affect the main factors in the pathogenesis of atherosclerosis and thrombosis: the integrity of the arterial wall, coagulability of the blood and quantity and quality of the circulating lipids (44). A recent clinical study (45) found that patients treated with peroral Mg for three months altered the composition of blood lipids in a way that, from a theoretical point of view, should give protection against atherosclerosis.

Mg and acute myocardial infarction

A catecholamine-induced hypomagnesaemia is known to occur during AMI (46). Mg binds to free fatty acids liberated during increased lipolysis (47). A reasonable explanation for the lowering of total serum during increased

Table 1. *Results of Mg supplementation during acute myocardial infarction.*

1. author	No. of patients	Treatment	Effect on	Mg	Placebo
Rasmussen (49, 50)	130	50 mM $MgCl_2$/24 h +12 mM MgCl2/24 h	Deaths/4 weeks Arrhythmias	7% 21%	19% 47%
Smith (51)	200	65 mM $MgSO_4$/24 h	Deaths/24 h Total cardiac events	1% 7%	7% 16%
Abraham (52)	94	10 mM $MgSO_4$/20 min	Potential lethal arrhythmias/24 h	15%	35%
Rasmussen (53)	270	50 mM $MgCl_2$/24 h +12 mM MgCl2/24 h	Deaths/1 year	20%	32%

Table 1 presents studies all indicating a positive effect of i.v. Mg infusion started on admission to the hospital. The last study (53) included all patients with suspected acute MI, while the others included only those with proven acute MI.

lipolysis may be an enhanced binding of Mg by free fatty acids within the adipocytes (4).

Hypomagnesaemia in patients with AMI on admission to hospital has been found to increase the incidence of severe arrhythmias, among those VF (48). To which extent this was also due to a pre-existing hypomagnesaemia is not known. Another study did not, however, find such a correlation (49).

Recently three small clinical studies (50-52) indicated a reduced mortality and less severe arrhythmias during the first days after AMI in those patients who received i.v. Mg supplementation when admitted to the hospital (Table 1). Further, in a one year follow up study, the mortality was lower, mainly due to a reduction in the first 30 days (53). The decrease in mortality has been considered to be mainly due to a reduction in lethal arrhythmias (22). On the basis of experimental studies we will now discuss the possibility that Mg status may also affect survival of the ischaemic myocardium.

III. Myocardial ischaemia and reperfusion. Role of Mg

It has been suggested that Mg supplementation early during AMI may reduce the infarct size (54). On the other hand, it has been suggested that chronic Mg deficiency may predispose to larger infarcts. We will briefly review experimental studies which may provide answers to these questions. Most of them are studies of global ischaemia resembling the conditions of electively induced ischaemia during open heart surgery.

Protective interventions during ischaemia and reperfusion

There is an important distinction between ischaemia, a reversible event, and necrosis or infarction which is irreversible. It has been shown that myocardial necrosis might be delayed by interventions both during regional and global ischaemia (55, 56).

Reperfusion, the reintroduction of blood and oxygen into the coronary circulation, may salvage reversibly injured myocytes but under certain conditions also induce a paradoxical extension of ischaemic damage (57). According to the latter view, interventions during reperfusion may also be important. The so-called reperfusion injury may be regarded in two ways: as a final event of dying cells or as an event by which certain unfavourable cellular changes may endanger an otherwise reversibly injured myocardium.

Cardioplegic solutions for myocardial protection during global ischaemia in open heart surgery have three principal goals: 1. rapid induction of diastolic ischaemic arrest before cellular energy stores are depleted; 2. reduction or delay of ischaemic injury; and 3. prevention of cellular injury at the onset of reperfusion. Whereas concomitant hypothermia is undoubtedly a major factor behind the second goal, the chemical composition of cardioplegic solutions is of importance in achieving all three goals. Research into the use of cardioplegic infusates during cardiac surgery has resulted in the investigation of compounds which may limit ischaemic injury.

Since Mg is an important i.c. cation, and since the concentration of this ion may decrease both in myocardial tissue and in plasma during ischaemia/reperfusion (47, 58), Mg has been suggested as being a protective agent, not only for protection against arrhythmias, but also for protection of the ischaemic myocardium.

The importance of e.c. Mg during ischaemia and reperfusion

K based cardioplegic solutions with high Mg administered to rats prior to total, global ischaemia improved ischaemic and post-ischaemic function (59) and metabolism (56) (Fig. 2). About 15-20 mM was found to be optimal (60). This finding was the basis for advocating 16 mM Mg in the cardioplegic solution during open heart surgery (56). This effect could be due to effects of high Mg immediately prior to ischaemia, during ischaemia, at the onset of reperfusion or of a combination.

We have demonstrated in recent studies that early reperfusion of the ischaemic heart in the presence of Mg elevation improved the recovery of cardiac function and metabolism (61, 62). In a concentration dependent manner Mg elevation increased post-ischaemic coronary flow rate (Fig. 3) and improved the recovery of energy metabolism, as assessed by ATP (Fig. 4) creatine phosphate, and of i.c. pH (62).

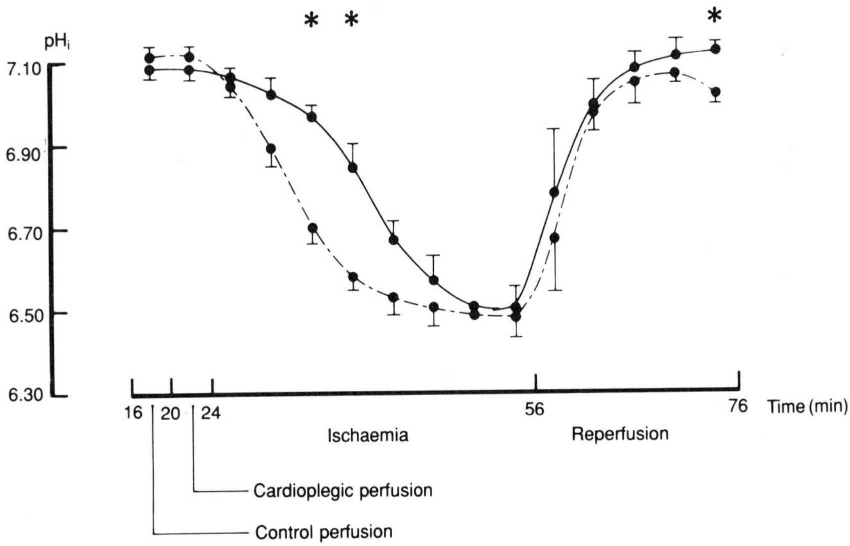

Fig. 2. *Changes in myocardial i.c. pH during control perfusion, global ischaemia and reperfusion of isolated rat hearts (60). The data are derived from ^{31}P NMR obtained over 4 min sampling periods and are expressed in pH units. The continuous and strippled lines represent the results from hearts being perfused (20-24 min) with high K cardioplegic solutions containing respectively 15 mM and 0 Mg. Points and bars represent means ±SE. The asterix indicates significant intergroup differences.*

On the other hand, perfusing isolated rat hearts with Mg-free solutions during reperfusion and subtotal global ischaemia reduced the myocardial tolerance to ischaemia (61,62). Electrophysiological instability was prominent in the groups perfused with 0 mM Mg. The experimental model may have some clinical relevance since some cardiac centres use a Mg-free cardioplegic solution (56) and since serum Mg is reduced after AMI (46) and open heart surgery (63).

Mechanisms of protective action by Mg during ischaemia and reperfusion

The protective role of Mg during ischaemia and reperfusion seems to be multifactorial, which should not be surprising in the light of the numerous tasks of the ion. Table 2 summarizes possible factors, some being confirmed by experimental studies, while others are rather hypothetical. Some of these factors may mainly influence the heart only during ischaemia or during reperfusion, while others are probably important during both ischaemia and reperfusion.

Since a former study found no protection of high Mg during ischaemia in the isolated rabbit heart (64), it was concluded that ischaemic protection

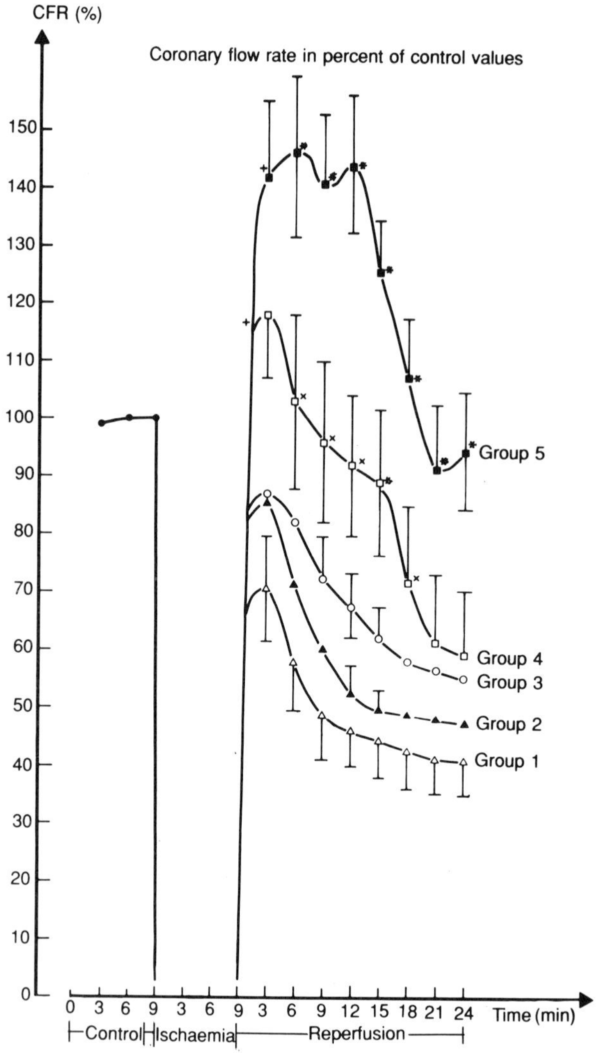

Fig. 3. *Changes in coronary flow rate during control perfusion, global ischaemia and reperfusion of isolated rat hearts (62). Coronary flow rate is presented in % of values obtained during 6-9 min of control perfusion as assessed by ^{31}P-NMR. Points and bars represent means ±SE. Groups 1-3: 0, 0.6 and 2.4 mM during the entire reperfusion period. Groups 4 and 5 received 15 mM Mg, and group 5 also high Ca during the first 12 min of reperfusion. * Significantly different from all other groups. x Significantly different from groups 1 and 2. + Significantly different from groups 1 to 3.*

in the rat heart was due to the pronounced Ca-Mg antagonism in this particular species leading to a more rapid introduction of diastolic arrest prior to ischaemia (64). However, there is experimental data to suggest that Mg may have a beneficial influence upon cellular metabolism during ischaemia, an effect not easily related to e.c. Ca-Mg antagonism. Thus, the addition of 15 mM of Mg to a cardioplegic solution containing 15 mM of K caused a delay in the development of cellular acidosis (60) (Fig. 2), probably the result of a retarded glycolysis.

During reperfusion there is experimental evidence for the assumption that high Mg improves coronary flow (62) (Fig. 3) and reduces the incidence of

Table 2. *Some potential mechanisms of Mg as a myocardial protective agent during ischaemia and reperfusion.*

Reduced cardiac work load
- Negative inotropy and chronotropy?
- E.c. Ca antagonism?

Improvement in coronary flow
- Counteracting coronary arterial spasm?
- Reversal of myocardial contracture?
- E.c. Ca antagonism?
- Endothelial metabolic effects?

Antiarrhythmic effects
- Conservation of i.c. K^+?
- Prevention of i.c. Na^+ overload?
- Prevention of i.c. Ca^{++}?

Modifying reperfusion injury
- E.c. Ca^{++} antagonism?
- Reduced generation or toxicity of oxygen radicals?

Improvement in recovery of metabolism
- I.c. Mg^{++} conservation?
- Reduced mitochondrial uptake of Ca?
- Improvement in coronary flow?

VF (62). Furthermore, high Mg may normalize i.c. K (62, 65) and pH (62) and enhance the replenishment of ATP (62) (Fig. 4). One may speculate that high e.c. Mg decreases the influx of Ca, which is prone to occur during reperfusion or leads to more i.c. Mg being available for cell function during reperfusion.

Myocardial Mg during ischaemia and reperfusion

Experimental studies have shown that an obvious loss of Mg occurs during post-ischaemic reperfusion and hypoxic perfusion, while the extent of Mg loss during total ischaemia is more uncertain (58, 66, 67). In recent NMR experiments (62) we were able to recognize a marked increase in i.c. free Mg during ischaemia from 0.5 mM to about 2.5 mM and a gradual return to a normal value during reperfusion (Fig. 5). These results are in contrast to a formerly established view that free i.c. Mg does not rise during myocardial ischaemia (4, 8). A rise in i.c. free Mg during myocardial ischaemia may favour conditions for a potential net cellular loss of Mg during reperfusion (4).

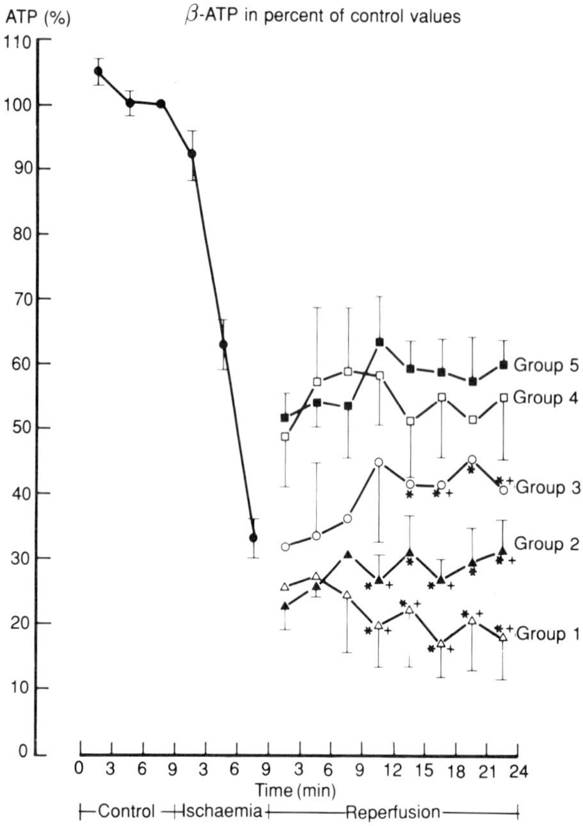

Fig. 4. *Changes in myocardial β-ATP during control perfusion, global ischaemia and reperfusion of isolated rat hearts (62). β-ATP is presented in % of values obtained during 6-9 min of control perfusion as assessed by* ^{31}*P-NMR. Points and bars represent means ±SE. Groups 1-3: 0, 0.6 and 2.4 mM during the entire reperfusion period. Groups 4 and 5 received 15 mM Mg, and group 5 also high Ca, during the first 12 min of reperfusion. *Significantly different from group 5. +Significantly different from group 4.*

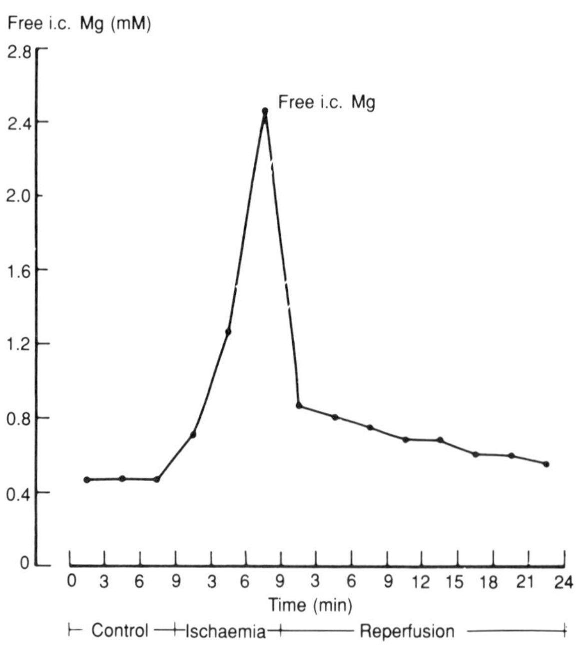

Fig. 5. *Changes in calculated i.c. free Mg in mM during control perfusion, global ischaemia and reperfusion of isolated rat hearts (62). The calculated i.c. free Mg is expressed in mM and is based on an accurate measurement of the chemical shift difference between the α-phosphate and β-phosphate resonances of i.c. ATP using the method described by Gupta et al (70).*

The effect of magnesium deficiency upon the infarct size

We have above indicated a positive role of acutely elevated e.c. Mg in myocardial protection as it appears from experimental studies. Experimental studies have also indicated that a pre-existing Mg deficiency state increases the ischaemic injury. A former experimental study demonstrated that Mg deficiency sensitizes the heart to catecholamine-induced damage (68). Doses of adrenaline mimicking acute systemic stress induced massive myocardial Ca overload, Mg loss and scattered necrosis in Mg deficient rats (68). These changes could be prevented by Mg supplementation.

We recently demonstrated that post-ischaemic cardiac function was impaired in isolated hearts from rats subjected to a Mg deficiency state by low dietary intake (69) or furosemide medication (70). This finding, that chronic Mg deficiency reduces the myocardial tolerance to ischaemia in spite of any reduction in myocardial tissue Mg concentration, is in accordance with a study of Mg deficient beagle dogs (71). Coronary artery ligation induced a higher ratio of necrotic muscle volume compared to the muscle volume at risk, than was found in control animals. Thus, another explanation for the positive correlation between chronic Mg deficiency and ischaemic heart disease may be suggested in addition to increased risk of arrhythmias, coronary vascular spasm and atherosclerosis: a pre-existing hypomagnesaemia may increase the myocardial vulnerability to ischaemia.

Possible mechanisms of reduced tolerance to ischaemia by chronic Mg deficiency

The finding of no reduction in myocardial tissue Mg (69-71) does not rule out the presence of small and/or compartmentalized losses of Mg from i.c. sites or from local pools in the sarcolemma in Mg deficient animals. Such compartmentalized losses of Mg may, through secondary effects, impair the myocardial tolerance to a subsequent period of ischaemia. Another explanation of the reduced ischaemic tolerance by Mg deficiency may be related to a low e.c. Mg. Since acute normalization of e.c. Mg did not improve the post-ischaemic recovery of hearts from Mg deficient rats (69), it is likely that the reduction in post-ischaemic recovery was not related to the low e.c. Mg per se, but rather to secondary, chronic changes in the myocardium.

One such secondary change which finds support from the recent experiment (69) and two later studies (71, 72), may be a rise in myocardial Na. This was the only demonstrated electrolyte alteration in hearts of Mg deficient rats (69) and the first electrolyte change to occur in hearts of Mg deficient hamsters (72). In the latter species, an early rise in tissue Na was later followed by Ca overload, Mg depletion and cardiac necrosis. In the study of myocardial infarct size in beagle dogs (71) a rise in Ca and specially in Na was also detected in non-infarcted areas, but there was no parallel decrease in Mg nor K.

A high i.c. Na may activate Na/Ca counter transport resulting in increased i.c. Ca. This may favour the production of transient depolarization with the tendency to repetitive arrhythmias (22) and make the myocardium more vulnerable to ischaemia.

Conclusions with clinical implications

Both epidemiological, experimental and clinical studies have indicated that Mg deficiency may modulate the events of cardiovascular diseases in an unfavourable manner. Since cardiac patients are at high risk of developing Mg deficiency because of diuretic treatment, hyperaldosteronism and malnutrition (73), it seems reasonable to be aware of and optimize Mg status in such patients. Patients on loop blocking diuretics or thiazides should, in addition, receive a K-and Mg-sparing diuretic.

An assessment of total Mg status is possible in hospitalized patients for instance by giving i.v. $MgSO_4$ 30 mmol over eight hours and sample Mg in urine 24 hours from the start. Normally, more than 80% of Mg is excreted, so a retention of more than 50% indicates a total Mg depletion in a patient in a stable phase (74). These Mg balance studies may be a good indicator of i.c. Mg status, which is important for normal cardiac function (73).

A poor correlation is found between serum Mg and Mg loading tests (75), and between serum Mg and Mg in skeletal muscle (73). However, serum Mg, the only easily available Mg measurement, should also be more frequently undertaken in cardiac patients, since experimental studies cited above demonstrate the importance of e.c. Mg upon the heart.

The question whether Mg should be used for treatment during AMI is still not solved. Exerimental studies may, however, indicate a beneficial effect of Mg during myocardial ischaemia and reperfusion. The superiority of Mg is its multifactorial effects: it may have both antiarrhythmic, vasodilating and anti-ischaemic properties.

Although three clinical studies have found less lethal arrhythmias when Mg was given during AMI, these studies are small. A multicentre-study should be performed and both arrhythmias, mortality and infarct size be recorded in patients with evolving AMI. Mg therapy should be combined with an established therapeutic principle, such as fibrinolysis, which may reperfuse ischaemic myocardium with this protective ion.

References

1. Zwillinger L. Über die Magnesiumwirkung auf das Herz. Klin Wochenschr 1935; 14: 1429-31.
2. Aikawa JK. Magnesium: Its biologic significant. Boca Raton: CRC Press, Inc. 1981.
3. Wacker EC. Magnesium and man. Cambridge Massachusetts: Harvard University Press, 1980.
4. Department of clinical chemistry, RiT: Analysis and investigations. University Hospital of Trondheim, 1985.
5. Ebel H, Günther T. Magnesium metabolism: A review. J Clin Chem Biochem 1980; 18, 257-70.
6. Kroll MH, Elin RJ. Relationships between magnesium and protein concentrations in serum. Clin Chem 1985; 31: 244-6.
7. Polimeni PI, Page E. Magnesium in heart muscle. Circ Res 1973; 33: 367-74.
8. Gupta RK, Gupta P, Yushok WD, Rose ZB. On the noninvasive measurement of intracellular free magnesium by 31P NMR spectroscopy. Physiol Chem Phys Med NMR 1983; 15: 265-88.
9. Garfinkel L, Altschuld RA, Garfinkel D. Magnesium in cardiac energy metabolism. J Moll Cell Cardiol 1986; 18: 1003-13.
10. Cittadini A, Scarpa A. Intracellular Mg^{2+} homeostasis of Ehrlich ascites tumor cells. Arch Biochem Biophys 1983; 227: 202-9.
11. Wu ST, Pieper GM, Salhany JM, Eliot RS. Measurement of free magnesium in perfused and ischaemic arrested heart muscle. A quantitative phosphorus-31 nuclear magnetic resonance and multiequilibria analysis. Biochemestry 1981; 20: 7399-7403.
12. Whang R, Welt RG. Observations in experimental magnesium depletion. J Clin Invest 1963; 42: 305-13.
13. Günther T. Wasser und Electrolytverteilung in einiger Organen von Mg-arm ernährten Ratten. Klin Biochem 1970; 8: 65-8.
14. Schilling K, Bornig H, Comme, Hoppe H. Effects of magnesium dependent cell membrane alterations on the transport of K^+ in Ehrlich ascites tumor cells. Acta Biol Med 1979; 38: 1101-14.
15. Skou JC. Further investigations on a Mg^{++}- and Na^+-activated adenosin-triphosphatase, possibly related to the active, linked transport of Na^+ and K^+ across the nerve membrane. Biochem Biophys Acta 1960; 42: 6-23.
16. Ryan MP. The role of magnesium in potassium deficiency. In: Whelton PK, Whelton A, Walker WG, eds. Potassium in cardiovascular and renal medicine – arrhythmias, myocardial infarction and hypertension. New York: Marcel Dekker, Inc., 1986: 23-42.
17. Dyckner T, Wester PO. Relation between potassium, magnesium and cardiac arrhythmias. Acta Med Scand 1981; (suppl. 647): 163-9.
18. Iseri LT, French JH. Editorial: Magnesium: Nature's physiologic calcium blocker. Am Heart J 1984; 108: 188-93.
19. Altura BM, Turlapaty PDMV. Withdrawal of magnesium enhances coronary artery spasms produced by vasoactive agents. Br J Parmacol 1982; 649-659.
20. Shine KJ. Myocardial effects of magnesium. Am J Physiol 1979; 237: H413-23.
21. Shine KJ, Douglas AM. Magnesium effects on ionic exchange and mechanical function in rat ventricle. Am J Physiol 1974; 227: 317-24.
22. Wester PO. Editorial note: Magnesium – effects on arrhythmias. Int J Cardiol 1986; 12: 181-3.
23. Gahni MF, Rabah M. Effect of magnesium chloride on electrical stability of the heart. Am Heart J 1977; 94: 600-2.
24. Sharper AG. Soft water, heart attacks and strokes. JAMA 1974; 230: 130.

25. Chipperfield B, Chipperfield JR. Magnesium and the heart. Am Heart J 1977; 93: 679-82.
26. Seelig MS. Magnesium deficiency in the pathogenesis of disease. New York: Plenum Press Medical Books, 1980.
27. Karppanen H. Epidemiological studies of on the relationship between magnesium intake and cardiovascular diseases. Artery 1981; 9: 190-9.
28. Behr G, Burton P. Heart muscle magnesium. Lancet 1973; 2: 450.
29. Lehr D. Magnesium and cardiac necrosis. Mag.-Bull 1981; 1a: 178-91.
30. Loeb HS, Petras RJ, Gunnar RM, Tobin JR. Paroxysmal ventricular fibrillation in two patients with hypomagnesemia. Circulation 1968; 37: 210.
31. Iseri LT, Freed J, Bures AR. Magnesium deficiency and cardiac disorders. Am J Med 1975; 58: 837-46.
32. Iseri LT. Magnesium and dysrythmias. Mag Bull 1986; 8: 223-9.
33. Seller RH, Banach S, Namey T, Neff M, Swartz C. Cardiac effect of diuretic drugs. Am Heart J 1975; 89: 493-500.
34. Iseri LT. Potassium, magnesium and digitalis toxicity. In: Whang R, ed. Potassium: Its biologic significance. Boca Raton: C.R.C. Press, 1983: 125-36.
35. Shine KJ, Douglas AM. Magnesium effects on ionic exchange and mechanical function in rat ventricle. Am J Physiol 19744; 227: 317-24.
36. Borchgrevink PC,Ryan MP. Effects of magnesium on 86Rubidium in a human atrial cell line. Br J Pharmacol 1988; 9: 379-83.
37. Nadler JL, Goodson S, Rude RK. Evidence that prostacyclin mediates the vascular action of magnesium in humans. Hypertension 1987; 9: 379-83.
38. Winkler AW, Smith PK, Hoff HE. Intravenous magnesium sulfate in the treatment of nephritic convulsions in adults. J Clin Invest 1942; 21: 207-16.
39. Altura BM, Altura BT. Magnesium and vascular tone and reactivity. Blood Vessels 1978; 15: 5-16.
40. Altura BM, Altura BT, Gedrowald A, Ising H, Günther T. Magnesium deficiency and hypertension: correlation between magnesium deficient diets and micro-circulatory changes in situ. Science 1984; 223: 1315-8.
41. Dyckner T, Wester PO. Effect of magnesium on blood pressure. Br Med J 1983; 286: 1847-51.
42. Cohen L, Kitzes R. Magnesium sulphate in the treatment of variant angina. Magnesium 1984; 3: 46-9.
43. Crawford T, Crawford MD. Prevalence and pathological changes of ischaemic heart disease in a hard water and in a soft water area. Lancet 1967; i: 229-32.
44. Rayssiguier Y. Magnesium, lipids and vascular diseases. Magnesium 1986; 5: 182-90.
45. Rasmussen HS, Aurup P, Goldstein K, et al. Influence of magnesium substitution therapy on blood lipid composition in patients with ischaemic heart disease 1989; 149: 1050-3.
46. Abraham AS, Eylath U, Weinstein M, Czaczkes E. Serum magnesium levels in patients with acute myocardial infection. N Engl J Med 1977; 296: 862-7.
47. Flink EB, Brick JE, Shane SR. Alterations of long-chain free fatty acid and magnesium concentrations in acute myocardial infarction. Arch Intern Med 1981; 141: 441-3.
48. Dyckner T. Serum magnesium in acute myocardial infarction. Relation to arrhythmias. Acta Med Scand 1980; 207: 59-67.
49. Rasmussen HS, Suensson M, McNair P,Nørregård P, Balsløv S. Magnesium infusion reduces the incidence of arrhythmias in acute myocardial infarction. A double-blind, placebo-controlled study. Clin Cardiol 1987; 10: 351-6.
50. Rasmussen HS, Nørregaard P, Lindeneg O, McNair P, Backer V, Balsløv S. Intravenous magnesium in acute myocardial infarction. Lancet 1986; 1: 234-6.
51. Smith LF, Heagerty AM, Bing RF, Barnett DB. Intravenous infusion of magnesium

sulphate after acute myocardial infarction:effects of arrhythmias and mortality. Int J Cardiol 1986; 12: 175-80.
52. Abraham AS, Rosenmann D, Kramer M, et al. Magnesium in the prevention of lethal arrhythmias in acute myocardial infarction. Arch Intern Med 1987; 147: 753-5.
53. Rasmussen HS, Grønbæk M, Cintin C, Balsløv S, Nørregård P, McNair P. One-year death rate in 270 patients with suspected acute myocardial infarction, initially treated with intravenous magnesium or placebo. Clin Cardiol 1988; 11: 377-81.
54. Morton BC, Smith FM, McKibbon TJ, Nair RC, Poznanski WJ. Magnesium therapy in acute myocardial infarction. Mag Bull 1981; 3,1a: 192-94.
55. Opie LH. Myocardial infarct size. Part 1. Basic considerations. Am Heart J 1980; 100: 355-72.
56. Hearse DJ, Braimbridge MV, Jynge P. Protection of the ischaemic myocardium: "Cardioplegia". New York: Raven Press, 1981.
57. Hearse DJ. Editorial: Reperfusion of the ischaemic myocardium. J Mol Cell Cardiol 1977; 9: 605.
58. Shen AC, Jennings RB. Myocardial calcium and magnesium in acute ischaemic injury. Am J Pathol 1972; 67: 417-40.
59. Hearse DJ, Stewart DA, Braimbridge MV. Myocardial protection during ischaemic cardiac arrest. The importance of magnesium in cardioplegic solutions. J Thorac Cardiovasc Surg 1978; 75: 877-85.
60. Jynge P, Borchgrevink PC, Espe E, Schie Bergan A, Krane J. Magnesium in cardioplegic solutions as assessed by 31p NMR spectroscopy. Mag Bull 1986; 8: 148-55.
61. Borchgevink PC, Øksendal AN, Jynge P. Acute extracellular magnesium deficiency and myocardial tolerance to ischaemia. J Am Coll Nutr 1987; 6: 125-30.
62. Borchgrevink PC, Schie Bergan A, Bakøy O, Jynge P. Magnesium and reperfusion of the ischaemic heart as assessed by ^{31}P NMR. Am J Physiol 1989; 256: H195-204.
63. Holden MP, Ionescu MI, Wooler GH. Magnesium in patients undergoing open-heart surgery. Thorax 1972; 27: 212-8.
64. Behrson MM, Shine KI, Sterman WD. Effect of increased magnesium on recovery from ischaemia in rat and rabbit hearts. Am J Physiol 1982; 242: H89-93.
65. Jennings RB, Reimer KA, Steensbergen C. Myocardial ischaemia revisited. The osmolar load, membrane damage, and reperfusion. Editorial comment. J Mol Cell Cardiol 1986; 18: 769-80.
66. Seelig MS, Heggtveit A. Magnesium interrelationships in ischaemic heart disease: a review. Am J Clin Nutr 1974; 27: 59-79.
67. Polimeni PI, Page E. Further observations on magnesium transport in rat ventricular muscle. Rec Adv Stud Card Struct Metabol 1974; 4: 217-32.
68. Vormann J, Fisher G, Classen HG, Thöni H. Influence of decreased magnesium supply on the cardiotoxic effects of epinephrine in rats. Arzneim Forsch/ Drug Res 1983; 33: 205-10.
69. Borchgrevink PC, Jynge P. Acquired magnesium deficiency and myocardial tolerance to ischaemia.J Am Coll Nutr 1987; 6: 355-63.
70. Borchgrevink PC, Jynge P. Prolonged diuretic administration and myocardial tolerance to ischaemia. Pharmacol Toxicol 1987; 61: 254-9.
71. Chang C, Varghese J, Downey J, Bloom S. Magnesium deficiency and myocardial infarct size in the dog. J Am Coll Cardiol 1985; 5: 280-9.
72. Chang C, Bloom S. Interrelationship of dietary Mg intake and electrolyte homeostasis in hamsters: 1. Severe Mg deficiency, electrolyte homeostasis and myocardial necrosis. J Am Coll Nutr 1985; 4: 173-85.
73. Dyckner T, Wester PO. Potassium/magnesium depletion in patients with cardiovascular disease. Am J Med 1987; 82 (3a): 11-7.

74. Dyckner T, Wester PO. Magnesium deficiency. Guidelines for diagnosis and substitution therapy. Acta Med Scand 1982; (suppl 661): 37-41.
75. Gullestad L, Søyland E, Kjekshus J,Aase O, Bjørnstad P. Magnesium deficiency. Tidskr Nor Lægeforen 1987; 107: 1751-4.

Myocardial dysfunction

10

Myocardial contractility during chronic ischaemia

PER THAYSSEN

Left ventricular systolic function is determined by preload, afterload and contractility. In the intact organism these three determinants interact, which makes it difficult to define the precise individual influence of the three on the current state of left ventricular function (LVF). This has been very difficult especially for contractility, mainly due to problems with definition and measuring techniques.

In the simple muscular model (Fig. 1A) contractility is the changes during contraction defined by interrelated variables of muscle force, velocity and length. This means, that at a given load there is an unique velocity of shortening, but changes in load will change both the velocity of shortening and the shortening itself. Based on this, *Sonnenblick* (1) defined myocardial contractility as "the entire spectrum of mechanical activity as far as it can be assessed".

Later, *Strobeck and Sonnenblick* (2) redefined myocardial contractility as "changes in cardiac function that are independent of alterations in preload and afterload or both". This in contrast to the term "ventricular performance", which is the change in cardiac function induced by alterations in preload and afterload.

During chronic ischaemia, e.g. ischaemic heart disease, several factors are changed compared to the normal situation (Fig. 2). On the cellular level, the consequence of chronic ischaemia has not been exactly defined, but oxygen deprivation, disturbed calcium homeostasis and ATP-depletion have been proposed as causes of the contractile failure (3). Simultaneously structural changes occur due to the disease itself with loss of contractile muscular fibres (e.g. acute myocardial infarction (AMI)), local or diffuse fibrosis and/or hypertrophy/dilatation. Both the cellular and structural changes will cause functional changes, involving both systolic (preload, af-

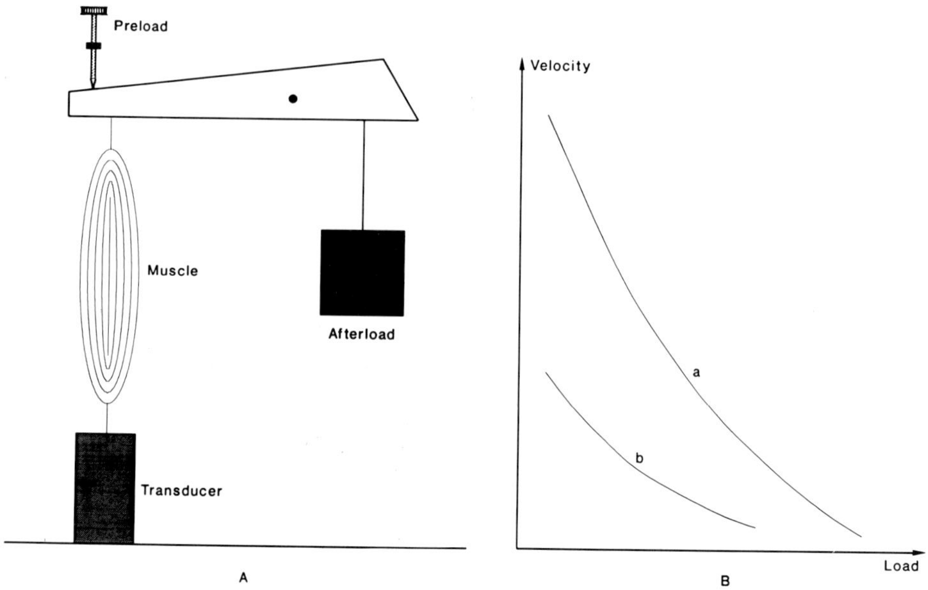

Fig. 1. *Panel A shows the simple muscular model for testing the influence of preload and afterload on contraction. Panel B shows schematically a constructed example of the force-velocity relationship in a normal muscle (A) and a muscle from an animal with cardiac failure (B).*

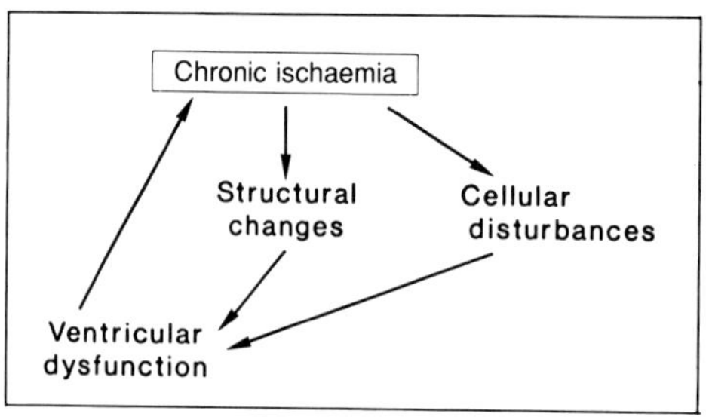

Fig. 2. *The vicious circle between chronic ischaemia and ventricular dysfunction (for further explanation: see text).*

terload and contractility) and diastolic (reduced ventricular compliance, disturbed relaxation) determinants and changed myocardial oxygen balance, partly by reducing coronary perfusion (increased heart rate and preload) and partly by increasing oxygen demand (increased heart rate and contractility). With time this vicious circle may lead to further deterioration of LVF.

Myocardial contractility

This consists of two phases, *isovolumic phase contractility* and *ejection phase contractility*. The former is the mechanical muscular activity performed during the isovolumic period from the closure of the atrioventricular valves to the opening of the semilunar valves, the latter, the mechanical activity during the ejection phase from the opening to the closure of the semilunar valves. Contractility in both phases can be altered by pharmacological intervention and are coupled to myocardial relaxation (4, 5).

One of the main problems with myocardial contractility is how to meassure it in human beings. In normal persons, but especially patients with ischaemic heart disease, the various measures of contractility depend on prerequisites such as ventricular geometry, mode of contraction and relaxation (4, 6, 7), factors that are heavily influenced by the cause of chronic ischaemia. In addition, many of the methods used for contractility measurements depend on the loading condition (7-9) giving rise to many problems in having a precise measure of myocardial contractility. Due to this, the purpose of this review has been to evaluate some of the concepts and invasive methods used for contractility measurements.

Experimental studies

The basic concepts in contractility arise from studies on isolated muscle strips, evaluated in an experimental situation as shown in Fig. 1A. By changing separately both preload and afterload, the regularity between these and contractility, measured as tension or force (isometric phase) and velocity of shortening (ejection phase), have been studied, showing that increase in afterload results in decreased velocity of contraction for an unchanged maximal force, while increase in preload increases force and probably also velocity. The property of the contractile element is usually evaluated from a force velocity relation (Fig. 1B) as shift of the curve or change in the course of the curve (10).

Both preload and afterload can be controlled in animal models and experiments.

In such studies, it has been shown, that measures of ejection phase contractilty (mean ejection rate) are rather insensitive to changes in afterload, while much more sensitive to alterations in preload (11, 12).

Correspondingly, measures of isovolumic phase contractility (maximum velocity of pressure rise) are sensitive to both preload and afterload (13).

Thus, in experimental studies on normal cardiac muscles, measurements of contractility during both the isovolumic and ejection phases are able to reflect changes in contractility, but are dependent on the loading conditions.

Methods for evaluation of myocardial contractility in human beings

In the intact human organism it is not possible to control either preload or afterload when evaluating myocardial contractility. Therefore, measurements of contractility can only be judged correctly when the influence of either preload or afterload on the method used are known, other prerequisites must also be considered carefully, frequently not being fulfilled in a number of diseases causing chronic ischaemia.

Isovolumic phase contractility

dp/dt-indices. These are calculated from recordings of pressure rise (mmHg/sec) during the isovolumic phase of the cardiac cycle. Only recordings obtained by a tip-transducer manometer can be used, being undamped with a true frequency response without any phase delay.

The most commonly used indices are (Fig. 3):

1) *dp/dt_{max}:* the peak pressure rise during the isovolumic period (14).
2) *$dp/dt_{max}/P$:* dp/dt_{max} divided by either ventricular end-diastolic pressure (EDP) or pressure at dp/dt_{max} minus EDP (15, 16).
3) V_{max} determined as the Y-axis intercept for the linear regression using ($dp/dt/(K \times Pt)$) as the ordinate and Pt as the abscissa. K is the serial-

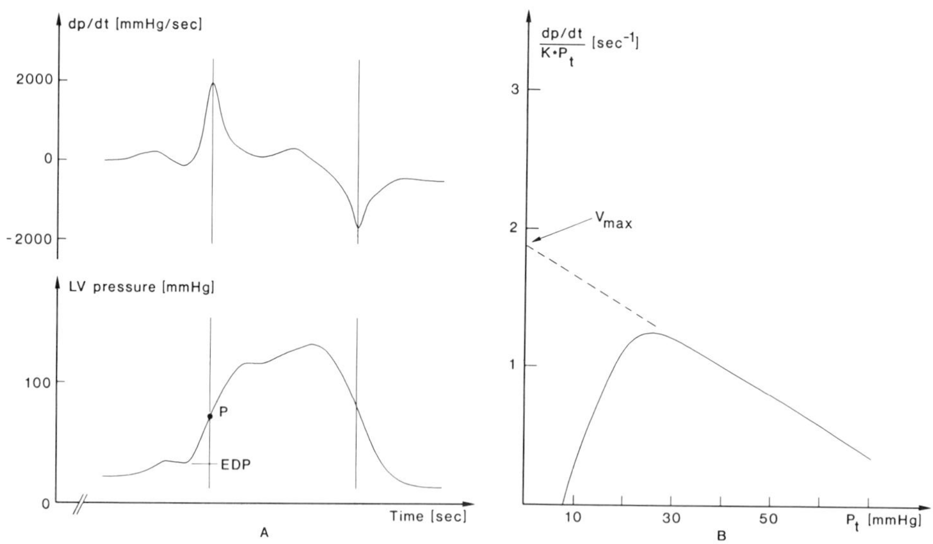

Fig. 3. *Panel A shows at the bottom the left ventricular pressure curve and at the top the differentiated left ventricular pressure curve defining dp/dt_{max}. EDP = end-diastolic pressure. P = left ventricular pressure at dp/dt_{max}.*

elastic constant known from animal studies, e.g. 32 (17), and Pt the instantaneous pressure (18).

Limitations: All indices are capable of reflecting alterations in isovolumic contractility (19), but in particular dp/dt_{max} and V_{max} are influenced to various degrees by heart rate, preload and afterload, being increased by increases in heart rate and preload, and reduced by decrease in afterload (7, 8, 12-14, 20). However, they seem useful in reflecting acute changes in a given patient (8, 21).

Attempts at correcting dp/dt_{max} for the influence of preload have been tried, by dividing dp/dt_{max} with a) EDP (15), b) pressure rise at dp/dt_{max} (13) and c) end-diastolic circumference (22). Such corrections may be useful with regard to normal ventricles, but in the case of ischaemic heart disease, changes in geometry and stiffness of the serial-elastic components have to be taken into account as well as the ventricular dilatation, which does not always represent the sarcomere stretch under these circumstances (8, 9).

Clinical implications: A problem for the evaluation of the indices as expressions of left ventricular contractility is the influence of ongoing medical treatment. It is known that in patients with ischaemic heart disease propranolol reduces $dp/dt_{max}/P$ and V_{max}, while this is not the case with verapamil (23-25). Digoxin has been shown to increase $dp/dt_{max}/P$ (26).

This must be taken into account if one is looking for the "true" state of isovolumic contractility in the individual patient.

Dp/dt indices and V_{max} have been shown to be able to discriminate between patients without significant coronary stenoses and normal EF compared to patients with severe coronary artery disease and reduced EF (27), but generally there is a considerable overlapping between normal subjects and patients with varying degrees of coronary artery disease (25, 28) and no significant correlation seems to exist between EF or either $dp/dt_{max}/P$ or V_{max} (27).

Bussmann et al (29), using stress-test, showed in patients with coronary artery disease, that the increase in dp/dt_{max} during exercise was inversely correlated to EDP and severity of angina pectoris as an expression of reduced contractile reserve in these patients.

Only little information regarding a prognostic value of dp/dt-indices is available. Although an increase in V_{max} from a level below normal limits before by-pass surgery to a level within normal range 12 months after by-pass surgery could be demonstrated, no information regarding cardiac events or death during or after by-pass surgery were obtained from preoperative measurements (25).

Thus, isovolumic contractility indices are difficult to use for the identification of the state of myocardial contractility in patients with chronic ischaemia. Still, for acute interventions during which preload and afterload can be controlled, they are sensitive measures of changes in the inotropic state.

Ejection phase contractility

The basis for measurements of contractility during ejection is the fact, that during this period the ventricle pumps out a given volume of blood to the aorta against a given resistance in a given time. Thus, one has to deal with a 3-dimensional function, which from a practical point of view is very difficult to describe. Therefore most measures of ejection phase contractility are based on only one or two of the three dimensions (volume – pressure – time) and with this being limited in giving a true picture of myocardial contractility during this phase.

Most methods are based on volume-calculations or pressure-volume relationship and with this methodological problems arise, predominantly due to discrepancies between the actual geometry of the ventricle and the theoretical model being used for the volume calculations. Further, the inter-relations between contractility and the other determinants of LVF, especially preload, afterload and relaxation disturbances, together with regional wall motion abnormalities have to be taken into account before the exact contractile state can be defined in a given patient. In many studies this is not the case and the results are therefore more a measure of LVF than of contractility itself.

Ejection fraction (EF)

This parameter of ejection phase contractility is usually used as a measure of LVF. It is based on volume calculations only, being stroke volume corrected for end-diastolic volume (EDV). In daily routine it is determined from volume calculations either from left ventriculography in the 30° right anterior oblique projection, isotope ventriculography (Multiple gated pool scanning) or echocardiography (four-chamber view). Assuming that the left ventricle is a rotational elipsoid, the end-systolic volume (ESV) and EDV are estimated on the basis of the area-length method and EF calculated as (30, 31)

$$EF = (EDV - ESV)/EDV)) \times 100$$

In the case of isotope ventriculography, the volume is based on the number of counts as described in another chapter of this book.

Limitations: EF can be determined with an acceptable reproducibility (coefficient of variation 5-10% (32)). Although being of great clinical value, it has considerable limitations as a contractility index of the left ventricle.

Firstly, the index depends on heart rate due to disproportional changes in EDV and ESV by increasing heart rate (33).

Secondly, despite the cause of ventricular dilatation, the calculation of ventricular volumes becomes more and more problematic with increasing volumes due to a worse "fit" to the theoretical elipsoid model. This results in a considerably reduced reliability in the calculation of EF (31). Thirdly, regional wall motion abnomalities may affect the reliability of the calculation, either in hyperkinesia or hypokinesia, if they are located to the circumference making the basis for end-systolic and end-diastolic measurements (34).

Lastly, reliable measurements can only be carried out on the left ventriculography if it is technically sufficient (sufficient contrast medium) and without arrhythmias (e. g., atrial fibrillation, ventricular ectopic beats).

It it also a problem, that EF is not independent of preload and afterload. Thus, an increased preload in itself may induce a reduced EF, while a decrease in afterload will increase EF, depending on the degree of impaired LVF (9, 35).

Calculation of EF during exercise gives additional information about LVF, but not specifically on left ventricular ejection phase contractility (36).

Clinical implications: During the last 2 decades a number of studies have been carried out on EF and LVF and it has been shown to be one of the most usefull parameters of the functional state and prognosis. It is essential to realize the above mentioned limitations, when evaluating clinical studies on EF as an expression of ejection phase contractility.

One must therefore be careful using this parameter as a measure of contractility, rather it is a parameter of the overall combined changes in left ventricular function due to changes in preload, afterload and contractility.

However, if preload and afterload are taken into account, EF reflects a reduced contractility with time in patients with ischaemic heart disease (37). In contrast to this, no definite correlation between EF and number of coronary artery stenoses can be demonstrated, probably because of compensatory alterations in preload and afterload (25, 38). It has also been shown in several studies, that EF is related to the extension of chronic regional ischaemia, although it might be normal with milder degrees of regional wall dysfunction (38). This may be due to the manner in which EF is measured, but can also be caused by compensatory hyperactivity in other regions of the left ventricular wall (9, 39). The latter problem has to some extent been overcome by regional analysis of ventricular wall motion, especially in patients with myocardial infarction (40). Perhaps the most important information, that one can gain from EF is the prognosis, where it has been useful in predicting survival (40, 41), and prognosis during and after AMI and coronary bypass surgery (42).

Although EF contains much clinically relevant information, it is rather problematic to use the index as a measure of ejection phase contractility partly due to methodological reasons and partly due to the dependence on preload and afterload.

Pressure-volume relations

During recent years much effort has been carried out to find indices and/or expressions of ejection phase contractility based on the systolic part of the pressure-volume relation (Fig. 4), the looped curve formed by simultaneous recordings of left ventricular volume (ventriculography, contrast or isotope) along the X-axis and pressure along the Y-axis.

The creation of such pressure-volume loops are technically difficult and therefore two approaches have been taken, a simple one based on the instantaneous ratio between pressure and ESV, and a more complicated one based on several pressure-volume loops in the same individual under different loading conditions (e.g., exercise).

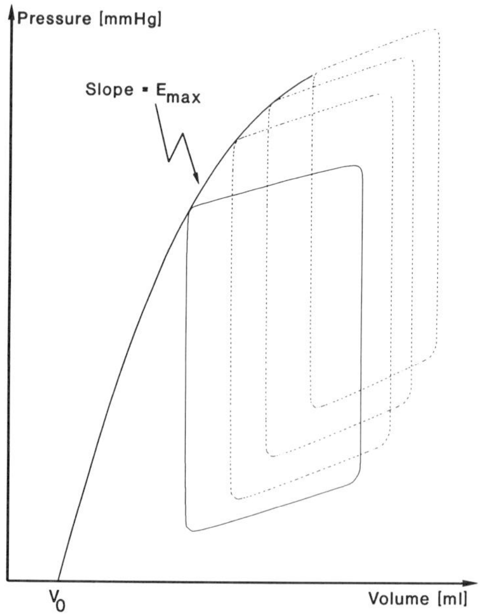

Fig. 4. *Shows schematically the basis for calculation of E_{max} and V_o based on 4 pressure-volume loops in the same individual under various conditions. The dark line represents the calculated line for which E_{max} is the slope, while V_o is the intercept between this line and the volume axis.*

End-systolic pressure-volume relation

From several pressure volume loops within the same patient under different loading conditions isochronal lines are constructed according to Sagawa's model of time-varying elastance (43). The maximum slope of these lines is called E_{max} and the intercept of this line with the X-axis is called V_0.

Limitations: E_{max} reflects the ability of the ventricle to contract at different afterloads and with this reflects ejection phase contractility as it has been shown both in dog experiments and in human studies. Being relatively independent of preload (44), the index, however, depends on a variety of factors, including chamber geometry, architectural arrangement of muscle fibers, left ventricular mass and connective tissue elements (45). Further, it is to some extent influenced by afterload itself (46).

With regard to V_0, this point on the X-axis represents the theoretical volume for the completely unloaded ventricle. Some authors find, that this parameter changes with changes in the inotropic state (47), while others do not (48). This is probably because V_0 depends on the method of measurement used (49), and probably due to recent findings that the line for E_{max} is curved, and the bending highly affected by afterload (46).

Pressure to end-systolic volume ratio

A number of ratios have been proposed, but only end-systolic pressure to end-systolic volume *(ESP/EDV)* and peak systolic pressure to end-systolic volume *(PSP/EDV)* will be discussed here. As the background for calculating these ratios is one pressure and one volume determination, they are much simpler to obtain in clinical practice, and with PSP/EDV it can be assessed non-invasively.

Limitations: ESP/EDV is calculated as the maximum value obtained from simultaneous recordings of ventricular pressure and volume (50). It correlates significantly with E_{max} (50), but might be dependent on afterload (51), although *Merillon et al* (52) did not find any such influence. The latter authors, however, conclude that the ratio is more an index of pump function than of muscle function and with this not contractility.

PSP/EDV is determined from simultaneous recordings of peak ventricular pressure and EDV corrected for body surface area (53). The ratio correlates well to E_{max} and to EF during exercise in a curvilinear fashion (53). Due to the correlation to E_{max}, one might anticipate dependency on afterload.

Clinical implications: Little is known about the clinical value of indices based on the pressure-volume relation.

It is known, that ESV itself contains valuable prognostic information, most recently demonstrated in predicting mortality after AMI using multivariate analysis with log rank test and Cox proportional hazards model (54). In this study, increasing ESV was the only parameter, that was superior in predicting mortality compared to, for example, EF or EDV. One might therefore expect indices derived from this parameter to contain both functional and prognostic information.

In patients with ischaemic heart disease *Iskandrian et al* (53) showed, that the non-invasively determined SPS/ESV-ratio both at rest and during exercise demonstrated a greater number of patients with abnormal LVF, than did EF alone, also in patients with a normal coronary angiography.

In patients undergoing mitral valve or aortic valve replacement, the outcome of operation was clearly better preoperatively predicted by the (end-systolic stress)/ESV-ratio compared to EF, due to the dependency of the latter on afterload (55).

Thus, from a clinical point of view E_{max} and pressure/ESV-ratio's are less dependent on loading conditions than EF and with this are probably more sensitive measures of the contractile state. However, the clinical value of this has not yet been defined, but hopefully future research will clear up this field further.

Conclusion

Despite intensive research over many years, we still lack the ideal measure of myocardial contractility, which is a parameter independent of the loading conditions and diastolic LVF, and still able to reflect the level of the contractile state as well as changes induced by disease and/or medical intervention. Although myocardial contractility decreases with progressive chronic ischaemia, we are at the moment unable to state whether this is predominantly due to a decrease in isovolumic contractility or ejection phase contractility or equally in both. It may also be possible that with different manifestions of chronic ischaemia, different patterns of abnormalities in myocardial contractility are present. However, to clear up the exact changes of myocardial contractility during various conditions and disease we have to develop more simple and more precise methods for determinations of myocardial contractility than is the case at present.

References

1. Sonnenblick EH. Contractility in the intact heart: Progress and problems. Eur J Cardiol 1973; 3: 319-25.
2. Strobeck JE, Sonnenblick EH. Myocardial contractile properties and ventricular performance. In: Fozzard HA, Haber E, Jennings RB, Katz AM, Morgan HE, eds. The heart and cardiovascular system. New York: Raven Press, 1986; 31-49.
3. Hearse DJ. Oxygen deprivation and early myocardial contractile failure: A reassessment of the possible role of adenosine triphosphate. Am J Cardiol 1979; 44: 1115-21.
4. Rousseau MF, Pouleur H, Detry J-MR, Brasseur LA. Relationship between changes in left ventricular inotropic state and relaxation in normal subjects and in patients with coronary subjects and in patients with coronary artery disease. Circulation 1981; 64: 736-44.
5. Langer GA. Ionic basis of myocardial contractility. Ann Rev Med 1977; 28: 13-20.
6. Berning J. Examination of cardiac function by means of quantitated angiography. A reference method of left ventricular volumes, ejection and regurgitant fraction. Ugeskr Laeg 1982; 39: 2837-40.
7. Karliner JS. Assessment of isovolumic and ejection phase indices of left ventricular performance. Herz 1981; 6: 195-208.
8. Quinones MA, Gaasch WH. Influence of acute changes in preload, afterload, contractile state and heart rate on ejection and isovolumic indices of myocardial contractility in man. Circulation 1976; 53: 293-301.
9. Sonnenblick EH, Strobeck JE. Current concepts in cardiology: Derived indexes of ventricular and myocardial function. N Engl J Med 1977; 296, 978-82.
10. Spann JF, Buccino RA, Sonnenblick RH. Braunwald E. Contractile state of cardiac muscle obtained from cats with experimental produced ventricular hypertrophy and heart failure. Cir Res 1967; 21: 341-48.
11. Braunwald E, Sarnoff SJ, Stainsby WN. Determinants of duration and mean rate of ventricular ejection. Cir Res 1958; 6: 319-25.
12. Mason DT, Braunwald E, Covell JW, Sonnenblick EH, Ross J jr. Assessment of cardiac contractility. The relation between the rate of pressure rise and ventricular pressure during isovolumic systole. Circulation 1971; 44: 47-58.
13. Videbaek J. Eksperimentelle og kliniske undersøgelser af isometriske trykindices afledt af venstre ventrikels trykstigningshastighed. Copenhagen: Fadl's forlag, 1979. Thesis.
14. Gleason WL, Braunwald E. Studies on the first derivative of the ventricular pressure pulse in man. J Clin Invest 1962; 41: 80-91.
15. Reeves TJ, Hefner LL, Jones WB, Coghlan C, Prieto G, Carroll J. The hemodynamic determinants of the rate of change in pressure in the left ventricle during isometric contraction. Am Heart J 1960; 60: 745-61.
16. Veragut UP, Krayenbühl HP. Estimation and Quantification of myocardial contractility in the closed-chest dog. Cardiologia 1965; 47: 96-112.
17. Yeatman LA, Parmley WW, Sonnenblick EH. Effects of temperature on series elasticity and contractile element motion in heart muscle. Am J Physiol 1969; 217, 1030-4.
18. Mason DT, Spann JF jr., Zelis R. The maximum intrinsic velocity of the myocardium in man: Estimation from the rate of pressure rise and intraventricular pressure throughout isovolumic left ventricular systole. Circulation 1968; 38 (suppl. 6): 134-41.
19. Klinike WP, Christie LG, Nichols WW, et al. Use of catheter-tip velocity-pressure transducer to evaluate left ventricular function in man: Effects of intravenous propranolol. Circulation 1980; 61: 946-54.
20. Schmidt HD, Hoppe H. Influence of the contractile state of the heart on preload depen-

dence of the maximal rate of intraventricular pressure rise dP/dt_{max}. Cardiology 1978; 63: 112-25.
21. Urschel CW, Vokonus PS, Henderson AH, Liedtke AJ, Horwitz LD, Sonnenblick EH. Critical evaluation of indices of myocardial contractility derived from the isovolumic phase of contraction. Cardiology 1980; 65: 4-22.
22. Frank MJ, Levinson GE. An index of the contractile state of the myocardium in man. J Clin Invest 1968; 47: 1615-26.
23. Bourdillon PD, Canepa-Anson R, Rickards AF. Hemodynamic effects of intravenous metoprolol. Am J Cardiol 1979; 44: 1195-200.
24. Vincenzi M, Morlino T, Allegri P, et al. Changes in cardiovascular function induced by verapamil in healthy subject and in patients with ischaemic heart disease. Clin Cardiol 1981; 4: 15-21.
25. Thayssen P. Systolic and diastolic time intervals in ischaemic heart disease. Odense 1985. Thesis.
26. Johnson BF, Meeran MK, Frank A, Taylor SH. Systolic time intervals in measurement of inotropic response to drugs. Br heart J 1981; 46: 513-21.
27. Peterson KL, Karliner JS, Ross J jr. Profiles in congestive and hypertrophic cardiomyopathies. In: Grossman W, ed. Cardiac catheterisation and angiography. Philadelphia: Lea and Febiger, 1974.
28. Kreulen TH, Bove AA, McDonough MT. The evaluation of left ventricular function in man. A comparison of methods. Circulation 1975; 51: 677-83.
29. Bussmann W-D, Heeger J, Kaltenbach M. Contractile and relaxation reserve of the left ventricle. IV Patients with coronary heart disease. Z Kardiol 1978; 67: 28-40.
30. Dodge HT, Sandler H, Baxley WA, Hawley RR. Usefulness and limitations of radiographic methods for determining left ventricular volume. Am J Cardiol 1966; 18: 10-25.
31. Erbel R, Schweizer P, Krebs W, Meyer J, Effert S. Sensitivity and specificity of two-dimentional echocardiography in detection of impaired left ventricular function. Eur Heart J 1984; 5: 477-89.
32. Chon PF, Levine JA, Bergeron GA, Gorlin R. Reproducibility of the angiographic left ventricular ejection fraction in patients with coronary artery disease. Am Heart J 1974; 88: 713-20.
33. Ricci DR, Orlik AE, Alderman EL, Ingels NB jr., Daughters GT II, Stinson EB. Influence of heart rate on left ventricular ejection fraction in human beings. Am J Cardiol 1979; 44: 447-51.
34. Rackley CE. Quantitative evaluation of left ventricular function by radiographic techniques. Circulation 1976; 54: 862-79.
35. Rønsberg D, Benn M, Karsch KR, Kreuzer H, Neuhaus KL, Spiller P. The influence of afterload on the normal and ischaemic myocardium in the dog. Z Kardiol 1978; 67: 595-600.
36. Iskandrian AS, Hakki A-H. Radionuclide evaluation of exercise left ventricular performance in patients with coronary artery disease. Am Heart J 1985; 110: 851-6.
37. Markis JE, Joffee CD, Roberts BH, et al. Evolution of left ventricular dysfunction in coronary artery disease. Serial cineangiographic studies without surgery. Circulation 1980; 62: 141-8.
38. Feild BJ, Russell ROjr., Dowling JT, Rackley CE. Regional left ventricular performance in the year following myocardial infarction. Circulation 1972; 46: 679-89.
39. Rigaud M,Rocha P, Boschat J, Farcot JC, Bardet J, Bourdarias JP. Regional left ventricular function assessed by contrast angiography in acute myocardial infarction. Circulation 1979; 60: 130-9.
40. Reet van, Quinones MA, Porliner LR. Comparison of two-dimensional echocardiography with gated radionuclide ventriculography in the evaluation of global and regional

left ventricular function in acute myocardial function. J Am Coll Cardiol 1984; 3: 243-52.

41. Hammermeister KE, Dekouen TA, Dodge HT. Variables predictive of survival in patients with coronary disease. Circulation 1979; 59: 421-30.
42. Cohn LH, Collins JJ jr., Cohn PF. Use of augmented ejection fraction to select patients with left ventricular dysfunction for coronary revascularization. J Thorac Cardiovasc Surg 1976; 72: 835-40.
43. Suga H, Sagawa K. Instantaneous pressure-volume relationships and their ratio in the exercise supported canine left ventricle. Circ Res 1974; 35: 117-26.
44. Little WC, Freeman GL, O'Rourke RA. Simultaneous determination of left ventricular end-systolic pressure-volume and pressure-dimension relationships in closed-chest dogs. Circulation 1985; 71: 1301-8.
45. Kass DA, Manghan WL. From 'Emax'to pressure-volume relations: A broader view. Circulation 1988; 77: 1203-12.
46. Manghan WL, Sunagawa K, Burkhoff D, Sagawa K. Effect of arterial impedance changes on the end-systolic pressure-volume relation. Circ Res 1984; 54: 595-602.
47. Grossmann W, Braunwald E, Mann T, McLaurin LP, Green LH. Contractile state of the left ventricle in man as evaluated from end-systolic pressure-volume relations. Circulation 1977; 56: 845-52.
48. Mehmel HC, Stockins B, Ruffman K, Olhausen K, Schuler G, Kubler W. The linearity of end-systolic pressure-volume relationship in man and its sensitivity for assessment of left ventricular function. Circulation 1981; 63: 1216-22.
49. Marsh JD, Green LH, Wynne J, Cohn PF, Grossman W. Left ventricular end-systolic pressure-dimension and stress-length relations in normal human subjects. Am J Cardiol 1979; 44: 1311-7.
50. McKay RG, Arocsty JM, Heller GV, Royal HD, Warren SE, Grossman W. Assessment of the end-systolic pressure-volume relationship in human beings with the use of a time-varying elastance model. Circulation 1986; 74: 97-104.
51. Kono A, Manghan L, Sunagawa K, Hamilton K, Sagawa K, Weisfeldt ML. The use of left ventricular end-systolic pressure and peak pressure in the estimation of the end-systolic pressure-volumne relationships. Circulation 1984; 70: 1057-65.
52. Merillon JP, Neukirch F, Motte G, et al. The left ventricular end-systolic pressure-volume ratio. Studies during changes in load and inotropism in the human. Eur Heart J 1981; 2: 41-8.
53. Iskandrian AS, Heo J. Left ventricular pressure/volume relationship in coronary artery disease. Am Heart J 1986; 112: 375-81.
54. White HD, Norris RM, Brown MA, Brandt PWT, Whitlock RML, Wild CJ. Left ventricular end-systolic volume as the major determinant of survival after recovery from myocardial infarction. Circulation 1987; 76: 44-51.
55. Carabello BA, Spann JF. The uses and limitations of end-systolic indexes of left ventricular function. Circulation 1984; 69: 1058-64.

11

Regional contractility of the heart during acute ischaemia

JON LEKVEN

Cardiac muscle normally contracts homogenously and responds to the varying demands of everyday life in a well-orchestrated manner. When shortage of oxygen occurs, however, this balanced mode of activity is disturbed so that contraction abnormalities arise. Several pathophysiological aspects of coronary artery disease may be considered in this light: oxygen shortage may be temporary or permanent, be partial or total, or may be local or generalised.

Dilation

The most striking abnormality of cardiac muscle associated with oxygen shortage is myocardial dilation. This feature had been recognised in experimental animals for almost a century (1), and *Tennant and Wiggers* proved in 1935 that bulging was caused by coronary artery occlusion (2). Techniques were developed later to measure dilation accurately, in particular from the ultrasound transit-time between implanted piezo-electric crystals (3, 4). Fig. 1 shows developments that occur in a segment of about 11 mm within the left ventricle during progressive constriction of the supplying coronary artery. Dilation is clearly visible through this experiment and represents a general principle during coronary insufficiency. Although end-diastole is the traditional reference point for cardiac dimensions, it appears from Fig. 1 that dilation comprises the entire heart cycle.

Reduced myocardial shortening

Myocardial contraction normally occurs from slightly prior to ejection until the end of the systole. It appears from Fig. 1 that shortening of the myocar-

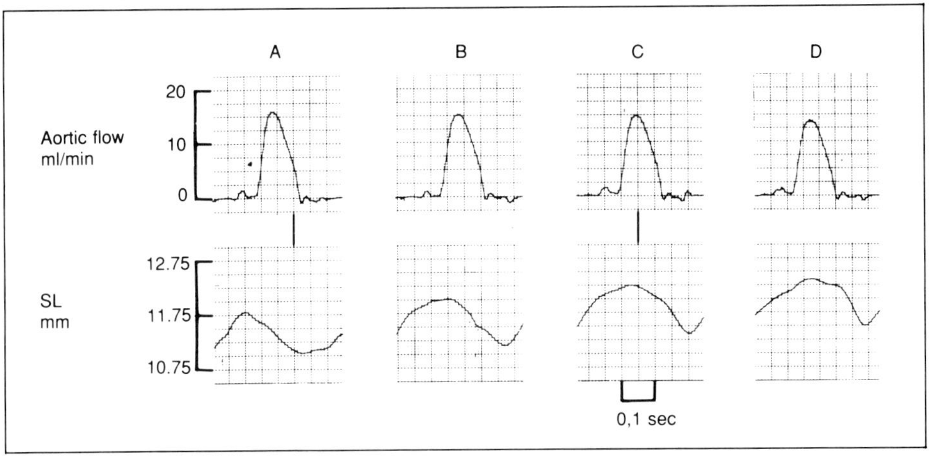

Fig. 1. *Development of myocardial contraction abnormality in a dog, from a control situation with undisturbed coronary flow (A), through stepwise tightening of the artery (B,C) until occlusion (D). All beats represent stable haemodynamic situations. SL = segment length. Adapted from Lekven and Kiil (51).*

dial segment gradually becomes affected during ischaemia. Although the total amplitude of movement is not changed to any great extent, less shortening takes place within the ejection period; during coronary occlusion there is virtually no systolic shortening. Characteristically, the ability to contract against a normal systolic pressure in the ventricle is compromised during ischaemia. Paradoxial elongation rather than contraction may even occur during the systole. Such segments obviously do not contribute very much to ventricular pumping. Actual shortening is delayed until pressure is low at the late relaxation phase and during diastolic filling.

Pressure-length loop analysis

Tyberg et al introduced in 1974 pressure-length loop analysis as a means of estimating the mechanical work of a region of the ventricle into which ultrasound crystals are implanted (5). Segment length recordings like the one in Fig. 1 are entered into a continuous X-Y function together with a high-fidelity left ventricular pressure recording. Such loops better visualise functional contraction because shortening is related to the actual pressure when the movement takes place. The area circumscribed by a loop that normally rotates in a counter-clockwise direction quantifies the generated external work of the segment. Fig. 2 shows the profound effects that occur following coronary ligation. Initially, segments give in at the completion of

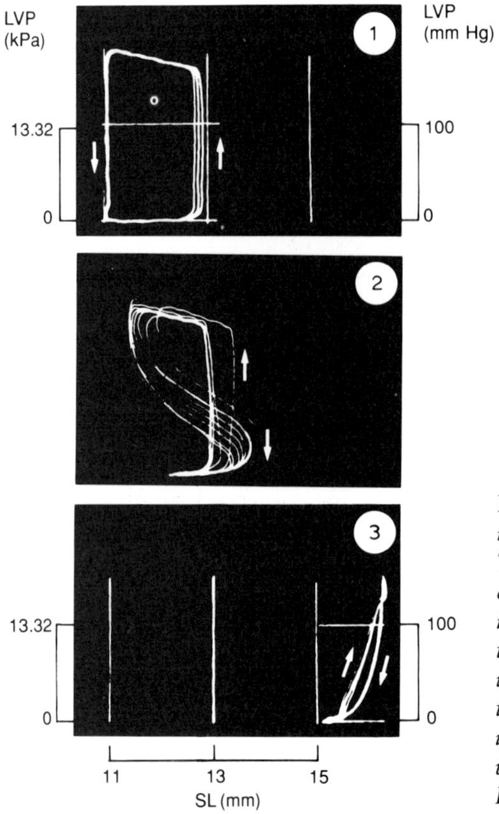

Fig. 2. *Development of contraction failure following coronary occlusion in a cat. Three superimposed normal beats rotate counter-clockwise (1). After 50 s the loop is transformed in shape and size, moved to the right (dilation) and rotates clockwise (3). Seven consecutive beats from the transition period indicate the initial failure at completion of systole (2). LVP = left ventricular pressure. SL = segment length. From Matre and Lekven (52).*

the systole (lower left corner of loops). Loops move to the right (dilation) and envelope much smaller areas. Also, loop rotation is reversed, indicating that external mechanical work is imposed *on* rather than being produced by the segment. Paradoxial bulging can thus be quantified.

The ability to complete the systole represents an essential part of cardiac function. Normally, the end-systolic relation of pressure-length loops, or pressure-volume loops, is linear provided there is a constant level of inotropy (6, 7). Two alterations occur during ischaemia. First, the slope of the relationship is reduced which is consistent with reduced contractility of the myocardium involved (8-10). Second, it has recently been suggested that the end-systolic pressure-segment relationship deviates from linearity at low pressures and that this effect may be ascribed to inadequate coronary perfusion (11-14).

Evolving ischaemia

Figure 2 shows that dramatic changes take place within the first minute of ischaemia. There is experimental evidence that these alterations proceed faster than electrocardiographic abnormalities (15, 16). Although depletion of cellular energy stores like ATP and creatine phosphate immediately follows the onset of oxygen shortage, the speed at which dilation and failure to shorten occur clearly exceeds these breakdown rates (17). Therefore, it is likely that the most sensitive mechanism is related to hampered release of calcium ions from the sarcolemma and sarcoplasmic reticulum that impairs normal interaction with the contractile proteins (18).

Functional derangements generally correlate with the severity and duration in later phases of ischaemia (19, 20). However, recovery is delayed because biochemical normalisation and replenishment do not readily occur (21). Impaired function may therefore persist for a long time even though revascularisation is established within the time limits for permanent structural damage not to occur; such tissue has been termed stunned myocardium (22). The first signs of cellular alterations can be observed by electron microscopy after 10 min of ischaemia (23). Exactly when permanent cellular damage occurs is a matter of debate, but ranges anywhere from 15-60 min in experimental animals at normothermia (24, 25), but myocytes at risk do not necessarily reach this critical point at the same time.

Non-uniformity

The myocardium has generally been considered to contract uniformly. In recent years, however, evidence has been accumulating that uniformity of contraction may represent a regulatory mechanism for mechanical performance; it is suggested that the vectorial contraction pattern is organised in such a way that some fibres, or layers of fibres, that "rest" during low-work conditions are called upon, or mobilised, when more work is needed (26-29). Such regulation depends on proper coronary circulation to all fibre layers. It has been demonstrated that reduced coronary flow disturbed this regulation so that non-uniformity occurred in studies of cross-oriented ultrasound crystals in a midwall position (14). Fig. 3 shows that a segment along muscle fibres was much less affected by ischaemia than a segment across the same fibres. Thus, the very structural organisation of fibre contraction is susceptible to ischaemic interference.

Much of ischaemic non-uniformity of contraction can be ascribed to subendocardial dysfunction (30-33). Although total blood flow in the left coronary artery was reduced by a modest 16% (Fig. 3), perfusion was markedly redistributed so that endocardial layers received only 46% of normal flow whereas epicardial flow remained essentially unchanged. It

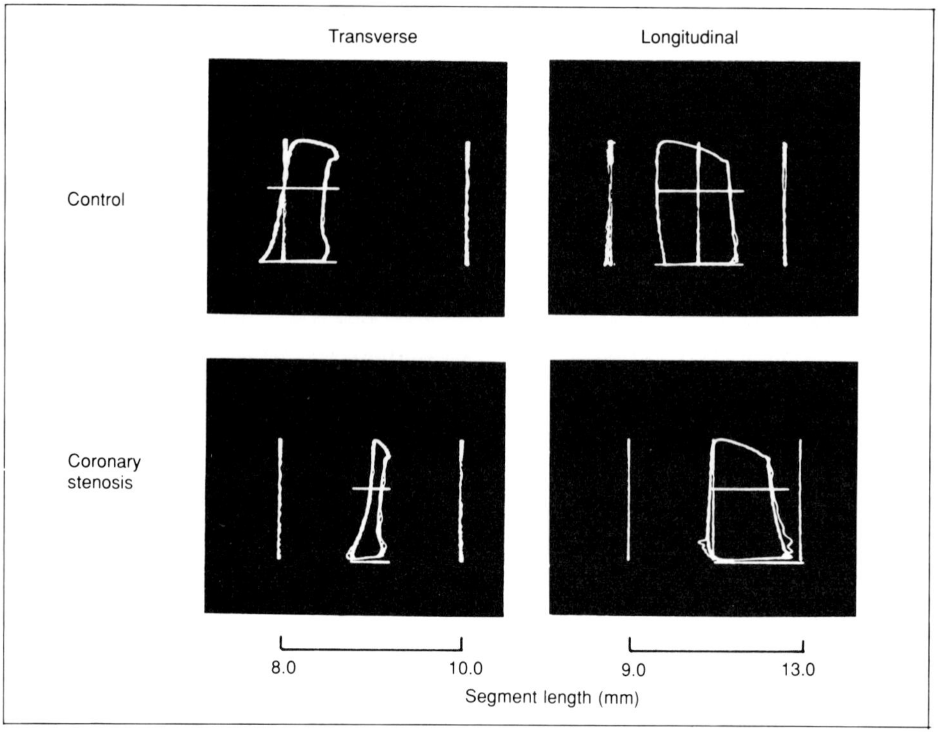

Fig. 3. *Pressure-length loops from cross-oriented segments in left ventricular midwall during coronary stenosis. One segment, longitudinal, runs along muscle fibres in the area; the other segment, transverse, runs across fibres. Adapted from Hexeberg (14).*

has been known for a long time that subendocardial infarcts are rather frequent, and may even go clinically undetected. Also, that patients with coronary artery disease show lower content of high-energy phosphates in inner muscle layers (34). *Buckberg et al* demonstrated in 1972 that frank endocardial ischaemia may arise even in hearts with normal coronary arteries (35). Thus, the endocardium is particularly susceptible to ischaemia because of uneven distribution of coronary blood flow across the ventricular wall (36). Maldistribution is most likely related to the coronary anatomy of end-arteries and the considerable extravascular tissue pressure imposed on these vessels (37).

Impact on global function

Dyssynchrony: It is possible that regions of the same ventricle might operate at different levels of inotropy or chronotropy (38-40). This obviously leads to improper coordination of the ventricular ejection effort. During ischaemia, such dissimilar contractile states certainly occur. When regions of the ventricle thus contract out of phase with the remaining myocardium, inefficient pumping must be expected. Pressure-length loop analysis is insensitive to phase shifts; a closer analysis of the experiment shown in Fig. 3 revealed worsening of dyssynchrony between the cross-oriented segments (14).

Compensation: Although functional disturbances might affect tissue that is not actually ischaemic, it has been shown that the left ventricle can compensate for up to 20% of coronary oxygen delivery with maintenance of pumping (8, 9, 40). This effect is dependant on increased left ventricular end-diastolic pressure (10), and can be interpreted as activation of the Frank-Starling mechanism in viable muscle of experimental animals (Fig. 4). Similar alterations in segment length have been verified by ultrasonometry in patients (41), and *Müller and Rørvik* observed in 1958 that the end-diastolic pressure in the left ventricle of patients rose during attacks of anginal pain (42).

Spatiality: It has, however, been a matter of debate exactly where such compensation takes place. Several studies show that normally perfused segments increase their shortening in the presence of regional ischaemia (43-46), whereas others failed to detect such changes (47-49). The zone close to an ischaemic region is of particular interest because one consequence of failing myocardium might be that adjacent healthy myocardium loses

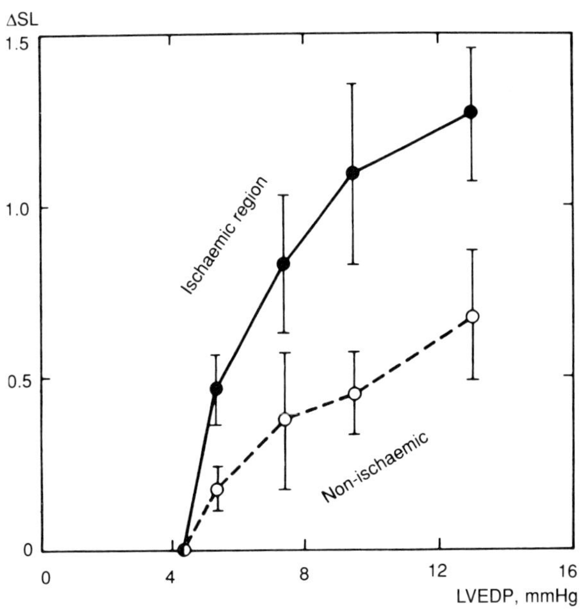

Fig. 4. *Relationship between segment dilation (ΔSL) and left ventricular end-diastolic pressure (LVEDP) for ischaemic and non-ischaemic regions of the same hearts.*

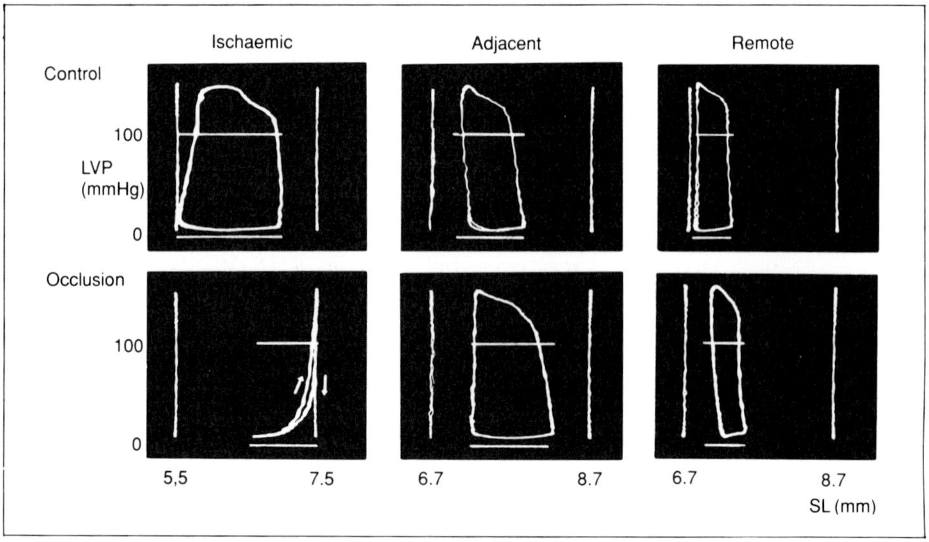

Fig. 5. *Pressure-length loops from three regions of a ventricle before and after coronary occlusion in a cat. All loops rotate counter-clockwise, except the lower left. LVP = left ventricular pressure. SL = segment length. From Matre et al (50).*

'foothold' for a pump-effective shortening. It is therefore possible that the net effect of regional ischaemia might exceed the proportional loss of active fibres. However, Fig. 5 provides an example where just this adjacent region was hyperactive (and hyperaemic) as a consequence of particularly strong Frank-Starling activation (50). Although this phenomenon has been observed by others (46), more studies are needed to resolve the intricate relationship between affected and unaffected regions of the ventricle in this respect.

Summary

Ischaemia very quickly leads to myocardial dilation and reduced systolic shortening. Actual shortening is delayed, impotent, and the tissue may even elongate during ejection. Contraction abnormalities arise from non-uniform contraction within and outside the primarily affected zones. Non-uniformity is phase-related as well as spatial, both with regard to lateral extension and wall depth. The functional impact of ischaemia may therefore exceed the proportional fraction of affected tissue, but compensatory mechanisms help maintain ventricular pumping to some extent.

References

1. Panum PL. Experimentelle Beiträge zur Lehre von der Embolie. Virchows Arch 1862; 25: 312-27.
2. Tennant R, Wiggers CJ. The effect of coronary occlusion on myocardial contraction. Am J Physiol 1935; 112: 351-61.
3. Rushmer RF, Franklin DL, Ellis RM. Left ventricular dimensions recorded by sonocardiometry. Circ Res 1956; 4: 684-8.
4. Bugge-Asperheim B, Leraand S, Kiil F. Local dimensional changes of the myocardium measured by ultrasonic technique. Scand J Clin Lab Invest 1969; 24: 361-71.
5. Tyberg JV, Forrester JS, Wyatt HL, Goldner SJ, Parmley WW, Swan HJC. An analysis of segmental ischemic dysfunction utilizing the pressure-length loop. Circulation 1974; 49: 748-54.
6. Grossman W, Braunwald E, Mann T, McLaurin LP, Green LH. Contractile state of the left ventricle in man as evaluated from end-systolic pressure-volume relations. Circulation 1977; 56: 845-52.
7. Sunagawa K, Maughan WL, Sagawa K. Effect of regional ischemia on the left ventricular end-systolic pressure-volume relationship of isolated canine hearts. Circ Res 1983; 52: 170-8.
8. Lekven J, Mjøs OD, Kjekshus JK. Compensatory mechanisms during graded myocardial ischemia. Am J Cardiol 1973; 31: 467-73.
9. Wyatt HL, Forrester JS, Tyberg JV, et al. Effect of graded reductions in regional coronary perfusion on regional and total cardiac function. Am J Cardiol 1975; 36: 185-92.
10. Koiwa Y, Nunokawa T, Ishide N, et al. The effect of graded coronary flow reduction in the left anterior descending and septal arteries on left ventricular function in the canine heart. Circulation 1980; 62: 745-55.
11. Sunagawa K, Maughan WL, Friesinger G, Guzman P, Chang MS, Sagawa K. Effect of coronary arterial pressure on left ventricular end-systolic pressure-volume relation of isolated canine hearts. Circ Res 1982; 50: 727-34.
12. Walley KR, Becker CJ, Hogan RA, Teplinsky K, Wood LDH. Progressive hypoxemia limits left ventricular oxygen consumption and contractility. Circ Res 1988; 63: 849-59.
13. Hexeberg E, Matre K, Lekven J. Nonuniform and nonlinear end-systolic pressure-length relations at low pressures. Cardiovasc Res 1990; under current revision
14. Hexeberg E. Uniformity of myocardial contraction in the anterior wall of feline left ventricles. Thesis. University of Bergen, 1989.
15. Lekven J, Ilebekk A, Fønstelien E, Kiil F. Relationship between ST-segment elevation and local tissue flow during myocardial ischaemia in dogs. Cardiovasc Res 1975; 9: 627-33.
16. Miller MM, Thorvaldson J, Ilebekk A, Lekven J. Myocardial ischemia. Relationship between local flow, function and ST-segment elevation. Eur J Cardiol 1979; 10: 7-18.
17. Jennings RB, Reimer KA, Hill ML, Mayer SE. Total ischemia in dog hearts in vitro. I. Comparison of high energy phosphate production, utilization and depletion, and of adenine nucleotide catabolism in total ischemia in vitro vs. severe ischemia in vivo. Circ Res 1981; 49: 892-900.
18. Katz AM. Effects of ischemia on the contractile processes of heart muscle. Am J Cardiol 1973; 32: 456-60.
19. Hearse DJ, Crome R, Yellon DM, Wyse R. Metabolic and flow correlates of myocardial ischaemia. Cardiovasc Res 1983; 15: 430-5.
20. Lekven J, Brunsting LA, Jessen ME, Abd-Elfattah AS, Doherty NE, Wechsler AS: Myocardial use during epinephrine administration to ischemically injured canine hearts. Circulation 1988; 78: III125-36.

21. Wechsler AS, Abd-Elfattah AS, Murphy CE, Salter DR, Brunsting LA, Goldstein JP. Myocardial protection. J Cardiac Surg 1986; 1: 271-306.
22. Braunwald E, Kloner RA. The stunned myocardium: Prolonged, postischemic ventricular dysfunction. Circulation 1982; 66: 1146-9.
23. Greve G. Across the border. An ultrastructural study of hearts with regional ischaemia. Thesis. University of Bergen, 1989.
24. Kloner RA, Braunwald E. Observations on experimental myocardial ischaemia. Cardiovasc Res 1980; 14: 371-95.
25. Spinale FG, Schulte BA, Crawford FA. Demonstration of early ischemic injury in porcine right ventricular myocardium. Am J Pathol 1989; 134: 693-704.
26. Brutsaert DL, Rademakers FE, Sys SU, Gillebert TC, Housmans PR. The heart as an integrated muscle and pump system: triple control and subdivision of the cardiac cycle. Acta Cardiol 1984; 39: 89-95.
27. Lew WYW, LeWinter MM. Regional comparison of midwall segment and area shortening in the canine left ventricle. Circ Res 1986; 58: 678-91.
28. Waldman LK, Nosan D, Villareal F, Covell JW. Relation between transmural deformation and local myofiber direction in canine left ventricle. Circ Res 1988; 63: 550-62.
29. Hexeberg E, Matre K, Birkeland S, Lekven J. Nonuniform shortening of the anterior wall of feline left ventricles. Am J Physiol 1989; 257: H1165-73.
30. Weintraub WS, Hattori S, Agarwal J, Bodenheimer MM, Banka VS, Helfant RH. The relationship between myocardial blood flow and contraction by myocardial layer in the canine left ventricle during ischemia. Circ Res 1981; 48: 430-8.
31. Gallagher KP, Osakada G, Hess OM, Koziol JA, Kemper WS, Ross J Jr. Subepicardial segment function during coronary stenosis and the role of myocardial fiber orientation. Circ Res 1982; 50: 352-9.
32. Hattori S, Weintraub WS, Agarwal JB, Bodenheimer MM, Banka VS, Helfant RH. Contrasting ischemic contraction patterns by zone and layer in canine myocardium. Am J Physiol 1982; 243: H852-5.
33. Prinzen FW, Arts T, van der Vusse GJ, Coumans WA, Reneman RS. Gradients in fiber shortening and metabolism across ischemic left ventricular wall. Am J Physiol 1986; 250: H255-64.
34. Jones RN, Peyton RB, Sabina RL, et al. Transmural gradient in high-energy phosphate content in patients with coronary artery disease. Ann Thorac Surg 1981; 32: 546-53.
35. Buckberg GD, Fixler DE, Archie JP, Hoffman JIE. Experimental subendocardial ischemia in dogs with normal coronary arteries. Circ Res 1972; 30: 67-81.
36. Kjekshus JK. Mechanism for flow distribution in normal and ischemic myocardium during increased ventricular preload in the dog. Circ Res 1973; 33: 489-99.
37. Hoffman JIE. A critical review of coronary reserve. Circulation 1987; 75: I6-11.
38. Noble MIM, Trenchard MD, Guz A. Left ventricular ejection in conscious dogs. II. Determinants of stroke volume. Circ Res 1966; 19: 148-52.
39. Ilebekk A, Lekven J, Kiil F. Left ventricular asynergy during intracoronary isoproterenol infusion in dogs. Am J Physiol 1980; 239: H594-600.
40. Boden WE, Liang CS, Apstein CS, Hood WB. Experimental myocardial infarction. XVI. The detection of inotropic contractile reserve with post extrasystolic potentiation in acutely ischemic canine myocardium. Am J Cardiol 1978; 41: 523-30.
41. Chitwood WR, Hill RC, Sink JD, Kleinemann LH, Sabiston DC Jr., Wechsler AS. Measurement of global ventricular function in patients during cardiac operations using sonomicrometry. J Thorac Cardiovasc Surg 1980; 80: 724-35.
42. Müller O, Rørvik K. Haemodynamic consequences of coronary heart disease. With observations during anginal pain and on the effect of nitroglycerine. Br Heart J 1958; 20: 302-10.

43. Theroux P, Franklin D, Ross J Jr, Kemper WS. Regional myocardial function during acute coronary artery occlusion and its modification by pharmacologic agents in the dog. Circ Res 1974; 35: 896-908.
44. Sasayama S, Gallagher KP, Kemper WS, Franklin D, Ross J Jr. Regional left ventricular wall thickness early and late after coronary occlusion in the conscious dog. Am J Physiol 1981; 240: H293-9.
45. Molaug M, Geiran O, Kiil F. Compensatory cardiac mechanisms evoked by septal ischemia in dogs. Am J Cardiol 1983; 51: 201-6.
46. Lew WY, Chen Z, Guth B, Covell JW. Mechanisms of augmented segment shortening in nonischemic areas during acute ischemia of the canine left ventricle. Circ Res 1985; 56: 351-8.
47. Kerber RE, Marcus ML, Ehrhardt J, Wilson R, Abboud FM. Correlation between echocardiographically demonstrated segmental dyskinesis and regional myocardial perfusion. Circulation 1975; 52: 1097-104.
48. Wyatt HL, Forrester JS, da Luz PL, Diamond GA, Chagrasulis R, Swan HJC. Functional abnormalities in nonoccluded regions of myocardium after experimental coronary occlusion. Am J Cardiol 1976; 37: 366-72.
49. Lima JAC, Becker LC, Melin JA, et al. Impaired thickening of nonischemic myocardium during acute regional ischemia in the dog. Circulation 1985; 71: 1048-59.
50. Matre K, Hexeberg E, Grong K, Lekven J. Local myocardial function following coronary occlusion in cats. Effect on non-ischaemic regions. Clin Physiol 1987; 7: 511-23.
51. Lekven J, Kiil F. Myocardial function in general and regional left ventricular ischaemia in dogs at control and high aortic blood pressure. Cardiovasc Res 1975; 9: 373-83.
52. Matre K, Lekven J. Measurement of cardiac pressure-length loops using an improved sonomicrometer. Accuracy and effect of respiration. J Biomed Eng 1983; 5: 110-6.

12

Assessment of cardiac function by radionuclide cardiography

POUL FLEMMING HØILUND-CARLSEN,
NIELS GADSBØLL

Routine assessment of cardiac function?

Why do many heart patients leave hospital without having undergone a quantitative examination of the pumping ability of their heart? The electrocardiogram and the chest X-ray are for other reasons important routines, but they tell us little about cardiac function. The physical examination includes a search for certain symptoms and signs of cardiac dysfunction, but it seems that clinicians often disagree on the presence or absence of these signs (1). This calls for methods, preferably quantitative, by which right and left ventricular function can be reliably assessed.

This chapter is devoted to a description of radionuclide cardiography in general and to its possible use in ischaemic heart disease including acute myocardial infarction (AMI). Some of the variables measured are explained with comments on reliability and possible clinical usefulness. Radionuclide methods for the detection and evaluation of ischaemic heart disease are mentioned only briefly, as they are not the main issue here. At the end we summarize what is in our opinion some of the advantages and benefits of radionuclide ventriculography in assessment of cardiac function.

Radionuclide ventriculography

Every so-called noninvasive method in nuclear cardiology involves intravenous injection of a radiopharmaceutical, external recording by gamma camera or more simple detectors of the radioactivity transmitted from the structure of interest and a succeeding computerized processing of the data acquired. Two main principles are available for the determination of ventricular ejection fraction and volume: the first-pass and the equilibrium techniques.

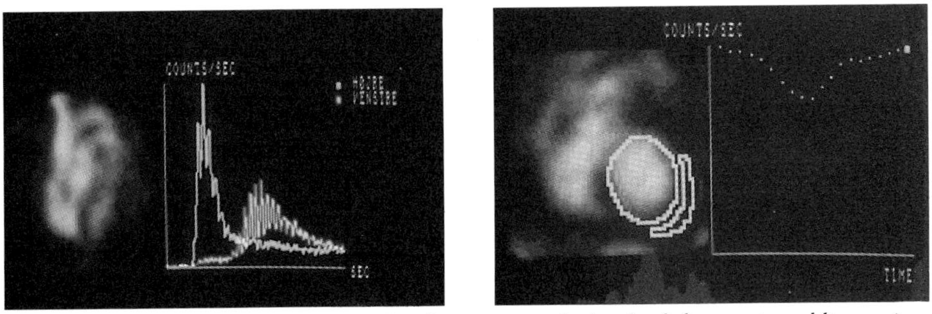

Fig. 1. Left panel: *Time sequence of a first-pass study in the left anterior oblique view. The picture to the left is composed of several frames to show both ventricles separated by the interventricular septum. The ventricular time-activity curves demonstrate that the bolus passage of the ventricles is composed of a dextrophase (yellow curve) and a levophase (blue curve) separated in time.* Right Panel: *Equilibrium study in the left anterior oblique view showing (left) the heart with left ventricular and background regions of interest and (right) the background subtracted ventricular time-activity curve. In the example chosen the LVEF is 0.25.*

First-pass technique: The first passage of an intravenously injected bolus of radioactivity through the central circulation, from the time it enters the right atrium until it leaves the left ventricle through the aorta, is recorded with a time resolution (often 20-40 frames per second) high enough to display, with little distortion, the cyclic changes of radioactivity within the right and left ventricles (Fig. 1, left panel). The level of radioactivity in end-diastole and end-systole is used to calculate the ejection fraction (2). The area under the entire passage curve allows determination of forward stroke volume and cardiac output and the calculation of ventricular volume (3, 4).

Equilibrium technique: Autologous red blood cells tagged with ^{99m}Tc are injected intravenously. A few minutes later, after complete mixing with the circulating blood ("equilibrium"), ECG-syncronized acquisition is performed of the intraventricular changes in radioactivity during a series of often several hundred successive heart beats. The popular term for this type of acquisition is MUGA, which is an abbreviation of multigated acquisition. The MUGA principle can be used in first-pass studies too, but it requires a fairly regular heart rhythm with less than, say, 20% ectopic beats. With higher degrees of arrhythmia, measurements will become increasingly imprecise or even impossible. In such cases only the first-pass technique, with measurements on every single beat, is applicable. The equilibrium study allows creation by computer of an "average" heart beat and an "average" left ventricular time-activity curve which is in principle proportional to the ventricular time-volume curve (Fig. 1, right panel). The ejection fraction is easily calculated from the radioactivity in end-diastole and end-systole (2,

Table 1. *Some functional variables obtainable by radionuclide ventriculography: normal values at rest and detectable changes at repeat determination.*

Variable	Abbreviation	Dimension	Normal range [1])	Significant change [2])
RV ejection fraction	RVEF	–	0.55-0.75 [3])	>0.09
RV end-diastolic volume	RVEDV	ml	80-180	>20% [4])
RV end-diastolic volume index	RVEDVI	ml/m^2	50-90	>20% [4])
LV ejection fraction	LVEF	–	0.55-0.75	>0.05
LV end-diastolic volume	LVEDV	ml	80-180	>20%
LV end-diastolic volume index	LVEDVI	ml/m^2	50-90	>20%
LV end-systolic volume	LVESV	ml	30-70	>20%
LV end-systolic volume index	LVESVI	ml/m^2	15-40	>20%
LV stroke volume	LVSV	ml	55-115	>20%
LV stroke volume index	LVSVI	ml/m^2	30-50	>20% [4])
Cardiac output	CO	l/min	3.4-5.8	>20% [4])
Cardiac index	CI	l/min.m^2	2.0-4.0	>20% [4])
LV systolic pressure/volume ratio	SP/V	mmHg/ml	1.7-4.5	>25% [4])
LV peak ejection rate	PER	EDV/s	2.4-3.8	>20% [4])
LV peak filling rate	PFR	EDV/s	2.4-3.9	>20% [4])

Abbreviations: RV = right ventricular; LV = left ventricular.

1) Observed 95% range in 30 healthy adult volunteers, 14 women and 16 men; rounded off figures.

2) A significant change in a *measured* value means that the difference between two measurements is so big that the *true*, but unknown, value of a patient has changed with 95% probability.

3) Measured by first-pass technique using separate end-diastolic and end-systolic regions of interest.

4) Approximate figures; thorough calculation of more exact figures has not been made.

5), whereas volume determination requires calibration with the radioactivity per ml in a simultaneously drawn sample of peripheral blood as well as correction for the individual degree of radiation attenuation dependent on left ventricular depth within the chest (6, 7).

A series of variables may be measured or calculated. Some of these are listed in Table 1 and explained in brief below.

Right ventricular ejection fraction (RVEF): is determined by first-pass technique. It is done differently in various laboratories, from either a single, fixed diastolic ventricular region of interest or from separate diastolic and systolic regions, the latter procedure taking into account that atrial activity is partly included in the fixed ventricular region of interest during systole. With separate diastolic and systolic regions of interest, values for the ejection fractions are higher, and values for RVEF are in normal subjects of approximately the same size as values for left ventricular ejection fraction (Table 1) (2).

Right ventricular end-diastolic volume: may, in the abscense of valve incompetence or intracardiac shunting, be calculated as stroke volume divided by RVEF.

Left ventricular ejection fraction (LVEF): is determined by first-pass or equilibrium technique, the latter method having higher precision (8).

Left ventricular end-diastolic volume: may also be determined by either technique, the latter being more "direct" and reliable. Once this volume is obtained a series of other variables such as end-systolic volume, stroke volume and cardiac output are easily calculated from knowledge of ejection fraction and heart rate. In contrast to measurement by the first-pass principle, stroke volume and cardiac output determined by the equilibrium technique represent total left ventricular ejection, i.e. the sum of antegrade and retrograde flow. This difference in technique may be used to quantitate mitral regurgitation noninvasively (9).

Left ventricular systolic pressure/volume ratio: is the ratio of systolic cuff blood pressure and end-systolic volume, an approximation to the invasively obtained end-systolic pressure/volume ratio which is thought to be a load-independent index reflecting myocardial contractility (10).

Left ventricular peak ejection rate and peak filling rate: are the maximal velocities of blood displacement out of and into the ventricle in systole and diastole. Conventionally, both measures are often expressed in proportion to the end-diastolic volume times second^{-1}. With the radionuclide technique, this is convenient because measurements can be made from changes in radioactivity alone, without performing the more cumbersome determination of ventricular volume. The interpretation and clinical relevance of these variables are as yet not entirely clear (11, 12).

Reliability and relevance

Among the many requirements to be fulfilled for a method to gain general acceptance some of the fundamental ones are reliability and relevance.

Reliability: For a method to be reliable it should be accurate and precise, i.e., it should measure the "true" quantity we want to examine, and it should do this with "sufficiently" little bias. Without accuracy, precision is irrelevant and vice versa. For a discussion of these concepts the readers are referred elsewhere (13, 14). They are mentioned here to call attention to the fact that many methods common in cardiology have never been subject to a more critical evaluation of their reliability when giving answers to questions like: If we measure variable x once in a patient, what is, with 95% probability, the true quantity of the patient? And, at repeat determination, how great should the difference between the measured values be for us to believe that there has been an actual change in the true, but unknown, value of the patient? Once accuracy, or for practical purposes agreement with a suitable reference, has been established, the degreee of acceptable imprecision should be decided on. The choice is arbitrary and should be made *a priori* for any new method based, as has been proposed, upon judgment of what is clinically relevant (15), recognizing again that clinical relevance is difficult to determine if we do not have objective measurements to rely upon.

Every new method in medicine is faced with this dilemma: It must have something to "do" with the clinical course of patients to become regarded as "relevant" or "important". But if agreement with clinical judgment is 100% or 0% there is little need for the new method. Thus, the span between these extremes is the one at disposal for a promising new method. The exact place to be occupied by the new method is difficult to define as it may be constantly moving in step with the appearance of new evidence and new uses.

There are marked discrepancies between clinical manifestations of heart failure and radionuclide measures of ventricular function (1). This fact can hardly be used to discredit either approach. Similar inconsistency exists between clinical findings and measures traditionally regarded as absolutely "true", as for instance the pulmonary capillary wedge pressure (1, 16). The implication is that clinical judgment and objective measurements are complimentary methods. How and to what degree they supplement each other are objects for investigation. An example: The presence of clinical signs of heart failure post AMI is not concordant with the reduction in global ventricular function represented by decreases in LVEF (Fig. 2) (17). Similar disagreement between left ventricular ejection fraction and exercise capacity has been demonstrated several times (18).

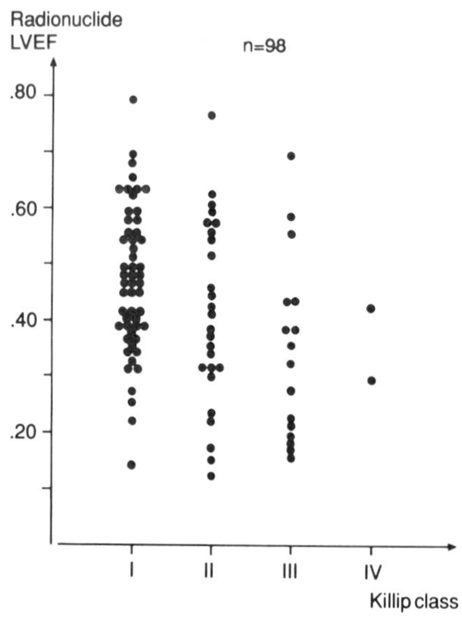

Fig. 2. *Relationship between the degree of clinical heart failure (Killip class I to IV) observed during admission and radionuclide left ventricular ejection fraction in the second week after AMI in 98 patients. The figure is based on data from Gadsbøll et al (17).*

Radionuclide ventriculography in ischaemia and infarction

An early use of radionuclide ejection fraction was in the detection of ischaemia provoked by physical exercise. The theoretical background for this was the demonstration in animal studies of regional wall motion abnormalities appearing earlier, during artificial ischaemia, than ECG changes. If sufficiently widespread regional changes would conceivably express themselves as an exercise-induced decrease in LVEF, as they did in patients as demonstrated for the first time in 1977 (19). However, a reduction in LVEF is not a consequence of ischaemia alone, but is brought about by almost any kind of myocardial injury, whether traumatic, inflammatory, ischaemic or metabolic. Over the years there has been a decline in the use of exercise radionuclide ventriculography in the diagnosis of ischaemic heart disease (20, 21). It has become clear that not all patients with ischaemia show a depression of LVEF during exercise, and also, that a number of subjects with normal coronary arteries do not respond to exercise with an increase in LVEF (22-24). Another type of radionuclide examination, namely myocardial scintigraphy, with either ^{201}thallium or the newer ^{99m}Tc-isonitriles and single photon emission tomography, has become the method of choice in the detection of ischaemia (Fig. 3) (25).

The present trend for the use of radionuclide ventriculography is quantitation of ventricular function in the description of natural history, as guidance for therapy and for the prediction of disease outcome.

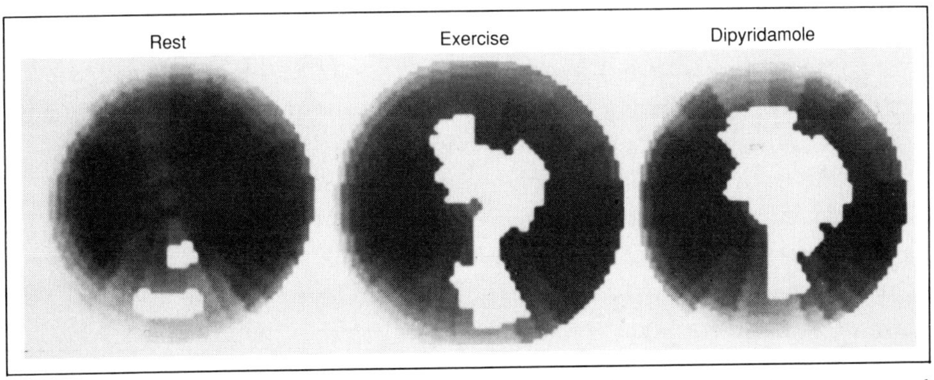

Fig. 3. *Bull's eye display of myocardial scintigraphy with ^{99m}Tc-isonitrile in a patient with ischaemic heart disease. The myocardium of the left ventricle is shown as a hemisphere with the apex in the centre and the base making up the periphery. Each of the concentric circles represents a tomographic slice made perpendicular to the long axis of the ventricle. On each scintigram the anterior wall of the ventricle is at the top and the septum is to the left. At rest there are minimal areas of hypoperfusion (shown in white) in the inferior wall. During exercise or coronary vasodilation following intravenous infusion of dipyridamole large perfusion defects appear close to the apex in the anterior and lateral regions. By courtesy of F. Pedersen.*

Ischaemia: There is little solid knowledge of ventricular function during acute ischaemia, mainly because of technical difficulties in the registration during attacks of pain. There is reason to believe that acute ischaemia leads to early appearance of regional wall motion abnormalities with consequent asynchronous and eventually incomplete contraction, reflected by an acute increase in end-systolic volume when compensatory increases in contractility of unaffected myocardium is no longer sufficient to maintain stroke volume. In the acute phase, the Starling mechanism has probably little to offer. How this line of events is governed and exactly which quantity is the regulated one is still unknown. What are the functional disturbances during silent ischaemia and whether they differ from those associated with angina, these are some of the questions to be answered in the future.

Infarction: In early AMI a substantial number of patients have a reduction not only in LVEF, but also in RVEF (26, 27). However, there is often some recovery of an initially reduced RVEF, whereas a depression in resting LVEF is more permanent (26-30). On hospital discharge approximately two thirds of patients with first AMI have a decrease in LVEF. About one third of these also have a decrease in RVEF, one tenth of all patients have a decrease in RVEF only, and one fourth have entirely normal ejection fractions. A depressed RVEF is more than twice as frequent in the presence of an inferior infarction compared to an anterior infarction. In the former condition there is, in general, a higher LVEF and a more favourable prognosis than the latter condition (30).

Almost every patient with AMI and a decrease in LVEF has, on discharge, an enlargement of the left ventricular end-systolic volume, whereas only two thirds have an increased end-diastolic volume also (Fig. 4). Patients with anterior infarction have similar end-diastolic volumes as patients with inferior infarction, but larger end-systolic volumes (31). A year after first AMI, surviving patients have in general fewer clinical and radiological signs of heart failure, but a 20-25% increase in end-diastolic and end-systolic volume as well as in stroke volume. The increases in volume are greater in patients with clinical manifestations of heart failure than in those without, but are not reflected by changes in LVEF (32).

The early finding of a frequent decrease in peak filling rate (expressed in terms of end-diastolic volumes filled into the ventricle per second (PFR EDV/s)) in patients with coronary artery disease (33) signalled a new interest in the diastolic properties of the heart. It has been proposed that patients may develop symptoms of heart failure because of diastolic rather than systolic left ventricular dysfunction (34-37). There are controversies as to what is the right way of assessing diastolic function (12, 38, 39), and PFR

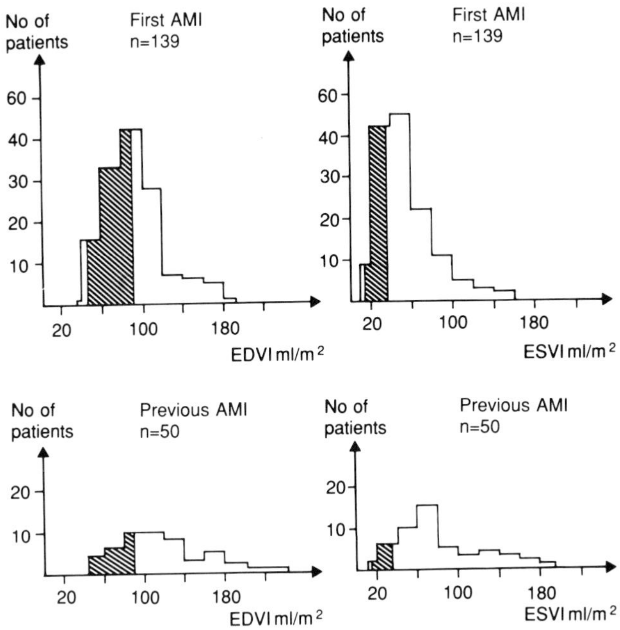

Fig. 4. *Left ventricular end-diastolic and end-systolic volume index (EDVI and ESVI) in the second week after AMI in 139 patients with first and 50 patients with previous infarction. From Gadsbøll et al (31) with permission.*

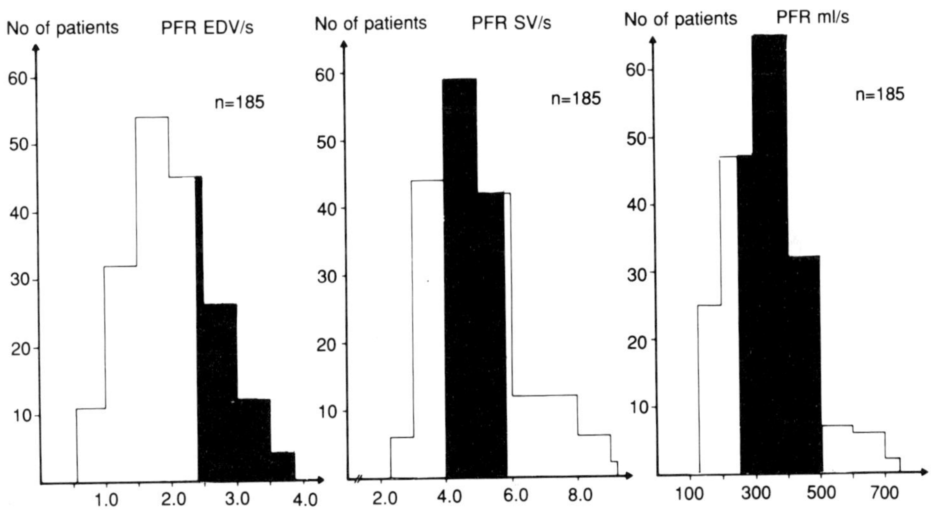

Fig. 5. *Left ventricular peak filling rate expressed in end-diastolic volumes per second (PFR EDV/s), in stroke volumes per second (PFR SV/s), and in actual millilitres of blood per second (PFR ml/s) in 185 patients in the second week after AMI. From Gadsbøll et al (12) with permission.*

may be expressed in relation to end-diastolic volume (PFR EDV/s) or stroke volume (PFR SV/s) or it may be given in actual millilitres filled into the ventricle per second (PFR ml/s). The number of patients with AMI having a decreased PFR on discharge varies greatly according to the way of expressing

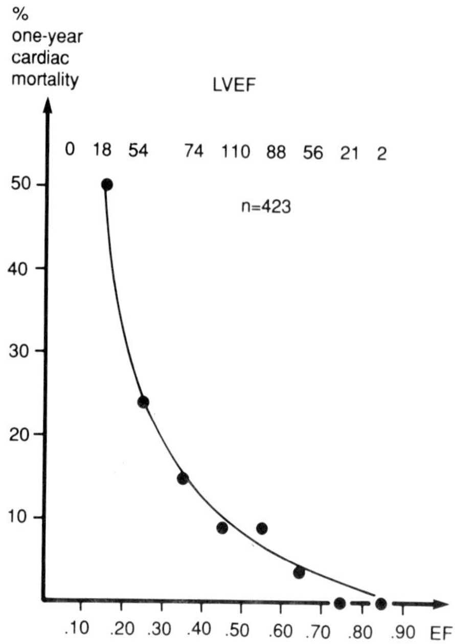

Fig. 6. *Relationship between predischarge LVEF and one-year cardiac mortality in 423 patients with AMI. From Gadsbøll et al (30) with permission.*

PFR (Fig. 5) (12). None of the three expressions of PFR can be shown to have an association to heart failure independent of left ventricular size or of measures of left ventricular function (12).

Many of the radionuclide variables have prognostic implications, but none of them provide independent prognostic information with regard to one-year survival after AMI that is more powerful than that obtained by a combination of clinical signs of heart failure and radionuclide LVEF – see also Fig. 6 (1, 12, 31).

Conclusion: Radionuclide ventriculography provides practically noninvasively a series of functional variables including ejection fraction, ventricular volumes, systolic pressure/volume ratio, peak ejection and peak filling rates. Some have become very popular, but the pathophysiology and clinical relevance of old and new functional variables is not fully understood. Radionuclide ventriculography is not the method of choice in the diagnosis of ischaemic heart disease. It could be in the quantitation of the functional disturbances brought about by acute and chronic ischaemia. So far, it has been used mostly in the description of natural history and for prognostication, whereas the obvious application as guidance for therapy of ischaemic heart failure has been somewhat overlooked.

References

1. Gadsbøll N, Høilund-Carlsen PF, Nielsen GG, et al. Symptoms and signs of heart failure in patients with myocardial infarction: Reproducibility and relationship to chest X-ray, radionuclide ventriculography and right heart catheterization. Eur Heart J 1989; 10: 1017-28.
2. Marving J, Høilund-Carlsen PF, Chræmmer-Jørgensen B, Gadsbøll N. Are right and left ventricular ejection fractions equal? Ejection fractions in normal subjects and in patients with first acute myocardial infarction. Circulation 1985; 72: 502-14.
3. Alazraki NP, Schelbert HR, Verba JW, Brock G, Johnson AD, Ashburn WL. Utilization of the radionuclide angiogram for determination of cardiac output and ejection fraction. J Nucl Biol Med 1975; 19: 127-34.
4. Kelbæk H, Hartling OJ, Skagen K, Munck O, Henriksen O, Godtfredsen J. First-pass radionuclide determination of cardiac output: an improved gamma camera method. J Nucl Med 1987; 28: 1330-34.
5. Strauss HW, Zaret BL, Hurley PJ, Natarajan TK, Pitt B. A scintiphotographic method for measuring left ventricular ejection fraction in man without cardiac catheterization. Am J Cardiol 1971; 28: 575-80.
6. Links JM, Becker LC, Shindledecker JG, et al. Measurement of absolute left ventricular volume from gated blood pool studies. Circulation 1982; 65: 82-90.
7. Høilund-Carlsen PF, Marving J, Rasmussen S, Haunsø S, Fog Pedersen J. Accuracy of absolute left ventricular volumes and cardiac output determined by radionuclide cardiography. Int J Cardiol 1984; 6: 505-25.
8. Høilund-Carlsen PF, Lauritzen SL, Marving J, et al. The reliability of measuring left ventricular ejection fraction by radionuclide cardiography: evaluation by the method of variance components. Br Heart J 1988; 59: 653-62.
9. Kelbæk H, Aldershvile J, Svendsen JH, Folke K, Nielsen SL, Munck O. Combined first passage and equilibrium radionuclide cardiographic: determination of stroke volume for quantitation of valvular regurgitation. J Am Coll Cardiol 1988; 11: 769-73.
10. Suga H, Sagawa K, Shoukas AA. Load independence of the instantaneous pressure-volume ratio of the canine left ventricle and effects of epinephrine and heart rate on the ratio. Circ Res 1973; 32: 314-22.
11. Iskandrian AS, Heo J, Segal BL, Askenase A. Left ventricular diastolic function: evaluation by radionuclide angiography. Am Heart J 1988; 115: 924-9.
12. Gadsbøll N, Høilund-Carlsen PF, Badsberg JH, et al. Left ventricular peak filling rate, heart failure and one-year survival in patients with acute myocardial infarction. Eur Heart J (submitted).
13. Collé R. Accuracy requires precision: a comment on understanding and using statistics in nuclear medicine. J Nucl Med 1980; 21: 290-1.
14. Høilund-Carlsen PF. [On the determination of ventricular ejection fractions by radionuclide cardiography (Thesis)]. Copenhagen: Private edition, 1988.
15. Bland JM, Altman DG. Statistical methods for assessing agreement between two methods of clinical measurement. Lancet 1986; i: 307-10.
16. Stage P, Movild B, Hesse B, Steinmetz E. Pulmonary congestion in chronic heart disease: Pulmonary, clinical and hemodynamic relationships. Acta Radiol Diagn 1976; 17: 417-24.
17. Gadsbøll N, Høilund-Carlsen PF, Nielsen GG, et al. Interobserver agreement and accuracy of bedside estimation of right and left ventricular ejection fraction in acute myocardial infarction. Am J Cardiol 1989; 63: 1301-7.
18. Franciosa JA. Exercise testing in chronic congestive heart failure. Am J Cardiol 1984; 53: 1447-50.

19. Borer JS, Bacharach SL, Green MV, Kent KM, Epstein SE, Johnston GS. Real-time radionuclide cineangiography in the noninvasive evaluation of global and regional left ventricular function at rest and during exercise in patients with coronary-artery disease. N Engl J Med 1977; 296: 839-44.
20. Rozanski A, Diamond GA, Berman D, Forrester JS, Morris D, Swan HJC. The declining specificity of exercise radionuclide ventriculography. N Engl J Med 1983; 309: 518-22.
21. Koss JH, Grunwald AM, Bodenheimer MM. Value of nuclear techniques in assessing the patient with suspected anginal syndrome. In: Kotler MN, Steiner RM, Brest AN, eds. Cardiac imaging: new technologies and clinical applications. Cardiovasc Clin 1986; 17/1: 243-6.
22. Gibbons RJ, Lee KL, Cobb FR, Jones RH. Ejection fraction response to exercise in patients with chest pain and normal arteriograms. Circulation 1981; 64: 952-7.
23. Iskandrian AS, Hakki A-H. Radionuclide evaluation of exercise left ventricular performance in patients with coronary artery disease. Am Heart J 1985; 110: 851-6.
24. Peperstraete B, Decoodt P, Paternot J, Dumont N, Verhas M, Telerman M. Predictors of the variation of the ejection fraction during exercise in patients with and without coronary heart disease. Clin Cardiol 1987; 10: 243-8.
25. West DJ, Najm YC, Mistry R, Clarke SE, Fogelman I, Maisey MN. The localization of myocardial ischaemia with technetium-99m methoxy isobutyl isonitrile and single photon emission computed tomography. Br J Radiol 1989; 62: 303-13.
26. Reduto LA, Berger HJ, Cohen LS, Gottschalk A, Zaret BL. Sequential radionuclide assessment of left and right ventricular performance after acute transmural myocardial infarction. Ann Int Med 1978; 89: 441-7.
27. Nemerovski M, Shah PK, Pichler M, Berman DS, Shellock F, Swan HJC. Radionuclide assessment of sequential changes in left and right ventricular function following first acute transmural myocardial infarction. Am Heart J 1982; 104: 709-17.
28. Marmor A, Geltman EM, Biello DR, Sobel BE, Siegel BA, Roberts R. Functional response of the right ventricle to myocardial infarction: Dependence on the site of left ventricular infarction. Circulation 1981; 64: 1055-111.
29. Hirsowitz GS, Lakier JB, Marks DS, Tennyson GL, Goldberg AD, Goldstein S. Sequential radionuclide angiographic assessment of left and right ventricular performance and quantitative thallium-201 scintigraphy following acute myocardial infarction. Am Heart J 1984; 107: 934-9.
30. Gadsbøll N, Høilund-Carlsen PF, Madsen EB, et al. Right and left ventricular ejection fractions: relation to one-year prognosis in acute myocardial infarction. Eur Heart J 1987; 8: 1201-9.
31. Gadsbøll N, Høilund-Carlsen PF, Badsberg JH, Marving J, Lønborg-Jensen H, Jensen BH. Left ventricular volumes in the recovery phase after myocardial infarction: relation to infarct location, left ventricular function and one-year cardiac mortality. Eur Heart J (in press).
32. Gadsbøll N, Høilund-Carlsen PF, Badsberg JH, et al. Late ventricular dilatation in survivors of acute myocardial infarction. Am J Cardiol 1989; 64: 961-6.
33. Bonow RO, Bacharach SL, Green MV, et al. Impaired left ventricular diastolic filling in patients with coronary artery disease: assessment with radionuclide angiography. Circulation 1981; 64: 315-23.
34. Dougherty AH, Naccarelli GV, Gray EL, Hicks CH, Goldstein RA. Congestive heart failure with normal systolic function. Am J Cardiol 1984; 54: 778-82.
35. Soufer R, Wohlgelernter D, Vita NA, et al. Intact systolic left ventricular function in clinical congestive heart failure. Am J Cardiol 1985; 55: 1032-6.
36. Harizi RC, Bianco JA, Alpert JS. Diastolic function of the heart in clinical cardiology. Arch Intern Med 1988; 148: 99-109.

37. Kessler KM. Heart failure with normal systolic function. Update of prevalence, differential diagnosis, prognosis, and therapy. Arch Intern Med 1988; 148: 2109-11.
38. Friedman BJ, Plehn JF. Noninvasive analysis of ventricular diastolic performance: in quest of a clinical tool. J Am Coll Cardiol 1988; 12: 944-6.
39. Plotnick GD, Vogel RA. Noninvasive evaluation of diastolic function: need for hemodynamically and clinically relevant variables. J Am Coll Cardiol 1989; 13: 1015-6.

13

Left ventricular diastolic dysfunction in myocardial ischaemia

RAGNAR DANIELSEN

Introduction

Myocardial ischaemia can be caused by impaired coronary blood flow and oxygen supply, increased oxygen demand, or a combination of these factors. Reduced oxygen supply to the myocardial cells leads to extensive biochemical and morphological changes. These changes, depending on the duration of ischaemia, result in widespread abnormalities of cardiac contraction, relaxation, electrical repolarisation, and to varying degrees of myocardial damage (1-2). Previously, studies mainly focused on left ventricular (LV) systolic dysfunction and the influence of ischaemia on LV performance. However, more recent studies during the last 10-15 years have increasingly high-lighted the importance of LV diastolic dysfunction as a consequence of myocardial ischaemia (3-7).

Metabolic and morphologic changes during ischaemia

Acute depriviation of oxygen delivery to the myocardial cells will after 10-15 seconds lead to a reduction in oxygen tension and high-energy phosphates such as creatine phosphate and ATP. Simultanously, myocardial metabolism changes from normally being aerobic over to an anaerobic state (1, 2). Nuclear magnetic resonance and positron emission tomographic techniques also can demonstrate ischaemic changes in the myocardium at an early stage (8, 9). The loss of high-energy phosphates from the myocardium causes functional disturbances of the ATP dependent natrium-potassium pump in the cell membrane, with potassium leaking out of the cell and the intracellular accumulation of hydrogen ions, lactate and harmful metabolites

(10-12). These metabolic changes reduce the escape of calcium ions from the sarcoplasmic reticulum, in addition to other disturbances in calcium metabolism, leading to abnormalities in both myocardial contraction and relaxation (3). Loss of enzymes becomes evident with increased duration of ischaemia, as a sign of irreversible damage to the cell membrane. Subsequently, the metabolic changes result in widespread morphological abnormalities in the myocardium, where electronic microscopy has revealed mitochondrial abnormalities at an early stage of ischaemia (12). More prolonged ischaemia results in myofibrillar oedema, reduced glycogen content, accumulation of fatty granula, and finally signs of irreversible myocardial necrosis (12, 13).

Basic physiology

Contraction of the myocardium is initiated by an increase in the intracellular calcium concentration in the vicinity of the sarcoplasmic reticulum. This leads to the release of large amounts of calcium from the sarcoplasmic reticulum, which reacts with the contractile proteins of the myofibrils thus causing contraction (14). Ischaemia most likely reduces the release of calcium ions from the sarcoplasmic reticulum. A possible mechanism is reduced sensitivity of the sarcoplasmic reticulum to calcium, due to an increased concentration of hydrogen ions and a reduction in pH, secondary to the ischaemia induced metabolic acidosis. Another possible mechanism is competition between the calcium and the hydrogen ions for the receptor on the troponin molecule. The final result is impaired myocardial contractility (14).

Relaxation after myocardial contraction is a complex energy dependent process which is a prerequisite for the LV pressure decay in the early diastole and the subsequent LV filling and volume increase (3, 5). Energy is needed to pump calcium from its active location on the contraction regulating troponin protein, back into the sarcoplasmic reticulum. The reduced calcium concentration in the vicinity of the myofibrillar proteins leads to a halt of the actin-myosin interaction, resulting in relaxation. It has been estimated that about 15% of the energy requirements of the heart are needed for this process (3). Catecholamines can stimulate the uptake of calcium into the sarcoplasmic reticulum and thus enhance myocardial relaxation as well as contractility (3, 15).

LV diastolic function is also influenced by many internal and external factors in a complex interplay. *Internal factors* can be both active and energy dependent (excitation-contraction-relaxation cyclus), or based on potential energy (recoil and atrial pressure). Others are determined by LV myocardial and chamber stiffness (viscoelastic properties) (3, 5). *External factors* influencing LV diastolic filling are interaction with right ventricular function, the pericardium, and the amount of blood in the coronary circulation, amongst others (16, 17).

Invasive studies

Changes in LV negative dp/dt. LV relaxation can be described by indexes such as the isovolumic relaxation time constant *tau*, and the peak LV pressure decay after completed contraction (peak -dp/dt) (18). A reduction in peak -dp/dt during experimentally induced ischaemia in dogs is one of the first measurable changes and can be demonstrated 15-30 seconds before a reduction in peak +dp/dt, or fractional shortening occurs (3). The use of peak -dp/dt, however, does have its limitations, as experimental studies have shown it to be dependent on both afterload, assessed as systolic aortic pressure, and on end-diastolic fibre lenght. A prolongation of the isovolumetric relaxation period is observed during acute ischaemia concomitantly with a reduction in peak -dp/dt. Incomplete relaxation during acute ischaemia also contributes to increased myocardial stiffness, and consequently to reduced LV compliance and increased LV diastolic pressure (3). In addition, the configuration of the -dp/dt curve may give information about early and mid LV diastolic relaxation abnormalities (19).

Pressure-volume relations. LV diastolic dysfunction during ischaemia can be assessed by the curvilinear relation between pressure and volume (4). "Chamber or volume stiffness" is defined as dp/dv, that is as the ratio between change in pressure (dp) for a given change in volume (dv) (Fig. 1). Conversely, "compliance" or "distensibility" represents the reciprocal of

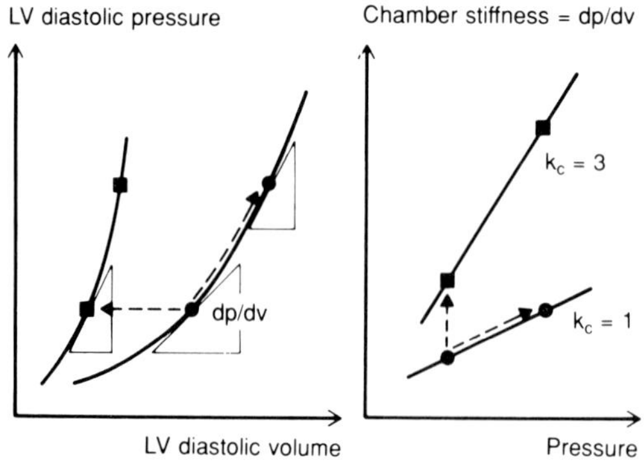

Fig. 1. Left panel: *Left ventricular (LV) diastolic pressure - volume relations and the definition of LV chamber stiffness (dp/dv).* Right panel: *The relation between chamber stiffness and LV pressure and the definition of the chamber stiffness constant (Kc). A left-ward shift of the pressure-volume curve leads to an increase in dp/dv (Adapted from reference 4).*

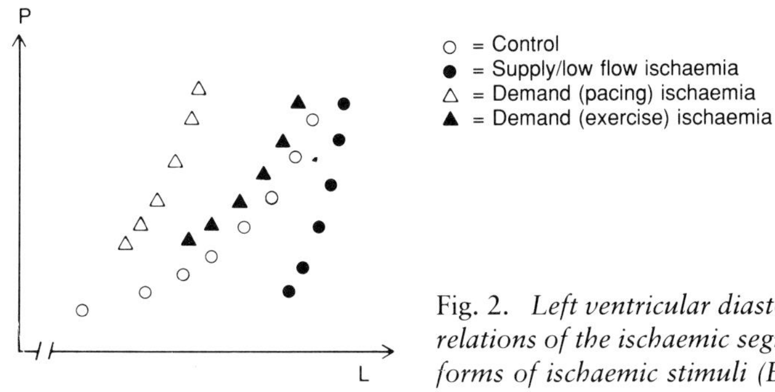

Fig. 2. *Left ventricular diastolic pressure (P) -length (L) relations of the ischaemic segment provoked by different forms of ischaemic stimuli (Based on reference 20).*

chamber stiffness, namely dv/dp. The module of chamber stiffness, on the other hand, is defined as the slope of the linear relation between chamber stiffness (dp/dv) and pressure. Therefore, chamber stiffness and compliance are related to the module of chamber stiffness, and a direct function of LV filling pressure (4). The concept "myocardial (muscle) stiffness" , however, differs from chamber stiffness and is derived from stress-strain calculations on the LV wall (4, 18). Although most researchers agree that acute ischaemia causes increased "myocardial stiffness", its assessment requires more complex and time consuming analysis than evaluation of chamber stiffness (17, 20, 21). When acute ischaemia leads to considerable myocardial infarction, LV dilatation and right displacement of the pressure-volume curve are a necessary mechanism of physiological adaptation to avoid pulmonary oedema (4, 6). Consequently, global LV compliance is not reduced. Conversely, global LV acute ischaemia without dilatation will cause upward and left displacement of the pressure-volume curve. This indicates considerable reduction in LV compliance, and may lead to a large increase in diastolic pressure and pulmonary oedema (4, 6). The term "stiff heart" has been used in extreme cases of reduced LV compliance due to acute ischaemia (22). It is characterized by a restrictive LV diastolic filling pattern, while LV systolic function and ejection fraction are generally normal (6). Thus, clinical studies have shown that approximately 40% of patients who develop acute pulmonary oedema secondary to myocardial infarction have an almost normal ejection fraction (23).

Pressure-length relations. Assessment of the change in LV pressure (dp) for a given alteration in segment radius length (dl) demonstrates a curvilinear relation (dp/dl). It resembles dp/dv and can be obtained from LV angiograms or by echocardiography (24). Neither dp/dv nor dp/dl, however, can distinguish between increased "stiffness" due to changes in the muscle fibres or those secondary to increased LV wall thickness or geometrical alterations

(25). Changes induced in the pressure-length relation by acute ischaemia depend on the method used to provoke the ischaemia (Fig. 2). In ischaemia secondary to decreased oxygen supply, as during acute coronary occlusion, the changes in the pressure-lenght relation from the ischaemic segment differ greatly from those induced by ischaemia due to increased oxygen demand, as during atrial pacing or exercise (20, 26). Acute myocardial ischaemia induced in dogs by coronary occlusion mainly causes a rightward displacement of the LV pressure-lenght curve from the ischaemic segment (20). In man, however, coronary occlusion during balloon dilatation may give a different response, with more upward displacement of the pressure-lenght curve. Such changes may be due to the combined effects of LV myocardial fibrosis and ischaemia (27). Conversely, ischaemia induced by atrial pacing displaces the pressure-length curve from the ischaemic segment upward and to the left, consistent with a considerable increase in dp/dl (20). Exercise provoked ischaemia, however, only causes a slight upward shift of the early diastolic pressure-length relation from the ischaemic segment, while the mid and late diastolic parts are mostly similar to controls (20, 28).

The difference in pressure-length curves obtained during differently induced ischaemia is secondary to their dissimilar physiologic response. This relates to differences in heart rate, venous return, arterial systolic blood pressure, peripheral dilatation, catecholamines, contractility, and to LV geometrical and structural changes (17, 20, 21, 25). Furthermore, the LV pressure-length relation from an ischaemic segment differs greatly from that of a non-ischaemic segment, or a global LV measure such as the pressure-volume curve (20,28-30). For a more complete evaluation of LV response to acute ischaemia it may therefore be of value to record pressure-volume or length relations throughout the cardiac cycle. This facilitates assessment of the close interaction between LV diastolic and systolic function (25).

Noninvasive studies

Radionuclide ventriculography. Several studies have demonstrated LV diastolic abnormalities in patients with coronary artery disease analysing time-derived volume curves constructed from radionuclide angiography data, both at rest and post-exercise (31-33). The most common finding is a reduction in LV early peak filling rate and an increase in the time-interval from end-systole to the point of the peak filling rate. Such changes have been reported both in patients with impaired and normal ejection fractions at rest, but a reduced peak filling rate was more prominent in those with a low ejection fraction (32). In one study, abnormalities of the afore mentioned LV diastolic variables were not related to the number of coronary arteries affected, age, heart rate, LV end-diastolic dimension, nor whether the ejection fraction increased or decreased during exercise (32). Others have pointed out the importance of interpreting radionuclide LV diastolic variables in relation to heart rate (33). In many radionuclide studies the majority of patients with coronary artery disease have received beta-blocker treatment, which influences heart rate and LV relaxation, thus confounding evaluation of the results (32-34). A reduction in LV peak filling rate has also been demonstrated during atrial pacing in patients with coronary artery disease (35). Some authors suggest that these LV diastolic abnormalities are secondary to irreversible myocardial damage due to both silent and clinically manifest ischaemia (32). Interestingly, isotope studies conducted during balloon dilatation of stenotic coronary arteries have shown clear improvement in variables of LV diastolic function measured before and after dilatation, together with an increase in exercise ejection fraction (36).

Digitized echocardiography. Conventional M-mode recordings of mitral valve movements along with registration of the LV posterior wall gives some qualitative information about LV diastolic function (37). However, computer analysis of digitized M-mode echocardiograms gives more exact quantitative information on time derived LV diastolic wall motion changes (38). In patients with coronary heart disease and regional myocardial dysfunction, asynergy is demonstrated as an increase in LV dimension during the isovolumic relaxation period, which itself is often prolonged (39). A reversal of the time relation between the opening of the mitral valve and the peak thinning rate of the LV posterior wall after systolic contraction has also been demonstrated (40). Others have revealed a reduced peak rate of LV distension and dimension increase in early diastole, concomitant with an increase in the atrial contribution to filling in late diastole (41). Although such changes are often considered to indicate LV ischaemia, the variables assessed may be influenced by several factors. These include age, heart rate, changes in preload and afterload, increased LV wall thickness from various causes, LV systolic function, and many cardioactive drugs (40, 42-46). Therefore, when evaluating LV diastolic function, the potential influence of such factors has to be considered.

Doppler echocardiography. Registration of the diastolic transvalvular mitral velocity spectrum by pulsed-wave Doppler is increasingly used to assess LV diastolic function in various heart diseases (47). The velocity spectrum across the mitral valve reflects the atrioventricular diastolic pressure difference, which is again influenced by many factors. These include left atrial and LV compliance, preload, the mode of LV early diastolic relax-

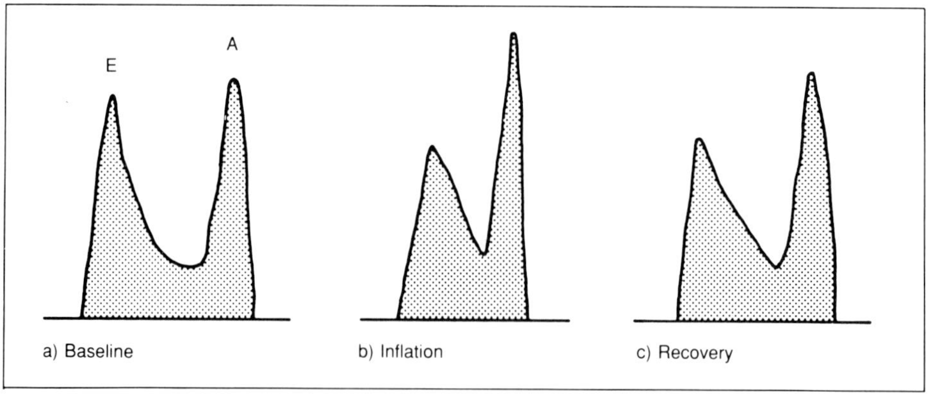

Fig. 3. *Schematic presentation of changes in the Doppler mitral velocity spectrum during myocardial ischaemia induced by balloon dilatation of a left coronary artery stenosis, and the recovery phase (Based on reference 52).*

ation and changes in the isovolumic relaxation period, heart rate, and atrial contraction late in diastole (48). In patients with coronary artery disease, the importance of the left atrial contribution to LV diastolic filling has long been recognized from invasive studies (14, 49), but is particularily easy to demonstrate noninvasively by Doppler. Compared to normal controls, patients with coronary artery disease are reported to have a reduced peak early (E) filling velocity, augmented late diastolic filling with an increase in peak atrial (A) filling velocity, and a reduced E/A ratio (48). Others, have further demonstrated that in patients with coronary artery disease and normal LV relaxation, increased chamber stiffness was positively associated with increased peak E velocity and a decreased atrial contribution to filling (50). Conversely, increased impairment of LV relaxation was characterized by a decrease in peak E velocity and increased filling during atrial systole (50). Potentiation of this abnormal pattern has been observed in patients during myocardial ischaemia induced by atrial pacing, who developed electrocardiographic signs of ischaemia, but not in those who did not (51).

Myocardial ischaemia, provoked during balloon dilatation of coronary artery stenosis, induces changes in the mitral velocity spectrum already after 15-20 seconds of occlusion. These are characterized by a reduced peak E velocity, increased peak A velocity, and a reduced E/A ratio, provided the occlusion time is not too long (30-50 sec) (52, 53) (Fig. 3). If, however, the occlusion time is more prolonged (60 sec) LV diastolic pressure increases further. This results not only in a reduced peak E velocity, but also in "pseudo-normalization" of the velocity profile by a decrease in the peak A velocity and inconsiderable changes in the E/A ratio (54). The severity of LV diastolic dysfunction is also greater in patients with stenosis of the left anterior descending coronary artery than in those with lesions of the circumflex branch or the right coronary artery (54).

Although the transvalvular mitral velocity spectrum gives valuable information about LV diastolic pathophysiologic changes, the abnormalities that have been related to coronary artery disease and ischaemia are not specific (48). Similar changes have been associated with increased age (55), and reported in various primary and secondary cardiomyopathies (56). Furthermore, in addition to heart rate, preload and afterload, changes in the mitral velocity spectrum are also influenced by catecholamines and several cardioactive drugs (47, 57-60). Therefore, from a clinical point of view, conclusions regarding LV diastolic function assessed by mitral velocity recordings should be accepted with caution.

Conclusion

Evaluation of LV diastolic function by noninvasive techniques has made great progress during the last 10-15 years. Although demonstration of LV diastolic abnormalities has increased our pathophysiologic understanding of different heart diseases, the practical clinical use of assessing LV diastolic function is still disputed (61). Whereas cardiac catheterization was previously the "gold standard" for assessing cardiac function, it has increasingly been replaced by noninvasive methods. Further development of these techniques will probably enable the use of integrated noninvasive ultrasound methods that give information regarding cardiac morphology, function and myocardial perfusion in one procedure (62).

References

1. Tennant R, Wiggers CJ. The effect of coronary artery occlusion on myocardial contraction. Am J Physiol 1935; 112: 351-61.
2. Maroko PR, Kjekshus JK, Sobel BE, et al. Factors influencing infarct size following experimental coronary artery occlusions. Circulation 1971; 43: 67-82.
3. Grossman W, McLaurin LP. Diastolic properties of the left ventricle (Review). Ann Int Med 1976; 84: 316-26.
4. Gaasch WH, Levine HJ, Quinones MA, Alexander JK. Left ventricular compliance: Mechanisms and clinical implications. Am J Cardiol 1976; 38: 645-53.
5. Brutsaert DL, Rademakers FE, Sys SU. Triple control of relaxation: implications in cardiac disease. Circulation 1984; 69: 190-6.
6. Pantely GA, Bristow JD. Ischemic cardiomyopathy. Progr Cardiovasc Dis 1984; 27: 95-114.
7. Armstrong WF. Echocardiography in coronary artery disease. Progr Cardiovasc Dis 1988; 30: 267-88.

8. Kavanaugh KM, Aisen AM, Fechner KP, Chenevert TL, Dunham WR, Buda AJ. Regional metabolism during coronary occlusion, reperfusion, and reocclusion using phosphorus[31] nuclear magnetic resonance spectroscopy in the intact rabbit. Am Heart J 1989; 117: 53-9.
9. Brunken RC, Kottou S, Nienbar CA, et al. PET detection af viable tissue in myocardial segments with persistent defects at Tl-201 SPECT. Radiology 1989; 172: 65-73.
10. Reimer KA, Loew JE, Rasmussen MM, Jennings RB. The wavefront phenomenon of ischemic cell death. I. Myocardial infarct size vs. duration of coronary occlusion in dogs. Circulation 1977; 56: 786-93.
11. Reimer KA, Jennings RB. The "wavefront phenomenon" of myocardial ischemic cell death. II. Transmural progression of necrosis within the framework of ischemic bed size (myocardium at risk) and collateral flow. Lab Invest 1979; 40: 633-44.
12. Braunwald E, Kloner RA. The stunned myocardium: prolonged, postischemic ventricular dysfunction. Circulation 1982; 66: 1146-9.
13. Jodalen H, Stangeland L, Grong K, Vik-Mo H, Lekven J. Lipid accumulation in the myocardium during acute regional ischaemia in cats. J Mol Cell Cardiol 1985; 17: 973-80.
14. Braunwald E, Sonnenblick EH, Ross J. Mechanisms of cardiac contraction and relaxation. In: Braunwald E, ed. Heart Disease. A textbook of cardiovascular medicine. Philadelphia: WB Saunders Company, 1988: 383-425.
15. Blaustein AS, Gaasch WH. Myocardial relaxation. VI. Effects of beta-adrenergic tone and asynchrony on LV relaxation rate. Am J Physiol 1983; 244 (Heart Circ Physiol 13):H417-22.
16. Janicki JS, Weber KT. The pericardium and ventricular interaction, distensibility, and function. Am J physiol 1980; 238 (Heart Circ Physiol 7):H494-503.
17. Sys SU, Brutsaert DL. Is stiffness increased during ischaemia? Am J Cardiol 1989; 63: 83E-6E.
18. Mirsky I. Assessment of diastolic function: suggested methods and future considerations. Circulation 1984; 69: 836-41.
19. Kumada T, Katayama K, Matsuzaki M, Kusukawa R, Nakamura Y, Kawai C. Usefulness of negative dp/dt upstroke pattern for assessment of left ventricular relaxation in coronary artery disease. Am J Cardiol 1989; 63: 60E-4E.
20. Krayenbuehl HP, Hess OM, Nonogi H. Om whether there is a true increase in myocardial stiffness during myocardial ischaemia. Am J Cardiol 1989; 63: 78E-82E.
21. Ross J. Is there a true increase in myocardial stiffness with acute ischaemia? Am J Cardiol 1989; 63: 87E-91E.
22. Dodek A, Kassebaum DG, Bristow JD. Pulmonary edema in coronary artery disease without cardiomegaly. Paradox of the stiff heart. N Engl J Med 1972; 286: 1347-50.
23. Warnowiaz MA, Parker H, Cheitlin MD. Prognosis of patients with acute pulmonary edema and normal ejection fraction after acute myocardial infarction. Circulation 1983; 67: 330-4.
24. Momomura S, Bradley AB, Gossman W. Left ventricular diastolic pressure-segment length relations and end-diastolic distensibility in dogs with coronary stenosis. An angina physiology model. Circ Res 1984; 55: 203-14.
25. Caroll JD, Hess OM, Hirzel HO, Turina M, Krayenbuehl HP. Effects of ischaemia, bypass surgery and past infarction on myocardial contraction, relaxation and compliance during exercise. Am J Cardiol 1989; 63: 65E-71E.
26. Paulus WJ, Grossman W, Serizawa T, Bourdillon PD, Pasipoularides A, Mirsky I. Different effects of two types of ischaemia on myocardial systolic and diastolic function. Am J Physiol 1985; 248 (Heart Circ Physiol 17): H719-28.
27. Wijns W, Serruys PW, Slager CJ, et al. Effect of coronary occlusion during percutaneous

transluminal angioplasty in humans on left ventricularchamber stiffness and regional diastolic pressure-radius relations. J Am Coll Cardiol 1986; 7: 455-63.
28. Nonogi H, Hess OM, Bortone AS, Ritter M, Carroll JD, Krayenbuehl HP. Left ventricular pressure-lenght relation during exercise-induced ischaemia. J Am Coll Cardiol 1989; 13: 1062-70.
29. Tebbe U, Scholz H, Kreuzer H, Neuhaus L. Changes in left ventricular diastolic function during exercise in patients with coronary artery disease. Europ Heart J 1987; 8 (suppl G): 21-8.
30. Greenberg MA, Menegus MA. Ischemia-induced diastolic dysfunction: New observations, new questions. J Am Coll Cardiol 1989; 13: 1071-2.
31. Iskandrian AS, Heo J, Segal BL, Askenase A. Left ventricular diastolic function: evaluation by radionuclide angiography. Am Heart J 1988; 115: 924-9.
32. Bonow RO, Bacharach SL, Green M, et al. Impaired left ventricular diastolic filling in patients with coronary artery disease: Assessment with radionuclide angiography. Circulation 1981; 64: 315-23.
33. Mancini GBJ, Slutsky RA, Norris SL, Bhargava V, Ashburn WL, Higgins CB. Radionuclide analysis of peak filling rate, filling fraction, and time to peak filling rate. Response to supine bicycle exercise in normal subjects and patients with coronary artery disease. Am J Cardiol 1983; 51: 43-51.
34. Polak JF, Kemper AJ, Bianco JA, Parisi AF, Tow DE. Resting early peak diastolic filling rate: A sensitive index of myocardial dysfunction in patients with coronary artery disease. J Nucl Med 1982; 23: 471-8.
35. Aroesty JM, McKay RG, Heller GV, Royal HD, Als AV, Grossman W. Simultaneous assessment of left ventricular systolic and diastolic dysfunction during pacing-induced ischaemia. Circulation 1985; 71: 889-900.
36. Bonow RO, Kent KM, Rosing DR, et al. Improved left ventricular diastolic filling in patients with coronary artery disease after percutaneous transluminal coronary angioplasty. Circulation 1982; 66: 1159-67.
37. Feigenbaum H. Echocardiographic evaluation of left ventricular diastolic function. J Am Coll Cardiol 1989; 13: 1027-9.
38. Gibson DG, Brown D. Measurements of instantaneous left ventricular dimension and filling rate using echocardiography. Br Heart J 1973; 35: 1141-9.
39. Upton MT, Gibson DG, Brown DJ. Echocardiographic assessment of abnormal left ventricular relaxation in man. Br Heart J 1976; 38: 1001-9.
40. Upton MT, Gibson DG. The study of left ventricular function from digitized echocardiograms. Progr Cardiovasc Dis 1978; 20: 359-84.
41. Lawson WE, Brown EJ, Swinford RD, Proctor C, Cohn PF. A new use for M-mode echocardiography in detecting left ventricular diastolic dysfunction in coronary artery disease. Am J Cardiol 1986; 58: 210-13.
42. Danielsen R, Nordrehaug JE, Vik-Mo H. Digitized echocardiographic measurements of left ventricular function: reproducibility and physiological factors influencing the method. Clin Physiol 1987; 7:411-21.
43. Danielsen R, Nordrehaug JE, Vik-Mo H. Importance of adjusting left ventricular diastolic peak filling rate for heart rate. Am J Cardiol 1988; 61: 489-91.
44. Bahler RC, Vrobel TR, Martin P. The relation of heart rate and shortening fraction to echocardiographic indexes of left ventricular relaxation in normal subjects. J Am Coll Cardiol 1983; 2: 926-33.
45. Hanrath P, Mathey DG, Siegert R, Bleifeld W. Left ventricular relaxation and filling pattern in different forms of left ventriclar hypertrophy: An echocardiographic study. Am J Cardiol 1980; 45: 15-23.
46. Suwa M, Hirota Y, Kawamura K. Improvement in left ventricular diastolic function

during intravenous and oral diltiazem therapy in patients with hypertrophic cardiomyopathy: An echocardiographic study. Am J Cardiol 1984; 54: 1047-53.
47. Labovitz AJ, Pearson AC. Evaluation of left ventricular diastolic function: Clinical relevance and recent Doppler echocardiographic insights. Am Heart J 1987; 114: 836-51.
48. Appleton CP, Hatle LK, Popp RL. Relation to transmitral flow velocity patterns of left ventricular diastolic function: New insights from a combined hemodynamic and Doppler echocardiographic study. J Am Coll Cardiol 1988; 12: 426-40.
49. Hamby RI, Noble WJ, Murphy DH, Hoffman I. Atrial transport function in coronary artery disease: relation to left ventricular function. J Am Coll Cardiol 1983; 4:1011-7.
50. Stoddard MF, Pearson AC, Kern MJ, Ratcliff J, Mrosek DG, Labovitz AJ. Left ventricular diastolic function: Comparison of pulsed Doppler echocardiography and hemodynamic indexes in subjects with and without coronary artery disease. J Am Coll Cardiol 1989; 13: 327-36.
51. Iliceto S, Amico A, Marangelli V, D'Ambrosio G, Rizzon P.Doppler echocardiographic evaluation of the effects of atrial pacing-induced ischaemia on left ventricular filling in patients with coronary artery disease. J Am Coll Cardiol 1988; 11: 953-61.
52. Labovitz AJ, Lewen MK, Kern M, et al. Evaluation of left ventricular systolic and diastolic dysfunction during transient myocardial ischaemia produced by angioplasty. J Am Coll Cardiol 1987; 10: 748-55.
53. DeBruyne B, Lerch R, Meier B, et al. Doppler assessment of left ventricular diastolic filling during brief coronary occlusion. Am Heart J 1989; 117: 629-35.
54. Bowman LK, Cleman MW, Cabin HS, Zaret BL, Jaffe CC. Dynamics of early and late left ventricular filling determined by Doppler two-dimensional echocardiography during percutaneous transluminal coronary angioplasty. Am J Cardiol 1988; 61: 541-5.
55. Kou LC, Quinones MA, Rokey R, Sartori M, Abinader EG, Zoghbi WA. Quantification of atrial contribution to left ventricular filling by pulset Doppler echocardiography and the effect of age in normal and diseased hearts. Am J Cardiol 1987; 59: 1174-8.
56. Lorell BH, Grossman W. Cardiac hypertrophy: the consequences for diastole. J Am Coll Cardiol 1987; 9: 1189-93.
57. Held AC, Lavine SJ. Effect of upright exercise on left ventricular diastolic filling in normal subjects. Am J Cardiol 1988; 62: 488-9.
58. Choong CY, Herrmann HC, Weyman AE, Fifer MA. Preload dependence of Doppler-derived idexes of left ventricular diastolic function in humans. J Am Coll Cardiol 1987; 10: 800-8.
59. Myreng Y, Ihlen H, Nitter-Hauge SL. Effects of beta-adrenergic blockade on left ventricular relaxation and filling dynamics in coronary artery disease: a pulsed Doppler echocardiographic study. Eur Heart J 1988; 9: 1167-74.
60. Myreng Y, Myhre E. Effects of verapamil on left ventricular relaxation and filling dynamics in coronary artery disease:A study by pulsed Doppler echocardiography. Am Heart J 1989; 117: 870-5.
61. Devereux RB. Left ventricular diastolic dysfunction: Early diastolic relaxation and late diastolic compliance. J Am Coll Cardiol 1989; 13: 337-9.
62. Martin RP. Myocardial contrast echocardiography: A light in the (heart of) darkness. J Am Coll Cardiol 1989; 13: 857-9.

14

Myocardial dysfunction during exercise

KAI ANDERSEN

Ischaemic myocardial dysfunction

Systolic myocardial dysfunction may be defined as inadequate myocardial contraction. It may be a result of coronary artery disease (1-4), primary myocardial disease (5) or ventricular pressure or volume overload (6, 7).

Inadequate contraction occurs during blood supply incommensurate with metabolic demands (8) with consequently reduced or abolished shortening or even elongation of myocardial fibres during systole (9). Thus, ischaemic dysfunction of left ventricular myocardium implies impairment of systolic wall thickening (9-11) and motion (1, 10, 11).

Impairment of wall thickening is the hallmark of myocardial ischaemia, and consequently occurs in insufficiently perfused ventricular regions supplied by obstructed coronary arteries (9-11). Systolic wall thickening is reduced or abolished (9, 11), and even wall thinning may occur during severe ischaemia (9, 12).

Systolic emptying of the left ventricle is normally associated with wall motion towards the centre of the ventricular cavity. Thus, myocardial dysfunction during ischaemia may be reflected by decreased, abolished or inverse wall motion (2, 10, 11). Such abnormalities of wall motion are designated as hypokinesis, akinesis and dyskinesis, respectively (Fig. 1). However, wall motion abnormalities may also occur in normally perfused areas adjacent to ischaemic regions and may be attributed to a tethering effect (12, 13). The size of an ischaemic area may therefore be overestimated if determined by wall motion abnormalities alone. In addition, pathologic wall motion patterns may occur due to abnormal ventricular depolarization (14) despite preserved wall thickening. Motion of the interventricular septum is also frequently abnormal in patients having undergone cardiac surgery but without concomitant impairment of septal thickening (15).

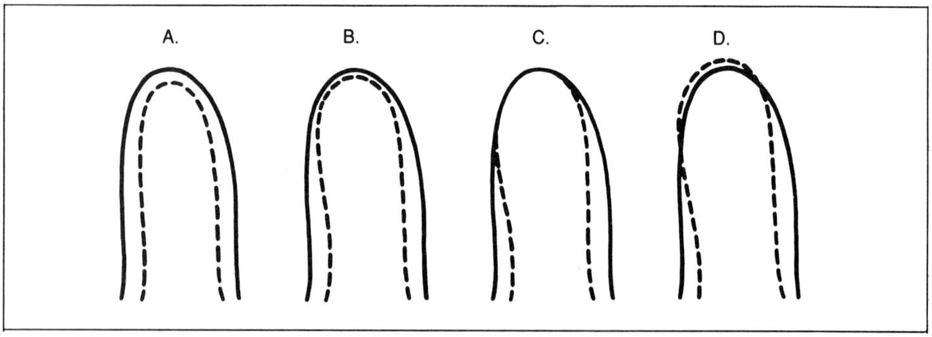

Fig. 1. *End-diastolic (——) and end-systolic (– – –) outlines of left ventricular endocardium in the echocardiographic four-chamber view during normal wall motion (A), hypokinesis (B), akinesis (C) and dyskinesis (D).*

Assessment of myocardial function during exercise

Contrast ventriculography. Exercise-induced wall motion abnormalities have been demonstrated by contrast ventriculography performed during cardiac catheterization (1). The method is invasive and will only be employed if catheterization is indicated for diagnostic or therapeutic purposes anyhow.

Radionuclide ventriculography. Radionuclide ventriculography has been established as a useful non-invasive method for the assessment of left ventricular wall motion during exercise (2, 3, 16). This method may detect changes in endocardial outlines, but without simultaneous assessment of wall thickness. Global left ventricular function may be assessed by the exercise response of left ventricular volume and ejection fraction (2, 3, 17).

Echocardiography. Regional (3, 4, 18) and global left ventricular function can be determined by echocardiography at rest, during or immediately after exercise (3, 4, 19). The method allows assessment of both wall motion (3,4,19) and thickening (3, 18). The reproducibility of left ventricular dimensions may be enhanced if echocardiographic measurements are standardized with regard to transducer position (20) and respiratory phases (21). Measurements may vary with respiration due to motion of the heart relative to the ultrasound beam and to physiologic variations in left ventricular volume and function (21). Thus, comparison of measurements at rest and during exercise should be made at end-expiration since forced respiration usually prohibits inspiratory recordings during exertion.

Echocardiography has several advantages such as ease of access, low cost, and no adverse effects. The main limitation of exercise echocardiography has been technically unsatisfactory recordings in some subjects (18, 19). Adequate studies may be possible in more than 85% of patients suspected of having coronary artery disease, when using modern echocardiographic equipment (22).

Assessment of wall motion. Regional wall motion may be assessed visually or by quantitative analysis of changes in endocardial outlines. Quantitative analysis may be performed by a fixed or floating reference system (23, 24). The former implies merely superimposing end-diastolic outlines, and consequently the overall motion of the heart may contribute to the observed wall motion (23). The latter method may mask wall motion abnormalities while correcting for the change in position of the heart during systole (24). Thus, no particular reference system has been found superior to others (23). However, a fixed reference system is usually employed in radionuclide ventriculography and contrast ventriculography.

Exercise response indicating myocardial dysfunction

Regional left ventricular function. Left ventricular wall thickening and motion normally increases during exertion (18, 25, 26) with increased ventricular performance in response to augmented oxygen demands of exercising tissues. Myocardial dysfunction due to exercise-induced ischaemia would thus be indicated by no change or reduction in wall motion and thickening from rest to exercise (18, 25, 26).

Global left ventricular function. Exercise-induced myocardial dysfunction of sufficient severity or extension may affect the global left ventricular performance. Before abnormal function can be determined, the normal left ventricular response to exercise should be defined. Cardiac output normally increases due to augmentation of heart rate and stroke volume (27-29) concomitantly with an increase in ejection fraction (17, 30). However, it is not clear whether stroke volume increases through augmentation of end-diastolic volume (the Frank-Starling mechanism) (31) or increased systolic emptying (17, 32), or both (29, 30). Findings during maximal semisupine exercise have indicated an increase in stroke volume as a result of augmented ventricular emptying without concomitant dilatation (33, 34). In young healthy men, the Frank-Starling mechanism does not seem to be operative to a greater extent during exercise than at supine rest. These findings are in agreement with those of others (17, 32, 35) and are also in keeping with the lack of a substantial increase in left ventricular filling pressure during maximal supine exercise (36). However, conflicting results of left ventricular dilatation during exertion have also been reported (29-31).

Myocardial dysfunction during exercise might be suggested by increased end-diastolic volume and unchanged or reduced ejection fraction. This is in agreement with ventricular dilatation and depressed ejection fraction response during exercise in patients with coronary artery disease (17, 30, 32). End-diastolic volume may be augmented by an increase of both non-ischaemic and ischaemic segment lengths but with varying pressure/length relationships during the course of the diastole (25). The ejection fraction is depressed as a result of impaired myocardial shortening in ischaemic regions.

However, the response to exercise may vary with body posture (29, 30), gender (37) and age (38, 39). Stroke volume increases from rest to mild exercise in the upright position mainly through an initial increase in end-diastolic volume (29, 30). A further augmentation of stroke volume may occur with increasing work loads through increased systolic emptying (29, 30). In women, the increase in the end-diastolic volume has been found to be more pronounced than in men concomitantly with no increase in ejection fraction from rest to maximal exercise (37). The ejection fraction response to exertion declines with increasing age (38, 39), and the Frank-Starling mechanism may play a part in the elderly for augmentation of stroke volume during exercise (39, 40). Left ventricular response to exertion is also influenced by drugs that alter ventricular loading conditions. Ventricular filling pressure (36) and end-diastolic dimension increase with exercise during beta-blockade in normal subjects (33), while systolic emptying at maximal exercise seems to increase with drug-induced reduction in afterload (33, 34). Accordingly, methodologic and physiologic aspects should be taken into account before an exercise response of global ventricular function is considered as abnormal.

Clinical importance of myocardial dysfunction during exercise

Detection of coronary artery disease. Coronary artery disease can be disclosed by myocardial dysfunction during exercise (2-4). This can be achieved by assessment of regional (2-4) and global left ventricular function (2, 3) by radionuclide angiography (2, 3) and echocardiography (3, 4). Visualization of wall motion abnormalities has been found to have a high sensitivity and specificity in detecting coronary artery disease (2-4). However, the degree of diagnostic ability depends on the selection of patients for the test procedure (41). Global ventricular dysfunction during exercise may also identify patients with coronary artery disease (2, 3), although this response is less specific. A lack of increase in ejection fraction might even be normal in elderly persons (38, 39).

Assessment of myocardial function during exercise will probably not be a screening method for detection of ischaemic heart disease. However, these methods are very useful when electrocardiographic findings during exercise are ambiguous or cannot be interpreted with regard to ischaemia (22) due to the influence of drugs, abnormal ventricular depolarization or left ventricular hypertrophy (42).

Assessment of prognosis. Myocardial dysfunction during exercise is of prognostic importance in patients with coronary artery disease (16, 19, 43). Exercise echocardiography has been shown to identify a majority of patients with cardiac events subsequent to myocardial infarction (43). The predictive ability of exercise echocardiography seems to be superior to that of routine treadmill exercise testing (19, 43). Consequently, the patients with such findings seem to need a more aggressive therapeutic approach than those without.

High-risk lesions such as left main (44) or proximal left anterior descending coronary artery disease (45) may also be disclosed by myocardial dysfunction, if the blood supply to the interventricular septum is taken into account (46). Septal motion and thickening decreased significantly during exercise-induced ischaemia in patients with such specific lesions while increasing in those without (26). However, the predictive ability of this method in less selected patients remains to be shown.

Assessment of functionally important coronary artery lesions. Coronary angiography accurately locates coronary artery stenoses but may be insufficient in assessing their functional importance. This may be due to variability of angiographic assessment, varying luminal geometry and presence or absence of collaterals (47, 48).

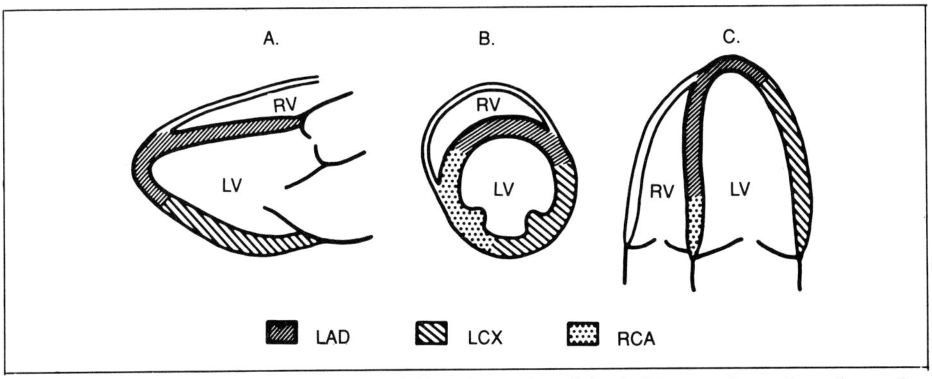

Fig. 2. *Schematic depiction of regional blood supply of the left ventricle in the echocardiographic parasternal long-axis (A), short-axis (B) and apical four-chamber views (C). LV = left ventricle. RV = right ventricle. LAD = left anterior descending coronary artery. LCX = left circumflex artery. RCA = right coronary artery.*

The functional significance of a stenosis can be disclosed through detection of localized myocardial dysfunction during exercise, thereby identifying the obstructed artery at the same time. In order for this to be possible it is necessary to take into consideration the regional blood supply by the major coronary arteries (Fig. 1) (49) although it should be borne in mind that there is a considerable overlap between regions sub-served by left circumflex and right coronary arteries (50). Such information on the functional significance of a stenosis may be of particular importance for the choice of treatment with coronary angioplasty or bypass surgery.

Summary

Myocardial dysfunction due to ischaemia may be precipitated by exercise in a ventricular region supplied by an obstructed coronary artery, often resulting in global ventricular dysfunction. Regional as well as global left ventricular dysfunction during exercise can be detected non-invasively by echocardiography and radionuclide ventriculography. This is clinically important for detection of coronary artery disease when electrocardiographic findings during exercise testing are ambiguous, for risk stratification of patients with coronary artery disease, and for assessment of the functional importance of coronary artery stenoses.

References

1. Sharma B, Taylor SH. Localization of left ventricular ischaemia in angina pectoris by cineangiography during exercise. Br Heart J 1975; 37: 963-70.
2. Borer JS, Bacharach SL, Green MV, Kent KM, Epstein SE, Johnston GS. Real-time radionuclide cineangiography in the noninvasive evaluation of global and regional left ventricular function at rest and during exercise in patients with coronary-artery disease. N Engl J Med 1977; 296: 839-44.
3. Limacher MC, Quinones MA, Poliner LR, Nelson JG, Winters WL, Waggoner AD. Detection of coronary artery disease with exercise two-dimensional echocardiography. Description of a clinically applicable method and comparison with radionuclide ventriculography. Circulation 1983; 67: 1211-8.
4. Armstrong WF, O'Donnell J, Dillon JC, McHenry PL, Morris SN, Feigenbaum H. Complementary value of two-dimensional exercise echocardiography to routine treadmill exercise testing. Ann Intern Med 1986; 105: 829-35.
5. Feild BJ, Bazley WA, Russell RO Jr, et al. Left ventricular function and hypertrophy in cardiomyopathy with depressed ejection fraction. Circulation 1973; 47: 1022-31.
6. Croke RP, Pifarre R, Sullivan H, Gunnar R, Loeb H. Reversal of advanced left ventricular dysfunction following aortic valve replacement for aortic stenosis. Ann Thorac Surg 1977; 24: 38-43.
7. Bonow RO, Picone AL, McIntosh CL, et al. Survival and functional results after valve replacement for aortic regurgitation from 1976 to 1983: impact of preoperative left ventricular function. Circulation 1985; 72: 1244-56.

8. Weber KT, Janicki JS. Interdependence of cardiac function, coronary flow, and oxygen extraction. Am J Physiol 1978; 235:H784-93.
9. Sasayama S, Franklin D, Ross J Jr, Kemper WS, McKown D. Dynamic changes in left ventricular wall thickness and their use in analyzing cardiac function in the conscious dog. A study based on a modified ultrasonic technique. Am J Cardiol 1976; 38: 870-9.
10. Hauser AM, Gangadharan V, Ramos RG, Gordon S, Timmis GC, Dudlets P. Sequence of mechanical, electrocardiographic and clinical effects of repeated coronary artery occlusion in human beings: echocardiographic observations during coronary angioplasty. J Am Coll Cardiol 1985; 5:193-7.
11. Alam M, Khaja F, Brymer J, Marzelli M, Goldstein S. Echocardiographic evaluation of left ventricular function during coronary artery angioplasty. Am J Cardiol 1986; 57: 20-5.
12. Guth BD, White FC, Gallagher KP, Bloor CM. Decreased systolic wall thickening in myocardium adjacent to ischemic zones in conscious swine during brief coronary artery occlusion. Am Heart J 1984; 107: 458-64.
13. Kerber RE, Marcus ML, Wilson R, Ehrhardt J, Abboud FM. Effects of acute coronary occlusion on the motion and perfusion of the normal and ischemic interventricular septum. An experimental echocardiographic study. Circulation 1976; 54: 928-35.
14. Feigenbaum H. Echocardiography. Philadelphia: Lea & Febiger, 1986: 230-9.
15. Force T, Bloomfield P, O'Boyle JE, et al. Quantitative twodimensional echocardiographic analysis of motion and thickening of the interventricular septum after cardiac surgery. Circulation 1983; 68: 1013-20.
16. Pryor DB, Harrell FE Jr, Lee KL, et al. Prognostic indicators from radionuclide angiography in medically treated patients with coronary artery disease. Am J Cardiol 1984; 53: 18-22.
17. Manyari DE, Melendez LJ, Driedger AA, Cradduck TD, MacDonald AC, Kostuk WJ. Left ventricular function and volume during supine exercise in subjects with coronary artery disease. J Appl Physiol 1981; 50: 636-42.
18. Mason SJ, Weiss JL, Weisfeldt ML, Garrison JB, Fortuin NJ. Exercise echocardiography: detection of wall motion abnormalities during ischemia. Circulation 1979; 59: 50-9.
19. Applegate RJ, Dell'Italia LJ, Crawford MH. Usefulness of two-dimensional echocardiography during low-level exercise testing early after uncomplicated acute myocardial infarction. Am J Cardiol 1987; 60: 10-4.
20. Popp RL, Filly K, Brown OR, Harrison DC. Effect of transducer placement on echocardiographic measurement of left ventricular dimensions. Am J Cardiol 1975; 35: 537-40.
21. Andersen K, Vik-Mo H. Effects of spontaneous respiration on left ventricular function assessed by echocardiography. Circulation 1984; 69: 874-9.
22. Armstrong WF. Exercise echocardiography: ready, willing and able. J Am Coll Cardiol 1988; 11: 1359-61.
23. Clayton PD, Jeppson GM, Klausner SC. Should a fixed external reference system be used to analyze left ventricular wall motion? Circulation 1982; 65: 1518-21.
24. Moynihan PF, Parisi AF, Feldman CL. Quantitative detection of regional left ventricular contraction abnormalities by twodimensional echocardiography. I. Analysis of methods. Circulation 1981; 63: 752-60.
25. Nonogi H, Hess OM, Bortone AS, Ritter AM, Carroll JD, Krayenbuehl HP. Left ventricular pressure-length relation during exercise-induced ischemia. J Am Coll Cardiol 1989; 13: 1062-70.
26. Andersen K, Vik-Mo H, Hoff PI. Left main or proximal left anterior descending coronary artery disease: detection by echocardiographic evaluation of interventricular septal function during exercise. Clin Physiol 1986; 6:269-80.

27. Thadani U, Parker JO. Hemodynamics at rest and during supine and sitting bicycle exercise in normal subjects. Am J Cardiol 1978; 41: 52-9.
28. Stenberg J, Åstrand P-O, Ekblom B, Royce J, Saltin B. Hemodynamic response to work with different muscle groups, sitting and supine. J Appl Physiol 1967; 22: 61-70.
29. Poliner LR, Dehmer GJ, Lewis SE, Parkey RW, Blomqvist CG, Willerson JT. Left ventricular performance in normal subjects: a comparison of the responses to exercise in the upright and supine positions. Circulation 1980; 62: 528-34.
30. Steingart RM, Wexler J, Slagle S, Scheuer J. Radionuclide ventriculographic responses to graded supine and upright exercise: critical role of the Frank-Starling mechanism at submaximal exercise. Am J Cardiol 1984; 53: 1671-7.
31. Weiss JL, Weisfeldt ML, Mason SJ, Garrison JB, Livengood SV, Fortuin NJ. Evidence of Frank-Starling effect in man during severe semisupine exercise. Circulation 1979; 59: 655-61.
32. Sharma B, Goodwin JF, Raphael MJ, Steiner RE, Rainbow RG, Taylor SH. Left ventricular angiography on exercise. A new method of assessing left ventricular function in ischaemic heart disease. Br Heart J 1976; 38: 59-70.
33. Andersen K, Vik-Mo H. Role of the Frank-Starling mechanism during maximal semisupine exercise after oral atenolol. Br Heart J 1982; 48: 149-55.
34. Andersen K, Vik-Mo H. Increased left ventricular emptying at maximal exercise after reduction in afterload. Circulation 1984; 69: 492-6.
35. Crawford MH, White DH, Amon KW. Echocardiographic evaluation of left ventricular size and performance during handgrip and supine and upright bicycle exercise. Circulation 1979; 59: 1188-96.
36. Sorensen SG, Ritchie JL, Caldwell JH, Hamilton GW, Kennedy JW. Serial exercise radionuclide angiography. Validation of count-derived changes in cardiac output and quantitation of maximal exercise ventricular volume change after nitroglycerin and propranolol in normal men. Circulation 1980; 61: 600-9.
37. Higginbotham MB, Morris KG, Coleman RE, Cobb FR. Sex-related differences in the normal cardiac response to upright exercise. Circulation 1984; 70: 357-66.
38. Port S, Cobb FR, Coleman RE, Jones RH. Effect of age on the response of the left ventricular ejection fraction to exercise. N Engl J Med 1980; 303: 1133-7.
39. Rodeheffer RJ, Gerstenblith G, Becker LC, Fleg JL, Weisfeldt ML, Lakatta EG. Exercise cardiac output is maintained with advancing age in healthy human subjects: cardiac dilatation and increased stroke volume compensate for a diminished heart rate. Circulation 1984; 69: 203-13.
40. Mann DL, Denenberg BS, Gash AK, Makler PT, Bove AA. Effects of age on ventricular performance during graded supine exercise. Am Heart J 1986; 111: 108-15.
41. Bairey CN, Rozanski A, Berman DS. Exercise echocardiography: ready or not? J Am Coll Cardiol 1988; 11: 1355-8.
42. Sheffield LT. Exercise stress testing. In: Braunwald E, ed. Heart disease. A textbook of cardiovascular medicine. Philadelphia: WB Saunders Company, 1988: 223-41.
43. Ryan T, Armstrong WF, O'Donnell JA, Feigenbaum H. Risk stratification after acute myocardial infarction by means of exercise two-dimensional echocardiography. Am Heart J 1987; 114: 1305-16.
44. Takaro T, Hultgren HN, Lipton MJ, Detre KM, and participants in the study group. The VA Cooperative Randomized Study of Surgery for Coronary Arterial Occlusive Disease. II. Subgroup with significant left main lesions. Circulation 1976; 54 (suppl. III): III-107-17.
45. European Coronary Surgery Study Group. Long-term results of prospective randomised study of coronary artery bypass surgery in stable angina pectoris. Lancet 1982;ii:1173-80.

46. James TN, Burch GE. Blood supply of the human interventricular septum. Circulation 1958; 17: 391-6.
47. Klocke FJ. Measurements of coronary blood flow and degree of stenosis: current clinical implications and continuing uncertainties. J Am Coll Cardiol 1983; 1:31-41.
48. Pitt B, Kalff V, Rabinovitch MA, et al. Impact of radionuclide techniques on evaluation of patients with ischemic heart disease. J Am Coll Cardiol 1983; 1:63-72.
49. Feigenbaum H. Echocardiography. Philadelphia: Lea & Febiger, 1986: 465-8.
50. Stamm RB, Gibson RS, Bishop HL, Carabello BA, Beller GA, Martin RP. Echocardiographic detection of infarct-localized asynergy and remote asynergy during acute myocardial infarction: correlation with the extent of angiographic coronary disease. Circulation 1983; 67: 233-44.

Coronary syndromes

15

Stable and unstable coronary syndromes

KRISTIAN THYGESEN,
HANS ERIK BØTKER,
JAN RAVKILDE

Ischaemic heart disease is the overall term generally used for syndromes having coronary atherosclerosis as the pathological basis. Atherosclerosis normally progresses slowly for decades, however in persons with risk factors, the process may accelerate and manifest itself clinically somewhat earlier. Coronary atherosclerosis can be asymptomatic or silent, but also symptomatic, producing chest pain, heart failure, rhythm disturbances or sudden coronary death. The recognition of this variety of clinical expressions of ischaemia has led to a greater appreciation that ischaemic syndromes may overlap each other and at times even demonstrate interaction (Fig. 1).

The principal cause of myocardial ischaemia is an oxygen imbalance in the myocardial tissue due to interchangeable and varying contribution of the following: atherosclerotic lesions, vasoreactivity and dynamic thrombus activity. However, the clinical expression of ischaemia is not always directly related to individual pathologic mechanisms. Some patients with stable angina may present with unstable angina following a change in the underlying plaque morphology; both patients with stable and unstable angina may also have episodes of silent ischaemia during their disease (1).

Stunned and hibernating myocardium

The sequence of myocardial ischaemic events is shown in Fig. 2. Ischaemia results within seconds in changes in the left ventricular function and electrocardiographic changes appear shortly thereafter (2). The indirect clinical expressions of systolic and diastolic dysfunction include fatigue and dyspnoea. The extent of dysfunction and the rate of recovery are both related to the extent of myocardial ischaemia (3).

It is now apparent that viable myocardial tissue that has been subjected to

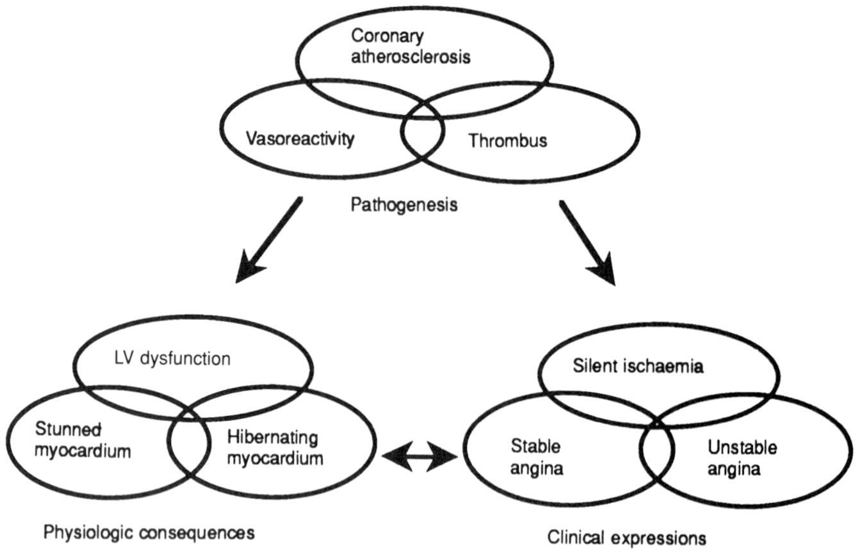

Fig. 1. *Pathogenetic and pathophysiologic mechanisms in clinical expressions of myocardial ischaemia.*

ischaemia may demonstrate relatively prolonged alteration in function and contribute to overall left ventricular dysfunction. Two such altered states of the myocardial tissue include the "stunned myocardium" and the "hibernating myocardium" (4, 5).

Myocardial stunning refers to periods of severe ischaemia associated with ultrastructural, biochemical and functional abnormalities that persist for hours to days after perfusion has been re-estabilished. While the stunned myocardium is a transient postischaemic contractile dysfunction, the hiber-

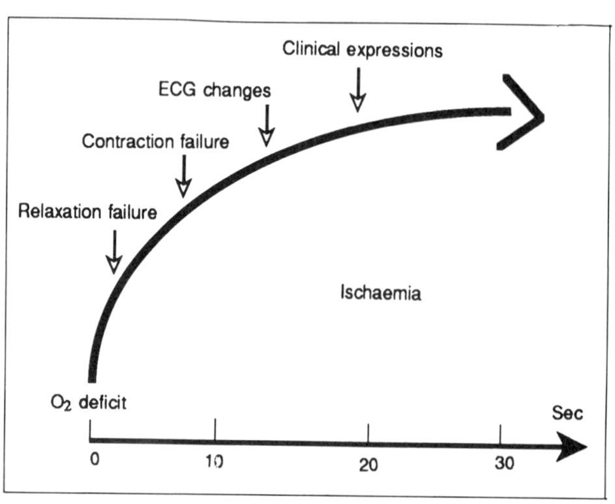

Fig. 2. *Sequence of events during the development of myocardial ischaemia.*

nating myocardium in contrast is a chronicly depressed contractile function that may persist from months to years. Hibernating myocardium may occur without angina pectoris and even without electrocardiographic changes of ischaemia. Such left ventricular dysfunction may be the sole clinical manifestation of myocardial ischaemia (6).

Stable coronary syndrome

The stable coronary syndrome comprises the static ischaemic entities, chronic stable angina pectoris and silent myocardial ischaemia. Stable myocardial ischaemia is the result of atherosclerotic obstructive lesions that inhibit the coronary blood supply. The degree of potential flow reduction is modulated by local vasoreactivity; this frequently occurs in patients with otherwise typical stable angina pectoris. Ischaemic attacks in patients with stable angina most frequently occur as a response to increased myocardial oxygen demand, brought about by physical activity, anxiety or exposure to cold (1).

There is considerable evidence that chronic stable angina is associated with exercise induced silent myocardial ischaemia as well as spontaneous silent myocardial ischaemia (7). However, silent ischaemia can also occur in persons with totally asymptomatic coronary artery disease. Further, silent ischaemia may occur after myocardial infarction (MI) and prior to sudden coronary death (8).

Unstable coronary syndrome

The mechanisms underlying unstable myocardial ischaemia differ considerably from those for stable ischaemia. In contrast to a supposed relatively fixed coronary stenosis in the latter condition there is evidence of an acute evolving arterial lesion leading to a reduction in coronary blood flow in unstable ischaemia. The final clinical outcome of the acute ischaemic event is dependent not only upon the degree of luminal obstruction but also on the duration of the hindrance and the degree to which collaterals are able to compensate for the impeded perfusion. Various clinical syndromes have been directly attributed to unstable ischaemia or are described as developing in association with unstable ischaemic attacks; we prefer to term these: unstable coronary syndrome, comprising unstable angina pectoris and acute MI.

One limitation to the usefulness of the clinical description is the inadequacy of symptom presentation to reflect accurately the underlying pathophysiology. Unstable angina is a very heterogeneous condition, thus the limitation is particularly emphasized for this clinical entity, whereas acute MI is related to the underlying coronary thrombosis to a very high degree. The distinction between stable and unstable ischaemia according to the definition given above is more closely related to the pathophysiology of the lesions involved than the classic clinical description of stable and unstable angina pectoris. However, clinical classifications still provide the most useful method for routinely defining functional, prognostic and therapeutic outcomes for myocardial ischaemia.

Unstable angina pectoris

A broad spectrum of patients with ischaemic heart disease varying widely in cause, severity, prognosis and responsiveness to therapy are assigned to the clinical entity unstable angina. A separation into subgroups of unstable angina is necessary in order to provide a precise basis for diagnosing, treating and studying these patients. Such classification implies a distinction between patients who suffer from unstable angina due to unstable ischaemia and patients who suffer from unstable angina due to aggravation of stable angina. The former group includes patients who develop symptoms in the absence of extracardiac conditions (primary unstable angina) and following acute MI (postinfarction unstable angina). The latter group includes patients who develop symptoms in the presence of extracardiac conditions that intensify myocardial ischaemia (secondary unstable angina) (9). Such conditions reduce myocardial oxygen supply or increase myocardial oxygen demand and include anaemia, infection, fever, hypotension, uncontrolled hypertension, tachyarrhythmia, emotional stress, thyrotoxicosis, and hypoxaemia secondary to respiratory insufficiency.

Not only the clinical description but also several other variables have been employed in order to predict the clinical outcome and response to therapy in patients with unstable angina (Table 1). ST-segment elevation during chest pain in unstable angina may occur but is rather unusual. It has been shown that thrombolytic therapy is effective in reducing the severity of the stenosis and in improving the acute clinical condition in patients with ST-segment elevation during bouts of chest pain (10). Even so, an ECG is rather insensitive for predicting the degree of ischaemia, the response to therapy and the clinical outcome (10, 11).

The presence of a biochemical marker of thrombus formation in unstable angina could serve to identify patients with an intracoronay thrombus and thus indicate the need for thrombolytic therapy. The data on platelet acti-

Table 1. *Predictive variables for outcome and treatment response in unstable angina pectoris.*

ECG changes	
	ST-segment elevation during chest pain
	Reversible or sustained T-wave inversion
Biochemical markers of thrombus formation	
	Thromboxane metabolites
	Fibrinopeptide A
	D-dimer and fibrin monomer
Biochemical markers of minimal myocardial tissue necrosis	
	Myoglobin
	Creatine kinase MB-subunit
	Myosin light chains
Coronary angiography	
	Intracoronary thrombus
	Complex coronary morphology

vation is difficult to interpret because of problems when sampling and the short half-life of most vasoactive substances secreted by activated platelets. However, significant increases in urinary metabolites of thromboxane were found in patients with unstable angina following episodes of chest pain (12). Similar findings have not been made when measuring markers indicating activation of the fibrinolytic system such as fibrinopeptide A and D-dimer and fibrin monomer (13, 14). Therefore, the importance of biochemical indicators, especially in the peripheral blood, for the identification of a dynamic thrombus in unstable angina remains controversial.

A high risk subgroup for developing coronary events such as MI, heart failure and death has been identified using markers of ischaemically damaged myocardial tissue in patients with unstable angina (15, 16). These patients suffered from minor myocardial necrosis although not diagnosed as having an acute MI according to the WHO-criteria (11, 16). Furthermore, highly sensitive CK-MB measurements in patients with stable, unstable angina and MI not only identify patients with unstable angina having minor myocardial necrosis, but they also demonstrate a continuum from MI to unstable angina with regard to the amount of ischaemic myocardial damage (11). Thus, these ischaemic tracers are not restricted in their application to conventional MI. They are able to reflect – in time and degree – a broad spectrum of ischaemic damage to the myocardium. It has as yet not been determined, whether the difference between no and minimal enzyme release reflects differentiation between stable and unstable ischaemic conditions.

Progression of stenosis has commonly been found in patients who underwent sequential coronary arteriography, before and after the onset of unstable angina. This progression is often precipitated by plaque rupture and in some cases, superimposed by thrombosis (17, 18). The demonstration of intracoronary thrombosis is dependent on the timing of angiography. The appearance is frequent (roughly 40 to 50%) if patients undergo angiography within 24 hours following the onset of symptoms, but the frequency decreases thereafter (19-22). These coronary thrombi are strongly predictive of both cardiac events and the outcome (20).

Acute myocardial infarction

Chest pain, evolving ECG-changes and elevated plasma enzymes still remain the corner-stones for establishing a diagnosis of acute MI. The chest pain is variable in intensity and typically lasts for more than 30 minutes. The ECG is subject to a number of characteristic changes during the evolution of a MI. The deviation of the ST-segment and inversion of T waves in connection with reduction of the amplitude or loss of the R wave and appearance of an abnormal Q-wave indicate MI ("transmural infarction"). However, isolated ST deviations and T wave changes may occur without the development of Q-waves ("subendocardial infarction") (23). Injured myocardial cells release enzymes which exceed the normal plasma range 4-6 hours after MI. These peak a number of hours later; e.g., total creatine kinase (CK) normally peaks about 24 hours after onset (24). Curves of changes in the amplitude of the Q

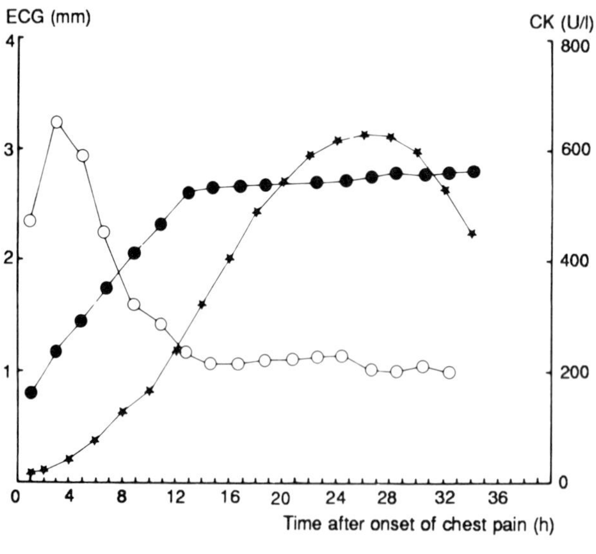

Fig. 3. *Changes in ECG and plasma CK concentration after onset of MI. (open circles: ST-elevation, closed circles: Q-wave amplitude, asterisk: plasma CK concentration).*

wave and plasma CK concentration initially run a parallel course, inasmuch as MI can first be recognized in the ECG and after a delay of some hours in the plasma enzymes. (Fig. 3).

The changes in the QRS complex following an acute MI are usually completed within 12-15 hours with a range from 8 to 48-72 hours (23). It is noteworthy that evolution of MI is a stepwise process in about one-third of patient (25). It has been observed experimentally that cells within an ischaemic region become injured irreversibly and electrically silent at different times. This is reflected in changes in the Q and R waves. A broad time range is seen in the evolution of acute MI because of factors such as collateral flow, energy depletion, wall tension, spontaneous recanalisation and reocclusion (23, 25, 26).

Q-wave and non-Q-wave infarction

As there is an imperfect correlation between the pathologic and ECG findings, it has been suggested, that the terms transmural and subendocardial infarction be avoided, when referring to the ECG pattern of MI and that the more appropiate terms of Q-wave and non-Q-wave MI be employed (27).

The ECG criteria for the differential diagnosis of Q-wave and non-Q-wave infarction present no difficulties. Serial ECG's show early ST-segment elevation followed by the development of pathologic Q-waves (i.e. $\geq$30 msec) in the case of Q-wave infarction, while in non-Q-wave infarction the serial ECG changes must be restricted to the ST-segment and/or the T-waves (28). Non-Q-wave infarction has mainly been characterized by ST-segment depression and/or T-wave inversion, but recent studies indicate, that between 30-40% of acute non-Q-wave infarctions present with ST-segment elevation (29, 30). These changes in diagnostic approach, greater sensitivity of diagnostic methods, together with the possible impact of therapeutic intervention, have increased the incidence of non-Q-wave infarction from 25-30% to more than 40% (28, 31).

Coronary arteriographic studies of non-Q-wave infarctions show that one-fourth of these patients have a completely occluded infarct-related vessel within 24 hours. The percentage of patients with complete occlusion rose to approximately 40% within one week (32). In contrast, about 80% of patients with Q-wave infarction have complete coronary occlusion within the first 24 hours, inasmuch as the frequency of complete occlusion fell from 85% within 0-6 hours to 64% within 12-24 hours (33). It has been assumed that non-Q-wave infarction is caused by complete thrombotic occlusion, but the latter is transient, either because of unsustained spasm (which may be necessary for clot stabilization) or because of an inherently more active fibrinolytic system, which leads to early lysis. This reflow theory is the likely mechanism in the majority of such infarctions (28).

Myocardial reperfusion

Recognition of myocardial reperfusion, both spontaneous as well as that occuring as a result of thrombolytic therapy, is important in the management of patients with MI. Angiography is the acknowledged standard for demonstrating coronary occlusion and recanalization, but catheterization facilities are rarely available and in any case, the majority of cardiologists do not like to carry out this procedure during the acute phase. Therefore, physicians must rely on non-invasive markers of reperfusion including clinical observations such as lessening of chest pain, regression of ST-segment changes, appearance and disappearance of cardiac rhythm disturbances and analysis of cardiac related time-activity plasma enzyme curves (34-37).

However, new biochemical markers for assessing myocardial reperfusion and injury have been developed in recent years. These belong to the contractile proteins of heart muscle. Markers such as myosin light chains and myosin heavy chains are of value in estimating infarct size, irrespective of coronary reperfusion (38-40). Distinct kinetic differences of troponin-T serum levels of patients treated with thrombolytic therapy have been observed in a recent multicentre study, indicating that troponin-T may be used as a non-invasive marker of reperfusion (Fig. 4) (41). Thus, the new

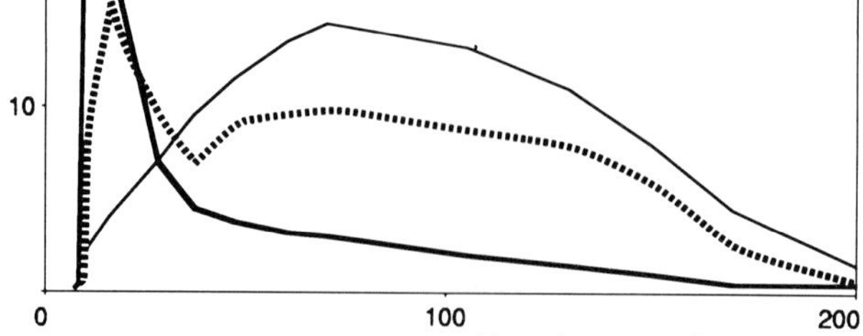

Fig. 4. *Changes in serum concentration of Troponin-T in three patients with MI given thrombolytic therapy. The curves illustrate examples of early (thick line), late (dotted line) and non-reperfusion (thin line). Relative concentrations are depicted.*

indicators appear promising for estimating infarct size and as non-invasive markers of spontaneous or induced reperfusion.

Conclusion

The stable coronary syndrome comprises chronic angina pectoris and silent myocardial ischaemia, while unstable coronary syndrome includes unstable angina pectoris and acute MI. However, the clinical expression of ischaemia does not always reflect the underlying pathological mechanisms, and as a consequence ischaemic syndromes may overlap and even be subdivided. Biological markers indicate that unstable angina pectoris represents both stable as well as unstable myocardial ischaemia. These markers can also be used for monitoring infarct development, for estimation of infarct size, and for assessing myocardial reperfusion (biochemical angiography).

References

1. Vetrovec GW. Changing concepts in the pathophysiology of myocardial ischaemia. Am J Cardiol 1989; 64: 3F-9F.
2. Hauser AM, Gangadharan V, Ramos RG, Gordon S, Timmis GC. Sequence of mechanical, electrocardiographic and clinical effects of repeated coronary artery occlusion in human beings: echocardiographic observation during coronary angioplasty. J Am Coll Cardiol 1985; 5: 193-7.
3. Plotnick GD, Becker LG, Fisher ML. Changes in left ventricular function during recovery from upright bicycle exercise in normal persons and patients with coronary artery disease. Am J Cardiol 1986; 58: 247-51.
4. Braunwald E, Kloner RA. The stunned myocardium: prolonged, postischemic ventricular dysfunction. Circulation 1982; 66: 1146-9.
5. Braunwald E, Rutherford JD. Reversible ischemic left ventricular dysfunction: evidence for the hibernating myocardium. J Am Coll Cardiol 1986; 8: 1467-70.
6. Kloner RA, Przyklenk K, Patel B. Altered myocardial states. The stunned and hibernating myocardium. Am J Med 1989; 86 (suppl lA): 14-22.
7. Mulcahy D, Keegan J, Crean P, et al. Silent myocardial ischaemia in chronic stable angina. A study of its frequency and characteristics in 150 patients. Br Heart J 1988; 60: 417-23.
8. Gottlieb SO, Weisfeldt ML, Ouyang P, Mellits ED, Gerstenblith G. Silent ischemia as a marker for early unfavorable outcomes in patients with unstable angina. N Eng J Med 1986; 314: 121-9.
9. Braunwald E. Unstable angina. A classification. Circulation 1989; 80: 410-4.
10. Gotoh K, Minamino T, Katoh O, et al. The role of intracoronary thrombus in unstable angina: angiographic assessment and thrombolytic therapy during ongoing anginal attacks. Circulation 1988; 77: 526-34.
11. Bøtker HE, Ravkilde J, Søgaard P, Jørgensen PJ, Hørder M, Thygesen K. Gradation of unstable angina on basis of a sensitive method for creatine kinase MB isoenzyme determination in serum. 1990 (submitted).

12. Fitzgerald DJ, Roy L, Cartella F, Fitzgerald GA. Platelet activation in unstable coronary disease. N Engl J Med 1986; 983-9.
13. Theroux P, Latour J-G, Leger C, DeLara J. Fibrinopeptide A and platelet factor levels in unstable angina pectoris. Circulation 1987; 75: 156-62.
14. Alexopoulos D, Stump D, Deshmuhk P, et al. Inability of thrombosis related markers to distinguish between unstable and stable angina pectoris. J Am Coll Cardiol 1989; 13 (suppl A): 15A.
15. Katus HA, Diederich KW, Hoberg E, Kübler W. Circulating cardiac myosin light chains in patients with angina at rest:Identification of a high risk subgroup. J Am Coll Cardiol 1988; 11: 487-93.
16. Isakov A, Shapira I, Burke M, Almong C. Serum myoglobin levels in patients with ischemic myocardial insult. Arch Intern Med 1988; 148: 1762-5.
17. Moise A, Theroux P, Taeymans Y, et al. Unstable angina and progression of atherosclerosis. N Engl J Med 1983; 309: 685-9.
18. Ambrose JA, Winters SL, Stern A, et al. Angiographic morphology and the pathogenesis of unstable angina pectoris. J Am Coll Cardiol 1985; 5: 609-16.
19. Capone G, Wolf NM, Meyer B, Meister SG. Frequency of intracoronary filling defects by angiography in unstable angina pectoris at rest. Am J Cardiol 1985; 56: 403-.
20. Freman MR, Williams AE, Chisholm RJ, Armstrong PW. Intracoronary thrombus and complex morphology in unstable angina. Circulation 1989; 80: 17-23.
21. Vetrovec GW, Cowley MJ, Overton H, Richardson DW. Intracoronary thrombus in syndromes of unstable myocardial ischaemia. Am Heart J 1981; 102: 1202-8.
22. Breshnahan DR, Davies JL, Holmes DR Jr, Smith HC. Angiographic occurence and clinical correlates of intraluminal coronary artery disease of intraluminal coronary artery thrombus: Role of unstable angina. J Am Coll Cardiol 1985; 6: 285-9.
23. Thygesen K. Assessing acute myocardial infarction by electrocardiography. Odense: Odense University Press, 1981.
24. Hørder M, Petersen PH, Thygesen K, Nielsen BL. Plasma enzymes in myocardial infarction. An appraisal of quantitative, clinical and pathophysiological information. Scand J Clin Lab Invest 1981; 41: 41-7.
25. Sederholm M, Grottum P, Erhardt L, Kjekshus J. Quantitative assessment of myocardial ischemia and necrosis by continous vectorcardiography and measurement of creatine kinase release in patients. Circulation 1983; 68: 1006-12.
26. Hackett D, Davies G, Chierchia S, Maseri A. Intermittent coronary occlusion in acute myocardial infarction: value of combined thrombolytic and vasodilator therapy. N Engl J Med 1987; 317: 1055-9.
27. Spodick DH. Q wave infarction versus S-T infarction. Nonspecificity of electrocardiographic criteria for differentiating transmural and nontransmural lesions. Am J Cardiol 1983; 51: 913-5.
28. Gibson RS. Non-Q-Wave myocardial infarction: Diagnosis, prognosis, and management. In: O'Rourke RA, Crawford MH, eds. Current problems in cardiology. Chicago: Year Book Medical Publishers, Inc, 1988; 13(1): 1-72.
29. Ogawa H, Hiramori K, Haze K, et al. Classification of non-Q-wave myocardial infarction according to electrocardiographic changes. Br Heart J 1985; 54: 473-8.
30. Huey BL, Gheorghiade M, Crampton RS, et al. Acute non-Q-wave myocardial infarction associated with early ST segment elevation: Evidence for spontaneous reperfusion and implications for thrombolytic trials. J Am Coll Cardiol 1987; 9: 18-25.
31. Goldberg RJ, Gore JM, Alpert JS, et al. Non-Q-wave myocardial infarction: Recent changes in occurence and prognosis – a community wide perspective. Am Heart J 1987; 113: 273-9.

32. DeWood MA, Stifter WF, Simpson CS, et al. Coronary arteriographic findings soon after non-Q-wave myocardial infarction. N Engl J Med 1986; 315: 417-23.
33. Dewood MA, Spores J, Notske R, et al. Prevalence of total coronary occlusion during the early hours of transmural infarction. N Eng J Med 1980; 303: 897-902.
34. Ganz W, Geft J, Maddahi J, et al. Nonsurgical reperfusion in evolving myocardial infarction. J Am Coll Cardiol 1983; 1: 1247-53.
35. Hackworthy RA, Vogel MB, Harris PJ. Relationship between changes in ST segment elevation and patency of the infarct-related coronary artery in acute myocardial infarction. Am Heart J 1986; 112: 279-84.
36. Cercek B, Lew AS, Laramee P, et al. Time course and characteristics of ventricular arrhythmias following reperfusion in acute myocardial infarction. Am J Cardiol 1987; 60: 214-8.
37. Ong L, Reiser P, Coromilas J, Scherr L, Morrison J. Left ventricular function and rapid release of creatine kinase MB in acute myocardial infarction. Evidence for spontaneous reperfusion. N Engl J Med 1983; 309: 1-6.
38. Isobe M, Nagai R, Ueda S, et al. Quantitative relationship between left ventricular function and serum cardiac myosin light chain I levels after coronary reperfusion in patients with acute myocardial infarction. Circulation 1987; 76: 1251-61.
39. Katus HA, Diederich KW, Schwarz F, Uellner M, Scheffold T, Kübler W. Influence of reperfusion on serum concentrations of cytosolic creatine kinase and structural myosin light chains in acute myocardial infarction. Am J Cardiol 1987; 60: 440-5.
40. Léger J, Bouvagnet P, Pau B, Roncucci R, Léger J-J. Levels of ventricular myosin fragments in human sera after myocardial infarction, determined with monoclonal antibodies to myosin heavy chains. Eur J Clin Invest 1985; 15: 422-9.
41. Gerhardt W, Katus H, Hamm C, et al. Clinical value of troponin-T in diagnosis and monitoring of coronary heart disease – results of a multicenter study. (Abstract) XIV International Congress of Clinical Chemistry. San Francisco, 1990.

16

Silent ischaemia and angina pectoris

KENNETH EGSTRUP

Manifestations of asymptomatic coronary artery disease have been known for many years as for acute myocardial infarction (1) and during exercise testing (2), but the use of ambulatory electrocardiographic monitoring during unrestricted daily life has stimulated the interest in assessment of silent myocardial ischaemia, especially in patients with stable angina pectoris. The first reports of ischaemic episodes out-of-hospital were noted in the sixties, but more systematic analysis of ischaemia with or without symptoms were performed about 10 years later with comparison of exercise testing, coronary arteriography and ischaemic episodes obtained by ambulatory monitoring (3-5). There is now substantial evidence that episodes of transient ST-segment depression detected during ambulatory monitoring, with or without symptoms, represent episodes with myocardial ischaemia. During cardiac catheterization, increased left ventricular end-diastolic pressures (6) and increased myocardial oxygen extraction (7) have been reported with ST-segment change without symptoms. Myocardial perfusion assessed by positron tomography using a short-lived cation, rubidium 82, during spontaneous ischaemic episodes has shown regional uptake defects independent of symptoms and with the same regional perfusion defect during symptomatic and asymptomatic ischaemia (8, 9). Furthermore, ambulatory registration of pulmonary artery pressure with a transducer-tipped catheter has noted, that episodes with ischaemia detected by ambulatory monitoring are accompanied by a rise in pulmonary artery diastolic pressure, independent of symptoms (10, 11).

Assessment of transient myocardial ischaemia with ambulatory monitoring (Holter monitoring)

The main use for Holter monitoring has, for many years, been the detection of arrhythmias, although ST-T-changes during an anginal attack were first described in 1961 (12). An increasing number of studies have utilized ambulatory monitoring for detection of transient ischaemic episodes during subsequent years and due to a great day to day variation in ischaemia the monitoring time has been extended up to 72 hours. In most studies, ST-segment depression has been considered significant if the depression was horizontal or downsloping with a magnitude of 1 mm or more measured 60 or 80 msec after the J-point and each episode lasting 1 minute or more (13-15). Low frequency response has been given as a requirement for reliable ST-segment analysis and the use of a frequency modulated Holter recorder has therefore been advocated, but there are now several studies that have documented the validity of amplitude modulated recorders by simultaneous recordings during exercise testing (16, 17). Ambulatory monitoring normally utilizes 2 bipolar leads and CM5 is most commonly recorded, and this lead has been found valid in detecting subendocardial ischaemia (18), and further, the use of a V3-like lead seems to increase the detection of ischaemic changes (17). The use of a 12-lead precordial mapping system during exercise testing may identify the position for the exploring electrode during ambulatory monitoring, and may increase the possibility to detect maximal shifts in the ST-segment (16).

The evaluation of ST-segment changes is cumbersom and time consuming even with the use of computer assisted programmes. Therefore systems, which analyse in real time are under development, but there are still unsolved problems concerning the long-term memory and the reliability of the systems.

Characteristics of silent ischaemia

Prevalence: The occurrence of silent ischaemia in asymptomatic middle-aged men has been estimated to about 2.5% (19, 20), and the corresponding number after myocardial infarction has been noted to about 20% (21). Ambulatory monitoring has mainly been used in patients with symptomatic coronary artery disease as angina pectoris, and silent ischaemia has been found in 60 to 100% of these patients (22-24).

Description of silent ischaemia: With the use of ambulatory monitoring, several studies have now noted that the majority of ischaemic episodes during daily life are not associated with symptoms (3, 8, 13, 23, 25), and indicate that about 75% of all ischaemic episodes are silent (Fig. 1). It has even been noted, that asymptomatic ST-segment deviation is often surprisingly prolonged and even high grade ST-segment depression is seen. There is a considerable overlap between symptomatic and asymptomatic episodes

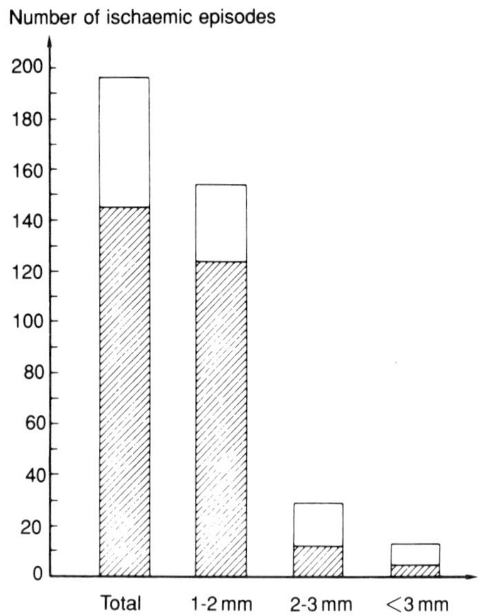

Fig. 1. *Frequency and magnitude of total and silent ischaemic episodes (hatched bars) obtained during ambulatory monitoring (reproduced with permission from Acta Med Scand).*

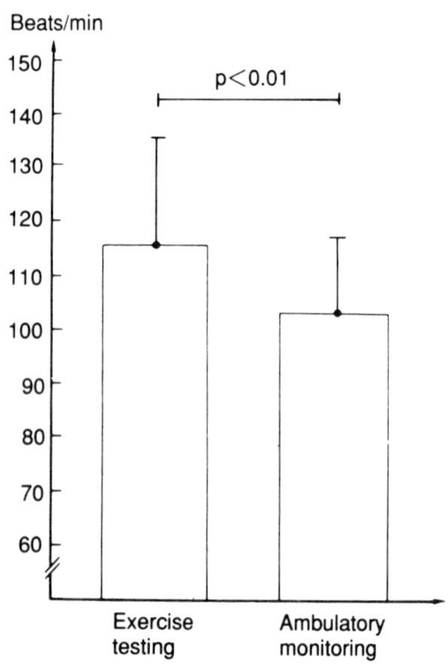

Fig. 2. *Heart rate at onset of ischaemia during exercise testing and ambulatory monitoring (mean±SD) (reproduced with permission from Acta Med Scand).*

and it must be concluded, that angina pectoris is an insensitive parameter of total ischaemic activity. The symptom angina is subjective and as such highly variable, and it has been found that only about 50% of episodes, identified by the patients as typical angina, are accompanied by transient ST-segment changes (26) (Table 1).

Ambulatory ischaemia is detected at a heart rate significantly lower than the heart rate during exercise induced ischaemia (23) (Fig. 2), and ischaemic

Table 1. *Relationship between anginal pain and ST segment change.*

	Group 1 N = 10	Group 2 N = 15	Group 3 N = 35	Group 4 N = 35	Total
No of episodes of anginal pain	18	29	68	80	195
No of episodes of ST segment change	8(44%)	10(35%)	30(44%)	46(58%)	94(48%)

(%) = episodes of both pain and ST segment change.
Group 1: positive exercise test; Group 2: positive coronary arteriography; Group 3 and 4: positive exercise test and coronary arteriography.

episodes occur often during low-level physical activity (27, 28), during smoking (29) and mental stress (9). Intra-arterial monitoring of the blood pressure has demonstrated considerable variation in relation to ischaemic episodes during daily life (30), and as the heart rate is one of the major determinants of myocardial oxygen consumption, it may indicate, that reduction in myocardial oxygen supply is responsible for transient ischaemic episodes. On the other hand, it has also been noted, that transient ischaemia is often preceded by an increase in heart rate (8, 13), and that the heart rate during ischaemia is 23% higher than the 24 hours mean heart rate (31). Thus the development of transient myocardial ischaemia may therefore be secondary to a complex interplay between reduction in myocardial oxygen supply and increased myocardial oxygen demand; this concept of a dynamic pathophysiology is supported by identification of a substance with a short half-life produced locally by the endothelium (endothelium derived relaxing factor), which dilates the coronary arteries (32) and by quantitative angiographic studies of the luminal area of coronary stenosis during exercise (33).

Circadian variation: A diurnal variation has been described for cardiac diseases, as the onset of myocardial infarction is noted with the highest frequency in the morning (34); the same pattern being found for sudden cardiac death (35). A similar daily rhythm has been observed for transient ischaemic episodes detected by ambulatory monitoring (Fig. 3) with the highest frequency of ischaemia in the morning, but also a lesser peak in the evening (23, 36, 37). This pattern is similar to the daily rhythm in heart rate (37), plasma catecholamines (38), platelet aggregability (39), arterial blood pressure (40), and the tone in epicardial coronary arteries (41). This may indicate a possible link between various forms of coronary artery disease, but the mechanisms that increase the occurrence of myocardial infarction and sudden cardiac death in the morning may not be the same as those involved in the pathophysiology of transient myocardial ischaemia during daily life.

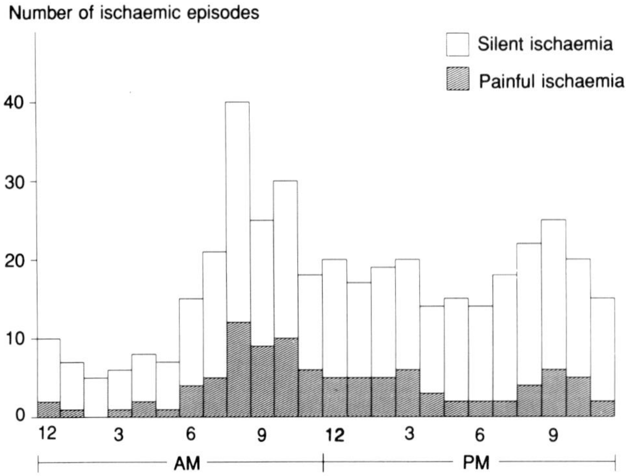

Fig. 3. *Circadian variation of transient ischaemic episodes.*

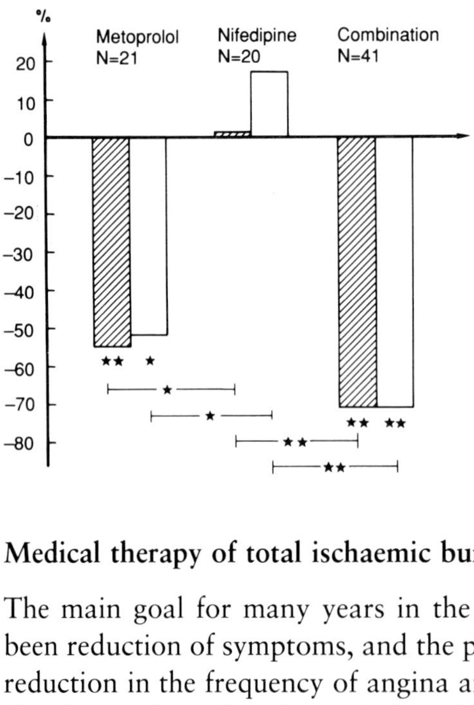

Fig. 4. *Changes (%) in frequency of total ischaemia and asymptomatic ischaemic episodes during treatment with metoprolol, nifedipine and their combination compared with placebo. Number of episodes at baseline (placebo) = 0%. Hatched bars denote all ischaemic episodes and open bars silent ischaemia.* * = $p < 0.05$ *and* ** $p < 0.01$ *compared with baseline (placebo) (reproduced with permission from American Heart Journal).*

Medical therapy of total ischaemic burden

The main goal for many years in the management of angina pectoris has been reduction of symptoms, and the primary objective for success has been reduction in the frequency of angina and use of nitroglycerin. But based on the observations that the majority of ischaemic episodes are silent and the increasing evidence that silent myocardial ischaemia may be associated with an adverse prognosis in patients with coronary artery disease (20, 21, 42, 46), it seems advisable to abolish not only symptomatic ischaemic episodes but total ischaemic activity.

Beta-adrenoceptor blocking drugs: Several studies have documented the effect of beta-blockers on total ischaemic activity and the results are ho-

Table 2. *Favourable effects of combined treatment with beta-blockers and calcium-blockers.*

I Improved antiischaemic effects.
   1) Decrease in angina frequency and nitroglycerin consumption.
   2) Increased exercise time, time to angina and time to ST-segment depression.
   3) Decreased total ischaemic activity during daily life.
   4) Effective in effort-induced angina and mixed angina.

II Positive haemodynamic profile.
   1) Reduction in reflex tachycardia induced by nifedipine.
   2) Prevention of exercise-induced vasoconstriction.
   3) Reduction of systemic and coronary vascular resistance induced by beta-blockade.
   4) Increased antegrade collateral flow by decreased preload and decreased end-diastolic pressure.

III Reduced side-effects due to lower doses of each drug and possible positive haemodynamic interplay.

mogeneous. Propranolol, atenolol, labetalol and metoprolol (Fig. 4) have all reduced the frequency and duration of all ischaemic episodes (47-52). Although the number of enrolled patients in some of the studies is small, the results are uniform and indicate that beta-receptor blockade is effective in the therapy of total ischaemic activity. The effect seems to be mediated through a reduction in myocardial oxygen demand as the effect parallels the reduction in heart rate (52).

Calcium channel blocking drugs: This group of drugs is more inhomogeneous and the number of studies that have assessed the effect of verapamil and diltiazem are limited, but the existing results indicate that they are effective (53, 54). This is in contrast to the effect of nifedipine where the effect has been variable, as some studies have noted a failing effect or even an increase in the frequency of ischaemia during therapy with nifedipine (47, 52) (Fig. 4). The absence of effect of nifedipine has been ascribed to reflex tachycardia with baromediated increase in plasma catecholamines, but even a coronary steal phenomenon may be of major importance (55).

Combined therapy: The combined treatment with beta-blockers and calcium channel blocking drugs may have an additive effect, as it has been noted for the combination of metoprolol or propranolol and nifedipine (47, 48, 52) and propranolol and verapamil (53, 56), the later combination should be employed with caution, especially in patients with impaired left ventricular function or with constant or intermittent conductive defects (57). The possible favourable effects of combined therapy are shown in Table 2.

Effect on circadian variation: As it has been noted, beta-blockers are effective in reducing total ischaemic activity but it has also been noted during

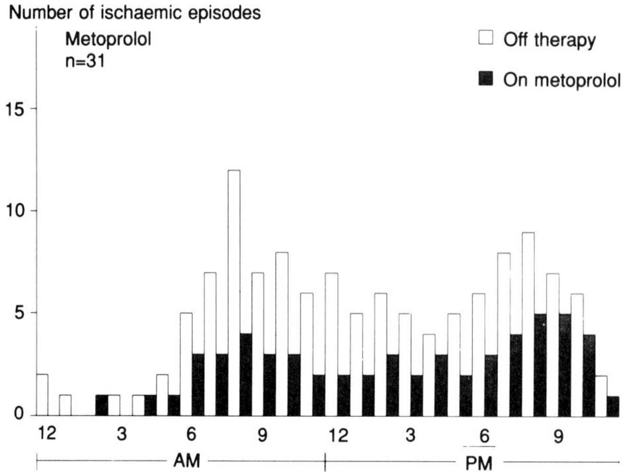

Fig. 5. *Circadian variation of transient ischaemia during therapy with metoprolol.*

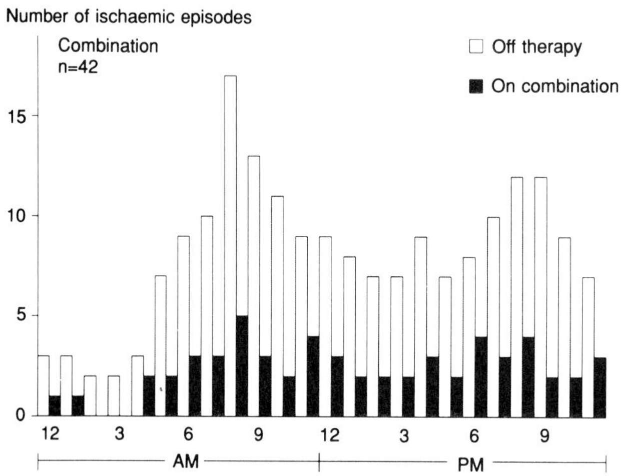

Fig. 6. *Circadian variation of transient ischaemia during combined therapy with metoprolol and nifedipine.*

therapy with metoprolol (51, 58) and atenolol (37), that these drugs are most effective in the morning where the frequency of ischaemia is highest and with attenuation of the morning peak (Fig. 5). The use of nifedipine in monotherapy has not influenced the circadian rhythm (37), whereas combined therapy with metoprolol and nifedipine seems to attenuate both the morning and the evening increase in ischaemic activity (Fig. 6). These observations may have implications for future medical strategy with focus on drugs or combination of drugs with various effects through the day and maximal pharmacologic effect that corresponds to the time of increase in ischaemic activity.

Summary

In the recent years substantial evidence has accumulated, that silent ischaemia in patients with coronary artery disease, as detected by ambulatory monitoring, represents episodes with myocardial ischaemia. Ambulatory monitoring, therefore, provides the possibility of detecting and describing transient ischaemia during daily life in selected patients with coronary artery disease and with this method it has been noted, that the majority of ischaemic episodes are silent, often prolonged and displaying a circadian variation similar to the onset of myocardial infarction and sudden death. The pathophysiology of ambulatory ischaemia seems complex and may change through the day.

With antianginal therapy it has been possible to reduce total ischaemic activity and studies employing beta-adrenoceptor blocking drugs have all been effective, whereas the effect of the calcium channel blocker nifedipine seems variable. Combined therapy may have additional favourable effects. Antiischaemic therapy has shown effect on the circadian variation of transient ischaemia, which may point forward to increased understanding and better therapy of the total ischaemic burden.

References

1. Margolis JR, Kannel WB, Feinleib M, Dawber TR, McNamara PM. Clinical features of unrecognized myocardial infarction – silent and symptomatic. Eighteen year follow-up: The Framingham Study. Am J Cardiol 1973; 32: 1-7.
2. Ellestad MH. Stress Testing: principles and practice. Philadelphia: FA Davis, 1975: 85-176.
3. Wolf E, Tzivoni D, Stern S. Comparison of exercise tests and 24-hour ambulatory electrocardiographic monitoring in detection of ST-T changes. Br Heart J 1974; 36: 90-5.
4. Stern S, Tzivoni D. Early detection of silent ischaemic heart disease by 24-hours electrocardiographic monitoring of active subjects. Br Heart J 1974; 36: 481-6.
5. Stern S, Tzivoni D, Stern Z. Diagnostic accuracy of ambulatory ECG monitoring in ischemic heart disease. Circulation 1975; 52: 1045-9.
6. Maseri A, Mimmo R, Chierchia S, Marchesi C, Pesola A, L'Abbate A. Coronary artery spasm as a cause of acute myocardial ischaemia in man. Chest 1975; 68: 625-33.
7. Chierchia S, Lazzari M, Freedman B, Brunelli C, Maseri A. Impairment of myocardial perfusion and function during painless myocardial ischemia. J Am Coll Cardiol 1983; 1: 924-30.
8. Deanfield JE, Selwyn AP, Chierchia S, et al. Myocardial ischaemia during daily life in patients with stable angina: its relation to symptoms and heart rate changes. Lancet 1983; 2: 753-8.
9. Deanfield JE, Kensett M, Wilson RA, et al. Silent myocardial ischaemia due to mental stress. Lancet 1984; 2: 1001-5.
10. Levy RD, Cunningham D, Shapiro LM, Wright C, Mockus L, Fox KM. Continuous ambulatory pulmonary artery pressure monitoring. A new method using a transducer tipped catheter and a simple recording system. Br Heart J 1986; 55: 336-43.

11. Levy RD, Shapiro LM, Wright C, Mockus L, Fox KM. Haemodynamic response to myocardial ischaemia during unrestricted activity, exercise testing and atrial pacing assessed by ambulatory pulmonary artery pressure monitoring. Br Heart J 1986; 56: 12-8.
12. Holter NJ. New method for heart studies. Science 1961; 134: 1214-20.
13. Chierchia S, Smith G, Morgan M, et al. Role of heart rate in pathophysiology of chronic stable angina. Lancet 1984; 2: 1353-7.
14. Levy RD, Shapiro LM, Wright C, Mockus L, Fox KM. Syndrome X: the haemodynamic significance of ST segment depression. Br Heart J 1986; 56: 353-7.
15. Quyyumi AA, Mockus LJ, Wright CA, Fox KM. Mechanisms of nocturnal angina pectoris: Importance of increased myocardial oxygen demand in patients with severe coronary artery disease. Lancet 1984; 1: 1207-9.
16. Egstrup K. The relationship between ST-segment deviation projected to the front of the chest during exercise and simultaneous Holter monitoring. Eur Heart J 1988; 9: 412-7.
17. Tzivoni D, Benhorin J, Gavish A, Stern S. Holter recording during treadmill testing in assessing myocardial ischemic changes. Am J Cardiol 1985; 55: 1200-3.
18. Quyyumi AA, Crake T, Mockus LJ, Wright CA, Rickards AF, Fox KM. Value of the bipolar lead CM5 in electrocardiography. Br Heart J 1986; 56: 372-6.
19. Eriksen J, Enge J, Forfang K, Storstein O. Falsepositive diagnostic tests and coronary angiographic findings in 105 persumably healthy males. Circulation 1976; 54: 371-6.
20. Eriksen J, Thaulow E. Follow-up of patients with asymptomatic myocardial ischemia. In: Rutishauser W, Roskamm H, eds. Silent myocardial ischemia. Berlin: Springer-Verlag, 1984: 156-64.
21. Mickley H, Pless P, Egstrup K, Rokkedal J, Møller M. Silent ischemia is a predictor of severe angina pectoris after first myocardial infarction. (Abstr). Eur Heart J 1988; 9: 314.
22. Cohn PF. Prognosis and treatment of asymptomatic coronary artery disease. J Am Coll Cardiol 1983; 1: 959-64.
23. Egstrup K. Transient myocardial ischaemia during ambulatory monitoring out of hospital in patients with chronic stable angina pectoris. Acta Med Scand 1988; 224: 311-8.
24. Quyyumi AA, Wright CA, Mockus LJ, Fox KM. How important is a history of chest pain in determining the degree of ischaemia in patients with angina pectoris? Br Heart J 1985; 54: 22-6.
25. Schang SJ, Pepine CJ. Transient asymptomatic ST segment depression during daily activity. Am J Cardiol 1977; 39: 396-402.
26. Egstrup K. The sensitivity of the symptom angina pectoris as a marker of transient myocardial ischaemia in chronic stable angina. Acta Med Scand 1987; 222: 301-6.
27. Campbell S, Barry J, Rebecca GS, et al. Active transient myocardial ischemia during daily life in asymptomatic patients with positive exercise tests and coronary artery disease. Am J Cardiol 1986; 57: 1010-6.
28. Carboni GP, Lahiri A, Cashman P, Raftery EB. Ambulatory heart rate and ST-segment depression during painful and silent myocardial ischemia in chronic stable angina pectoris. Am J Cardiol 1987; 59: 1029-34.
29. Deanfield JE, Shea MJ, Wilson RA, Horlock P, de Landsheere CM, Selwyn AP. Direct effects of smoking on the heart: silent ischemic disturbances of coronary flow. Am J Cardiol 1986; 57: 1005-9.
30. Davies AB, Bala Subramanian V, Cashman P, Raftery EB. Simultaneous recording of continuous arterial pressure, heart rate, and ST segment in ambulant patients with stable angina pectoris. Br Heart J 1983; 50: 85-91.
31. Lee DD, Kimura S, DeQuattro V. Noradrenergic activity and silent ischaemia in hypertensive patients with stable angina pectoris: Effect of metoprolol. Lancet 1989; 1: 403-6.

32. Griffith TM, Edwards DH, Collins P, Lewis MJ, Henderson AH. Endothelium derived relaxant factor. J Royal Coll Phys Lond 1985; 19: 74-9.
33. Gage JE, Hess OM, Murakani T, Ritter M, Grimm J, Krayenbuehi HP. Vasoconstriction of stenotic coronary arteries during dynamic exercise in patients with classic angina pectoris: reversibility by nitroglycerin. Circulation 1986; 73: 865-76.
34. Muller JE, Stone PH, Turi ZG, et al. Milis Study Group. Circadian variation in the frequency of onset of acute myocardial infarction. N Engl J Med 1985; 21: 1315-22.
35. Ludmer PL, Alymer GZ, Muller JE. Circadian variation of sudden cardiac death. J Am Coll Cardiol 1986; 7: 209 A.
36. Rocco MB, Barry J, Campbell S, et al. Circadian variation of transient myocardial ischemia in patients with coronary artery disease. Circulation 1987; 75: 395-400.
37. Mulcahy D, Cunningham D, Crean P, et al. Circadian variation of total ischaemic burden and its alteration with antianginal agents. Lancet 1988; 2: 755-9.
38. Turton NB, Deegan T. Circadian variations of plasma catecholamines, cortisol, and immunoreactive insulin concentrations in supine subjects. Clin Chim Acta 1974; 55: 389-97.
39. Tofler GH, Buzinski D, Schafer AI, et al. Concurrent morning increase in platelet aggregability and the risk of myocardial infarction and sudden cardiac death. N Engl J Med 1987; 316: 1514-8.
40. Millar-Graig MW, Biskop CN, Raftery EB. Circadian variation of blood pressure. Lancet 1971; 1: 795-7.
41. Fugita M, Fraklin D. Diurnal changes in coronary blood flow in conscious dogs. Circulation 1987; 76: 488-91.
42. Egstrup K. Asymptomatic myocardial ischemia as a predictor of cardiac events after coronary artery bypass grafting for stable angina pectoris. Am J Cardiol 1988; 61: 248-52.
43. Gottlieb SO, Weisfeldt ML, Ouyang P, Mellitz ED, Gerstenblith G. Silent ischemia as a marker for early unfavorable outcomes in patients with unstable angina. N Engl J Med 1986; 314: 1214-9.
44. Nadamee K, Intarachot V, Josephson M, Rieders D, Mody F, Singh B. Prognostic significance of silent myocardial ischemia in patients with unstable angina. J Am Coll Cardiol 1987; 10: 1-9.
45. Rocco M, Nabel E, Campbell S, et al. Prognostic importance of myocardial ischemia detected by ambulatory monitoring in patients with stable coronary artery disease. Circulation 1988; 78: 877-84.
46. Tzivoni D, Weisz G, Gavish A, Zin D, Keren A, Stern S. Comparison of mortality and myocardial infarction rates in stable angina pectoris with or without ischemic episodes during daily activities. Am J Cardiol 1989; 63: 273-6.
47. Egstrup K. Effects of metoprolol, nifedipine and their combination on total ischemic activity in effort and mixed angina. A randomized double-blind study. Am J Noninvas Cardiol 1989; 3: 290-6.
48. Lynch P, Dargie H, Krikler S, Krikler D. Objective assessment of antianginal treatment: a double-blind comparison of propranolol, nifedipine, and their combination. Br Med J 1980; 2: 184-7.
49. Quyyumi AA, Wright C, Mockus L, Fox KM. Effect of partial agonist activity in beta-blockers in severe angina pectoris. Br Med J 1984; 2: 951-3.
50. Quyyumi AA, Wright C, Mockus L, Shackell M, Sutton GC, Fox KM. Effects of combined alpha and beta adrenoceptor blockade in patients with angina pectoris. A double-blind study comparing labetalol with placebo. Br Heart J 1985; 53: 47-52.
51. Imperi GA, Lambert CR, Coy K, Lopez L, Pepine CJ. Effects of titrated beta blockade

(metoprolol) on silent myocardial ischemia in ambulatory patients with coronary artery disease. Am J Cardiol 1987; 60: 519-24.

52. Egstrup K. Randomized double-blind comparison of metoprolol, nifedipine and their combination in chronic stable angina. Effects on total ischemic activity and heart rate at onset of ischemia. Am Heart J 1988; 116: 971-8.
53. Bala Subramanian V, Bowles MJ, Davies AB, Raftery EB. Combined therapy with verapamil and propranolol in chronic stable angina. Am J Cardiol 1982; 49: 125-32.
54. Bala Subramanian V, Bowles MJ, Khurmi NS, Davies AB, Raftery EB. Randomized double-blind comparison of verapamil and nifedipine in chronic stable angina. Am J Cardiol 1982; 50: 696-703.
55. Schulz W, Jost S, Kober G, Kaltenbach M. Relation of antianginal efficacy of nifedipine to degree of coronary arterial narrowing and to presence of coronary collaterals vessels. Am J Cardiol 1985; 55: 26-32.
56. Johnson SM, Mauritson DR, Corbett JR, Woodward W, Willerson JT, Hillis LD. Doubleblind, randomized, placebocontrolled comparison of propranolol and verapamil in the treatment of patients with stable angina pectoris. Am J Med 1981; 71: 443-51.
57. Reddy PS, Kritsky BF, Steinfeld M. The hemodynamic effects of intravenous verapamil in patients on chronic propranolol therapy. Am Heart J 1984; 107: 97-101.
58. Willich SN, Pohjola-Sintonen S, Bhatia S, et al. Suppression of silent ischemia by metoprolol without alteration of morning increase of platelet aggregability in patients with stable coronary artery disease. Circulation 1989; 79: 557-65.

17

Prognostic significance of silent ischaemia

J. ERIKSSEN,
E. THAULOW,
G. ERIKSSEN

Notwithstanding different pathophysiologic mechanisms silent ischaemia (SI) is observed in a high proportion of the population as indicated in Table 1.

When myocardial perfusion pressure for various reasons falls below 50-55 mmHg, subendocardial perfusion becomes inadequate and anaerobic metabolism is initiated (2), followed rapidly by a cascade of biochemical and functional myocardial aberrations. Provided the ischaemic stimulus is sufficiently severe, prolonged and extensive these functional aberrations may be sufficiently severe to give rise to clinically significant symptoms and signs. However, during the progression of ischaemia, pain is a relatively late clin-

Table 1. *Groups of subjects among whom SI is detected.*

1. Totally asymptomatic subjects in whom the exercise – ECG (or other tests) indicates the presence of ischaemic heart disease (Cohn type I)*).
2a. Subjects with a previous, known MI in whom signs of ischaemia are elicited e.g. during an exercise test in the absence of angina pectoris (Cohn type II)*).
2b. Apparently normal subjects in whom at least one routine ECG is normal prior to the development of unequivocal signs of MI in subsequent routine ECGs, provided no symptoms between the last normal and the first pathologic ECG suggest the presence of an acute episode of MI.
3. Subjects with clinical angina pectoris in whom episodes of SI are detected (Cohn type III)*).
4. Previously asymptomatic subjects who are successfully resuscitated after circulatory arrest, who are asymptomatic afterwards but present objective signs of SI during e.g. stress testing or Holter monitoring.
5. Subjects awaiting major surgery for e.g. peripheral atherothrombotic disease or heart valve surgery in whom routine testing (performed because of high surgical risk) reveals SI.

*) Classification according to *Cohn* (1).

Table 2. *Some methods used for detecting myocardial ischaemia.*

A: Invasive methods (with/without pharmacologic interventions)

During rest/exercise/ambulatory/pacing: – Right/left heart catheterization with pressure monitoring
- Coronary sinus catheterization (measurement of lactate, etc.)
- Contrast ventriculography
- Intracardiac ECG registration

B: Noninvasive methods: (with/without pharmacologic intervention)
- Magnetic resonance
- Positron emission tomography
- Thallium scintigraphy
- Echocardiography (rest and exercise or dipyridamol stress testing)
- Electrokymography/cardiokymography
- Holter monitoring
- Resting/exercise ECG testing
- Others

C: Combined methods from A and/or B

ical event, almost invariably preceded by detectable functional aberrations as shown with a variety of invasive and non-invasive techniques.

As long as symptoms of angina – or angina equivalents – are absent, SI is said to be present if other tests (Table 2) signify the presence of ischaemia. Among these tests some data have recently been published on the value of using e.g. echocardiography to detect SI (3-5), but the bulk of the evidence about the significance of SI is derived from stress ECG-testing, Holter monitoring and thallium 201 scintigraphy.

In the present synopsis the main emphasis therefore will be paid to data derived from exercise testing, Holter monitoring and thallium 201 scintigraphy. Patients with SI were divided into 5 groups. Detailed data on subjects from groups 4 and 5 in Table 1 are almost non-existent, and the discussion will therefore focus on current knowledge about subjects belonging to subgroups 1, 2a, 2b and 3.

Silent ischaemia in totally asymptomatic subjects

Numerous studies in apparently healthy subjects have documented the negative prognostic impact of a positive exercise ECG stress test (6-11). However, considering all confounding variables which can cause significant ST-depression in the absence of true ischaemia (12), the lack of validation of the positive stress tests in these population studies makes it difficult to assess the true prevalence and significance of SI in asymptomatic subjects.

Only a few groups of investigators have applied coronary angiography to validate a positive stress test in asymptomatic subjects and these limited studies have emphasized the high number of false positive stress tests among asymptomatic subjects (13-15).

Available follow-up data suggest that SI detected during exercise testing in middle aged men carries an adverse prognosis (6, 7, 17). After an observation period of 13 years in one study the relative risk of cardiac morbidity and mortality was increased three to four fold in subjects with true SI as compared to apparently healthy age counterparts with a negative exercise stress test (18).

Similar findings are observed in a 4-5 year follow-up study of healthy volunteers participating in a screening programme at John Hopkins Hospital (19); 407 subjects underwent both a symptom-limited treadmill exercise ECG test and Thallium 201 stress test. Subjects with both tests positive had a 7-fold increased relative risk of developing a coronary event during a period of 4 1/2 years compared to subjects with both tests negative (19). Subjects with one test positive had an intermediately increased risk. Since subjects who have both a positive exercise ECG and thallium test very probably have coronary artery disease (CAD), these data strongly support the limited angiographic studies mentioned above.

This notion is further corroborated in a recently published study from Malmø (20). In this study routine 24 hours Holter monitoring showed a high frequency of positive Holter tracings among subjects aged 68 years. The short term prognostic impact of a positive Holter finding was very grave in this community based study (20).

Thus, in the absence of decisive studies we have to conclude from the limited available experience that SI significantly increases the risk of cardiac morbidity and mortality when encountered in asymptomatic middle aged and old subjects.

Silent ischaemia in patients with a previous myocardial infarction (MI)

Although the best risk stratification of patients with a previous MI can be made from knowledge of the extent of myocardial damage and of angiographically verified coronary atheromathosis, knowledge of whether or not SI is present or absent adds important information (21-26).

As noted in Table 1 an ECG-proven MI may have been clinically recognized or not. Although patients who have unequivocal signs of MI in the ECG do not necessarily have SI at the time they are investigated, one can at least conclude confidently that they must have had a severe episode of

SI when their asymptomatic MI developed. It may therefore be of interest to compare the prognosis in subjects without clinical as compared to those with a symptomatic MI.

Long term epidemiological studies have unequivocally shown that a considerable number of apparently healthy subjects develop ECG signs of MI which have escaped clinical detection, and hence is only detected on routine ECG recordings (21, 27). In fact experience from e.g. the Framingham study has suggested that approximately one third of ECG proven MI's are clinically undetected, and that one half of these are completely silent clinically (21, 27). It has further been shown that the long term prognosis in such subjects is almost identical to that of subjects with clinically recognized MI (21, 27). ECG signs of a previous, asymptomatic MI should therefore give rise to similar therapeutic considerations as in symptomatic subjects, all factors equal. Or rephrased: A silent episode of MI appears to be as malignant as a clinical episode.

A host of diagnostic techniques have been used to assess the prognosis in patients with a recent, clinically diagnosed MI. Of the tests used to detect various aberrations caused by myocardial ischaemia, exercise testing, thallium 201 scintigraphy, Holter monitoring and isotope-ventriculography are the most popular and widely used. The majority of prognostic data, however, which aim at searching for post MI silent ischaemia are related to exercise test and Holter monitoring findings. Both tests indicate that individuals with positive stress tests and positive Holter findings – regardless of whether or not they have symptoms – have far poorer prognosis than patients without these findings (22-26). Less is known about the long term significance of other tests searching for signs of ischaemia post MI.

On average, the risk of dying within one year increases by a factor of three among subjects with exercise induced ST-depression compared with subjects without (22-26). Limited experience with Holter monitoring and thallium 201 scintigraphy are in agreement with these stress test-findings (28-30).

As a conclusion, patients with asymptomatic MI's have as poor a prognosis as patients with symptomatic MI's. In the latter, the presence of SI observed during exercise ECG stress testing, thallium scintigraphy and Holter monitoring worsen the prognosis significantly at least in the year following the tests.

Silent ischaemia in patients with angina pectoris

It is well known that patients with clinical angina may often have a positive exercise ECG stress test without angina. Moreover, in those in whom the test finally is terminated because of angina, significant ST depression often precedes the development of angina by minutes.

Holter monitoring has drastically changed out concept of the pathophysiologic mechanisms involved in the development of myocardial ischaemia during daily life. It has for instance been shown convincingly that 2/3 to 3/4 of episodes of ST-depression are observed during periods when the patient is totally unaware of the presence of ischaemia (31). Although symptomatic ischaemic episodes are, on average, of moderately longer duration, are slightly more pronounced and involve more myocardial mass (as evidenced by both invasive and noninvasive ambulatory monitoring) (32-34), a very wide overlap exists in pathophysiologic aberrations during symptomatic and asymptomatic episodes (32-34). Holter monitoring has shown that the increase in heart rate and blood pressure during spontaneous symptomatic and asymptomatic ischaemia is modest when compared to that observed when ischaemia is elicited by stress testing (31). This suggests that many ischaemic episodes during daily life are caused by a decrease in oxygen supply rather than to an increased oxygen demand. Vasomotion (read: intermittent vasospasm) is thought to be responsible for this phenomenon. This explanation seems plausible in view of the well-known reaction of atheromatotic vessels to various stimuli (2). Thus, a host of physiologic stimuli may cause vascular spasm in slightly/moderately diseased coronary vessels, even when such stimuli elicit a vasodilatory response in normal vessels (2). Regardless of the mechanisms involved, SI detected during Holter monitoring and stress testing adversely affects the prognosis in subjects with stable angina (31, 35, 38). In a recent study, the great majority of cardiac events took place among subjects with positive Holter findings whereas subjects with only a positive stress test had a far better prognosis (35). A positive Holter test may therefore be a more ominous sign than a positive stress ECG test only. (It is well known that some 60% of subjects with a positive stress test have a positive Holter test, and it has been suggested that very few subjects with a negative stress test have a positive Holter test) (31).

A special case relates to patients with unstable angina pectoris. ECG monitoring of such subjects during their stay in the coronary care unit reveals that a sizeable proportion of such patients have prolonged periods with severe but SI (39-42). Such patients – even when completely asymptomatic – have a far poorer prognosis than those without SI (39-42). Moreover, the longer the periods of ischaemia, the worse the prognosis (42). Similar findings have been suggested by others (41).

Conclusion

SI detected with conventional stress ECG testing and Holter monitoring carries a poor prognosis when encountered both in subjects with angina pectoris and unstable angina pectoris.

Implications

In view of the severe aberrations in cardiac physiology observed both during prolonged periods of both symptomatic and asymptomatic ischaemia (31, 34), it has been suggested that treatment should be aimed not only at reducing symptoms, but at alleviating all ischaemic episodes ("total ischaemic burden") (27, 43, 44). The mere focusing on symptomatic treatment of angina pectoris is probably outdated.

Although information on the significance of SI is rapidly expanding in patients with known coronary heart disease (angina and previous MI), knowledge of the prevalence, incidence and significance of SI in the asymptomatic population is only slowly emerging. Moreover, follow up data from studies using techniques other than stress testing, Holter monitoring and thallim-scintigraphy are only beginning to emerge.

The resource problem related to screening for SI in the asymptomatic population has recently attained considerable attention. Most investigators seem to favour the view that cost-effectiveness is low when conventional techniques are applied in asymptomatic populations with an estimated low prevalence of advanced CAD (6, 7, 45, 46). However, more research is needed to be able to provide guide-lines for when and how to search for SI in asymptomatic subjects.

References

1. Cohn PF. Asymptomatic coronary artery disease: Pathophysiology, diagnosis, management. Mod Concepts Cardiovasc Dis 1981; 50: 55-60.
2. Brown BG, Smith BH. Regulation of myocardial perfusion in ischemic heart disease. Role of dynamic coronary stenosis. In: Singh BN, ed. Silent myocardial ischemia and angina. New York: Pergamon Press, 1988: 16-27.
3. Armstrong WF. Echocardiography in coronary artery disease. Prog Cardiovasc Dis 1988; 30: 267.
4. Jaarsma W, Visser CA, van Eenig MJ, et al. Prognostic implications of regional hypokinesia and remote asynergia of noninfarcted myocardium. Am J Cardiol 1986; 58: 394-8.
5. Picano E, Severt S, Michelassi C, et al. Prognostic importance of dipyridamole-echocardiography in coronary artery disease. Circulation 1989; 80: 450-7.

6. Sox HC. Exercise testing in suspected coronary artery disease. Dis Month 1985; 31: 3-93.
7. Froelicher VF, Duarte GM, Oakes DF, Klein J, Dubach PA, Janosi A. The prognostic value of the exercise test. Dis Month 1988; 34: 677-735.
8. Falcone C, de Servi S, Poma E. Clinical significance of exercise-induced silent ischemia in patients with coronary artery disease. J Am Coll Cardiol 1987; 9: 295-9.
9. Bonow RO, Bacharach SL, Green MV, LA Freniere RL, Epstein SE. Prognostic implications of symptomatic versus asymptomatic (silent) myocardial ischemia by exercise in mildly symptomatic and asymptomatic patients with angiographically documented coronary artery disease. Am J Cardiol 1987; 50: 778-83.
10. Assei ME, Walters GL, Dendrikx GH, Carabello BA, Usher BW, Spann JF jr. Incidence of acute myocardial infarction in patients with exercise-induced silent myocardial ischemia. Am J Cardiol 1987; 59: 497-500.
11. Mark DB, Hlatky MA, Califf RM. Painless exercise ST-deviation on the treadmill: Long term prognosis. J Am Coll Cardiol 1989; 14: 885-92.
12. Erikssen J, Myhre E. False positive exercise tests: A misnomer? Int J Cardiol 1984; 6: 263-8.
13. Froelicher VF, Yanowitz FG, Thompson AL. The correlation of coronary angiography and electrocardiographic response to maximal treadmill response in 76 asymptomatic men. Circulation 1973; 48: 597-604.
14. Borer JS, Bensike JF, Redwood DR, et al. Limitation of the electrocardiographic response to exercise in predicting coronary artery disease. N Engl J Med 1975; 293: 367-72.
15. Erikssen J, Enge I, Forfang K, Storstein O. False positive diagnostic tests and coronary angiographic findings in 105 presumably healthy males. Circulation 1976; 54: 371-6.
16. Erikssen J. Prognostic value of silent ischaemia during long-term follow-up of patients with coronary artery disease. Hertz 1987; 12: 359-68.
17. Erikssen J, Cohn PF, Thaulow E, Mowinkel P. Silent myocardial ischaemia in middle-aged men. Long term clinical course. In: Arnim Th v., Maseri A, eds. Silent ischaemia. Current concepts and management. Darmstadt: Steinkopf Verlag, 1987: 45-51.
18. Erikssen J, Thaulow E, Cohn PF. Long term prognostic of fifty totally asymptomatic middle-aged men with silent myocardial ischemia and angiographically documented coronary artery disease. (Abstract). Circulation 1987; 76 (suppl 9): 77.
19. Fleg JL, Gerstenblith G, Zonderman AB, et al. Prevalence and prognostic significance of exercise-induced silent myocardial ischemia detected by thallium scintigraphy and electrocardiography in asymptomatic volunteers. Circulation 1990; 81: In press.
20. Hedblad B, Juul Møller S, Swensson K, et al. Increased mortality in men with ST-segment depression during 24h ambulatory long-term ECG recording: Results from prospective population study "Men born in 1914" from Malmø, Sweden. Eur Heart J 1989; 10: 149-58.
21. Kannel WB, Cupples LA. Silent myocardial infarction. In: Singh BN, ed. Silent myocardial ischemia and angina. New York: Pergamon Press, 1988: 174-82.
22. Theroux P, Wates DD, Halphen C, Debasiex CC, Mizzala HF. Prognostic value of exercise testing after myocardial infarction. N Engl J Med 1979; 301: 341-5.
23. Davidsen DM, Debusk R. Prognostic value of a single exercise test 3 weeks after an uncomplicated myocardial infarction. Circulation 1980; 61: 236-42.
24. Jespersen CM, Kassis E, Edeling CJ. The prognostic value of maximal exercise testing soon after myocardial infarction. Eur Heart J 1985; 6: 769-72.
25. Krone RJ, Gillespie JA, Wild FM, Miller JP, Moss AJ. Low level exercise testing after myocardial infarction: Usefulness in enhancing clinical risk stratification. Circulation 1985; 71: 80-9.

26. Weiner DA. Predischarge exercise testing after myocardial infarction. Prognostic and therapeutic features. Cardiovasc Clin 1985; 15: 95-104.
27. Kannel WB. Detection and management of patients with silent myocardial ischemia. Am Heart J 1989; 117: 221-6.
28. Deedwania PC. Silent myocardial ischaemia and its relationship to acute myocardial infarction. Cardiol Clin 1986; 4: 643-58.
29. Hung J, Goris ML, Nash E, et al. Comparative value of maximal treadmill testing, exercise thallium myocardial perfusion scintigraphy and exercise radionuclide ventriculography for distinguishing high and low risk patients soon after myocardial infarction. Am J Cardiol 1984; 53: 1221-7.
30. Gibson RS, Watson DD, Craddock GB. Prediction of cardiac events after uncomplicated myocardial infarction: A prospective study comparing predischarge exercise thallium – 201 scintigraphy and coronary angiography. Circulation 1983; 68: 321-36.
31. Deanfield J. Characteristics of silent and symptomatic ischemia in chronic stable angina. Comparison with unstable and vasospastic angina. In: Singh BN, ed. Silent myocardial ischemia and angina. New York: Pergamon Press, 1988: 104-11.
32. Chierchia S, Lazzasi M, Freedman MB, Brunelli C, Maseri A. Impairment of myocardial perfusion and function during painless myocardial ischemia. J Am Coll Cardiol 1983; 1: 924-30.
33. Hirtzel HO, Leutwyler R, Krayenbuhl HP. Silent myocardial ischemia: Hemodynamic changes during dynamic exercise in patients with proven coronary artery disease despite absence of angina pectoris. J Am Coll Cardiol 1985; 6: 275-84.
34. Levy R, Shapiro LM, Mochus L, Fox K. The hemodynamic significance of asymptomatic ST-depression assessed by ambulatory pulmonary artery monitoring. Br Heart J 1986; 56: 526-30.
35. Ricco MB, Nabel EG, Cambell S, et al. Prognostic importance of myocardial ischemia detected by amulatory monitoring in patients with stable coronary artery disease. Circulation 1988; 78: 877-84.
36. Weiner DA, Ryan TJ, Mc Cabe CH, et al. Prognostic importance of a clinical profile and exercise test in medically treated patients with coronary artery disease. J Am Coll Cardiol 1984; 3: 722-9.
37. Bonow RO, Kent KM, Rosing SR, et al. Exercise induced ischemia and preserved left ventricular function. N Engl J Med 1984; 311: 1339-45.
38. Tzivoni D, Weiss G, Gavish A, Lin D, Keren A, Stern S. Comparison of mortality and myocardial infarction in stable angina pectoris with and without ischemic episodes during daily activities. Am J Cardiol 1989; 63: 223-6.
39. Johnson SM, Mauritson DS, Winniford MD, et al. Continous electrocardiographic monitoring in patients with unstable angina pectoris. Identification of high risk subgroup with severe coronary disease, variant angina and/or impaired early prognosis. Am Heart J 1982; 103: 4-16.
40. Nademanee K, Interachot V, Piontek M, Mody FV, Josephson MA, Singh BN. Silent myocardial ischaemia on Holter: Has it clinical significance? Circulation 1984; 70(suppl III): 452.
41. Nademanee K, Interachot V, Josephson MA, Rieders D, Mody FV, Singh BN. Prognostic significance of silent myocardial ischemia in patients with unstable angina pectoris. J Am Coll Cardiol 1987; 10: 1-9.
42. Gottlieb SO, Weisfeldt ML, Ouyand P, Mellits ED, Gerstenblith G. Silent ischemia as marker for early infavourable outcomes in patients with unstable angina. N Engl J Med 1986; 314: 1214-9.
43. Kowalchuk GJ, Nesto RW. Silent ischemia. Mechanisms and rationale for therapy. Am J Med 1989; 86 (suppl IA): 9-13.

44. Cohn PF. Total ischemic burden. Implications for prognosis and therapy. Am J Med 1989; 86 (suppl IA): 6-8.
45. Cohn PF. Clinical importance of silent myocardial ischemia in asymptomatic subjects. Circulation 1990; 81: In press.
46. Sox HC, Littenberg B, Garber AM. The role of exercise testing in screening for coronary artery disease. Ann Int Med 1989; 110: 456-69.

18

Acute chest pain and prognostic aspects

JAN KYST MADSEN

Admissions to coronary care units (CCU) are primarily due to acute chest pain. In almost all cases, the main suspicion is acute myocardial infarction (AMI) or at least a suspicion strong enough to justify an admission, so that AMI may be ruled out.

However, to have AMI or not to have AMI is not the only aspect of acute chest pain. There are several diagnostic possibilities in patients without AMI, e.g., unstable angina pectoris, stable angina pectoris, non-cardiac chest pain or cardiac pain of non-coronary origin (1-7). The prognosis during admission and following discharge varies considerably depending on the diagnosis.

The purpose of the present chapter is to describe the diagnostic possibilities and the prognosis after discharge of these subgroups, and further to outline the clinical consequences.

Acute myocardial infarction

Acute myocardial infarction is the final diagnosis in approximately one half of all admitted patients. This proportion may vary from institution to institution, but seems rather constant in hospitals in the Western world. The diagnosis is based on changes in coronary enzymes and ECG and despite minor differences the diagnostic criteria are internationally accepted.

The in-hospital mortality in AMI patients is 10-15%, and the one year mortality is 5-10%. The mortality, however, is falling with the increased use of medical intervention e.g., thrombolysis, beta-blockers, calcium antagonists and ACE inhibitors. Mechanical intervention with coronary by-pass surgery or PTCA has so far not shown any reduction in mortality or reinfarction following AMI.

Table 1. *Non-cardiac and non-coronary causes of chest pain in 975 patients admitted due to suspicion of AMI (6).*

Non-cardiac cause of chest pain		59
Pneumonia/pleuritis	12	
Pulmonary embolism	18	
Duodenal or ventricular ulcer	7	
Back pain	7	
Gall bladder stones	1	
Others	14	
Non-coronary cause of chest pain		51
Pericarditis	8	
Valve diseases	3	
Congenital heart diseases	3	
Cardiac arrhythmias	31	
Others	6	

Non-cardiac chest pain

A non-cardiac cause of chest pain is found in 5-20 % of CCU admissions (2-7). This proportion and the diagnosis is dependent on how extensively the patients are examined for a non-cardiac cause of chest pain. There are no available systematic examinations of the various organ systems that may cause chest pain. Routine observations usually identify pulmonary inflammation and embolism as the most common cause (6) (Table 1). Specific studies of esophageal diseases (8-10) or the thoracic facet syndrome (11) indicate that these entities may account for the chest pain in a considerable number of patients, which of course has therapeutic consequences. Other diagnoses include shingles, Tietze's syndrome, cervical radiculitis and aorta dissection. The latter being very important because of the consequences.

The overall mortality in patients with non-cardiac cause of chest pain, following discharge, is low (Table 2). However, the functional status after one or two years, or the prognosis in relation to the specific diagnosis is unknown. Further studies of the benefit of e.g., pulmonary scintigraphy, lung function tests, oesophagoscopy, oesophagus manometry, acid perfusion tests or physical examination of musculo-skeletal structures are underway to clarify the need of routine examinations.

Cardiac non-coronary chest pain

The majority of these patients have arrhythmias as the primary cause of chest pain (6, 7). Other diagnoses include cardiomyopathies, valve diseases

Table 2. *Standardized mortality rate* after one year in patients admitted due to suspicion of AMI, in whom this was not confirmed.*

Non-cardiac chest pain	1.5
Non-coronary chest pain	4.1
Coronary or possible coronary chest pain	3.1

* Standardized mortality rate is the number of observed deaths divided by the number of expected deaths in a population with the same age and sex distribution.

Table 3. *Prognosis one year after discharge in patients admitted with chest pain, without a non-cardiac or non-coronary cause of chest pain, i.e. patients with coronary or possible coronary chest pain.*

	Mortality	AMI morbidity	AMI or cardiac death
Dussia (1)	10%	–	–
Nordlander (2)	19%	7%	–
Madsen (3)	12%	–	–
Engby (4)	16%	10%	–
Madsen (5)	5%	7%	9%

or pericarditis (Table 1). As for the non-cardiac causes of chest pain, no studies with, for instance, consecutive echocardiography for diagnostic purposes have been performed. It is, however, likely that most non-coronary cardiac causes of chest pain are diagnosed, especially as the physicians in the CCUs already concentrate their attention on the heart.

The overall prognosis is poor (Table 2). This is to be expected as this category includes patients with valve diseases and cardiomyopathies. A study of the prognosis in relation to the specific diagnosis has not been performed.

Unstable angina pectoris

Unstable angina is usually defined as angina at rest with or without transient ST or T changes without development of Q waves or significant enzymatic changes.

Approximately 10% of unstable angina patients develops AMI or die during admission despite intensive treatment (12, 13). The treatment usually includes i.v. nitroglycerine, beta-blockers, calcium antagonists, long acting nitrates, aspirin, thrombolysis and in resistent cases coronary by-pass surgery or PTCA.

The risk of AMI or death one year after discharge is 10-20 % (5, 12, 13). Considerations regarding treatment are dealt with in the following paragraphs.

Angina or possible angina pectoris

This category includes several subgroups of patients who, without further examinations may be more or less distinguishable on discharge:

* patients with unstable angina pectoris that has been stabilized during admission
* patients with stable angina pectoris prior to admission for chest pain, but without unstable angina
* patients with previous AMI but no history of angina prior to or on admission, and no unstable angina during admission
* patients with no history of angina or AMI prior to admission with chest pain and no unstable angina during admission.

The risk of AMI or cardiac death one year after discharge in the entire patient population is between 9 and 20 % (1-5) (Table 3) (Fig. 1) and emphasizes the need of a closer examination of these patients.

It is important to emphasize that the impaired prognosis is not only due to a high proportion of patients with unstable angina. In one study (5) of

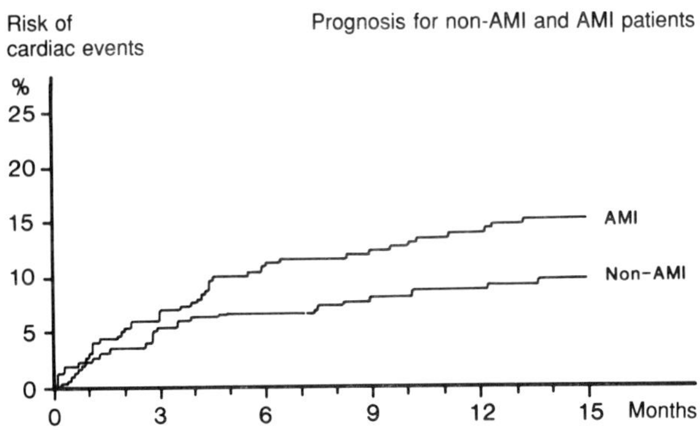

Fig. 1. *Risk of AMI or cardiac death in patients with confirmed AMI and patients without confirmed AMI and no non-cardiac or cardiac non-coronary cause of chest pain i.e. patients with coronary or possible coronary chest pain (non-AMI) (p=0.05) (5).*

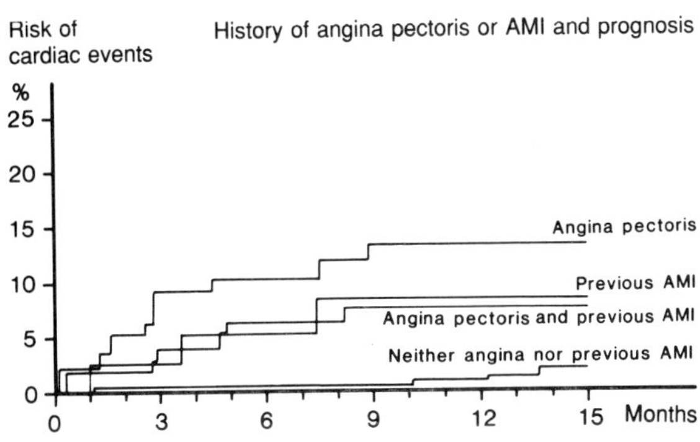

Fig. 2. *Risk of AMI or cardiac death following discharge, in relation to medical history (p=0.001) (5). The figure shows the risk in a Cox model including* normal *ST segment and T wave on admission only.*

Table 4. *History of ischaemic heart disease in patients admitted with chest pain, without AMI and with coronary or possible coronary chest pain.*

	Previous AMI	Angina pectoris
Dussia (1)	46%	–
Nordlander (2)	34%	69 %
Madsen (3)	29%	33 %
Engby (4)	38%	75 %
Madsen (5)	25%	36 %

Table 5. *Results of non-invasive investigations in patients admitted with chest pain, without AMI and with coronary or possible coronary chest pain (6, 15, 16).*

ECG at rest n=217	
Q wave	13%
Negative T wave	30%
ST depression	11%
Any abnormality	37%
Exercise ECG n=215	
ST depression	20%
Abnormal ST response	27%
Angina during exercise	23%
ECG, rest or exercise	
Abnormal at rest, during exercise or both	45%
Thallium scintigraphy n=158	
Persistent defect	30%
Transient defect	18%
Holter monitoring n=198	
Premature ventricular beats	65%
Pairs of PVBs	10%
Chest X-ray n=215	
Cardiomegaly	41%
Echocardiography n=136	
Mitral-septal separation >5mm	27%

257 patients, 14% had unstable angina, and accounted for only 23% of all later cases of AMI or cardiac death. This indicates that patients with unstable angina are not the only high-risk group.

A history of ischaemic heart disease is found in about one half of all patients (1-5). This proportion varies with age. In studies including elderly patients, more tend to have a history of AMI or angina. Other factors such as local admission practice and prevalence of coronary heart disease, probably have influence also.

Non-invasive investigations before discharge confirm that approximately 50% of patients have ischaemic heart disease (Table 5) (5, 6, 15, 16).

The prognosis is closely related to signs of ischaemic heart disease (Table 6). In figures 2 and 3 are shown the increased risk of AMI or cardiac death in relation to a history of AMI or angina (5) and to transient defects on thallium scintigraphy (16), respectively.

Multivariate analysis of variables including medical history, gender and ECG on admission identify two variables with independent, significant, prognostic information (5): a) previous AMI, angina or both, b) permanent or transient ST or T changes or intraventricular block on admission.

Multivariate analysis including results of non-invasive investigations and medical history, identify one variable with independent, significant, prognostic information, i.e., the combination of ECG at rest and during exercise. The risk of cardiac events was increased by a factor 12 in patients with an abnormal ECG at rest (Q wave, ST elevation or depression, negative T wave or intraventricular block) or an abnormal ST response during exercise, or both (Fig. 4) (15).

The variables in the latter multivariate analysis included a history of angina or previous AMI, ST-T abnormalities on admission, any abnormal-

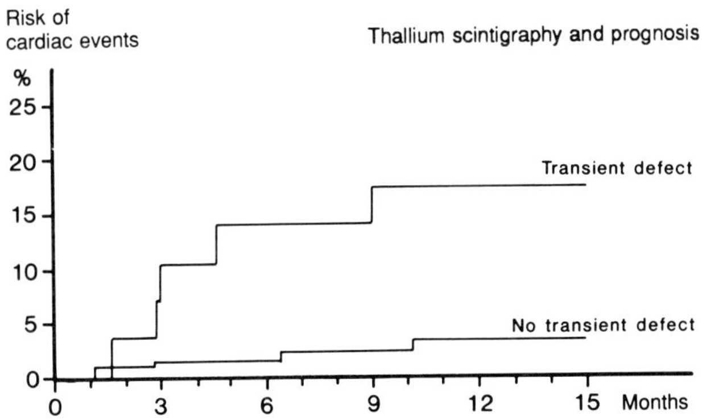

Fig. 3. *Risk of AMI or cardiac death in relation to thallium scintigraphy (p=0.001) (16).*

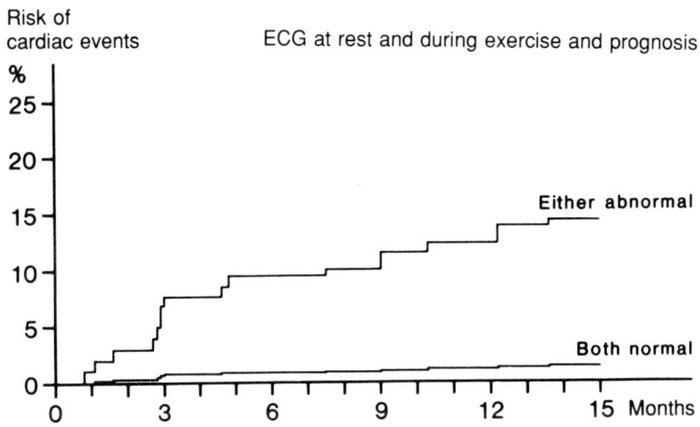

Fig. 4. *Risk of AMI or cardiac death in relation to ECG at rest and during exercise (se text) (p<0.001) (15).*

ity in the resting ECG, ST segment changes during exercise, combination of ECG at rest and during exercise, transient defects on thallium scintigraphy, mitral septal separation, relative heart volume and pairs of premature ventricular beats on Holter monitoring. The importance of left ventricular dysfunction may be underestimated, as more precise methods such as 2-D echocardiography and radionuclide cardiography have not been used. Furthermore, the importance of silent ischaemia has not been evaluated.

It may be concluded from these studies that patients without AMI and with no overt non-cardiac or non-coronary cause of chest pain can be divided into high- and low-risk patients on discharge:

* high-risk patients include all with signs of ischaemic heart disease, which for practical reasons may be defined as a history of angina or AMI, unstable angina during admission or an abnormal ECG at rest or during exercise.
* low-risk patients include patients without the above mentioned signs of ischaemic heart disease in their medical history, during admission or non-invasive investigations. The latter should as a minimum include an exercise test.

Management of low-risk patients

These patients have an excellent prognosis, although non-cardiac causes for their chest pain may be present. There are no studies available to indicate if further routine examinations are needed. The low-risk patients should be assured of the benign course of their chest pain in order to avoid cardiac neuroses and unnecessay consultations or admissions.

Management of high-risk patients

High-risk patients should be followed closely. These high-risk patients present themselves without population screening, and are usually highly motivated for intervention or treatment following the acute admission. Two studies of aspirin in patients with "unstable angina" included patients who resemble these high-risk patients (17, 18). These studies showed a considerable reduction in mortality and AMI morbidity. Consequently, aspirin, 150 or 300 mg per day should be prescribed for all high-risk patients.

Treatment with beta-blockers, calcium antagonists, and long acting nitrates should be given according to the symptoms, and patients should be referred to PTCA or coronary by-pass surgery following the usual practice. Risk factors should be controlled according to ordinary guidelines.

Table 6. *Risk of AMI or cardiac death after one year, in relation to medical history or results of non-invasive investigations in patients admitted with chest pain, without AMI and with coronary or possible coronary chest pain (5, 6, 15, 16).*

	Abnormality		
	present	not present	p*
Medical history			
Angina pectoris	18%	3%	<0.0001
Previous AMI	16%	6%	0.02
Angina, previous AMI or both	18%	1%	0.0001
Heart failure	12%	8%	0.43
ECG at rest n=217			
Q wave	11%	6%	0.24
Negative T wave	15%	3%	<0.001
ST depression	22%	5%	<0.01
Any abnormality	13%	3%	<0.0001
Exercise ECG n=215			
Abnormal ST response	14%	3%	0.009
Angina during exercise	12%	5%	0.009
ECG, rest or exercise			
Abnormal at rest, during exercise or both	13%	2%	<0.001
Thallium scintigraphy n=158			
Persistent defect	6%	6%	0.51
Transient defect	17%	2%	0.001
Holter monitoring n=198			
Premature ventricular beats	12%	4%	0.38
Pairs of PVBs	20%	5%	0.01
Chest X-ray n=215			
Cardiomegaly	12%	3%	0.03
Echocardiography n=136			
Mitral-septal separation >5mm	15%	4%	0.055

* log-rank test comparison of survival curves.

Conclusions

Patients admitted with chest pain without AMI and without a non-cardiac or cardiac non-coronary cause of chest pain have a considerable risk of AMI or cardiac death in the first year following discharge. The risk is almost the same as in AMI patients.

These patients should be evaluated for signs of coronary heart disease. This should as a minimum include a medical history, ECG at rest and during exercise.

A low-risk group with no signs of coronary heart disease can be assured of their excellent prognosis.

High-risk patients with a history of angina pectoris or myocardial infarction, unstable angina during admission, abnormal ECG at rest or during exercise can be identified. These patients should be treated with aspirin and followed closely with regard to the need for medical or surgical treatment of angina pectoris.

References

1. Dussia EE, Cromartie D, McCreaney J, Mead G, Wenger NK. Myocardial infarction with and without laboratory documentation – one year prognosis. Am Heart J 1976; 92: 148-51.
2. Nordlander R, Nyquist O. Patients treated in a coronary care unit without acute myocardial infarction. Br Heart J 1979; 41: 647-53.
3. Madsen JK, Hansen JF. The prognosis for patients admitted to a coronary care unit due to suspected acute myocardial infarction with and without confirmed diagnosis. Acta Med Scand 1982; 211: 453-7.
4. Engby B, Strunge P, Olsen J. The prognosis for patients referred with suspected acute myocardial infarction. Acta Med Scand 1985; 217: 465-71.
5. Madsen JK, Thomsen BL, Sørensen JN, Kjeldgaard K-M, Kromann-Andersen B. Risk factors and prognosis after discharge for patients admitted because of suspected acute myocardial infarctionnwith and without confirmed diagnosis. Am J Cardiol 1987; 59: 1064-70.
6. Madsen JK. Prognose for patienter indlagt på mistanke om akut myokardieinfarkt, men som fik diagnosen afkræftet. København: Eget forlag, 1988.
7. Ahnve S. Noninfarction cases without previously known ischemic heart disease admitted to a coronary care unit. Eur J Cardiol 1979; 9: 307-18.
8. Davies HA, Jones DB, Rhodes J. "Esophageal angina" as the cause of chest pain. JAMA 1982; 248: 2274-8.
9. Roberts R, Henderson RD, Wigle ED. Esophageal disease as a cause of severe retrosternal chest pain. Chest 1975; 67: 523-6.
10. Areskog M, Tibbling L, Wranne B. Non-infarction coronary care unit patients. Acta Med Scand 1981; 209: 51-7.
11. Bechgaard P. Segmentære thorakalsmerter hos patienter indlagt på koronarafdeling. Ugeskr Læger 1982; 144: 13-5.
12. Mulcahy R, Daly L, Graham L, et al. Unstable angina: Natural history and determinants of prognosis. Am J Cardiol 1981; 48: 525-8.
13. Mulcahy R, Awadhi AHA. Buitlor M, et al. Natural history and prognosis of unstable angina. Am Heart J 1985; 109: 753-8.
14. Olson HG, Lyons KP, Aronow WS, Stinson PJ, Kuperus, Waters HJ. The high-risk angina patient. Identification by clinical features, hospital course, electrocardiography and technetium-99m stannous pyrophosphate scintigraphy. Circulation 1981; 64: 674-84.
15. Madsen JK, Thomsen BL, Mellemgaard K, Hansen JF. Independent prognostic risk factors for patietns admitted because of suspected acute myocardial infarction without confirmed diagnosis. Prognosis after discharge in relation to medical history and non-invasive investigations. Eur Heart J 1988; 9: 610-8.
16. Madsen JK, Stubgaard M, Utne HE, et al. Prognosis and Thallium-201 scintigraphy in patients admitted with chest pain without confirmed acute myocardial infarction. Br Heart J 1988; 59: 184-9.

17. Lewis HD, Davis JW, Archiebald DG, et al. Protective effects of aspirin against acute myocardial infarction or death in men with unstable angina. N Engl J Med 1983; 309: 396-403.
18. Cairns JA, Gent M, Singer J, et al. Aspirin, sulfinpyrazone, or both in unstable angina. N Engl J Med 1985; 313: 1369-75.

19

Assessment of the extent of myocardial damage: Lessons from the thrombolytic era

PEER GRANDE,
PETER CLEMMENSEN

Myocardial reperfusion and myocardial salvage

It has been accepted for more than a decade that sudden and persistent thrombus formation in a subepicardial coronary artery is the most common cause of acute myocardial infarction (AMI). The size of the myocardial infarct is a key determinant of the functional status of the residual myocardium which in turn is the major predictor of both short- and long-term prognosis. Several interventions were created or gained routine status through the nineteen eighties as a means of reestablishing myocardial perfusion early after the interruption of coronary blood flow. Through controlled randomized clinical trials we experienced an improved survival in AMI patients treated with thrombolytic therapy (i.e., the ISIS-2, GISSI and ASSET trials). Clinical studies confirmed the findings of animal studies, that salvage of acutely jeopardized myocardium is confined to patients in whom myocardial perfusion is reestablished early (within 4-6 hours) after the onset of symptoms (1). The recent ISIS-2 trial showed a substantial reduction in mortality in patients treated with intravenous streptokinase. The effect of streptokinase was most prounced in patients admitted early after symptom onset, but a reduction in mortality of 38% was seen in the combined streptokinase and aspirin group even in patients admitted as late as 12-24 hours after the onset of symptoms.

Patients in the ISAM Study (2), who did not show signs of early reperfusion by non-invasive criteria, had significantly better left ventricular function if the infarct related artery was patent 1 month after the infarction. In the patients with late reperfusion, regardless of whether thrombolytic therapy was given or not, the mean ejection fraction was 56%, vs. 50% in those without reperfusion.

Late reperfusion of the culprit coronary artery may interfere with the natural post infarction remodelling of the left ventricle. The patent blood filled coronary artery bed may serve as a scaffold for the healing process. The remodelling results from infarct expansion, volume overload and dilation of the remaining viable myocardium. Late reperfusion of the infarct artery may prevent or limit this remodelling by a variety of mechanisms (3). Further, late reperfusion may affect the electrophysiological properties of the myocardium and improve the electrical stability, thus leading to a reduction in malignant arrhythmias.

Thus, new data indicate that also late reperfusion of an infarct related artery has a potential impact on the preservation of left ventricular function either by improvement, prevention of deterioration, or both, with subsequent improved survival of the treated patients.

Thrombolytic therapy is based on the main hypothesis that reperfusion of the infarct related artery results in salvage of the acutely jeopardized ischaemic myocardium, reduced myocardial infarct size, reduced deterioration in left ventricular function, and reduced mortality following AMI (3).

However, reperfusion does not result in myocardial salvage if the myocytes have been subjected to prolonged ischaemia resulting in necrosis. Also, it is now apparent that viable myocytes may demonstrate prolonged alterations in function following reperfusion and salvage. These alterations may contribute to the overall left ventricular dysfunction. Stunned myocardium refers to viable myocardium that has been salvaged by coronary reperfusion, yet exhibits prolonged but transient postischaemic contractile dysfunction, lasting hours to days (4). Hibernating myocardium refers to ischaemic myocardium supplied by a narrowed coronary artery, in which the myocytes remain viable but the contraction is chronically depressed (5). Both stunned and hibernating myocardium may follow reperfusion and myocardial salvage, thus depressing left ventricular function for shorter or longer periods of time.

Thus, reperfusion does not always result in myocardial salvage, and myocardial salvage does not always result in contractile myocytes. On the other hand, late reperfusion without salvage may result in improved left ventricular function. To elucidate these relationships, and to determine the success of thrombolytic therapy, electrocardiographic and enzymatic methods have been developed to assess the extent of myocardium at risk, the final myocardial infarct size and degree of reperfusion.

Characteristics of the serum CK-MB and myoglobin time activity curves for estimating reperfusion and final infarct size

Serum CK-MB and myoglobin for assessment of reperfusion

It is well-established that early intracoronary therapy resulting in reperfusion in AMI can alter the pattern of creatine kinase (CK) in blood. Changes include an abrupt and rapid increase in serum CK that result in a shortened time to peak concentration compared with non reperfused AMI (6). Three recent studies of intravenous thrombolysis have shown the same pattern (7-9). Using simple data from CK or the more cardiospecific isoenzyme CK-MB time activity curves, parameters as time to peak value and the rate of increase of serum CK or CK-MB have been proposed to identify reperfusion. However, as noted by several authors, there is a large overlap in these characteristics (6, 9).

We have recently published a study of isoforms of serum CK-MB (10), and others of CK-MM isoforms (11). Both CK-MB and CK-MM are present in one isoform in myocardial tissue. Circulating in the plasma, these isoforms undergo modifications by proteolysis, resulting in sequentional unidirectional conversion to two additional isoforms of each of the isoenzymes (MB1, MB2, MB3, and MM1, MM2, MM3). The ratio of both the MB and MM isoforms has been suggested to be dramatically changed in reperfusion, with fast deliberation of enzymes from cells to blood, compared to the non reperfused AMI. The use of these new isoforms may be valuable in the future, but these first reports need to be confirmed by others, and the techniques for analysis need to be faster and more simple.

Using a mono-compartment model, *Ong et al* (9) demonstrated that the appearance rate for CK-MB in blood almost completely separated 21 reperfused from 5 non reperfused patients who were angiographically studied 18 to 48 hrs after thrombolytic therapy. We used a modification of a multicompartment model (12) to determine CK-MB kinetics and identify reperfusion characteristics in a group of 29 patients with documented acute reperfusion (TIMI grade 3) compared to a group of 44 patients who received no thrombolytic therapy (13). An early rise and peak of serum CK-MB from frequent blood sampling were confirmed in patients with reperfusion (Fig. 1). The higher peak in this group results from a more uniform distribution of peak values about 10 hrs after the onset of symptoms. In the non reperfusion group, maximal mean CK-MB activity is reached at about 20 hrs after onset of symptoms. In this study we compared a number of curve characteristics from the two groups. The most significant differences were the appearance rate constant, and the time from rise to peak of CK-MB in

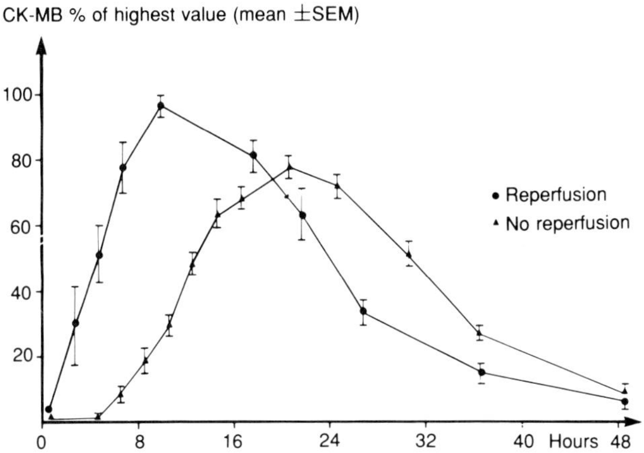

Fig. 1. *Serum CK-MB in patients with and without coronary reperfusion following acute myocardial infarction. Hours (= hours from start of symptoms).*

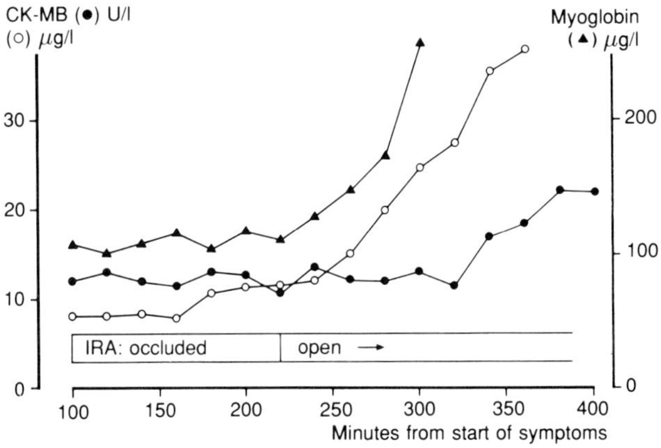

Fig. 2. *Serum CK-MB and myoglobin in one patient during opening of the occluded infarct related artery (=IRA), see text.*

blood. A cut-off level indicating reperfusion if appearance rate k1 >0.185 and the time index <16.5 hrs demonstrated overlapping values between the two groups in only 4 patients (k1), 2 patients (time index) and 6 patients (using the combination). This corresponds to a sensitivity of 86% (k1), 93% (time index) or 100% (combination), and a estimated specificity of 100% (k1), 100% (time index) or 89% (combination) (13).

Among the 29 patients with documented acute reperfusion and TIMI grade 3 flow, the times from onset of symptoms to time of treatment, respectively, time to reperfusion were related to the reperfusion characteristics. Both times correlated significantly negatively to k1 (r= –0.36 and –0.41) and positively to the time index (r=0.49 and 0.63). Thus, these indices not only reflect the presence or absence of coronary reperfusion, but also provide quantitative information as to the degree of reperfusion.

Release of intracellular macromolecules is considered a sign of irreversible ischaemia. This assumption is based on experimental data (14) and may be a simplification of a complex biological system. Fig. 2 shows an example of serum activity and concentration of CK-MB and myoglobin in one patient with AMI during opening of the infarct related artery with PTCA (15). Neither serum myoglobin nor CK-MB activity increases during 220 minutes of ischaemia. After coronary artery opening, myoglobin increases more rapidly than CK-MB. However, the more accurate and sensitive CK-MB mass assay identifies a slight release of CK-MB at about 180 minutes. Myoglobin has a molecular weight of 17,000, CK-MB of 85,000. This illustrates not only the well known early appearance of myoglobin compared to CK-MB in blood, but also that improved analytical techniques will make it possible to identify new pathophysiological information.

Myoglobin has been studied as a marker for early detection of successful reperfusion in patients with AMI by *Ellis et al* (16). Of 42 patients treated with streptokinase or r-tPA, coronary arteriography during the first 5 days showed reperfusion in 35 patients and persistent occlusion in 7. In the reperfusion group mean peak serum myoglobin occured 2 hrs after the start of therapy vs. 6 hrs in the non reperfusion group.

In a recent acute angiographic study of 60 patients with AMI, 32 patients showed TIMI grade 2-3 (open infarct related artery) after thrombolysis, and 17 had TIMI grade 0-1 (closed or nearly closed artery) after thrombolysis, but were opened to TIMI 3 by PTCA, whereas 11 had no attempts at opening the occluded artery (Fig. 3 and 4) (15). We demonstrated paralell characteristic changes in both serum myoglobin and CK-MB in the three groups. The earliest increase was seen in patients in TIMI grade 2-3 for both myoglobin and CK-MB, followed by a much higher increase for both substances in TIMI group 1-2 who were opened to TIMI 3 by PTCA.

The larger increase in the group who were initially TIMI 0-1, probably reflects larger infarcts due to initially failed thrombolysis. This study demonstrated that the most accurate and early predictor for the presence or absence of reperfusion was a peak serum myoglobin before or after 300 minutes. The predictive value of a positive test (early peak and reperfusion) was 1.0, and the predictive value of a negative test (later peak and no reperfusion) was 0.81 (15).

Further studies will be required to determine the true ability of these characteristics of the myoglobin and CK-MB activity curves to quantitate the coronary artery reperfusion flow. Furthermore, the now available reperfusion indices were developed for use when there has been sufficient time for the peak serum CK-MB or myoglobin to have occurred. Further studies of even more frequent sampling of the biochemical markers will be required to determine if the immediate effects of reperfusion on parameters such as

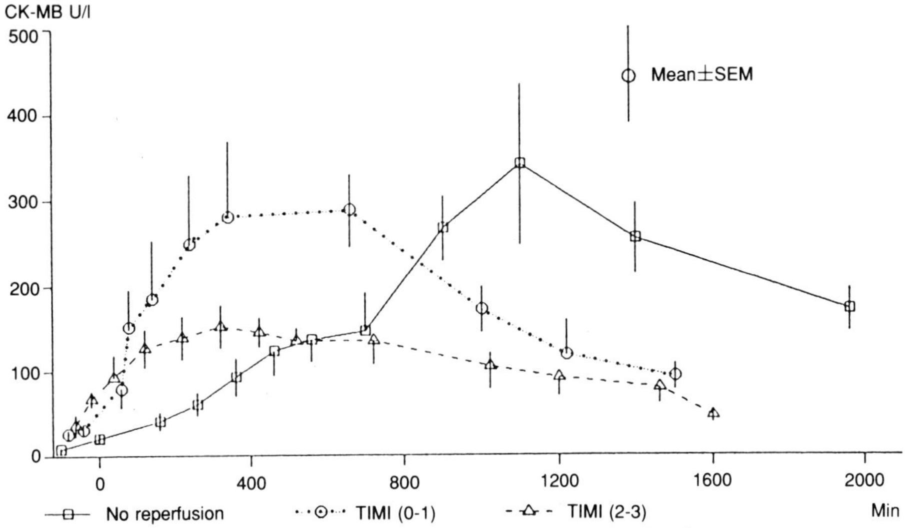

Fig. 3. *Serum CK-MB activity following acute myocardial infarction in patients with different flow in the infarct related artery, see text.*

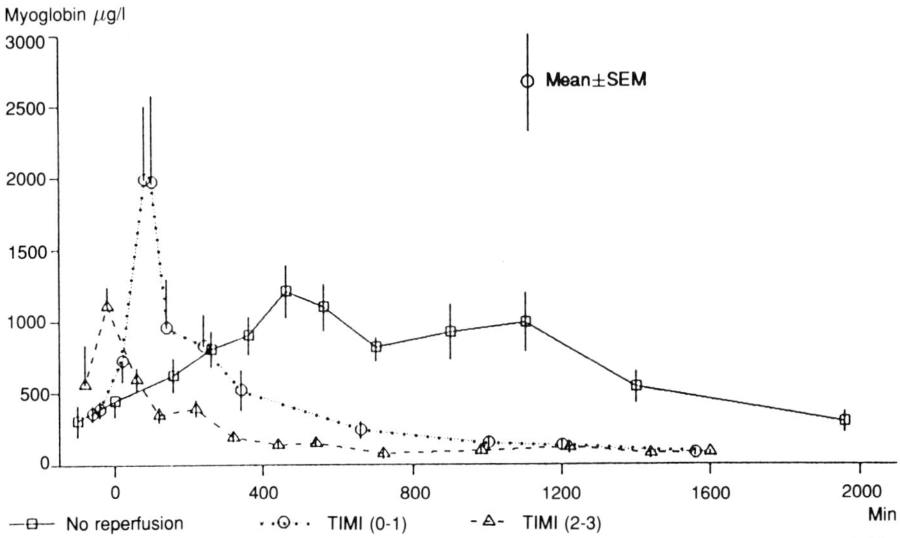

Fig. 4. *Serum myoglobin following acute myocardial infarction in patients with different flow in the infarct related artery, see text.*

k1 are sufficient to permit identification or quantification at an earlier point in time.

Serum CK and CK-MB for estimating infarct size in patients treated with thrombolytic therapy

Previous studies before the thrombolytic era, have demonstrated that both

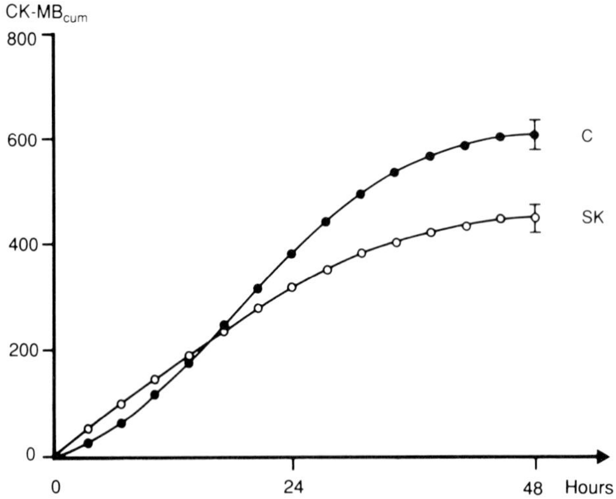

Fig. 5. *Cumulated serum CK-MB in two groups of patients with AMI. SK= patients treated with 1.5 mill Units of streptokinase for 1 hour; C= controls treated with placebo; see text.*

serum CK-MB (12) and QRS score (17) are usefull for estimating myocardial infarct size in man. When correlating the estimates from these methods to autopsy measurements, the coefficients of correlation were approximately r=0.80, and the standard error of estimate about 30%. Cardiac mortality, development of heart failure, arrhythmias and cardiac performance at rest and during exercise, also correlate to serum CK-MB estimated infarct size.

In experimental studies reperfusion changed the rate of appearance of CK and CK-MB in blood, which could effect the accuracy of esimated infarct size. The hypothesis was, that with very early reperfusion, an increase in the proportion of enzyme depleted from myocardium would occur and thus limit the time available for local proteolysis and inactivation of enzymes in the necrotic tissue. However, recently it has been demonstrated both in experimental and clinical studies that myocardial infarct size can be reliably estimated from serum CK and CK-MB in reperfused patients also.

Sobels group (18) demonstrated a very close correlation between enzymatically estimated and measured infarct size in dogs (r=0.92), and a similar close relationship between early CK estimated infarct size and infarct size delineated by positron emission tomography in patients with coronary reperfusion (r=0.93). Highly significant correlations between CK and CK-MB estimated infarct size and myocardial technetium tomography computed scans have also been demonstrated (r=0.89) (19).

In the Copenhagen part of the ISIS-2 trial 122 patients were randomized to streptokinase or placebo-streptokinase. Fig. 5 demonstrates a reduction in infarct size of approximately 25% in the streptokinase group (20).

ECG estimation of the extent of myocardium at risk of acute infarction and resulting infarct size

ST segment deviation for estimating the extent of myocardium at risk of acute infarction

In the present era one of the primary therapeutic goals in the management of patients with acute coronary occlusion is intervention aimed at restoring myocardial blood flow. The clinical decision to intervene must be made at the earliest possible moment in order to maximize the salvage of jeopardized myocardium.

The 12-lead ECG is the only immediately available clinical test which can identify, locate, and estimate the extent of the acute ischaemic injury. Clinical investigations have shown that the extent of acute myocardial injury as determined by ECG effects the outcome of reperfusion therapy (21, 22). *Mauri et al* showed that in the GISSI trial there was a progessive increase in mortality rate with increasing number of ECG leads involved in the infarction. Furthermore, streptokinase only reduced the mortality when the acute infarction extended over more than 3 leads (21). Recent studies have determined the relationship between the extent of acute ST segment changes on the initial ECG and both acute wall motion abnormalities and subsequent AMI size, estimated by either QRS score or CK-MB (17, 23-27). *Cohen et al* found significant correlations (r=0.89-0.96) between both the number of leads with new ST elevations, the sum of this elevation, and the extent of acute hypocontractility during controlled coronary occlusion via angioplasty balloon inflation (23). Two recent studies established the mathematical relationships between acute ST elevation and final QRS score (24, 26). They resulted in formulas for both anterior and inferior AMI, which predict the final QRS score estimated AMI size from the acute ST elevation in patients who do not receive infarct limiting therapy (Table 1). Although a highly significant correlation was established between predicted and final AMI size (r=0.65 and r=0.72, $p<0.0001$; for inferior and anterior AMI, respectively) these formulas should be used with caution in individual patients due to a considerable standard error of up to 38%. As these formulas

Table 1. *Formulas for predicting the final QRS score estimated per cent AMI size based on the acute ST segment deviation.*

Anterior % AMI size	=	3[1.5 (# leads with ST↑) – 0.4]
Inferior % AMI size	=	3[0.6(ΣST↑ II, III, aVF) + 2.0]
		+3[1.5(# non-inferior leads ST↑) – 0.4]

AMI = acute myocardial infarction; # = number; Σ= sum; ST↑ = ST segment elevation.

QRS criteria

Lead	Criteria	Points
I	Q > = 30 ms	1
	{R/Q < = 1	1
	{R < = 0.2 mV	1
II	{Q > = 40 ms	2
	{Q > = 30 ms	1
aVL	Q > = 30 ms	1
	R/Q < = 1	1
aVF	{Q > = 50 ms	3
	{Q > = 40 ms	2
	{Q > = 30 ms	1
	{R/Q < = 1	2
	{R/Q < = 2	1
V1		
Ant	Any Q '	1
	S > = 1.8 mV	1
Post	R/S > = 1	1
	{R > = 50 ms	2
	{R > = 1.0 mV	2
	{R > = 40 ms	1
	{R > = 0.6 mV	1
	S < = 0.3 mV	1
V2	{RV2 < = RV1 mV	1
Ant	{Any Q	1
	{R < = 10 ms	1
	{R < = 0.1 mV	1
Post	R/S > = 1.5	1
	{R > = 60 ms,	2
	{R > = 2.0 mV	2
	{R > = 50 ms	1
	{R > = 1.5 mV	1
	S < = 0.4 mV	1
V3	{Any Q	1
	{R < = 20 ms	1
	{R < = 0.2 mV	1
V4	Q > = 20 ms	1
	{R/Q < = 0.5	2
	{R/S < = 0.5	2
	{R/Q < = 1	1
	{R/S < = 1	1
	{R < = 0.7 mV	1
	{Notched R	1
V5	Q > = 30 ms	1
	{R/Q < = 1	2
	{R/S < = 1	2
	{R/Q < = 2	1
	{R/S < = 2	1
	{R < = 0.7 mV	1
	{Notched R	1
V6	Q > = 30 ms	1
	{R/Q < = 1	2
	{R/S < = 1	2
	{R/Q < = 3	1
	{R/S < = 3	1
	{R < = 0.6 mV	1
	{Notched R	1

Fig. 6. *Complete 54 criteria / 32 points Selvester QRS scoring system.*

quantitatively estimate the extent of acutely jeopardized myocardium prior to the initiation of therapy aimed at limiting AMI size, they might provide a basis for the decision to commence thrombolytic therapy and non-invasive evaluation of myocardial salvage. When the thus ST estimated amount of jeopardized myocardium is compared to some other non-invasive quantitative estimate of the extent of infarcted myocardium after the completion of intervention aimed at reducing AMI size, the difference between the two estimates represents the salvaged myocardium.

QRS score for estimating the size of myocardial infarcts

It is generally known, that the major determinants of immediate and long-term outcome of AMI are the size of the infarct and the functional status of the residual myocardium; thus, clinical methods that are able to estimate the extent of myocardial necrosis are needed. Furthermore, the recent interest in the limitation of AMI size by means of therapeutic intervention has prompted the evaluation of several clinical methods aimed at estimating the size of an AMI. One of the most extensively studied methods during the past decade for estimating AMI size is the QRS scoring system developed by *Selvester and coworkers* (17). The method is based on computer simulation of heart activation in the human torso, and resulted in a 54 criteria QRS scoring system (Fig. 6) using the 12-lead ECG for estimating AMI size. In this scoring system, which considers Q and R wave durations, R/Q or R/S amplitude ratios and R wave notch, a maximum of 32 points can be awarded from the 54 weighted criteria. Each of the 32 points represents approximately 3% infarcted left ventricular myocardium. In post-mortem studies the total number of points has been shown to correlate (r=0.80) positively with per cent AMI size for both anterior, inferior, and posterior AMI locations (17). This scoring system has also been shown to correlate inversely (r=–0.80, when combining anterior and inferior infarcts) with radionuclide left ventricular ejection fraction (28). The QRS score provides strong prognostic information by itself in patients with coronary artery disease. In a recent study, a QRS score of zero was associated with a 95% one year and 88% 5 year survival rate, whereas patients with a score of 10 or more had survival rates of 81% and 52%, respectively (29).

The Selvester QRS scoring system has proved to be a useful clinical descriptor and clinical investigational tool because it is in-expensive and simple and maximizes the prognostic information from the ECG.

ECG estimated myocardial reperfusion and salvage

In the thrombolytic era, the application of the standard ECG has expanded from a diagnostic test which identifies and localizes AMI, to a test which recognizes myocardial reperfusion and estimates the extent of myocardial salvage. Earlier studies showed that myocardial reperfusion following thrombolytic therapy is associated with an accelerated normalization of ST segment deviation as compared to non-reperfused patients (30). The altered speed of ST resolution following myocardial reperfusion has led to investigations of the predictive value of this ST shift in order to predict reperfusion (31-33). It should be pointed out that the outcome in these studies has been patency or occlusion of the infarct related artery following attempted thrombolysis, and that myocardial reperfusion per se was not measured. It is likely that a discrepancy exists between epicardial coronary patency and small vessel patency due to the various mechanisms behind the no reflow phenomenon. It is therefore important to realize that, although often used as such, myocardial reperfusion and infarct artery patency are not synonyms (see above).

Myocardial reperfusion or infarct artery patency can be reliably assessed using serial ECG recordings (31-33). *Krucoff and associates* found that achievement of a stable ST segment within 100 minutes after completed streptokinase infusion was 89% sensitive and 82% specific for the detection of reperfusion (32). Their method, however, was based on 3-lead Holter monitoring which is not routinely available and the detection of steady state requires continued ST segment measurements over a 24-48 hour period. These promising results have been confirmed in other prospective studies using the more readily available 12-lead standard ECG (31, 33). In the first study, a 50% reduction in ST elevation in the maximum deviated lead was 67% specific and 93% sensitive for infarct artery patency; and similar results were found in the larger study by our study group. In the latter study a reduction in ST elevation of only 20% after attempted thrombolysis achieved a high both positive and negative predictive value for identifying infarct vessel patency (88% and 80%, respectively) (33). Thus, of 100 patients treated with a thrombolytic agent with an 80% reperfusion rate, the above criteria would indicate that 26 patients should be subjected to emergency cardiac catheterization. Of the 26 patients, 16 non reperfused would be correctly identified. Only 4 patients without reperfusion, would be falsely considered as reperfused, and thus loose the opportunity of a rescue procedure.

Salvage of acutely jeopardized myocardium is the ultimate therapeutic goal of interventions directed toward re-establishing infarct related patency after coronary occlusion. It would therefore be clinically important if myocardial salvage could be identified non-invasively. Studies from the early thrombolytic era showed trends towards early (48 hours post admission) disappearance of Q waves and increase in R wave height which could be related to salvage in patients with myocardial reperfusion via the left anterior descending coronary artery (30). Myocardial salvage has also been

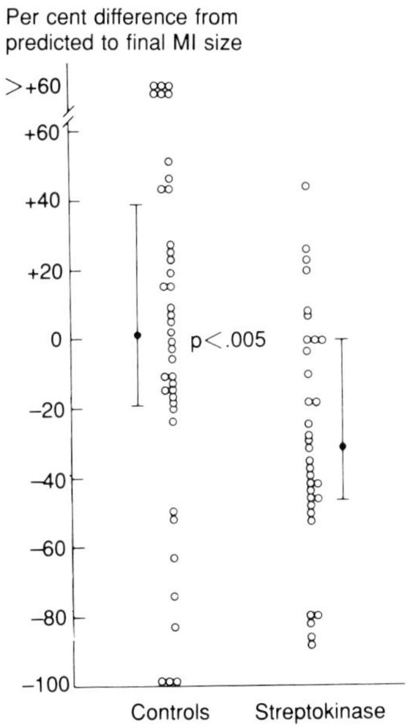

Fig. 7. *The relative % difference between electrocardiographic acutely ST predicted and final QRS score estimated AMI size in patients treated conservatively (left panel) and with intravenous streptokinase (right panel). For details see text.*

suggested by investigators comparing QRS changes between groups of patients with or without infarct artery patency. *Hackworthy et al* (34) found a significantly lower sum of Q waves in reperfused than in non-reperfused patients 24 hours after treatment. *Timmis et al* (35) found significantly more instances of non Q wave infarction among patients with either spontaneous or pharmacologically induced reperfusion. Recently, two investigations have suggested that myocardial salvage can be estimated non-invasively by the ECG employing comparison of the acute ST segment changes and the final AMI size estimated by the Selvester QRS score (36, 37). In a study by *Hogg et al* (36) a ST segment area (= area above the isoelectric line from the J point to the end of the T wave) was measured and compared in 30 patients with successful angiographic reperfusion and 35 control patients. Despite similar potential infarct sizes (=ST segment areas) acutely, the QRS at 48 hours was almost reduced by 50% in the reperfused group (mean 7.8 versus 4.1). A different approach using the formulas in Table 1 was applied by our study group in a placebo controlled study of intravenous streptokinase versus placebo. The predicted AMI size was determined from the acute ST segment elevation (Table 1) on the admission ECG and compared to the pre-discharge final QRS score estimated AMI size in each patient (37). Streptokinase was found to have a highly significant effect on the relationship between predicted and final AMI size. The "% difference" [=(final AMI size − predicted AMI size)/predicted AMI size × 100] between initial ST predicted and final QRS estimated AMI size was zero in the control group whereas in patients receiving intravenous streptokinase a median −32% difference occurred, indicating a 32% reduction in AMI size in this group (Fig. 7).

Thus, intensive ECG research during the past decade has resulted in methods based on quantitative analysis of the ST segment and QRS morphology, which enhances this old diagnostic tool to meet the needs of the thrombolytic era. Although the development of these methods is not entirely completed, they do provide the ability to non-invasively: 1) estimate the amount of acutely jeopardized myocardium; 2) indentify infarct related coronary artery patency following intravenous thrombolytic treatment; 3) estimate myocardial salvage by comparing ECG indices of the amount of myocardium acutely jeopardized with the amount of myocardium finally infarcted; and 4) estimate the final AMI size and thus provide information on left ventricular function, and subsequent patient prognosis.

Conclusion

A few simple non-invasive tests based on measurements of CK-MB and myoglobin in blood, and analysis of the standard 12 lead ECG gives the opportunity of assessing the major events of the evolving myocardial infarction treated with thrombolytic agents. The amount of myocardium at jeopardy may be assessed from ST changes in ECG; the success or failure of restoring blood flow in the infarct related artery may be assessed from both serum myoglobin and CK-MB data and from the ST changes in ECG; the myocardial salvage may be assessed by comparing initially ST predicted jeopardized myocardium and final QRS infarct size; and the final infarct size can be estimated from both serum CK-MB time activity curves and QRS score.

References

1. Simoons ML, Serruys PW, Brand MJMB, et al. Early thrombolysis in acute myocardial infarction: limitation of infarct size and improved survival. J Am Coll Cardiol 1986; 7: 717-28.
2. Schrøder R, Neuhaus KL, Linderer T, Brüggemann T, Tebbe U, Wegsceider K. Impact of late coronary artery reperfusion on left ventricular function one month after acute myocardial infarction (Results from the ISAM study). Am J Cardiol 1989; 64: 878-84.
3. Braunwald E. Myocardial reperfusion, limitation of infarct size, reduction of left ventricular dysfunction, and improved survival. Should the paradigm be expanded? Circulation 1989; 79: 441-4.

4. Braunwald E, Kloner RA. The stunned myocardium: prolonged postischemic ventricular dysfunction. Circulation 1982; 66: 1146-9.
5. Braunwald E, Rutherford JD. Reversible ischemic left ventricular dysfunction: evidence for the hibernating myocardium. J Am Coll Cardiol 1986; 8: 1567-70.
6. Gore JM, Roberts R, Ball SP, Montero A, Goldberg RJ, Dalen JE. Peak creatine kinase as measure of effectiveness of thrombolytic therapy in acute myocardial infarction. Am J Cardiol 1987; 59: 1234-8.
7. Garabedian HD, Gold HK, Yasda T, et al. Detection of coronary artery reperfusion with creatine kinase MB determination during thrombolytic therapy: correlation with acute angiography. J Am Coll Cardiol 1988; 11: 729-34.
8. Lewis BS, Ganz W, Laramee P, et al. Usefulness of a rapid initial increase in plasma creatine kinase activity as a marker of reperfusion during thrombolytic therapy for acute myocardial infarction. Am J Cardiol 1988; 62: 20-4.
9. Ong L, Coromilas J, Zimmerman JM, et al. A physiologically based model of creatine kinase MB release in reperfusion of acute myocardial infarction. Am J Cardiol 1989; 64: 11-5.
10. Christenson R, Ohman EM, Clemmensen P, et al. Characteristics of creatine kinase MB and MB isoforms in serum after reperfusion in acute myocardial infarction. Clin Chem 1989; 35: 2179-85.
11. Jaffe AS, Sertoa H, Grace A, Sobel BE. Diagnostic changes in plasma creatine kinase isoformes early after onset of myocardial infarction. Circulation 1986; 74: 105-9.
12. Grande P, Hansen BF, Christiansen C, Næstoft J. Estimation of acute myocardial infarct size in man by serum CK-MB measurements. Circulation 1982; 65: 756-64.
13. Grande P, Granborg J, Clemmensen P, Sevilla DC, Wagner NB, Wagner GS. Qualitative and quantitative indices of reperfusion in patients with acute myocardial infarction using characteristics of the CK-MB time activity curve. Circulation, submitted.
14. Ahmed SA, Williamson JR, Roberts R, Clark RE, Sobel BE. The association of increased plasma MB CPK activity and irreversible ischemic myocardial injury in the dog. Circulation 1976; 54: 187-93.
15. Grande P, Clemmensen P, Ohman EM, et al. Changes in serum myoglobin and CK-MB in patients with or without reperfusion after thrombolytic therapy for acute myocardial infarction. J Am Coll Cardiol, submitted.
16. Ellis AK, Little T, Masud ARZ, Liberman HA, Morris DC, Klocke FJ. Early noninvasive detection of successful reperfusion in patients with acute myocardial infarction. Circulation 1988; 78: 1352-7.
17. Selvester RH, Sanmarco ME, Solomon JC, Wagner GS. The electrocardiogram: QRS change. In: Wagner GS, ed. Myocardial infarction: Measurement and intervention development in cardiovascular medicine, vol. 14. The Hague: Martinus Nijhoff, 23-50.
18. Devries SR, Jaffe AS, Geltman EM, Sobel BE, Abendsheim DR. Enzymatic estimation of the extent of irreversible myocardial injury early after reperfusion. Am Heart J 1989; 117: 31-6.
19. Hasimoto T, Kambara H, Fudo T, et al. Early estimation of acute myocardial infarct size soon after coronary reperfusion using emission computed tomography with technetium-99m pyrophosphate. Am J Cardiol 1987; 60: 952-7.
20. Clemmensen P, Grande P, Petersen F, et al. Electrocardiograpic and enzymatic indicators of therapeutic success after intravenous streptokinase for acute myocardial infarction. Am Heart J, submitted.
21. Mauri F, Gasparini M, Barbonaglia L, et al. Prognostic significance of the extent of myocardial injury in acute myocardial infarction treated by streptokinase (the GISSI trial). Am J Cardiol 1989; 63: 1291-5.
22. Bar FW, Vermeer F, De Zwaan C, et al. Value of the admission electrocardiogram in

predicting outcome of thrombolytic therapy in acute myocardial infarction. Am J Cardiol 1987; 59: 6-13.

23. Cohen M, Scharpf SJ, Rentrop KP. Prospective analysis of electrocardiographic variables as markers for extent and location of acute wall motion abnormalities observed during coronary angioplasty in human subjects. J Am Coll Cardiol 1987; 10: 17.
24. Aldrich HR, Wagner NB, Boswick J, et al. Use of initial ST-segment deviation for prediction of final electrocardiographic size of acute myocardial infarcts. Am J Cardiol 1988; 61: 749-3.
25. Hindman NB, Schocken DD, Widmann M, et al. Evaluation of a QRS scoring system for estimating myocardial infarct size. V. Specificity and method of application of the complete system. Am J Cardiol 1985; 55: 1485-90.
26. Clemmensen P, Grande P, Wagner NB, Aldrich HR, Wagner GS. Initial ST segment elevation can predict the final electrocardiographic size of myocardial infarcts. J Am Coll Cardiol 1988; 11: 68A.
27. Yusuf S, Lopez R, Maddisson A, et al. Value of electrocardiogram in predicting and estimating infarct size in man. Br Heart J 1979; 42: 286-93.
28. Palmeri ST, Harrison DG, Cobb FR, et al. A QRS scoring system for assessing left ventricular function after myocardial infarction. N Engl J Med 1982; 306: 4-9.
29. Bounous ED, Califf RM, Harrell FE, et al. Prognostic value of the simplified Selvester QRS score in patients with coronary artery disease. J Am Coll Cardiol 1988; 11: 35-41.
30. Blanke H, Scherff F, Karsch KR, Levine RA, Smith H, Rentrop P. Electrocardiographic changes after streptokinase induced recanalization in patients with acute left anterior descending artery obstruction. Circulation 1983; 68: 406-12.
31. Hogg KJ, Hornung RS, Howie CA, Hocking N, Dunn FG, Hillis WS. Electrocardiographic prediction of coronary artery patency after thrombolytic treatment in acute myocardial infarction: use of the ST-segment as non-invasive marker. Br Heart J 1988; 60: 275-80.
32. Krucoff MW, Green CE, Satler LF, et al. Non-invasive detection of coronary artery patency using continuous ST-segment monitoring. Am J Cardiol 1986; 57: 916-22.
33. Clemmensen P, Ohman EM, Sevilla D, et al. Changes in standard electrocardiographic ST segment elevation predictive of successful reperfusion in evolving myocardial infarction. Submitted.
34. Hackworthy RA, Sorensen SG, Fitzpatrick PG, et al. Effect of reperfusion on electrocardiographic and enzymatic infarct size: Results of randomized multicenter study of intravenous anisoylated plasminogen streptokinase activator complex (APSAC) versus intracoronary streptokinase in acute myocardial infarction. Am Heart J 1988; 116: 903-13.
35. Timmis AD, Griffin B, Crick JCP, Nelson DJ, Sowton E. The effects of early coronary patency on the evolution of myocardial infarction: a prospective artertiographic study. Br Heart J 1987; 58: 345-51.
36. Hogg KJ, Lees KR, Hornung RS, Howie CA, Dunn FG, Hillis WS. Electrocardiographic evidence of myocardial salvage after thrombolysis in acute myocardial infarction. Br Heart J 1989; 61: 489-95.
37. Clemmensen P, Grande P, Saunamaki K, et al. Effect of intravenous streptokinase on the relationship between initial ST predicted and final QRS estimated size of acute myocardial infarcts. J Am Coll Cardiol. In press.

20

Right ventricular infarction

HENNING RUD ANDERSEN

The initial autopsy report on acute right ventricular infarction was published in 1930 by *Sanders* (1), but it was not until 1974 that *Cohn et al* (2) by invasive measurements recognized the haemodynamic characteristics associated with this infarct location. At the same time a Swedish study by *Erhardt* (3) reported the diagnostic value of an electrocardiographic bipolar right chest lead (CR4R) to give the non-invasive diagnosis. Since then, diagnosis, management and treatment of patients with right ventricular infarction have improved due to better pathophysiological understanding of this clinical syndrome.

Pathoanatomic findings

Coronary artery supply

Right ventricular infarction occurs when the blood supply to the right ventricle is interrupted. In anterior infarction, the infarct related coronary artery is the left anterior descending which supplies a small amount of the right ventricle near the septum, particularly in the apical region (4, 5). In posterior infarction, about 90% of right ventricular infarcts are caused by occlusion of the right coronary artery, and 10% by occlusion in the left circumflex coronary artery (4, 6). In patients, who are "right dominant", the right coronary artery supplies most of the anterior and all of the lateral and posterior right ventricle together with variable amounts of the posterior left ventricular wall. In patients, who are "left dominant", a small part of the posterior right ventricular wall near the septum is supplied by the left circumflex artery. Consequently, right ventricular infarction large enough to cause severe right ventricular dysfunction is caused by occlusion proximal in the right coronary artery, and is normally associated with some posterior left ventricular infarction (combined left and right ventricular infarction).

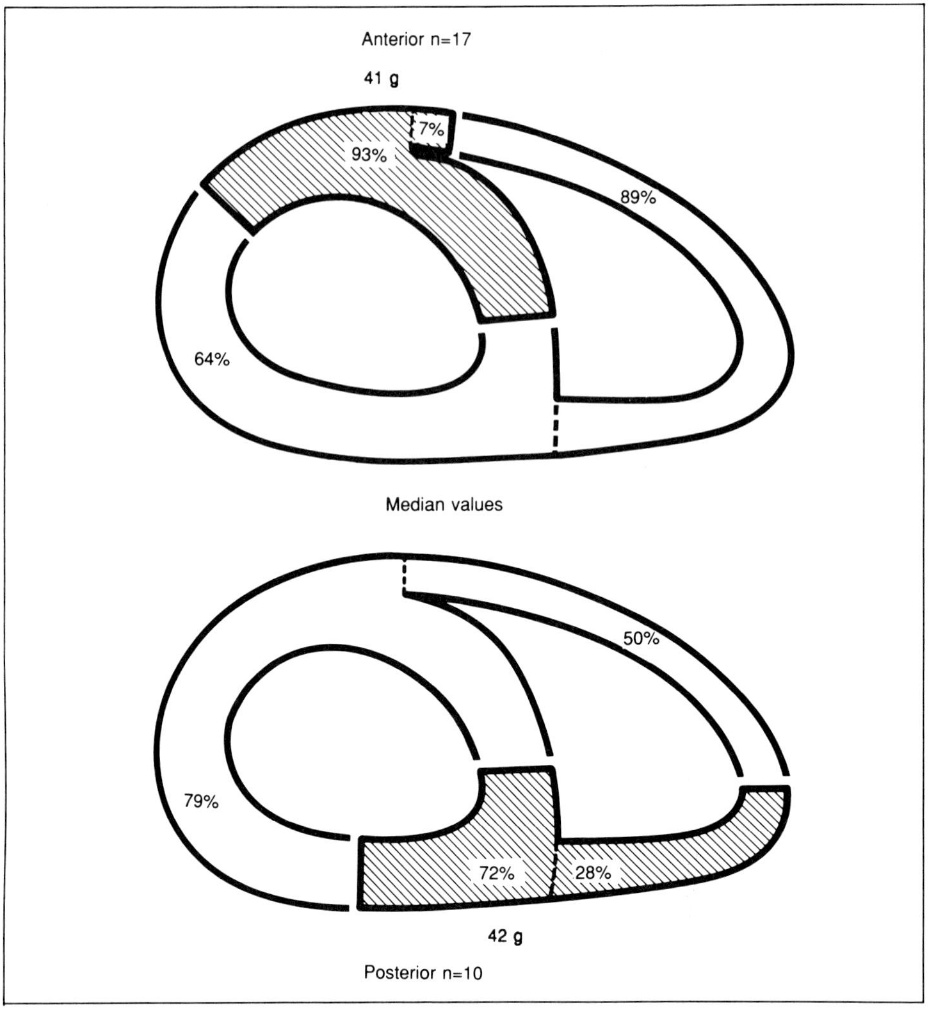

Fig. 1. *Outline illustrating the topography of right ventricular and left ventricular involvement in patients who died from their first anterior (n=17) or posterior (n=10) acute myocardial infarction. The hatched areas indicate infarct location. Percentages in the hatched areas indicate distribution of total infarction within each ventricle and percentages in non-hatched areas indicating the size of preserved myocardium in each ventricle. Although total infarct size was similar in the two groups (median 41 g versus 42 g), patients with posterior infarction had significantly larger right ventricular infarction (28% versus 7%, $p<0.01$) and smaller left ventricular infarction (72% versus 93%, $p<0.05$) and concomitantly more left ventricular myocardium intact (79% versus 64%, $p<0.05$), and less right ventricular myocardium intact (50% versus 89%, $p<0.01$).*

Frequency

Conflicting results on the frequency of right ventricular infarction have previously been reported indicating differences in study design, autopsy techniques and patient selection in these studies (7-9). Only a few prospective necropsy studies have been concerned with right ventricular infarction, and only one was confined to right ventricular infarction (4). We investigated 107 consecutive patients who died from coronary heart disease, and found a total of 214 infarcts (4). Isolated right ventricular infarct fibrosis was found in three patients, all due to occlusion of a right marginal branch. Combined left and right ventricular infarcts were found in 90 patients (84%), and isolated left ventricular infarcts were found in 17 patients (16%). A total of 85 anterior, 56 lateral, and 70 posterior left ventricular infarcts were found. The frequency of concomitant right ventricular infarction associated with these different sites, (combined left and right ventricular infarcts) were 64%, 7%, and 66%, respectively. Consequently, right ventricular involvement should be considered in about 2/3 of all patients with anterior or inferior/posterior infarction, but this is rare in patients with left lateral infarcts.

Infarct location and size

Right ventricular involvement is much larger in inferior/posterior than in anterior infarction (4, 5, 9). Consequently, when total infarct size (left plus right ventricular component) is similar in anterior and inferior/posterior infarction, a different infarct distribution exists between the two ventricles. We investigated 27 consecutive patients who died from their first acute myocardial infarction (MI) (anterior or inferior/posterior), (Fig. 1). Although total infarct size was equal in these two groups, patients with inferior/posterior infarcts had much larger right ventricular infarction and concomitant smaller left ventricular involvement with more left ventricular myocardium intact. This may explain the better prognosis after inferior/posterior than after anterior infarcts of apparently equal size (measured enzymatically) because preserved left ventricular function is a major determinant of post-infarct survival (10-13). Furthermore, severe right ventricular dysfunction caused by extensive right ventricular infarction is often present in patients with inferior/posterior infarction but is very rarely seen in patients with other infarct locations.

Clinical findings

Clinical presentation

Patients with haemodynamic important right ventricular infarction usually present with evidence of acute Q-wave inferior/posterior MI, often associated with advanced atrioventricular block. Elevation of the jugular venous

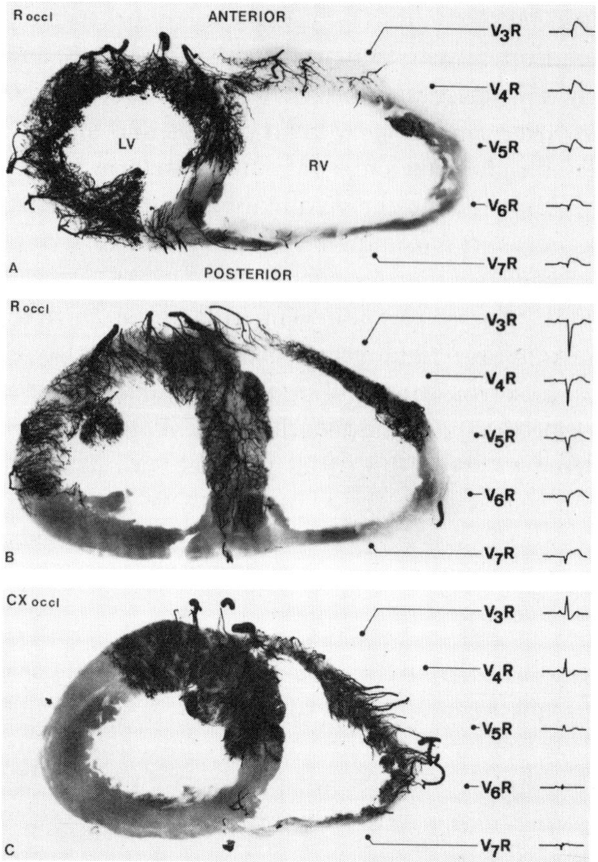

Fig. 2. *Inferior/posterior infarction. Right chest electrocardiogram (V_3R to V_7R) with corresponding necropsy angiograms of 1 cm thick transventricular slices showing poor contrast filling in infarcted myocardium. (A and B): posterior infarction caused by occluded right coronary artery (R occl) with extensive right ventricular (RV) infarction and concomitant minor (A) and larger (B) left ventricular (LV) infarction. (C): posterolateral infarct caused by occluded circumflex coronary artery (CX occl) with extensive left ventricular infarction and minor right ventricular infarction. Corresponding electrocardiograms show ST elevation in five leads (A), three leads (B), and one lead (C).*

pressure and concomitant arterial hypotension (with or without shock) is often present, together with signs of low cardiac output. In contrast to predominant left ventricular infarction with evidence of left ventricular dysfunction, the lungs are usually clear to auscultation, and the chest X-ray is free of signs of pulmonary oedema.

Electrocardiographic diagnosis

In 1949 *Myers et al* (14) investigated the electrocardiographic abnormalities in conventional electrocardiographic leads but did not find any specific changes associated with right ventricular infarction. In 1974, *Erhardt* (3) suggested that ST elevation ≥1 mm in the right chest lead CR4R was a good indicator of the extensive right ventricular infarction. Since then, many studies have evaluated the diagnostic value of various right chest leads. Most studies were limited to leads V_3R and V_4R, but we found that even large right ventricular infarction could be present without ST elevation in these leads, but it was present in V_5R, V_6R and V_7R as illustrated in Fig. 2B. A few studies have focused on lateral right chest leads V_5R and V_6R (15-18) and in two of these studies (17, 18) the lateral leads were most accurate.

Funk (17) found the highest diagnostic sensitivity and specificity for V_6R. We investigated the diagnostic accuracy of electrocardiographic right chest leads V_3R to V_7R by clinicopathologic correlation in 43 consecutive fatal cases (Table 1) (18). Sensitivity and positive predictive value reached 100% in V_6R and V_7R. The diagnostic accuracy differed with various infarct sites. It was low in anterior infarcts (sensitivity < 28%) but much higher in electrocardiographic inferior/posterior infarcts where specificity reached 100% in V_5R, V_6R and V_7R (Table 2).

The right chest leads do not add much to the diagnostic accuracy of the 12-lead electrocardiogram (19). Therefore, the risk of missing a diagnosis of acute MI if the right chest leads are not examined, is very small, but

Table 1. *Diagnostic accuracy (%) of right chest leads in 43 patients with or without right ventricular infarction.*

	Sensitivity	Specificity	Positive predictive value	Negative predictive value	Efficiency
ST elevation ≥ 1 mm in leads:					
V3R	37	81	77	43	53
V4R	33	86	82	44	53
V5R	26	94	88	43	51
V6R	33	100	100	47	58
V7R	41	100	100	50	63

Table 2. *Diagnostic accuracy (%) of right chest leads in 16 patients with electrocardiographic inferior/posterior infarction.*

	Sensitivity	Specificity	Positive predictive value	Negative predictive value	Efficiency
ST elevation ≥ 1 mm in leads:					
V3R	64	80	88	50	69
V4R	73	80	89	57	75
V5R	64	100	100	56	75
V6R	73	100	100	63	81
V7R	91	100	100	83	94

they are useful in determining the distribution of infarcts between the right and the left ventricle. Therefore, in patients with electrocardiographic inferior/posterior infarction, the right chest leads can differentiate those patients with extensive infarction of the right ventricle and minor infarction of the left ventricle (ST elevation in all leads V_3R to V_7R) from patients with predominantly left ventricular infarction (ST elevation in less than all leads V_3R to V_7R). This differentiation is of prognostic importance (20).

Other diagnostic procedures

Right ventricular performance can be assessed in patients using radionuclide angiography and two dimensional echocardiography (11, 21-23). A low right ventricular ejection fraction as demonstrated by radionucleide angiography, may indicate right ventricular infarction (11, 21). Abnormal wall motion and/or right ventricular dilatation shown by echocardiography, may also indicate right ventricular infarction (22). Furthermore, M-mode echocardiographic demonstration of early opening of the pulmonary valve due to atrial contraction indicates severe right ventricular dysfunction and highly increased right ventricular diastolic pressure (23). Myocardial scintigraphy may also be useful, but differing results have been reported (24).

Haemodynamics and therapeutic implications

The syndrome of predominant right ventricular dysfunction in patients with right ventricular infarction was first reported by *Cohn et al* in 1974 (2). The aetiology of shock in patients with extensive right ventricular infarction is caused by severe dysfunction of the right ventricle which is unable to generate sufficient pressure to propel blood through the pulmonary circulation and into the left ventricle. These patients suffer from a low-output syndrome despite an nearly intact left ventricle. The treatment of such patients is related not only to instituting appropriate therapy for severe pump failure but also to avoid inappropriate therapy. The goal of therapy is to increase left ventricular output. Therefore, a greater blood flow must be propelled into the left ventricle. This can be achieved by 1) minimizing the pulmonary vascular resistance (by good oxygenation), 2) increasing the pressure gradient favoring passive flow through the lungs (plasma infusion), and 3) increasing the contractile power in the right ventricle and atrium (dobutamine infusion) (25).

Treatment may be guided by measuring the left ventricular filling pressure which is often low in the untreated patient with right ventricular infarction and shock due to severe right ventricular dysfunction (2). In Contrast, measuring a high right ventricular filling pressure (venous engorgement and high central venous pressure) do not guide treatment because they do not reflect left ventricular dysfunction; and it may even lead the physician to choose inappropriate therapy (diuretics or nitroglycerin infusion) which further lowers left ventricular filling pressure.

Prognosis

Myocardial infarct size and left ventricular function are important determinants of prognosis after infarction (10, 12). It has been demonstrated that the size of infarction assessed enzymatically correlates with the degree of haemodynamic dysfunction of the left ventricle (26-28). Cardiac enzymes, however, may originate from both ventricles and the right ventricle may theoretically be the source of a considerable amount of these enzymes in inferior/posterior infarction. We investigated this in a clinico-pathologic study (29). The coefficients of correlation (r) between peak serum lactate dehydrogenase, and anatomically estimated infarct size were 0.88 for 24 anterior infarcts and 0.84 for 14 posterior infarcts. Exclusion of the right ventricular infarct component from the total infarct size altered the coefficient of correlation to 0.59 ($p=0.09$) in the posterior infarcts, but in anterior infarcts it remained unchanged (0.88). This indicates that infarcted right ventricle released a considerable amount of enzymes in posterior infarction, but not in anterior. Infarct size estimated enzymatically is probably an important predictor of prognosis when the released enzymes reflect left ventricular necrosis. If, however, the enzymes mainly reflect right ventricular necrosis, correlation between prognosis and infarct size estimated enzymatically may be poor (20, 29). Furthermore, this may explain why left ventricular infarct site (anterior versus inferior/posterior) is an independent predictor of survival in groups of patients with similar infarct size estimated enzymatically (10, 13, 20). In patients with inferior/posterior infarction, a better preserved left ventricular function is found because more of the infarct is located in the right ventricle (Fig. 1).

The relative importance of right and left ventricular dysfunction regarding long-term prognosis has recently been studied (11). It was concluded that patients with impaired right ventricular function had the same mortality as patients with normal right ventricular function, whereas left ventricular function was a major determinant of the one-year prognosis. This observation is in accordance with our study (20) where extensive right ventricular infarction diagnosed by ST elevation >1 mm in right chest leads V_3R to

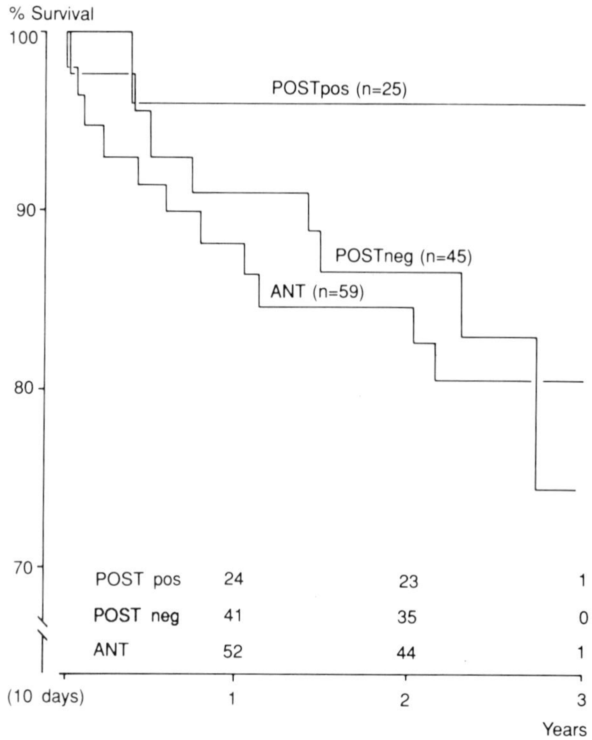

Fig. 3. *Cumulative survival for 129 patients who were alive 10 days after infarction. Statistical evaluation of differences between the curves gave: POSTpos versus ANT: p=0.08; POSTpos versus POSTneg: p=0.09; POSTpos versus ANT+POSTneg (not shown): p=0.05; POSTneg versus ANT: p=0.50. Numbers above the abscissa indicate patients at risk during follow-up. POSTpos=inferior/posterior infarction with ST elevation in all right chest leads V_3R to V_7R, (extensive right ventricular infarction and small left ventricular infarction); POSTneg=inferior/posterior infarction without ST elevation in all leads V3R to V7R (extensive left ventricular infarction); ANT=anterior infarction.*

V_7R predicted a good prognosis for patients alive 10 days after infarction, whereas patients without ST elevation in all these leads (predominantly left ventricular infarction) had a poorer prognosis (Fig. 3).

Conclusion

Right ventricular infarction is present in most patients with inferior/posterior infarction and can be diagnosed by right chest electrocardiography. Patients with extensive right ventricular infarction may develop cardiogenic shock due to severe dysfunction of the right ventricle, despite a nearly undamaged left ventricle. This condition needs appropriate and specific treatment to be reverted, however, the long term prognosis for those patients who survive the initial days after infarction is excellent.

References

1. Sanders AO. Coronary thrombosis with complete heart-block and relative ventricular tachycardia. A case report. Am Heart J 1930-31; 6: 820-3.
2. Cohn JN, Guiha NH, Broder MI, Limas CJ. Right ventricular infarction: Clinical and hemodynamic features. Am J Cardiol 1974; 33: 209-14.

3. Erhardt LR. Clinical and pathological observation in different types of acute myocardial infarction: a study of 84 patients deceased after treatment in a coronary care unit. Acta Med Scand 1974; 26(suppl): 1-78
4. Andersen HR, Falk E, Nielsen D. Right ventricular infarction. Frequency, size and topography in coronary heart disease: A prospective study comprising 107 consecutive autopsies from a coronary care unit. J Am Coll Cardiol 1987; 10: 1223-32.
5. Cabin HS, Soni K, Wackers TJ, Zaret BL. Right ventricular myocardial infarction with anterior wall left ventricular infarction: an autopsy study. Am Heart J 1987; 113: 16-23.
6. Ratliff NB, Hackel DB. Combined right and left ventricular infarction: pathogenesis and clinicopathologic correlation. Am J Cardiol 1980; 45: 217-21.
7. Wade WG. The pathogenesis of infarction of the right ventricle. Br Heart J 1959; 21: 545-54.
8. Harnarayan C, Bennett MA, Pentecost BL, Brewer BL. Quantitative study of infarcted myocardium in cardiogenic shock. Br Heart J 1970; 32: 728-32.
9. Isner JM, Roberts WC. Right ventricular infarction complicating left ventricular infarction secondary to coronary heart disease. Am J Cardiol 1978; 42: 885-94.
10. Hands MD, Lloyd BL, Robinson JS, Klerk N, Thompson PL. Prognostic significance of electrocardiographic site of infarction after correction for enzymatic size of infarction. Circulation 1986; 73: 885-91.
11. Gadsbøll N, Høilund-Carlsen PF, Madsen EB, et al. Right and left ventricular ejection fraction: relation to one-year prognosis in acute myocardial infarction. Eur Heart J 1987; 8: 1201-9.
12. Taylor GJ, Humphries JO, Mellits ED, et al. Predictors of clinical course, coronary anatomy and left ventricular function after recovery from acute myocardial infarction. Circulation 1980; 62: 960-70.
13. Stone PH, Raabe DS, Jaffe AS, et al. Prognostic significance of location and type of myocardial infarction: Independent adverse outcome associated with anterior location. J Am Coll Cardiol 1988; 11: 453-63.
14. Myers GB, Klein HA, Hiratzka T. Correlation of electrocardiographic and pathologic findings in infarction of the interventricular septum and right ventricle. Am Heart J 1949; 37: 720-70.
15. Bratt SH, Brugada P, De Zwaan C, Coenegracht JM, Wellens HJJ. Value of electrocardiogram in diagnosing right ventricular involvement in patients with an acute inferior wall myocardial infarction. Br Heart J 1983; 49: 368-72.
16. Croft CH, Nicod P, Corbett JR, et al. Detection of acute right ventricular infarction by right precordial electrocardiography. Am J Cardiol 1982; 50: 421-7.
17. Funk M. Diagnosis of right ventricular infarction with right precordial ECG leads. Heart & Lung 1986; 15: 562-71.
18. Andersen HR, Falk E, Nielsen D. Right ventricular infarction: diagnostic accuracy of electrocardiographic right chest leads V3R to V7R investigated prospectively in 43 consecutive fatal cases from a coronary care unit. Br Heart J 1989; 61: 514-20.
19. Andersen HR, Nielsen D, Falk E. Right ventricular infarction: diagnostic value of ST elevation in lead III exceeding that of lead II during inferior/posterior infarction and comparison with right chest leads V3R to V7R. Am Heart J 1989; 117: 82-6.
20. Andersen HR, Nielsen D, Falk E. Prognostic significance of right ventricular infarction diagnosed by ST elevation in right chest leads V3R to V7R. Int J Cardiol 1989; 23: 349-56.
21. Marving J, Høilund-Carlsen PF, Chræmmer-Jørgensen B, Gadsbøll N. Are right and left ventricular ejection fraction equal? Ejection fractions in normal subjects and in patients with first acute myocardial infarction. Circulation 1985; 72: 502-14.

22. Lopez-Sendon J, Coma-Canella I, Lombera F, et al. Diagnosis of ischemic right ventricular dysfunction by M-mode echocardiography. Eur Heart J 1982; 3: 230-7.
23. Coma-Canella I, Lopez-Sendon J, Oliver J. Premature pulmonic valve opening and inverted septal convexity in acute ischemic right ventricular dysfunction. Am Heart J 1981; 101: 684-5.
24. Nestico PF, Hakki AH, Felsher J, Heo J, Iskandrian AS. Implications of abnormal right ventricular thallium uptake in acute myocardial infarction. Am J Cardiol 1986; 58: 230-4.
25. Edwards D, Whittaker S, Prior A. Cardiogenic shock without a critically raised left ventricular end diastolic pressure: management and outcome in eighteen patients. Br Heart J 1986; 55: 549-53.
26. Strauss HD, Sobel BE, Roberts R. The influence of occult right ventricular infarction on enzymatically estimated infarct size, hemodynamics and prognosis. Circulation 1982; 66: 503-8.
27. Bleifeld W, Mathey D, Hanrath P, Buss H, Effert S. Infarct size estimated from serial serum creatine phosphokinase in relation to left ventricular hemodynamics. Circulation 1977; 55: 303-11.
28. Herlitz J, Hjalmarson Å, Waldenström J. Five-year mortality rate in relation to enzyme-estimated infarct size in acute myocardial infarction. Am Heart J 1987; 114: 731-7.
29. Andersen HR, Nielsen D, Falk E. Right ventricular infarction: larger enzyme release with posterior than with anterior involvement. Int J Cardiol 1989; 22: 247-55.

21

Diagnostic application of biochemical markers in acute myocardial infarction

MOGENS HØRDER,
WILLIE GERHARDT

Introduction

The clinical diagnosis of acute myocardial infarction (AMI) has been based on clinical signs and ECG findings for more than fifty years. During the 1950- and 1960ies enzyme determinations were introduced as supplementary support for the diagnosis. The enzymes in current use in the late sixties were aspartate aminotransferase (ASAT), lactate dehydrogenase (LD) and creatine kinase (CK) (1-3). The role of enzyme measurements was, however, not recognized by the WHO expert group who in 1971 recommended the criteria for the diagnosis of AMI (4). The changes of ECG were described in detail, whereas the diagnostic criteria for enzymes were few. Thus, it was not indicated which enzymes to measure, how to interpret changes; neither were technical reasons for erroneous results considered.

The lack of agreement about the application of biochemical markers in the evaluation and classification of AMI has resulted in different views of their value in the clinic. The aim of this chapter is therefore to review the kind of markers that are available as reliable tools to evaluate patients with suspected myocardial damage.

Emphasis will be laid on those markers that are in current use in clinical cardiology, i.e. mainly plasma enzymes. However, due to the rapid development of techniques for measuring non-enzymatic markers this new type will also be briefly discussed.

Pertinent properties of biochemical markers for myocardial ischaemia

Biochemical markers for myocardial damage: Sequential release of intracellular components may be used to describe the progression of the lack of integrity of the cell membrane of the myocardial cells (5). It is supposed that myocardial damage has a reversible phase followed by the irreversible phase in which the cell will end up as necrotic tissue. Very early in the reversible phase small molecules like the potassium ion and lactate leak out of the cell. It is only later, after 15-30 minutes, that bigger molecules like enzymes and proteins are released. Traditionally, this has been interpreted as if the myocardial damage is on its way to being irreversible. The more sensitive and specific assays now available may show that enzymes and proteins are released in minor quantities from cells in which the ischaemic damage is reversible.

The development of immunological based assay techniques has shown that not only enzymes and myoglobin, but also proteins that are more or less specific for the myocardial cell are released. It is therefore to be expected that a changing spectrum of markers will be available over the coming years being more and more specific for particular components of the myocardial cell. Table 1 shows those markers that are in use at present together with markers that may replace current markers.

Release of biochemical markers: It is not known in detail how enzymes are released from myocardial cells following ischaemia. The release of enzymes will always occur in cases where ischaemia leads to necrosis. They may, however, not reach the blood if the circulation of the myocardium is abnormal. It is not exactly known how enzymes and other markers reach the blood. Although experiments in dogs have shown that the markers are transported via the lymph this may not be the case for humans.

It has been found in animal experiments that leakage of cytosolic and mitochondrial enzymes show different patterns (6). Although liver cells were used in these experiments there is enough evidence to suggest that the same will be true for myocardial cells. It was found that on recirculation of ischaemic liver, mitochondrial ASAT (mASAT) did not leak into the circulation from ischaemic liver until most of the cytoplasmic ASAT had leaked out. This delayed leakage of mitochondrial enzymes was also consistent with the fact that the mitochondrial membranes maintained a diffusion barrier against matrix enzymes, even after anoxia for 2 h, when their oxidative phosphorylation capacity had been lost. These results indicate that mitochondrial enzymes are liberated into the blood only after appreciable disintegration of the cells, probably necrosis, and that the cumulative activity of mASAT in the blood should reflect the extent of necrosis in ischaemic organs better than that of cASAT.

Interpretations from the time curve and appearance function of biochemical markers in the blood: The time curves of changes of concentrations

Table 1. *Characteristics of biochemical markers.*

Marker	Isoform	Location in myocardium	Extramyocardial location	Release and turnover
CK	MB	cytosol	low in skeletal muscle	rapid
CK	MM	cytosol	high in skeletal muscle	rapid
LD	LD-1	cytosol	liver, erythrocytes	slow
ASAT	mASAT	mitochondria	liver	slow
Myoglobin	–	cytosol	high in skeletal muscle	rapid
Troponin	T	muscle thin filament	skeletal muscle	slow (and rapid?)
Myosin	light chain	muscle thick filament	skeletal muscle	rapid?

of markers in the blood show a certain variability. The time curve may be transformed to an appearance function which describes the net influx of marker into the blood. Recently the peak time of the time curve and the slope of the appearance function have been used to evaluate the effectiveness of thrombolytic therapy in AMI. It is now agreed by most authors that an earlier peak time and a steeper slope of the appearance curve indicate reperfusion (7).

It should be noticed that the estimation of infarct size from the cumulated appearance function of cytosolic enzymes may lead to over-estimation (8). In the absence of reperfusion, the extent of infarction can be estimated reasonably accurately by analysis of serial changes of CK or CK-MB activity, because the cumulative amount of CK appearing in plasma reflects the amount elaborated from the necrotic myocardium. However, reperfusion alters the rate of appearance of CK in plasma and may affect the accuracy of estimates of infarct size. Reasonable estimates can be made from analysis of the rate of increase of plasma CK activity early after recanalization because a substantial and consistent fraction of the total CK that will appear in plasma over 24 hours appears within one hour after recanalization. Thus, the rate of increase of plasma CK activity occurring within 2.5 hours of the time of recanalization correlates closely with infarct size measured independently one to two weeks later by positron emission tomography ($r = 0.93$).

Because thrombolysis is now used routinely, the estimation of infarct size from released markers should be based on non cytosolic markers, e.g.

mitochondrial-ASAT (9) or troponin (10). It is to be expected that the combined application of such markers with different location in the cell and different turnover after release will be valuable tools in the interpretation of the kind and extent of ischaemic damage of the myocardium.

Another interesting possibility seems to arise from the interpretation of the post-release breakdown of CK (11). This approach is based on the following considerations: The CK-MM isoenzyme in myocardium is a dimer composed of two M chains each of which exhibits a carboxy-terminal lysine. The tissue isoform (MM_3) undergoes post-translational modification while circulating in the plasma as a result of proteolysis, with liberation of lysine from two additional isoforms, MM_2 and MM_1, with the latter devoid of any carboxy terminal lysine on either of its M subunits. Conversion of MM_3 to MM_1 is unidirectional, sequential, time- and temperature-dependent. Because of the relatively rapid rate of conversion and relatively slow rate of liberation of CK-MM from tissue under physiological conditions, the prevailing circulating moiety in normal human subjects is MM_1. In cases of AMI, the ratio of MM_3 to MM_1 in plasma increases because of elaboration of MM_3 from the myocardium. However, the rate of rise of the ratio is relatively modest. Sudden washout of MM_3 into plasma results when recanalization occurs in vessels supplying myocardium that has already undergone some irreversible injury. Consequently, the rate of rise of MM_3 increases dramatically, and the rate of rise of the ratio of MM_3 to MM_1 in plasma markedly exceeds that seen with spontaneously evolving infarction. Accordingly, recanalization can be detected simply by analyzing sequential plasma samples and calculating the rate of change of MM_3 and the rate of increase of the ratio of MM_3 to MM_1. Analysis of such changes permits noninvasive detection of recanalization within 30 to 60 minutes with considerable accuracy.

Plasma enzymes in the diagnosis of acute myocardial disease

Choice of marker enzymes: CK and LD have gained general acceptance as enzymes of choice. A "normal", stable concentration of these two enzymes in a patient suspected of having AMI will, with high certainty, exclude myocardial damage. The development of reliable and simple techniques for measuring isoforms of these two enzymes has resulted in tests that combine high sensitivity with high specificity. The location of the various isoenzymes of CK and LD are shown in Table 1.

The analytical reliability of CK and LD and their isoenzymes can now be kept at a coefficient of variation of 5% or lower in clinical chemistry laboratories. This means that a significant change of enzyme concentrations

Table 2. *Decision limits for enzymatic markers of myocardial ischaemia and infarction.*

Marker		Decision Low	Decision High
CK (total)	U/l	150	210
CK-B residual	U/l	12	20
CK-MB enzymimmunoassay	μg/l	10	30
ASAT	U/l	40	60
ASAT-mitochondrial	U/l	3	10
LD-1	U/l	170	200

Enzyme concentrations (U/l) are according to the Scandinavian Committee on Enzymes (SCE). These are for CK and ASAT comparable to the international units of IFCC measured at 37° C. Values below the low limit indicate with high probability that neither ischaemia nor infarction has occurred. Values above the high limit indicate with high probability infarction.

Table 3. *Diagnostic reliabilities of enzymatic markers for myocardial infarction.*

Marker	Sensitivity	Specificity
CK (total)	0.98	0.74
CK-MB	0.99	0.98
LD-1	0.98	0.96
ASAT	0.98	0.80

Sensitivity is the proportion of subjects with infarction who have a positive test. Specificity is the proportion of subjects without the disease who have a negative test.

is approx 15% at values near to the decision limit, Table 2. The clinical, diagnostic reliability of these enzyme tests is shown in Table 3. The table is meant to serve only as a basis for comparison of the tests. The absolute clinical reliability depends on the prevalence of disease and on application within the proper time-window as will be discussed later.

Sources of error in the interpretation of concentrations of markers in the blood: Falsely negative results are unlikely, provided the analytical laboratory has a procedure for quality assurance but may occur due to non-appearance of the marker in the blood following lack of perfusion of the myocardium.

Falsely positive results may occur due to analytical and biological non specificity of the tests. CK-MB isoenzyme may be determined by electrophoresis, immunoinhibition (CK-B residual activity) chromatography and enzyme-immunoassay (ELISA). Electrophoresis and chromatography are both specific if the best techniques are used. They are, however, not suited for the routine laboratory and are not used now by many laboratories. The immunoinhibition technique is widely used. It will detect not only CK-MB but also CK-BB. Normally CK-BB occurs in very low concentrations in the blood. It may be found in detectable concentrations in a macroform, i.e.

a complex of CB-BB with an immunoglobulin. Clinically this is presented as an increased, and persistent concentration of CK-B residual activity that also represents a higher proportion of total CK than is found in patients with AMI. This source of error may be compensated for by an intelligent cooperation between the clinicians and the laboratory. In a few years the more specific enzyme-immunoassay will probably replace the immunoinhibition techniques. This will compensate for the false results due to analytical unspecificity. They cannot, however, compensate for errors due to biological unspecificity: CK-MB occurs in elevated concentrations in patients with high concentrations of CK due to trauma, necrosis and ischaemia of the skeletal muscle. The clinical situation will, however, in most cases prevent the clinician from misinterpretation of such false elevated CK-MB in terms of being indicative for AMI.

Leakage of CK-MB from myocardial cells without an infarct being present may occur in coronary angiography and other diagnostic manipulations of the heart. Clinical experience has shown that this will be interpreted as a positive result in a few cases only.

Finally, the occurrence of elevated CK-MB in angina pectoris should be mentioned. Using the immunoinhibition technique it is not possible to detect any significant changes. The more specific enzymeimmunotechnique has a lower limit of detectability. Therefore, changing values of CK-MB may be detected at the concentration interval of 10-30 μg/l, which is below the limit of 30 μg/l for the diagnosis of AMI (12). Clinically, such patients will present an unstable angina. It is therefore most probable that these patients have a minor infarct that will not be classified as such with the criteria used hitherto.

LD-1 may be falsely elevated also, and more often than CK-MB. The most frequent reason for this is haemolysis. Even minor haemolysis will lead to significant increase of LD-1. But LD-1 may also be elevated in patients suffering from congestion of the lungs, the liver and the pancreas. LD-1 is therefore not the marker of choice if more specific markers with the same kind of kinetic become available. Troponin seems to be a candidate to replace LD-1 (10).

Choice of time-window for measuring markers in the blood: The presence of markers in the blood in AMI is a dynamic process. It is therefore of decisive importance to optimize the time of blood drawing in a way that with high probability will detect any deviation of the marker concentration from the stable base line. To do so, the blood drawings should be placed in relation to the probable onset of infarction. Markers that have a rapid release and turnover will be detectable within a time-interval of few hours

(2-4) to 12-24 hours after onset of infarction. CK MB and myoglobin have such characteristics. Markers that show a slower release or turnover or both may be detectable for several days following infarction. LD-1 and troponin have such characteristics. It has now been shown that it is possible, with 3-4 blood drawings placed within a time window of 4-30 hours after onset of pain, to confirm or exclude with high probability an AMI. Further blood drawing is not needed for the diagnosis but may be used for estimation of infarct size. If the time of onset of suspected infarction is unknown, further blood drawing may also be needed.

Diagnostic power of biochemical markers: The values for the diagnostic reliability of various markers as shown in Table 3 are valid provided the markers are measured within the proper time-window. The positive and negative predictive values of a series of 3-4 measurements in a coronary care unit (CCU) will be very high, provided the proper marker and time-window are chosen. In general practice, in emergency rooms, in postoperative units and in departments of internal medicine and surgery the diagnostic power in terms of the positive predictive values of the test results will always be lower than in CCU's due to the much lower prevalences of the disease.

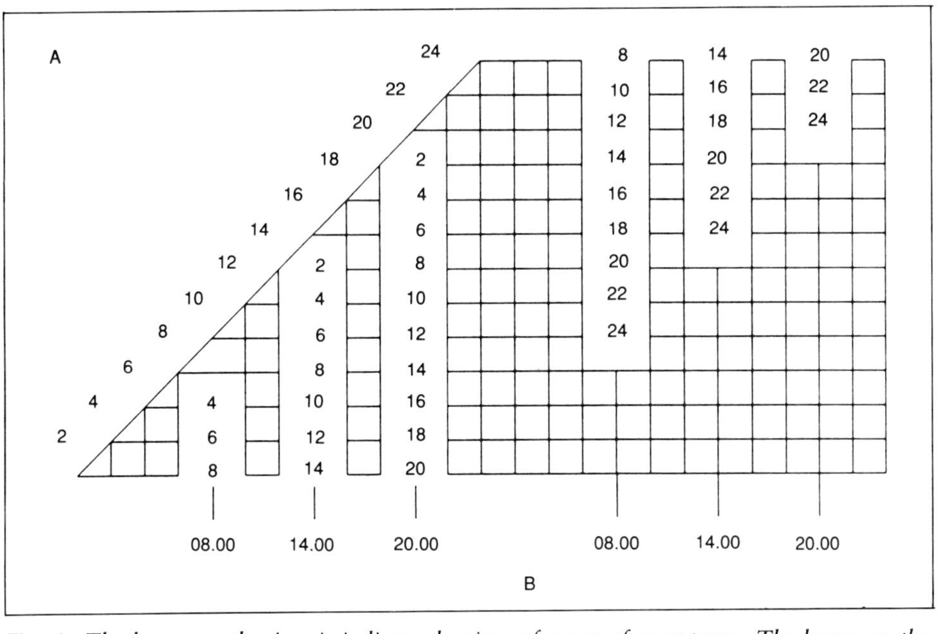

Fig. 1. *The hours on the A-axis indicate the time of onset of symptoms. The hours on the B-axis indicate the fixed hours at which blood drawing is performed thrice a day. In the diagram is seen the three occasions at which each patient will have blood drawn within a proper time-window.*

Practical clinical strategies

Choice of markers: One marker with rapid release and one marker with slower release and turnover (Table 1) will yield all necessary information. The present combination of highest diagnostic value is CK-MB and LD-1. Newer and more specific markers will probably replace LD-1 soon. More markers are unnecessary from a clinical point of view.

Time-window and number of blood drawings: Clinical experience has shown (13) that a reliable procedure of reasonable practicability is to place blood drawings at fixed hours during the day. An example is shown in Fig. 1. It is practical because the phlebotomists perform the blood drawing for all patients in one round and the laboratory can do the analysis either immediately or in one or two series during the day. All patients will have three measurements performed within time windows that are 4-16 as the earliest and 12-24 as the latest. This is a compromise that ensures a reliable clinical diagnostic procedure at lower costs and is therefore well-suited for most CCU's. If slow release markers are needed for evaluation of infarct size they should be measured once more a day in the one or two days following the first three measurements as shown in Fig. 1.

References

1. LaDue JS, Wroblewski F, Karmen A. Serum glutamic oxalacetic transaminase activity in human transmural myocardial infarction. Science 1954; 120: 497-9.
2. Wroblewski F, Ruegsegger P, LaDue JS. Serum lactic dehydrogenase activity in acute transmural myocardial infaction. Science 1956; 123: 1122-3.
3. Dreyfus JC, Schapira G, Resnias J, Scebat L. La créatinekinase sérique dans le diagnostic de l'infarctus yocardique. Rev Fr Etudes Clin Biol 1960; 5: 386-7.
4. Ischaemic Heart Disease Registers. Report of the fifth working group. København: WHO, 1971.
5. Hearse DJ. Cellular damage during myocardial ischaemia: Metabolic changes leading to enzyme leakage. In: Hearse DJ, DeLeiris J, eds. Enzymes in cardiology. Diagnosis and research. Chichester, John Wileys & Sons Limited, 1979.
6. Kamiike W, Fujukawa M, Koseki M, et al. Different patterns of leakage of cytosolic and mitochondrial enzymes. Clin Chem Acta 1989; 185: 265-70.
7. Zwaan CD, Willems GM, Vermeer F, et al. Enzyme tests in the evaluation of thrombolysis in acute myocardial infarction. Br Heart J 1988; 59: 175-83.
8. Bergmann SR, Sobel BE. Noninvasive assessment of the efficacy of coronary thrombolysis. In: Julian D, Kübler W, Norris RM, Swan HJC, Collen D, Verstraete M, eds. Thrombolysis in cardiovascular disease. New York: Marcel Dekker Inc, 1989: 141-61.
9. Panteghini M, Pagani F, Cuccia C. Effects of therapeutic coronary reperfusion on aspartate aminotransferase isoenzymes in sera of patients with acute myocardial infarction. Clin Chem 1989; 35: 909-12.
10. Gerhardt W, Katus H, Hamm C, et al. Clinical value of troponin-T in diagnosis and monitoring of coronary heart disease – results of a multicenter study. (Abstract) XIV International Congress of Clinical Chemistry. San Francisco, 1990.

11. Puleo PR, Perryman MB, Bresser MA, et al. Creatine kinase isoform analysis in the detection and assessment of thrombolysis in man. Circulation 1987; 75: 1162-8.
12. Bøtker HE, Ravkilde J, Søgaard P, Jørgensen PJ, Hørder M, Thygesen K. Gradation of unstable angina on basis of a sensitive method for creatine kinase MB isoenzyme determination in serum. Br Heart J (in press).
13. Engebretsen LF, Strømme JH, Skjæggestad Dørum H-P. Enzymstatus ved hjerteinfarkt. Tidskr Nor Lægeforen 1989; 109: 1276-9.

Arrhythmias and sudden death

22

The prehospital phase in acute ischaemic heart disease Primary arrhythmias and sudden death

TORBEN HAGHFELT

Epidemiology

Sudden coronary death (SCD) is one of the major causes of death in Scandinavia and other industrialized areas, the frequency being about 30 SCD per week per million inhabitants. Data collected in such countries indicate, that 25% of the patients suffering from heart attack die suddenly. Of those who die during the first 2 weeks after the event, approximately 40% die within one hour of the onset of symptoms, the vast majority of them before they reach hospital. Studies of patients who died suddenly and of prehospital resuscitated patients indicate, that 75-80% had some prior manifestation of cardiac disease, and in more than half of the remaining 20-25% cardiac arrest is due to acute myocardial infarction (AMI). The percentage dying suddenly without prior symptoms may be higher in younger age groups.

The occurrence of ischaemic heart disease (IHD) in Denmark has been increasing throughout recent years, and the mortality during the acute phase is very high, despite the advances made in the mean time. This applies especially to patients with acute ischaemic heart disease (AIHD) – including AMI. Thus, the incidence of AMI is around 4 per thousand (1, 2) and the total mortality in the acute phase (0-28 days) about 50%. More than one half of these deaths take place during the initial phase, often prior to hospitalization, inasmuch as 60-75% of all deaths from AMI occur <24 hours after the onset of symptoms, either in the form of instantaneous coronary death (ICD) (<15 minutes), or SCD (<24 hours).

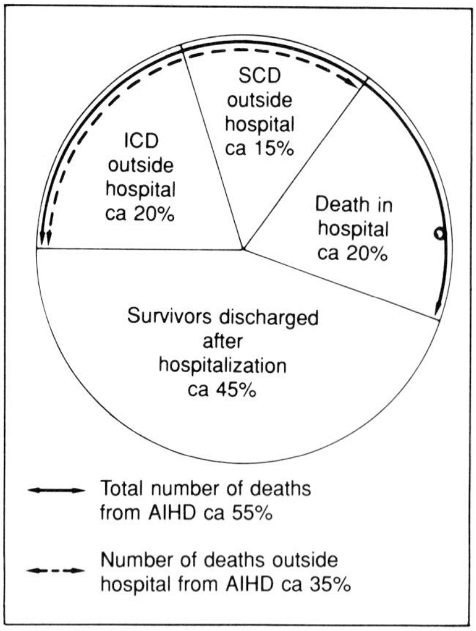

Fig. 1. *The prehospital course for patients with acute ischaemic heart disease (AIHD); (average figures from the literature (1, 52-54) ICD: Instantaneous coronary death, SCD: sudden coronary death).*

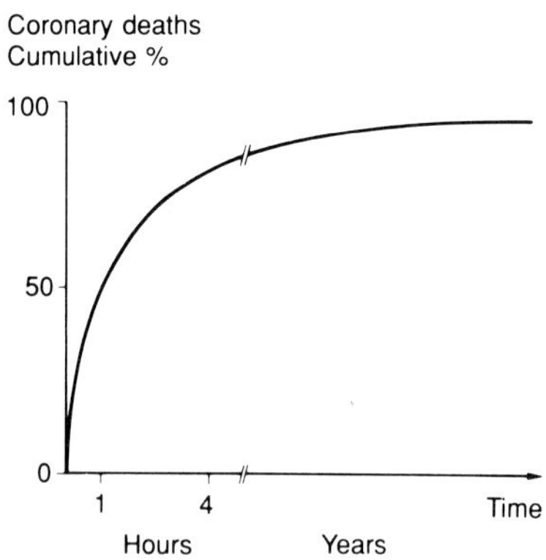

Fig. 2. *The cumulative (%) mortality of acute ischaemic heart disease (AIHD) in relation to the duration of symptoms (average figures from the literature) (1, 52-54).*

Fig. 1 shows a schematic survey of the course of AIHD during the prehospital and hospital phase. In respect of mortality from AIHD, there has been a real increase within recent years, which cannot be ascribed to changes in the age distribution of the population (3, 4). In this connection it is important to underline the fact that the the risk of lethal arrhythmias in patients with AIHD, without later verified AMI, is of importance (1, 4-6).

Fig. 2 shows the cumulative (percentage) mortality from AIHD in relation to the duration from the onset of symptoms. It is known from *Haghfelt's* thesis (1) that younger patients are more likely to be the subject of an attack of ICS or SCD than the elderly with AIHD, and that this applies in particular to patients with no or only a short history of IHD.

Pathology, pathogenesis, mechanism and occurrence of primary arrhythmias/SCD

Severe coronary atherosclerosis, often accompanied by stenosis, is the most common characteristic found in cases of SCD. There is, however, an ill-defined fraction of SCD, perhaps as large as about 20% that occurs in individuals exhibiting little or no coronary atherosclerosis. So from the point of view of its prevention, SCD should not be equated with coronary atherosclerosis. There are several mechanisms which could lead to SCD. Such factors include platelet-thrombus formation, sudden increases in myocardial oxygen demand, alteration of autonomic neural control, coronary spasms, changes in the cardiac conduction system and increased sensitivity of the myocardium to ischaemia. A particular problem, still incompletely resolved, is the role of platelet-thrombus formation in precipitating ventricular fibrillation (VF). Most occlusive thrombi are associated with visible structural changes in the atheromatous plaque (cracks and haemorrhages). The frequency of occlusive thrombi increases with the interval between the onset of symptoms and SCD.

Liberthson et al (7, 8) and *Dalen et al* (9) found in an autopsy study of 220 patients with SCD, *acute* coronary artery lesions (thromboses, plaque rupture or intramural haemorrhage) in the great majority as a single coronary affection. It was possible to demonstrate AMI with certainty at autopsy in about 1/4th. The most frequent finding was plaque rupture. Chronic coronary artery stenosis of more than 75% of the lumen in at least one of the large coronary arteries was found in approximately 90% of the patients and most frequently as 3 vessel disease, which was found in 2/3rds of the patients, while about 1/4th had 2 vessel disease.

The pathogenesis of primary tachyarrhythmias in patients with AMI is the infarcted area or myocardial ischaemia, in cases with atrial fibrillation, however, more often changes in the haemodynamic state. Hypercatecholaminaemia and other autonomic changes can also result in tachy- or brady-arrhythmias, especially in the first few hours of AMI.

It has been shown both by experimental studies and clinical investigations following the introduction of mobile coronary care units (MCCU), Holter-monitoring etc, that the mechanism of cardiac arrest during the prehospital phase with AIHD possibly leading to SCD, is primarily electrical instability and primary VF. The occurence of VF is particulary high in the very first minutes/hours after the onset of the acute myocardial episode. Both experimental and clinical studies have demonstrated that it is frequently a question of a potentially reversible arrhythmia, provided sufficient treatment can be commenced within a few – generally – 4-5 minutes (1, 10-13).

When VF develops, it may be the result of acute ischaemia or it may occur in the absence of acute ischaemia – for example in patients with severe congestive heart disease and scars of myocardial infarction or with ventricular aneurysm. VF may also develop in patients with severe bradycardia, electrolyte imbalance, drug intoxication, congenital abnormalities (for instance long QT-syndrome or in patients with overt or concealed accessory pathways). Better identification of the various clinical markers associated with each pathogenic mechanism is needed to assess the prevalence of the various causes of SCD, especially in apparently normal individuals.

In animals, experimentally-induced ischaemia and reperfusion of the myocardium both cause malignant ventricular arrhythmias. There is also a delayed phase of ventricular arrhythmias (6-24 hours) caused by the development of intrinsic automatic rhythm in surviving Purkinje fibres in the endocardial zone of the infarct. The same mechanism presumably operates in man. The importance of reperfusion in producing arrhythmias in man is, however, still controversial. The development of VF in some patients with IHD, but without signs of AMI, is considered to be caused by coronary spasm, and approximately 30% of VF episodes develop during painless ischaemia (14).

In the acute phase of AIHD there are, especially in the first hour, supraventricular or ventricular arrhythmias in more than 90% of patients. The incidence of tachyarrhythmias during the first 24 hours after AMI (15) is shown in Table 1.

The supraventricular arrhythmias are almost, without exception, the indirect result of the myocardial infarction itself. The most common forms are atrial flutter, atrial fibrillation and atrial tachycardia, nearly always secondary to heart failure and haemodynamic effect. The latter caused by dilatation of the left atrium, possibly due to infarction in the area supplied by the right coronary artery, with accompanying affection of the atrial structure.

The occurrence of ventricular arrhythmias or atrial flutter in patients with AMI produces more or less the same mortality, namely about 15%. How-

Table 1. *Primary tachyarrhythmias during the first 24 hours of AMI (incidence).*

Supraventricular tachycardia	24%
Supraventricular extrasystolia	24%
Atrial fibrillation	12%
Atrial flutter	3%
More than 5 ventricular extrasystolia/minute	21%
Ventricular tachycardia	13%
Ventricular fibrillation	5%

ever, the occurrence of ventricular tachycardia at the time of admission results in a mortality during the following four weeks of 30-35% (15). Patients who are admitted to hospital before 2-3 hours, have significantly more primary arrhythmias during the hospital phase than patients admitted later. This is in good agreement with the arrhythmia phases identified by *Bigger and Wit* (16) in experimental AMI. It has been shown that a high frequency of ventricular arrhythmias occurs in *arrhythmia phase I* (the first 2 hours after occlusion of a coronary artery). These have a prolonged transmission time (reduced potential rate in ischaemic/infarcted myocardial tissue), resulting in entry-block and later re-entry phenomenon. The occurrence of the re-entry phenomenon is reduced considerably during *arrhythmia phase II*. The cellular background is presumably a slower impulse-distribution brought about partly by the calcium canals, and partly by the cellular concentration of catecholamine (16). In addition, necrotic and ischaemic myocardial cells have an increased tendency to loose potassium. The increased extracellular potassium concentration thus brought about can result in the membrane potential being reduced, and increased secondary automaticity in the Purkinje fibres. The occurrence of the so-called "*late potentials*" can play a role in the increased occurrence of ventricular arrhythmias and VF during the very early hours of AIHD.

In a study from Belfast (17), performed during a 3 year period, 295 patients with AMI, were examined within one hour of onset of the symptoms, (in the prehospital phase). The 295 patients were alive when first seen or were successfully resuscitated. This study provided information regarding *primary arrhythmias* in the first hour during AIHD among patients, who did not suffer SCD; 58% had ventricular ectopics while primary VF (in the absence of significant left ventricular failure or cardiogenic shock) occurred in 10%. Sustained ventricular tachycardia and supraventricular dysrhythmia during the first hour (most frequently atrial fibrillation), occurred in only 2-3% each.

It was concluded that there is considerable evidence, that AMI is accompanied by an early rise in blood catecholamines, and that this response probably results from nervous reflexes arising from the site and boundary of the infarction. Patients with sympathetic overactivity are likely to have sinus tachycardia or tachyarrhythmias. Patients with evidence of parasympathetic overactivity often have sinus bradycardia and transient AV block of second or third degree, perhaps also transient hypotension with systolic blood pressure below 100 mmHg. Sympathetic overactivity occurs more frequently than parasympathetic overactivity in patients with anterior infarction, whereas the opposite is the case in patients with inferior or posterior infarction. The overall incidence of automatic disturbance among patients with inferior or posterior myocardial infarction was 93%, which was significantly higher than the 73% among patients with anterior myocardial infarction, and the incidence of autonomic disturbance was significantly lower in patients seen in the second half of the first hour compared to patients seen in the first half hour.

The fundamental properties of the myocardium, namely rhythmicity, conductivity and contractility may be suppressed by vago-overactivity. There could also be a depressed atrial contractility, during vago-overactivity. This can reduce stroke volume, cardiac output and coronary perfusion pressure, as well as elevating left atrial pressure and left ventricular end-diastolic pressure. Furthermore, it is now known that bradycardia can be a precursor of VF and thereby an important factor in the high early mortality from AMI. Malignant ventricular ectopics may appear in association with early bradycardia and hypotension and be abolished by increasing the heart rate and blood pressure. Tachycardia and sympathetic overactivity may also affect the VF threshold by increasing the oxygen demand of the myocardium.

Goldstein et al (18) performed an analysis of cardiac symptoms preceding cardiac arrest outside hospital. They found, that cardiac arrest was sudden (with either no symptoms or symptoms for less than one hour) in 71% of the patients examined, and non-sudden, which means cardiac arrest occurring after more than one hour of symptoms, in 29% of the patients. A history of cardiovascular disease was present in 85% of patients with sudden cardiac arrest and in 83% with non-sudden arrest. Cardiac arrest occurred without symptoms in 38% of the patients with sudden cardiac arrest and was the first expression of coronary artery disease in 4% of the entire study group. The study indicates that cardiac arrest usually occurs with symptoms and almost always in the setting of a history of cardiovascular disease.

Patients with previous AMI and accompanying reduced left ventricular function, patients with remaining ischaemia after AMI and/or angina pectoris, as well as patients with IHD and recurring ventricular tachycardia are at high risk of SCD (14).

Prehospital care

Despite more and more coronary care units all over the world, the community mortality from IHD still remains very high. Any reduction of mortality by coronary care is swamped by the large number of deaths in people suffering a heart attack, who do not reach hospital alive.

In Scandinavia, western Europe and USA it has been debated for many years, whether prehospital treatment does reduce mortality from AMI. However, irrespective of whether there is any survival advantage, patients wish for optimal diagnostic and treatment facilities, as well as skilled nursing, effective pain relief, effective resuscitation etc. including an optimal prehospital coronary care.

The experience from Belfast, Seattle, Miami and many other places, including Scandinavia, where MCCU's have been introduced, it is known that resuscitation from VF has been successfully carried out by doctors, ambulance personnel, emergency medical technicians, other types of paramedics, nurses and general practitioners. Experience with ambulance personnel suggests, that intensive training and frequent retraining is required, further, that primary resuscitation attempted by bystanders is very important, if professional personnel are to be successfull with advanced cardiac life support (ACLS).

The latest investigational results regarding prehospital conditions in AIHD in Denmark originate from a prospective study carried out in Odense in 1988 (19-21). This showed significantly better survival when using a rendez-vouz model (a physician car with transportable defibrillator equipment as compared to the conventional ambulance system/ambulances equipped with defibrillator, and manned by well-educated "technicians"). In addition, the investigation rendered probable the following:

1) That intensifying courses in cardiac arrest treatment of non-medical persons with no simultaneous increase in the knowledge, by both patients and relatives of warning symptoms, as well as the establishment of a better and more effective alarm system will in the future permit even better treatment results, irrespective of the ambulance model employed.
2) The better and more professional this prehospital treatment has been, the fewer are the cerebral injuries and sequelae after treatment of cardiac arrest during the prehospital phase.

An investigation (21) which included dementia and psychological testing of surviors of cardiac arrest outside of hospital thus showed a significant fall in the number of brain injuries in the period where the prehospital treatment was carried out with the participation of physicians (rendez-vous model with a physician car, or heart ambulance manned by physicians), as compared to the conventional ambulance system (without the participation of physicians in the prehospital phase). The fear of an increasing number of survivors with cerebral sequelae following anoxia after the introduction of various types of heart ambulances thus seems quite unfounded.

In the study from Odense (20) only about 5% of the cardiac arrest victims received cardiopulmonary resuscitation from bystanders, as compared to 17% in a Northern Ireland study (22) and 40% in Seattle where about 400.000 citizens took part in a community training programme (22). Because cardiopulmonary resuscitation training is time consuming and at least half of the victims have known IHD (22), it may be more rewarding to target relatives of cardiac patients for training. Consequently, training in basic life support (BLS) should be offered to relatives of cardiac patients. Such a policy would presumably give better survival among patients with cardiac arrest in the prehospital phase.

In Denmark 5-6.000 cases occur annually of potentially reversible cardiac arrest outside hospital. An optimal prehospital treatment, where all the steps in "the chain of survival" are improved, will presumably lead to an 5-10 fold increase in the survival percentage (patients without cerebral sequelae after anoxia), so that about 20 (40%) corresponding to more than 1.000 human lives would also be "saved" annually. The efforts should also be concentrated on a) education of the population in life-saving first aid and recognition of prodromal symptoms of AMI, and b) an effectivation of the alarm procedures. Experience from Danish studies, suggests the following outline for a country-wide prehospital cardiac arrest treatment:

a) Larger towns and cities with more than 100.000-200.000 inhabitants should have at least one physician ambulance, equipped with defibrillator and intubation equipment. In addition, defibrillator equipment in all acute ambulances. The physician ambulance can function as a rendezvous model.
b) Medium sized provincial towns should have all acute ambulances equipped with defibrillators, possibly with ad hoc help from the hospital by nurses/physicians.
c) In the rural areas and small towns help from general practitioners/physician clinics ad hoc would be the most expedient model. Further, all acute ambulances, should be equipped with a defibrillator.

The ambulance staff should attend obligatory courses in defibrillation techniques.

Early commencement of cardiopulmonary resuscitation and rapid definitive care (defibrillation) are each associated with a favourable outcome (23). The survival rate following VF may reach 70% under ideal conditions, in comparison with an average rate of about 30%.

As is known, the delay before BLS and ACLS in patients with cardiac arrest outside hospital is the major determinant of survival (the mortality increases by 4% for each minute until defibrillation is attempted) (24), therefore it is extremely important that bystanders give the correct alarm and start BLS as soon as possible. This will give the professionel team much better results with ACLS when they arrive at the scene of the accident.

The development in the area of defibrillators with *semi-automatic* or even *automatic* defibrillators during the last few years seems to improve further the results of VF treatment outside hospital, as these defibrillators can be used by ambulance drivers, paramedicals or even in some instances by laypersons. Only a few hours of training are required (25). In Denmark there has been good experience using *semi-automatic* defibrillators in the prehospital phase, also when used by ambulance drivers after very short courses. Concern regarding the possibility of patients receiving inappropriate shocks have proved unfounded, as available machines are 100% specific. That is also the reason why, in some places, automatic defibrillators have been placed in the homes of those at risk (26). Automatic defibrillators may also be able to save lives if placed in densely populated areas, such as office blocks, factories and airports (27).

While it is generally accepted, that prompt action can restore patients stricken with VF to their former state, and that the prognosis remains extremely poor following cardiac arrest outside hospital associated with asystole or electromechanical dissociation, it is possibly less widely appreciated, that the hospital mortality following prehospital *medical* management during the acute phase of AMI may be reduced and the long-term prognosis improved (28, 29). This phenomenon is likely to result from prevention of extension of the infarct secondary to the disturbances of heart rate, rhythm and blood pressure, which few patients escape. Clearly, a comprehensive prehospital strategy must take into account the need to deal effectively not only with VF, but also, if possible, with the other disturbances which frequently complicate the acute phase of infarction. Being in the *thrombolysis area* it has been shown that very early thrombolysis in patients with AIHD/AMI will further improve the prognosis in respect of the residual ventricular function and mortality (30-33). This suggests that the benefit of *thrombolytic therapy* may best be realized through prehospital-initiated treatment. However, before such treatment can be routinely offered in this setting, there are several important questions to be answered. How many patients with AMI utilize the prehospital care system? Can these patients be accurately and rapidly identified by paramedics working under field conditions? Does prehospital administration of thrombolytic therapy confer advantages without added risk over those realized, when treatment is initiated in a well-prepared emergency department? Will the frequency of reperfusion arrhythmias increase? Can treatment of inappropriate patients be avoided? – and finally will the benefit/risk ratio be favourable?

To date there are only a few reports of the administration of thrombolytic substances during the prehospital phase (34-36). The anticipated enhanced salutary effect on the extent of permanent myocardial injury and the left ventricular function has been confirmed in only two of these (34, 36). Ease of administration of the thrombolytic agent is of particular importance in the prehospital setting. Anisoylated plasminogen-streptokinase complex (APSAC) has the advantage that it is given as an intravenous bolus (37).

It is known with regard to prehospital *antiarrhythmic treatment*, that there are no reliable electrocardiographic predictors of VF. Consequently, all patients with AIHD must be considered potentially at risk. However, the risk is markedly time dependent, as primary VF rarely occurs 6 or more hours after the onset of symptoms. The clinical history combined with knowledge of the time of onset of symptoms, provides a readily available assessment of risk.

Investigating the potential of prophylactic antiarrhythmic therapy in the acute phase of AIHD is technically and ethically difficult. Few drugs are as attractive as lidocaine for use in infarct patients, and there has been a paucity of large, well-conducted investigations of other antiarrhythmic agents. None have yielded confirmed statistically significant positive results. The *ISIS-1 trial* demonstrated, however, that the administration of atenolol to patients with suspected infarction meeting the entry criteria was associated with a 53% reduction among patients entering the trial within 2 hours of onset of symptoms. A case can therefore be made for the cautious administration of a beta-blocking agent to suitable patients in the prehospital setting (38).

Very early prehospital management of shock, heart failure and bradycardia may also prevent further deterioration of the myocardium. However, prehospital interventions after one hour, appear to have had but little impact, and patients with AMI who arrive at hospital late (after the onset of symptoms) have higher mortality rates than those who come to hospital early (36, 39-41).

The future role of prehospital management of AIHD/AMI is far from clear. The availability of thrombolytic therapy, coronary angioplasty and emergency surgery will further complicate the prehospital triage of patients seen by emergency technicians. The use of additional technology is likely to be necessary (42), and will increase the already complex setting in which the prehospital health care provider must work. Prehospital administration of thrombolytic therapy will have to be shown to be both safe and more effective than rapid triage and transport to a well-prepared receiving facility in order to justify this approach. These yet unanswered questions are important areas for investigation, but the increasing sophistication at the present stage reinforces the belief that a second tier is required and that where possible this should be medical. A great deal more can be done to improve the outlook of the patients during the first hours than during the entire hospital phase.

It has been estimated from the literature that resuscitation by a MCCU would lead directly to the fall in community IHD-mortality of about 1%, and in Virginia, USA, a fall of 2% in community mortality was directly attributable to out-of-hospital resuscitation by mobile coronary care. Because AMI is such a common cause of death, especially as SCD, even a small reduction in mortality (in %) would save many lives. The only way to obtain a reduction in the mortality from AIHD is to intensify the prehospital treatment by introducing MCCU equipped with semi-automatic or automatic defibrillators and well educated ambulance personnel. Furthermore, it is necessary to get more and more layman to BLS-courses.

It seems possible, based on the newer results from the UK and USA, to resuscitate 100-400 per million inhabitants annually with an ideal prehospital care system, depending on local and geographical circumstances, and the educational level and interest of the public.

In the Scandinavian countries the optimal prehospital care system may obviously vary from place to place. There is a need of doctor-manned ambulances in larger cities, well-equipped (with semi- and fully-automatic defibrillators) ambulances in all places (manned with technicians/ambulance men educated in ACLS), and in certain places a "Life-flight" helicopter-service (43-47).

The cost-effectiveness of prehospital coronary care

There have been few reports on the cost of mobile coronary care, but available estimation suggests, that a cardiac ambulance operating from a hospital coronary care unit adds relatively little to the overall expense of providing coronary care. The cost per life saved by prehospital resuscitation therefore is not excessive and well within the range of costs that the community is prepared to pay for the treatment of other fatal conditions.

The cost of a saved life following out-of-hospital cardiac arrest resuscitated by specially trained ambulance personnel or by MCCU has been roughly estimated in several investigations, among others in a study from Sweden (48) and in studies from the USA (49-51). The average cost of an ambulance programme was estimated to be about 15.000 US dollars, which is only a moderately higher price than for a coronary artery by-pass operation.

Summary

SCD is one of the major causes of death in the Scandinavian countries as in other industrialized areas.

Despite advanced cardiac life support in more and more countries, the mortality from acute ischaemic heart disease is still very high in the first few hours after debut of symptoms, most often in the prehospital phase. Introduction of more and more sophisticated equipment in ambulances and of prehospital thrombolysis, prophylactic antiarrhythmic therapy has still not been able to reduce this high prehospital mortality. An increasing number of laymen courses concerning basic life support and how to react when cardiac symptoms appear, is needed. The cost effectiveness of prehospital coronary care seems favourable, so further initiatives are recommendable.

References

1. Haghfelt T. The prehospital phase in acute myocardial infarction. Odense: Eget forlag, 1976. Thesis.
2. Schroll M. Hjertesygdommens betydning for midaldrende danskere. Ugeskr Læg 1980; 142: 1173-6.
3. Jensen G. Epidemiology of chest pain and angina pectoris. Copenhagen: Eget forlag, 1983. Thesis.
4. Madsen JK. Ischaemic heart disease and prodromes of sudden cardiac death. Br Heart J 1985; 54: 27-32.
5. Adgey AAJ, Allen JD, Geddes JS, et al. Acute phase of myocardial infarction. Lancet 1971; 2: 501-3.
6. Adgey AAJ. Sudden death, ventricular fibrillation, ventricular defibrillation – historical review and recent advances. In: Adgey AAJ, ed. Acute phase of ischaemic heart disease and myocardial infarction. Hauge, 1982: 1-9.
7. Liberthson RR, Nagel EL, Hirschman JC, Nussenfeld SR, Blackbourne BD, Davis JH. Pathophysiologic observations in prehospital ventricular fibrillation and sudden cardiac death. Circulation 1974; 49: 790-5.
8. Liberthson RR, Nagel EL, Ruskin JN. Pathophysiology, clinical course and management of prehospital ventricular fibrillation and sudden cardiac death. In: Adgey AAJ ed. Acute phase of ischaemic heart disease and myocardial infarction. Hauge, 1982: 166.
9. Dalen JE, Ockene IS, Alpert JS. Coronary spasm, coronary thrombosis and myocardial infarction: A hypothesis concerning the pathophysiology of acute myocardial infarction. Am Heart J 1982; 104: 1119-24.

10. Eisenberg MS, Copass MK, Hallstrom AP, et al. Treatment of out-of-hospital cardiac arrests with rapid defibrillation by emergency medical technicians. N Engl J Med 1980; 302: 1379-83.
11. Lawrie DM, Higgens MR, Goodman MJ, Oliver MF, Julian DG, Donald KW. Ventricular fibrillation complicating acute myocardial infarction. Lancet 1968; 2: 523-5.
12. Lown B, Klein MD, Hershberg PI. Coronary and precoronary care. Am J Med 1969; 46: 705-7.
13. Wennerblom B, Ekström L, Holmberg S. Resuscitation of patients in cardiac arrest outside hospital. Comparison of two different organizations of mobile coronary care in one community. Eur Heart J 1984; 5: 21-6.
14. Oliver MF. Sudden cardiac death. WHO Scientific Group on Sudden Cardiac Death. Geneva, 1984.
15. Rehnqvist N. Arytmier i den tidiga fasen av akut hjärtinfarkt. I: Thygesen K, Kjekshus J, eds. Hjerteinfarkt. København: FADL's Forlag, 1985: 219-28.
16. O'Doherty M, Tayler DI, Quinn E, Vincent R, Chamberlain DA. Five hundred patients with myocardial infarction monitored within one hour of symptoms. Br Med J 1983; 286: 1405-8.
17. Adgey AAJ, Webb SW. In: Califf RM, Wagner GS, eds. Acute coronary care: principles and practice. Boston: Martinus Nijhoff, 1986: 87.
18. Goldstein S, Medendorp SV, Landis JR, et al. Analysis of cardiac symptoms preceding cardiac arrest. Am J Cardiol 1986; 58: 1195-8.
19. Larsen CF, Jørgensen HR, Nielsen JR, et al. Præhospital behandling. Ambulanceprojektet Odense. En prospektiv undersøgelse. Ugeskr Læg 1990, in press.
20. Nielsen JR, Lybecker H, Andersen C, et al. Hjertestop uden for hospital. Prospektiv undersøgelse af forskellige typer af udvidet præhospital behandling i Odense. Ugeskr Læg 1990, in press.
21. Nielsen JR, Gram L, Larsen CF, et al. Intensivering af præhospital hjertestopbehandling øger antallet af overlevende med god cerebral funktion. Ugeskr Læg 1990, in press.
22. Weaver WD, Cobb LA. Prehospital administration of thrombolytic therapy: Present and future. In: Cadliff RM, Mark DD, Wagner GS, eds. Acute coronary care in the thrombolytic era. Chicago: Year Book Medical Publishers, Inc. 1988: 103-13.
23. Weaver WD, Cobb LA, Hallstrom AP, Fahrenbruch C, Copass MK, Ray R. Factors influencing survival after out-of-hospital cardiac arrest. J Am Coll Cardiol 1986; 7: 752-7.
24. Weaver WD, Cobb LA, Hallstrom AP, et al. Considerations for improving survival from out-of-hospital cardiac arrest. Ann Emerg Med 1986; 15: 1181-6.
25. Weaver WD, Copass MK, Hill DL, Fahrenbruch C, Hallstrom AP, Cobb LA. Cardiac arrest treated with a new automatic external defibrillator by out-of-hospital first responders. Am J Cardiol 1986; 57: 1017-21.
26. Moore JE, Eisenberg MS, Andresen E, Cummins RO, Hallstrom A, Litwin P. Home placement of automatic external defibrillators among survivors of ventricular fibrillation. Ann Emerg Med 1986; 15: 811-2.
27. Chapman PJC, Chamberlain DA. Death in the clouds [Letter]. Br Med J 1987; 294: 181.
28. Pantridge JF. Prehospital coronary care. Q J Med 1970; 39: 621-2.
29. Grace WJ, Chadbourn JA. The mobile coronary care unit. Heart Lung 1974; 3: 736-41.
30. Vermeer F, Simoons ML, Baer FW, et al. Which patients benefit most from early thrombolytic therapy with intracoronary streptokinase? Circulation 1986; 74: 1379-89.
31. Reimer KA, Lower JE, Rasmussen MM, et al. The wavefront phenomenon of ischemic cell death: 1. Myocardial infarct size versus duration of coronary occlusion in dogs. Circulation 1977; 56: 786-94.

32. The I.S.A.M. Study Group. A prospective trial of intravenous streptokinase in acute myocardial infarction (I.S.A.M.): mortality, morbidity, and infarct size at 21 days. N Engl J Med 1986; 314: 1465-71.
33. Fine DG, Weiss AT, Sapoznikov D, et al. Importance of early initiation of intravenous streptokinase therapy for acute myocardial infarction. Am J Cardiol 1986; 58: 411-7.
34. Gotsman MS, Weiss AT, Fine DG, et al. Prehospital coronary thrombolysis: A new strategy in acute myocardial infarction [Abstract]. Ann Cardiol Angiol (Paris) 1987; 36: 57-8.
35. Villemant D, Barriot P, Riou B, et al. Achievement of thrombolysis at home in cases of acute myocardial infarction [Letter]. Lancet 1987; i: 228-9.
36. Koren G, Weiss AT, Hasin Y, et al. Prevention of myocardial damage in acute myocardial ischemia by early treatment with intravenous streptokinase. N Engl Med 1985; 313: 1384-9.
37. Ikram S, Lewis S, Bucknall C, et al. Treatment of acute myocardial infarction with anisoylated plasminogen streptokinase activator complex. Br Med J 1986; 293: 786-9.
38. ISIS-1 (First International Study of Infarct Survival). Collaborative Group. Randomised trial of intravenous atenolol among 16027 cases of suspected acute myocardial infarction. ISIS-1. Lancet 1986; ii: 57-66.
39. Cobb LA. A community's experience with pre-hospital emergency care, in Report of World Health Organization Working Group: The Development of Coronary Care in the Community. Brussels, WHO Annex II, 1979, 14-20.
40. Turi ZG, Stone PH, Muller JE, et al. Implications for acute intervention related to time of hospital arrival in acute myocardial infarction. Am J Cardiol 1986; 58: 203-9.
41. Moss AJ, Goldstein S. The pre-hospital phase of acute myocardial infarction. Circulation 1970; 41: 737-42.
42. Grimm P, Feldman T, Wilson GT, et al. Cellular phone transmission of 12-lead ECGs from ambulance to hospital, abstracted. Circulation 1986; 74 (suppl II): II-147.
43. Mackenzie JR. The role of the aero-medical helicopter. Hosp Aviat July 1984; 25-7.
44. Topol EJ, Fung AY, Kline E, et al. Safety of helicopter transport and out-of-hospital intravenous fibrinolytic therapy in patients with evolving myocardial infarction. Cath Cardiovasc Diagn 1985; 12: 151-5.
45. Bellinger RL, O'Callaghan WG, Simonton CA, et al. Safety and efficacy of emergency air transport in the management of patients with acute myocardial infarction. Circulation 1986; 74: II-147.
46. Bellinger RL, Califf RM, Mark DB, et al. Helicopter transport of patients during acute myocardial infarction. Am J Cardiol, in press.
47. Bellinger RL, Weber R, Califf RM. Helicopter transport of patients with acute ischemic syndromes. In: Acute Coronary Care 1987. Norwell, Mass: Martinus Nijhoff, 1986.
48. Jakobsson J, Nyquist O, Rehnqvist N, Norberg KA. Cost of a saved life following out-of-hospital cardiac arrest resuscitated by specially trained ambulance personnel. Acta Anaesthesiol Scand 1987; 31: 426-9.
49. Eisenberg MS, Copass MK, Hallstrom A, Cobb LA, Bergner L. Management of out-of-hospital cardiac arrest. JAMA 1980; 243: 1949-51.
50. Urban N, Bergner L, Eisenberg MS. The costs of a suburban paramedic program in reducing deaths due to cardiac arrest. Med Care 1981; 4: 379-92.
51. Acton J. Evaluating public programs to save lives: the cases of heart disease. Rand Corporation Report R 930 RC. Santa Monica: Rand Corporation, 1973.
52. Armstrong A. Edinburgh community study of acute coronary disease. In: Julian DG, Oliver MF, eds. Acute myocardial infarction. Edinburgh, 1968: 299.
53. Armstrong A, Duncan B, Oliver MF, et al. Natural history of acute coronary heart attacks. A community study. Br Heart J 1972; 34: 67-9.

54. McNeilly RH, Pemberton J. Duration of last attack in 998 fatal cases of coronary artery disease and its relation to possible cardial resuscitation. Br Med J 1968; 3: 139-41.

23

Electrical instability after myocardial infarction

MOGENS MØLLER,
PETER PLESS

Introduction

The development of new techniques in clinical electrophysiology, and especially the introduction of the invasive approach in studying arrhythmias, have provided new insights into the mechanisms of arrhythmogenesis. Despite these advances sudden cardiac death (SCD), however, remains a major community health issue.

Although most patients with SCD have coronary artery disease, about 50% of the sudden death victims have had no preceding symptoms before the lethal event. At the present time it is not possible to recognize this "unknown" high risk group. However, 30% of the patients dying suddenly have symptomatic coronary artery disease. An easy subgroup to identify is the patients with a previous myocardial infarction (MI), who have a 3-8% incidence of SCD in the first year following the infarction, and 2-4% in the following years as compared to lower than 1% in the general population.

Ambulatory ECG monitoring obtained during SCD has demonstrated that in 85% of the cases ventricular fibrillation (VF) is the terminal arrhythmia, in most cases preceded by ventricular tachycardia (VT) initiated by a ventricular ectopic beat with a long coupling interval.

The relevant questions therefore are 1) Does the pattern of ventricular ectopic beat (VEB) in postinfarction patients identify high risk groups, 2) Can electrical instability be detected by other methods, and can the methods alone or in combination identify high risk groups, and 3) How can VT and SCD be prevented?

Mechanism of arrhythmias

In general, the mechanism of cardiac arrhythmias can be divided into 3 categories: 1) disorders of impulse formation, 2) disorders of impulse conduction and 3) combination of both. From experimental studies it is known, that a combination of both disorders plays a major role in the mechanism of ventricular arrhythmias in the acute phase of MI.

The electrophysiological characteristics of the myocardium change immediately after occlusion of a coronary artery. The extracellular and intracellular resistance increase, and at the same time the amplitude and upstroke velocity of the action potential decrease. The consequences of these changes are a reduction in the conduction velocity. Later on during the ischaemic process, inhomogenous conduction and conduction block are observed, caused by cellular uncoupling. Furthermore, it has been observed that the recovery of excitability (the refractory period) is longer in the central ischaemic zone as compared to the borderzone, where even the refractory period may be shorter than in the normal myocardium. Thus, acute ischaemia causes an increase in the spatial dispersion of refractory periods within the ischaemic area (1, 2).

Immediate ventricular arrhythmias occuring within 5 minutes after occlusion of a coronary artery can be correlated to conduction delay and fragmentation of the electrogram recorded from the ischaemic subepicardium. Continuous fragmented activity extending from the QRS complex of a normally propagated sinus impulse to the beginning of premature ventricular depolarization can often be obtained. This so called "diastolic bridging" is not observed during the second peak incidence of arrhythmias - delayed early ventricular arrhythmias. These findings have been interpreted as indicating that immediate ventricular arrhythmias are reentrant in nature, caused by disorders of impulse conduction, whereas mechanisms such as enhanced automaticity, maybe related to the release of endogenous catecholamines, can explain the delayed early ventricular arrhythmias.

A variety of modulating factors further complicate the arrhythmogenesis of ventricular tachyarrhythmias. Enhanced activity of the sympathetic nervous system is a factor increasing the incidence of ischaemia-induced arrhythmias. The arrhythmogenic effect of increased sympathetic activity may be indirectly caused by an increase in the heart rate. The direct effect of sinus tachycardia is related to the delayed recovery of excitability of ischaemic cells, thus an increase in heart rate may induce electrical inhomogenity and thereby create zones of functional uni-directional block, one of the prerequisites for the re-entry phenomenon.

Early after depolarization (triggered activity) can induce premature ventricular complexes in the ischaemic cells. These can cause the re-entry phenomenon in the same way as an increase in heart rate, and thus trigger VF.

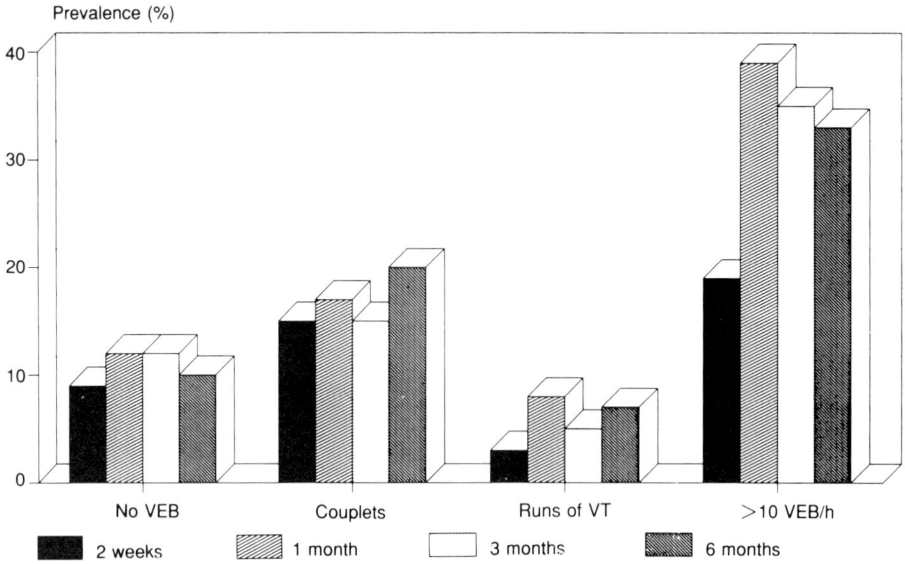

Fig. 1. *Prevalence of different types of ventricular arrhythmias during 24-hour ambulatory ECG recording performed 2 weeks, 1, 3 and 6 months after an acute MI in 100 consecutive patients (4).*

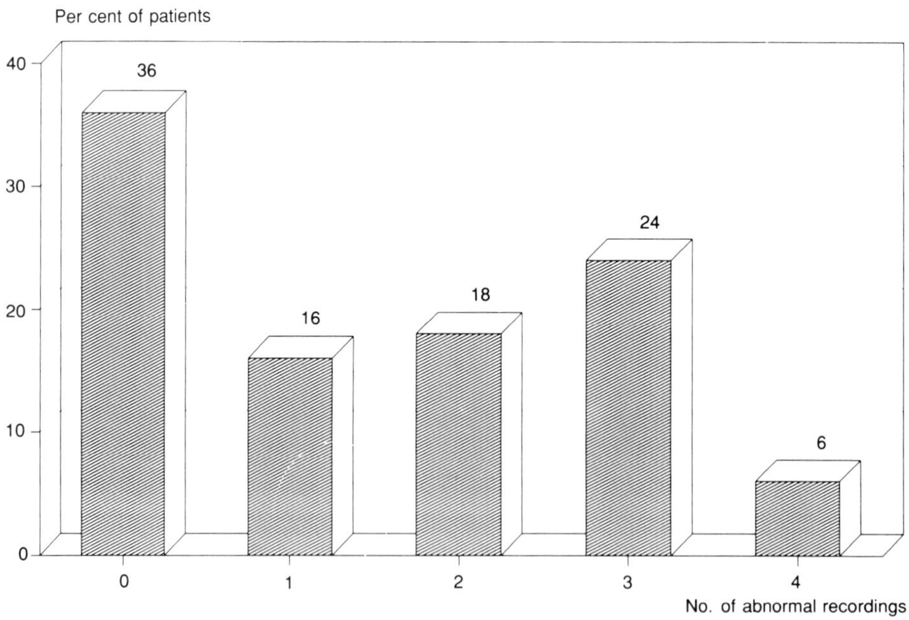

Fig. 2. *Number of abnormal 24-hour ECG recordings in 96 consecutive patients with 4 recordings performed 2 weeks and 1, 3 and 6 months after a first MI. Abnormal recording was defined when >10 VEB/hour or repetitive forms occurred (4).*

The substrate for the ventricular tachyarrhythmias in the chronic stage of MI may be a more or less well-defined anatomical re-entry circuit. The prerequisites for re-entry to initiate and perpetuate are uni-directional block and slow conduction. Further, the wavefront of excitation requires a proper balance between the conduction velocity and recovery of excitability of the tissue ahead of the wavefront in order to always find excitable tissue ahead (3).

Although the electrophysiologic mechanism for SCD in post-infarction patients is commonly caused by re-entry VT degenerating to VF, some post-infarction ectopic rhythms may be caused by focal discharge of ischaemic myocardial cells. The latter may be secondary to other mechanisms such as abnormal automaticity or triggered activity.

Ventricular arrhythmias after myocardial infarction

The prevalence of ventricular arrhythmias in the late hospital phase and 1, 3 and 6 months after a first MI is shown in Fig. 1 (4). The variability from time to time is considerable as illustrated in Fig. 2, as only 42% of the patients showed the same classification on all 4 recordings, when the criterion < 10 VEB/h and abscence of repetitive forms of VEB was used for a normal recording.

Prognostic significance of ventricular arrhythmias

Several large studies have demonstrated a significant prognostic importance of the ventricular ectopic activity in patients with a recent MI. Ventricular arrhythmias are an independent predictor of sudden as well as non-sudden cardiac death (Table 1), but it is reasonable to believe that ventricular arrhythmias are only one of several variables associated with an increased mortality in ischaemic heart disease. The study (5) included 940 men below the age of 66 years, and it is obvious from Table 1 that a well-defined

Table 1. *Prognostic significance of different types of VEB on Holter monitoring after MI (5).*

		Pts with SCD		Pts with non-SCD	
	No of pts	No	%	No	%
No VEB	470	17	3.6	13	2.8
Simple VEB	254	14	5.5	10	3.9
Complex VEB	216	23	10.6	20	9.3

high risk group could not be identified, as more than half of the diseased patients did not have complex arrhythmias. Patients without ventricular arrhythmias constituted a large, reasonably well-defined low risk group, but included approximately 30% of patients who died.

Autonomic tonus

In clinical practice the QTc interval and heart rate variability have been used to evaluate the tonus of the autonomic nervous system. QT prolongation is due to heterogenous prolongation of repolarization resulting in increased dispersion of refractory periods across the ventricle. Consequently, several studies have been performed in order to evaluate the relation between ventricular arrhythmias and the QTc interval and to describe the prognostic importance of the QTc interval with regard to SCD. In most studies a trend, and in some a significantly increased risk have been demonstrated (6, 7).

The mean, the maximum and the minimum heart rate during a 24-hour ambulatory ECG monitoring exhibit no relation to SCD. However, a simply derived parameter such as the standard deviation of all normal R-R intervals on a 24-hour Holter has been shown to be a strong predictor of SCD (8), probably because the parameter is reversely correlated to parasympathetic activity.

Signal averaged electrocardiogram

During invasive electrophysiologic studies of post-MI patients with spontaneous and/or inducible sustained VT it has been shown that the anatomic substrate for the reentry tachycardia seems to be present in regions where fragmented electrograms can be recorded, indicating an area with slow inhomogenous conduction. These delayed and fractionated potentials have been called "late potentials" (9). The amplitude of ventricular late potentials is in the low millivolt range using invasive recording methods, so these signals are not visible on the conventional ECG. However, using computer averaging techniques and appropriate amplification and filtering, these signals can be recorded from the body surface (10).

In general, late potentials are defined as high frequency, low amplitude fractionated activity appearing at the end of the QRS-complex and extending into the ST-segment. Examples of signal averaged ECG in patients with first MI are shown in Fig. 3.

Earlier studies have shown that patients with documented VT and/or VF have an incidence of late potentials ranging from 30-95%. The lowest incidence is found in patients with a history of VF outside acute MI and with no previous documented episodes of sustained VT. The highest incidence is found in patients with sustained VT and a cycle length greater than 225 msec (11, 12).

In patients with their first MI the prevalence of late potentials in the acute phase ranges from 14-55%. The reason for this variability is the timing

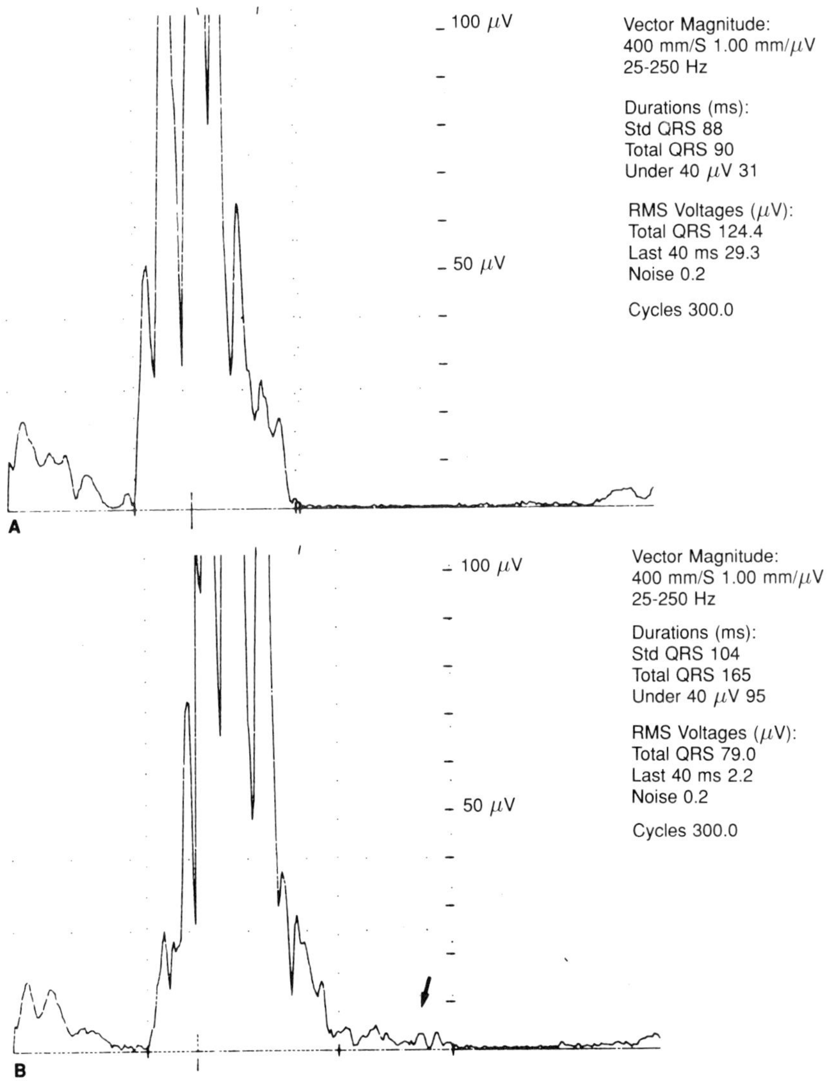

Fig. 3. *An example of two signal averaged electrocardiograms in patients with first MI.* A: *All quantitative signal averaged ECG variables are normal.* B: *The total duration of the signal averaged QRS and the duration of low amplitude signals < 40 µV are prolonged. The root mean square (RMS) voltage of the last 40 ms is 2.2 µV. Arrow points to the prominent late potentials.*

Table 2. *Prognostic value of the signal averaged ECG in predicting arrhythmic events after MI.*

Ref.	Author	No of pts.	Prevalence of LP	Sens.	Spec.	PPV
14	*Breithardt*, 1983	160	51%	73	51	10
15	*Denniss*, 1986	306	26%	66	78	24
16	*Kuchar*, 1987	200	39%	93	65	17
17	*Cripps*, 1988	159	24%	91	81	26
18	*Gomes*, 1989	115	42%	81	65	27

Ref, reference; LP, late potentials; Sens, sensitivity; Spec, specificity; PPV, positive predictive value.

of the recording in relation to the ischaemic event, as well as the criteria used in defining late potentials. The highest prevalence of late potentials is at the time of discharge. As might be expected from the very complex arrhythmogenesis in the acute phase of MI, the positive predictive value of late potentials in relation to in-hospital ventricular tachyarrhythmias is only about 15-27% (13). Only a few prospective studies concerning the prognostic significance of the signal averaged ECG in patients with acute MI have been published until now. Table 2 shows a summary of some of the results from these studies.

Comparison of the different studies is often very difficult, partly because of the different methods utilized in the averaging procedure, but also because no consensus exists in defining an abnormal signal averaged ECG. However, it can be stated that the signal averaged ECG in relation to arrhythmic events has a relatively high sensitivity, a lower specificity and a positive predictive value in the range of about 20-25%.

Electrophysiologic studies

It is well documented that VT can be induced by programmed electrical stimulation in more than 90% of patients with spontaneous episodes of VT and ischaemic heart disease,

Patients with a recent MI have a myocardial scar with the potency of unidirectional block and delayed conduction and the patients have an increased risk of ectopic ventricular activity – together increasing the risk of initiating VT on the basis of local reentry circuits. Therefore, it is reasonable to assume that programmed ventricular stimulation can be used to test the electrical instability of the myocardium and serve as a prognostic tool. The first report was published in 1978 (19) and later several conflicting papers have shown the difficulty in reaching a consensus of opinion with regard to study-population, stimulation protocol and end-points (20, 21). In the best conducted study (21) 165 patients from an infarct population of 341 patients were included (37 died before programmed ventricular stimulation, 139 had persistent ischaemia, uncontrolled heart failure or received cardioprotective medication). The assessed and non-assessed patients differed with regard to age, sex and anterior infarctions, but not with regard to diseased vessels and ejection fraction. The stimulation protocol included 1 and 2 ventricular extra-stimuli during pacing at 100 bpm from the right ventricular apex and outflow tract. Electrophysiologic end-point was VT of more than 10 seconds duration or VF.

Thirty eight (23%) of the 165 patients were found to be inducible. The inducible patients had more often a transmural infarction and a lower mean ejection fraction than the non-inducible, while the number of affected vessels did not differ. During a follow-up period of 1 year the results showed (Fig. 4) that non-inducibility identified a large group of patients with a very low risk of SCD and that inducibility identified a group with an approximately 20% risk of SCD.

Combination of methods for risk stratification

The important issue for the prevention of SCD after MI is to improve risk stratification. In recent years several studies have elucidated the importance of the prognostic information obtained from Holter monitoring, signal av-

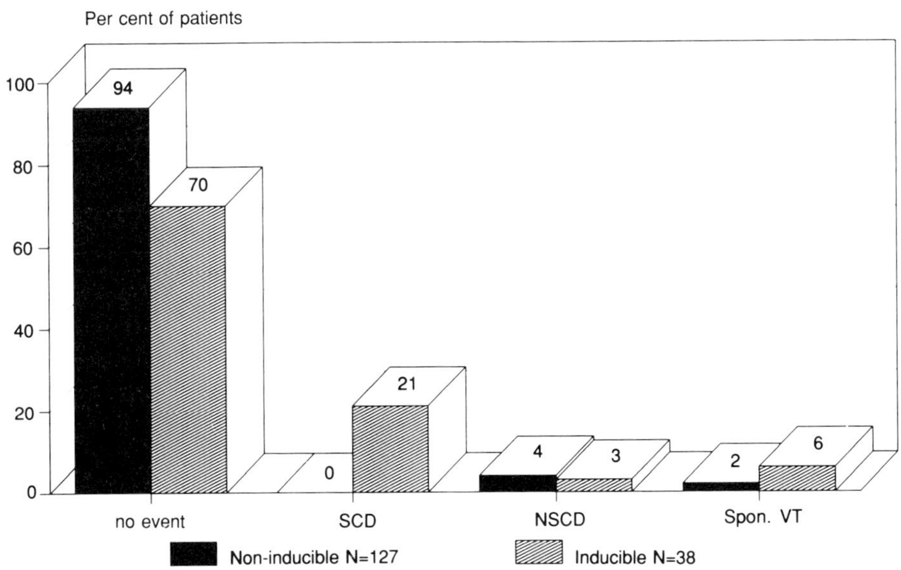

Fig. 4. *The predictive value of inducibility and non-inducibility during programmed ventricular stimulation in patients with an acute MI (20). SCD = sudden cardiac death. NSCD = non-sudden cardiac death. Spon. VT = spontaneous ventricular tachycardia.*

eraged ECG, exercise test, assessment of left ventricular function and programmed ventricular stimulation.

However, it must be emphasized that because of the very complex arrhythmogenesis involved in ventricular tachyarrhythmias each one of these methods has inherent limitations. Holter monitoring looks at the spontaneously occurring probable triggers – VEB, whereas late potentials on the signal averaged ECG indicate an area of delayed activation, but do not establish the presence of a re-entry circuit, and during programmed ventricular stimulation the induced arrhythmias are forced to occur as a result of artificial triggers (premature stimuli), however, the induced arrhythmias do not necessarily have to occur spontaneously. So, if we are going to improve the management of the post-MI patients it is necessary to use a combination of these methods in the risk stratification, and non-invasive procedures are obviously preferable from the clinical point of view.

In one of the early studies combining the results from the signal averaged ECG and programmed ventricular stimulation it could be demonstrated that patients with late potentials had a 4.4 times greater risk of developing sustained VT as compared to those without late potentials. The combined results of the signal averaged ECG and the invasive test point out a small subgroup of post-MI patients with an event rate of 33% during follow-up (22). In a more recent study from the *Westmead-Group* (23), 200 patients with MI were studied with programmed stimulation, signal averaging, ambulatory monitoring for 24 hours, assessment of left ventricular ejection fraction using radionuclide technique, and exercise testing. During follow-up (median 12 months) there were 9 end-points, consisting of sudden death and episodes of spontaneous VT or VF. Depending on the protocol used during the invasive test, the highest sensitivity found was in fact rather low – 56%, but with an acceptable positive predicitive value of 33%. The results from measurement of ventricular activation time at signal averaging did not appear as potent a predictor of arrhythmic events as programmed stimulation. Unfortunately, the results from the signal averaging are not comparable with results from other groups because of the special techniques used in this study to detect late potentials. The results from the Holter monitoring and assessment of left ventricular function did not appear to add any further prognostic information.

However, in other recent studies using multivariate analysis (16, 18) a triad of non-invasive tests comprising the signal averaged ECG, Holter monitoring and assessment of left ventricular ejection fraction were found to provide independent prognostic information. The combination of late potentials and frequent ectopics or late potentials and a reduced ejection

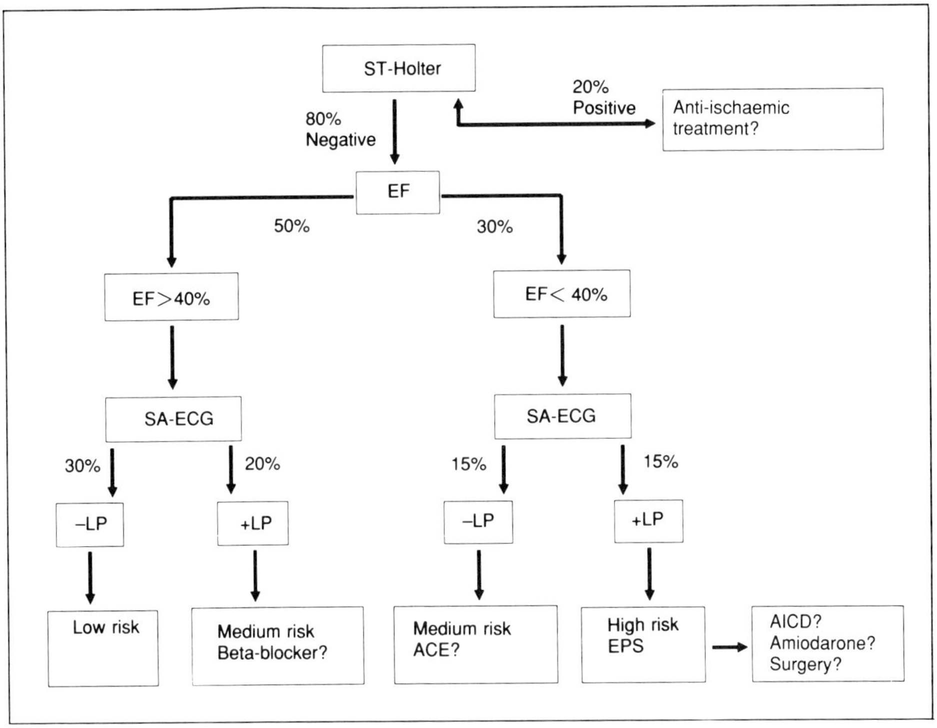

Fig. 5. *A proposal for a risk stratification algorithm in patients with acute MI. ST-Holter, Holter ST-segment monitoring; EF, assessment of left ventricular ejection fraction; SA-ECG, signal averaged electrocardiogram; –LP, late potentials absent; + LP, late potentials present; ACE, angiotensin converting enzyme inhibitor; EPS, electrical programmed stimulation; AICD, automatic implantable cardioverter-defibrillator.*

fraction significantly increase the positive predictive value for the prediction of arrhythmic events.

In Fig. 5 we have delineated a proposal for a risk stratification algorithm based on our personal experience, where Holter ST-segment monitoring is an integrated part of the initial evaluation (24).

Prevention of malignant ventricular arrhythmias and sudden cardiac death

Pharmacological intervention

The primary indication for medicamentel intervention in patients at risk of developing malignant ventricular arrhythmias and/or SCD is to control symptoms and reduce the probability of a lethal event.

Several studies have emphasized that frequent ventricular ectopic and non-sustained VT are associated with an increased risk of SCD. Therefore, a great deal of effort has been invested in secondary prevention trials of anti-arrhythmic therapy based on the assumption that suppression of the triggers (VEB) for re-entry tachycardia will decrease the incidence of sudden death. However, until now none of these prevention trials have been able to demonstrate any significant beneficial effect in the context of improved survival (25). On the contrary, the recent results published from the Cardiac Arrhythmia Suppression Trial (CAST) demonstrate that administration of a class 1 C anti-arrhythmic resulted in a higher mortality in patients with asymptomatic ventricular arrhythmias as compared to patients receiving placebo, even when class 1 C anti-arrhythmic suppressed ventricular ectopic activity during Holter monitoring (26). Preliminary results from the Canadian CAMIAT pilot study indicate that amiodarone may be of beneficial effect in improving survival of post-MI patients presenting with frequent or repetitive forms of VEB during Holter monitoring.

Beta-blockers have been found to reduce the total mortality and the SCD rate after MI by approximately 25% (27). The reason for the beneficial effect has not been clarified, but may depend on suppression of triggers that can induce re-entry tachycardia, interaction with the autonomic nervous system and an anti-ischaemic effect of importance for preventing a substrate for re-entry to occur.

Within the last five years the possibility of reducing the SCD rate by drugs other than beta-blockers has become evident. Several large studies have confirmed the effect of early thrombolytic therapy (28) and ACE-inhibitors may be of value in post-infarction patients with impaired left ventricular function (29).

Surgical intervention

The great majority of VT or VF detected on ambulatory ECG monitoring are not preceeded by detectable myocardial ischaemia. In general, the effect of revascularization on left ventricular function and ventricular arrhythmias is small if detectable (30). Patients with exercise induced ventricular tachyarrhythmias constitute a specific subgroup who should undergo coronary arteriography as PTCA or grafting may completely abolish the arrhythmias.

Patients with recurrent, sustained VT after MI may be candidates for arrhythmia surgery. The optimal candidate is the patient with inducible, sustained VT refractory to anti-arrhythmic drugs and with a well-defined left ventricular aneurysm. It is rather convincing that simple aneurysmectomy is not a reliable therapy, and in most centres surgery for VT is now performed with endocardial, peroperative mapping to identify the endocardial area with the earliest depolarization. This area is resected or encircled.

The operation should, if possible, be postponed until at least 2-3 months after the infarction, but even then the operative mortality is in the range of 10-20%. In experienced centres the results are promising (31), but to date no controlled studies have been carried out with regard to survival.

The implantable automatic antitachycardia pacemaker/cardioverter/defibrillator can be used in selected post-infarction patients. The device is not suitable for a more general prophylaxis of SCD after MI, but may be justified in a small well-defined high risk group (see Fig. 5).

Perspectives

The methods to identify the different risk groups after MI still have to be refined. It is necessary to continue the search for a combination of non-invasive tests that at the same time can stratify the patients and be used to monitor the effect of an interventional programme.

Probably no single drug can be used to prevent fatal ventricular arrhythmias in all patients without a potential of severe side-effects, and it will still be important to reduce infarct size and to prevent left ventricular dilatation after the infarction. Within a few years improved technology may make it possible to develop small, non-expensive and easy-to-implant electrical devices, which can be used for general prevention of SCD in larger high risk groups after acute MI.

References

1. Janse MJ, Kleber AG, Capucci A, Coronel R, Wilms-Schopman F. Electrophysiological basis for arrhythmias caused by acute ischemia. Role of the subendocardium. J Mol Cell Cardiol 1986; 18: 339.
2. El-Sherif N, Scherlag BJ, Lazzara R, Hope RR. Reentrant ventricular arrhythmias in the late myocardial infarction period. I. Conduction characteristics in the infarction zone. Circulation 1977; 55: 686-702.
3. Zipes DP. Electrophysiological mechanisms involved in ventricular fibrillation. Circulation 1975; 52 (suppl. III): 120-30.
4. Møller M. Ventricular arrhythmias following myocardial infarction. Incidence and prognostic importance studied by repeated 24-hour electrocardiographic monitoring. Odense University Press 1981 (thesis).
5. Moss AJ, Davis HT, DeCamilla J, Bayer LW. Ventricular ectopic beats and their relation to sudden and non-sudden cardiac death after myocardial infarction. Circulation 1979; 60: 998-1003.
6. Møller M. QT interval in relation to ventricular arrhythmias and sudden cardiac death in post myocardial infarction patients. Acta Med Scand 1981; 210: 73-7.
7. Ahnve A, Gilpin E, Madsen EB, Froelicher V, Henning H, Ross Jr T. Prognostic importance of QTc interval at discharge after myocardial infarction: a multicenter study of 865 patients. Am Heart J 1984; 108 (2): 395-400.

8. Kleiger RE, Miller JP, Bigger JT, Moss AJ, MPIP Research Group. Decreased heart rate variability and its association with increased mortality after acute myocardial infarction. Am J Cardiol 1987; 59: 256-62.
9. Josephson ME, Horowitz LN, Farshidi A, Spielman SR, Michelson EL, Greenspan AM. Sustained ventricular tachycardia: evidence for protected localized re-entry. Am J Cardiol 1978; 42: 416-24.
10. Berbari EJ, Scherlag BJ, Hope RR, Lazzara R. Recording from the body surface of arrhythmogenic ventricular activity during the ST segment. Am J Cardiol 1978; 41: 697-702.
11. Breithardt G, Becker R, Seipel L, Abendroth R-R, Ostermeyer J. Non-invasive detection of late potentials in man – a new marker for ventricular tachycardia. Eur Heart J 1981; 2: 1-11.
12. Simson MB. Identification of patients with ventricular tachycardia after myocardial infarction from signals in the terminal QRS complex. Circulation 1981; 64: 235-42.
13. Pless P, Mickley H, Møller M. Natural history of late potentials in the acute phase of myocardial infarction and relation to in-hospital ventricular tachyarrhythmias. Circulation 1989; 80 (suppl.): II-37.
14. Breithardt G, Schwarzmaier J, Borggrefe M, Haerten K, Seipel L. Prognostic significance of late ventricular potentials after acute myocardial infarction. Eur Heart J 1983; 4: 487-95.
15. Denniss AR, Richards DA, Cody DV, et al. Prognostic significance of ventricular tachycardia and fibrillation induced at programmed stimulation and delayed potentials detected on the signal-averaged electrocardiograms of survivors of acute myocardial infarction. Circulation 1986; 74: 731-45.
16. Kuchar DL, Thorburn CW, Sammel NL. Prediction of serious arrhythmic events after myocardial infarction: signal-averaged electrocardiogram, Holter monitoring and radionuclide ventriculography. J Am Coll Cardiol 1987; 9: 531-8.
17. Cripps T, Bennett ED, Camm AJ, Ward DE. High gain signal averaged electrocardiogram combined with 24 hour monitoring in patients early after myocardial infarction for bedside prediction of arrhythmic events. Br Heart J 1988; 60: 181-7.
18. Gomes JA, Winters SL, Martinson M, Machac J, Stewart D, Targonski A. The prognostic significance of quantitative signal-averaged variables relative to clinical variables, site of myocardial infarction, ejection fraction and ventricular premature beats: a prospective study. J Am Coll Cardiol 1989; 13: 377-84.
19. Greene ML, Reid PR, Schaeffer ASH. The repetitive ventricular response in man. A predictor of sudden death. N Engl J Med 1978; 299: 729-34.
20. Richards DA, Cody DV, Denniss AR, Russell PA, Young AA, Uther JB. Ventricular electrical instability: A predictor of death after myocardial infarction. Am J Cardiol 1983; 51: 75-80.
21. Marchlinski FE, Buxton AE, Waxman HL, Josephson ME. Identifying patients at risk of sudden death after myocardial infarction: Value of the response to programmed stimulation, degree of ventricular ectopic activity and severity of left ventricular dysfunction. Am J Cardiol 1983; 52: 1190-6.
22. Breithardt G, Borggrefe M, Haerten K. Role of programmed ventricular stimulation and noninvasive recording of ventricular late potentials for the identification of patients at risk of ventricular tachyarrhythmias after acute myocardial infarction. In: Zipes DP, Jalife J, eds. Cardiac electrophysiology and arrhythmias. New York: Grune and Stratton 1985: 553-61.
23. Rickards DA, Taylor A, Fahey P, et al. Identification of patients at risk of sudden death after myocardial infarction: The Continued Australian Experience. In: Brugada

P, Wellens HJJ, eds. Cardiac Arrhythmias: Where To Go From Here? Mount Kisco NY: Futura Publishing Company, Inc. 1987: 329-41.
24. Mickley H, Pless P, Nielsen JR, Møller M. Ambulatory ST-segment monitoring is superior to exercise testing in predicting subsequent ischaemic events after first myocardial infarction. J Amb Monitor 1990 (in press).
25. May GS, Eberlein KA, Furberg CD, Passamani ER, Demets DL. Secondary prevention after myocardial infarction: a review of long term trials. Progr Cardiovasc Dis 1982; 24: 331-52.
26. Cardiac Arrhythmia Suppression Trial (CAST) Investigators. Preliminary report: effect of encainide and flecainide on mortality in a randomized trial of arrhythmia suppression after myocardial infarction. N Engl J Med 1989; 321: 406-12.
27. Yusuf S, Peto R, Lewis J, Collins R, Sleight P. Beta-blockade during and after myocardial infarction: An overview of the randomised trials. Progr Cardiovasc Dis 1985; 27: 335-71.
28. Gruppo Italiano per lo Studio della Streptochinasi nell' Infarto Miocardico (GISSI). Long-term effects of intravenous thrombolysis in acute myocardial infarction: Final report of the GISSI study. Lancet 1987; 2: 871-4.
29. Concensus trial group. Effect of enalapril on mortality in severe congestive heart failure. Results of the Comparative North Scandinavian Enalapril Survival Study (CONSENSUS). N Engl J Med 1987; 316: 1429-35.
30. Møller M, Thayssen P, Alstrup P, Haghfelt T, Andersen Jr. PE. The effect of coronary artery bypass surgery on ventricular arrhythmias. Eur Heart J 1983; 4: 26-30.
31. Miller JM, Kienzle MG, Harken AH, Josephson ME. Subendocardial resection for ventricular tachycardia: predictors of surgical success. Circulation 1984; 70: 624-31.

24

Non-pharmacological treatment of malignant ventricular arrhythmias after myocardial infarction

POUL ERIK BLOCH THOMSEN,
OLE KROMANN,
PETER KILDEBERG PAULSEN

Introduction

A tremendous advance in the management of patients with ventricular tachycardia has been made during the last decade. This includes medical antiarrhythmic therapy guided by programmed electrical stimulation (1, 2) as well as *non-pharmacological* treatment i.e. arrhythmia surgery with mapping-guided subendocardial resection of the arrhythmogenic area (3, 4). The innovation and introduction of the automatic implantable cardioverter defibrillator into clinical practice was another major step forward in non-medical treatment of patients who had survived one or more attacks of "sudden cardiac death" (5-7).

In the following our present indications for non-pharmacological treatment of patients with ischaemic malignant ventricular arrhythmias will be reviewed. The electrophysiological and operative techniques will be discussed and the results of non-pharmacological treatment of 47 patients presented.

Selection of appropriate therapy

Empiric medical antiarrhythmic therapy of patients with ventricular tachycardia and/or ventricular fibrillation *(VT/VF)* after acute myocardial infarction (AMI) is associated with a poor clinical outcome. Thus, *Wellens* (8) found an 83% mortality after one year, and often the death was sudden, in patients who had experienced VT/VF less than 8 weeks after AMI. Similarly, a 47% mortality was reported after a mean follow-up of 2½ years when the first attack of VT/VF appeared more than 8 weeks after the AMI.

The introduction of invasive electrophysiology (9) has proved a basis for rational medical management of VT. In the cardiac electrophysiology laboratory, it is possible using programmed electrical stimulation to provoke the clinical arrhythmia in more than 90% of the patients suffering from sustained VT (10). In otherwise comparable patients without spontaneous VT, a sustained VT could only be induced in 3% of 443 patients (10).

After the clinical arrhythmia has been provoked and studied in the laboratory, serial drug-testing is performed and the stimulation protocol provoking the arrhythmia is repeated for each drug regimen. The ability of a certain drug regimen to prevent the initiation of a sustained VT by programmed stimulation has been shown in several studies to predict an excellent clinical outcome (11-13).

In contrast, patients in whom it was not possible to find a drug regimen which could prevent or improve the clinical arrhythmia in the laboratory was associated with a very poor prognosis (13). These patients are most often treated with Amiodarone, frequently in combination with a class 1 C drug and/or a beta-blocker. Life table analysis of these patients shows a cumulative percentage of *sudden cardiac death* of more than 70% after 3-4 years (13). These "non-responders" are the prime candidates for non-pharmacological treatment.

In our institution we try 2-3 different conventional antiarrhythmic drugs, often in combination and most often a class 1 A or C drug are combined with a beta-blocker. If the patient is still inducible in the laboratory by programmed electrical stimulation, we change to Amiodarone 1200 mg daily for 2 weeks. Then, if the patient is still inducible he or she is considered a candidate for non-pharmacological treatment of the ventricular arrhythmia, either arrhythmia surgery or implantation of the implantable cardioverter defibrillator.

Before the decision of the appropriate therapy is taken the patient undergoes left ventriculography and coronary angiography. In addition, 2-D echocardiography, MUGA, CT-scanning and lately NMR-scanning of the heart are performed to estimate left ventricular function, especially to differentiate between left ventricular aneurysm and dyskinesis/akinesis.

Our present indications for surgical treatment of VT are listed in Table 1. The reason for preferring patients with monomorphic VT is, that these

Table 1. *Indications for surgical treatment of ventricular tachycardia.*

1. Life-threatening arrhythmia
2. Medically refractory
3. Monomorphic ventricular tachycardia
4. Discrete anterior wall aneurysm
5. Fractional EF >0.40
6. One-vessel disease
7. Congestive heart failure due to aneurysm
8. Embolism from LV aneurysm
9. Per occasionem

Table 2. *Indications for the automatic implantable cardioverter defibrillator.*

Ventricular fibrillation
Polymorphic ventricular tachycardia
Medically refractory
No discrete aneurysm
Prohibitive left ventricular dysfunction
Failed arrhythmia surgery
Life-expectancy more than 1 year

Table 3. *Non-pharmacological treatment of ventricular tachycardia/fibrillation.*

Clinical data		
No. of pts.	47	(8F, 39M)
Age, years (mean, range)	56	(37-71)
Time from MI to surgery (months)	34	(2-88)
VT/VF	23/5	
VT+VF	19	
CL of VT/msec	290	(200-500)
No. of antiarrhythmics per patient	2.6	(0-7)
Amiodarone	15	
Heart failure (NYHA II-IV)	29	
LAD/CX/RC	42/14/18	
1,2,3-vessel disease	25/14/8	
Aneurysm (ant./inf./post.)	38/1/4	
EF (mean, range)	0.33	(0.15-0.61)
LVEDP/mmHg (mean, range)	22	(8-46)
Inducible VT preoperatively	42/47	

patients most often pre- and peroperatively show one "site of origin", which can be mapped easily. Monomorphic VT is furthermore most often seen in patients with a discrete anterior-wall aneurysm, whereas patients with left inferior-wall or posterior-wall aneurysms are more difficult to map because they often show polymorphic VT.

If fractional ejection fraction in patients with left ventricular aneurysm is less than 0.40 the operative risk is increased. These patients are considered candidates for the implantable cardioverter defibrillator. Our present indications for implanting the cardioverter defibrillator are listed in Table 2. Only patients identified as being at extremely high risk of dying from refractory arrhythmias *not* associated with AMI are considered candidates.

Patients with frequent attacks of malignant ventricular arrhythmias e.g. more than one attack per month are not candidates for obvious reasons. These patients are nowadays candidates for heart transplantation.

Material and methods

The series comprised 47 consecutively treated patients (Table 3), 39 males and 8 females with a mean age of 56 (range 37-71) years. All had had AMI 1 month to 88 months preoperatively. Nineteen had had attacks of both VF and VT, while 23 had only VT and 5 only VF. All but three received from one to seven antiarrhythmic drugs, without effect, including amiodarone in 15 cases. Twelve patients were in drug-resistant heart failure, including one with a ventricular septal defect severe enough to be an indication for surgery.

All patients underwent left ventriculography and coronary angiography. Left ventricular aneurysms were found in 43 of 47 cases including one patient with two aneurysms, 1 anterior, 1 inferior. Coronary angiography revealed more than 50% stenosis of the left anterior descending artery in 42 cases, of the circumflex artery in 14 and the right coronary artery in 18 cases. One-vessel disease was present in 25 cases, two-vessel disease in 14 and three-vessel disease in 8. The mean ejection fraction was 0.33 (range 0.15-0.61), and the mean left ventricular end-diastolic pressure 21 (range 8-46) mmHg. Two of the 47 patients who had poor global left ventricle function with an EF of 0.21 and 0.22 respectively were not considered candidates for arrhythmia surgery and were treated with the implantable cardioverter defibrillator.

The preoperative electrophysiologic study was performed as previously described (14). Electrode catheters were introduced percutaneously and positioned high in the right atrium, in the His bundle region and in the right ventricle. Programmed ventricular stimulation was carried out in the right ventricular apex (or outflow tract), and comprised pacing with a basic cycle length of 500 msec for 8 beats followed by single, double or triple ventricular extrastimuli with decreasing coupling intervals (Fig. 1). If the procedure failed to induce VT, the basic cycle length was decreased to 400

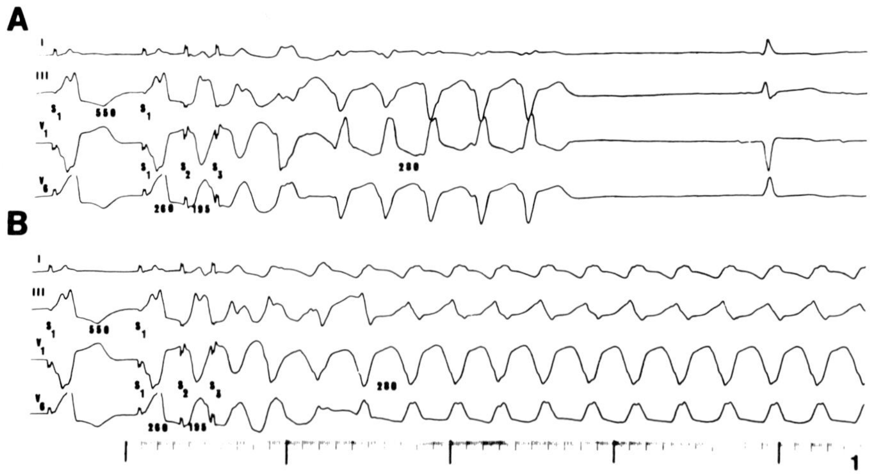

Fig. 1. *Precipitation of VT by programmed electrical stimulation. The standard electrocardiographic leads I, III, V_1 and V_6 are shown. S_1, S_2, S_3 are the pacestimulus artefacts. Right ventricular pacing with a basic cycle of S_1-S_2 = 550 ms is performed. Two extra pacing stimuli S_2 and S_3 are introduced in coupling intervals of S_1-S_2 = 260 msec and S_2-S_3 = 195 msec.* Upper panel A: *The first attempt results in a non-sustained VT of six beats.* Panel B: *The second attempt results in a monomorphic sustained VT with a cycle length of 280 msec and similar to the patients spontaneous VT.*

msec. Finally, if this stimulation procedure still did not provoke VT, burst pacing was employed, i.e. bursts of 8 beats with cycle lengths from 300 to 200 msec. Endocardial catheter mapping was not done routinely during the induced VT. The main purpose of the preoperaive electrophysiologic study was to identify the stimulation procedure resulting in VT identical to the spontaneous VT. The same procedure was thereafter used per- and postoperatively.

Operative procedure

Cardiopulmonary bypass was used and normothermia was secured by active warming. A pentapolar, specially designed reference electrode was sutured to the epicardium of the right ventricular outflow tract close to the interventricular septum and used to record a bipolar reference electrogram and for ventricular pacing. Simultaneously four electrocardiographic leads (I, III, V_1 and V_6) were recorded. VT was provoked with the above-described stimulation procedure and the aneurysm was incised (3). Using a specially designed exploring electrode with an interelectrode distance of 2 mm, bipolar electrograms were recorded from the endocardium at the borderline between

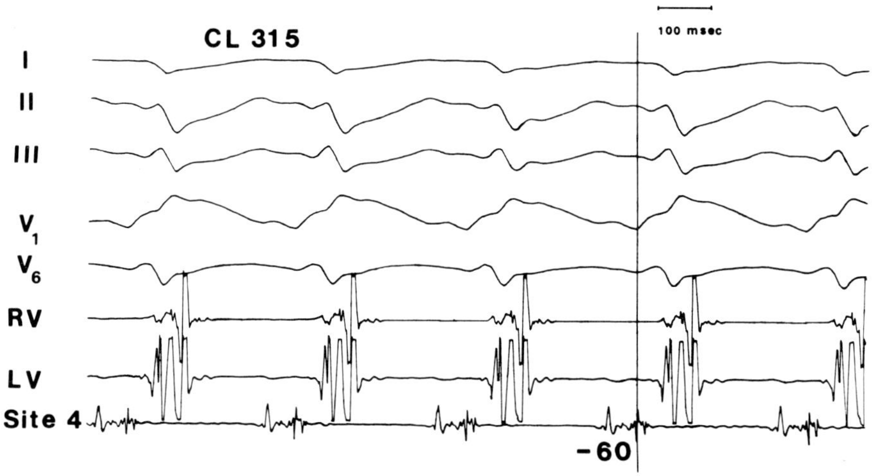

Fig. 2. *Peroperative endocardial mapping. The patient is on normothermic cardiopulmonary bypass with induced VT, cycle length (CL) 315 msec, analogous to the spontaenous VT. Standard leads I, II, III, V_1 and V_6. Two reference electrograms (RV and LV) are recorded epicardially on the right and left ventricle. After the aneurysm has been opened the exploring bipolar electrode is advanced round the margin of the aneurysm on the endocardium. At* Site *4 presystolic local electrograms are recorded 60 msec before the start of the QRS complex marked by the vertical line. Site 4 was therefore judged to be the site of origin of the VT.*

aneurysmal tissue and normal endocardium with the heart in sustained VT. Readings were noted round the clock at the borderline, with repetition several times. In this way *the area of earliest activation* during VT was located (Fig. 2).

If sustained VT could not be provoked by programmed stimulation, *pacemapping* was carried out (14): The bipolar exploring electrode was used to pace on the endocardium with a cycle length as close as possible to that of the spontaneous VT. The electrode was then moved around the margins of the aneurysm and recordings of the surface ECG were performed. The site at which pacing resulted in a QRS configuration most closely resembling the QRS of the spontaneous VT was considered to be the site of origin of the tachycardia.

After identification of the site of origin, aneurysmectomy was performed, followed by endocardial resection of a 10-15 cm^2 area around the point of earliest endocardial activation (3). The left ventricle was then closed and temporary pace wires were placed on the atrium and on the anterior wall of the right ventricle close to the interventricular septum. Coronary artery bypass grafting was performed only if the patient had angina pectoris with significant coronary artery stenosis or main stem lesion.

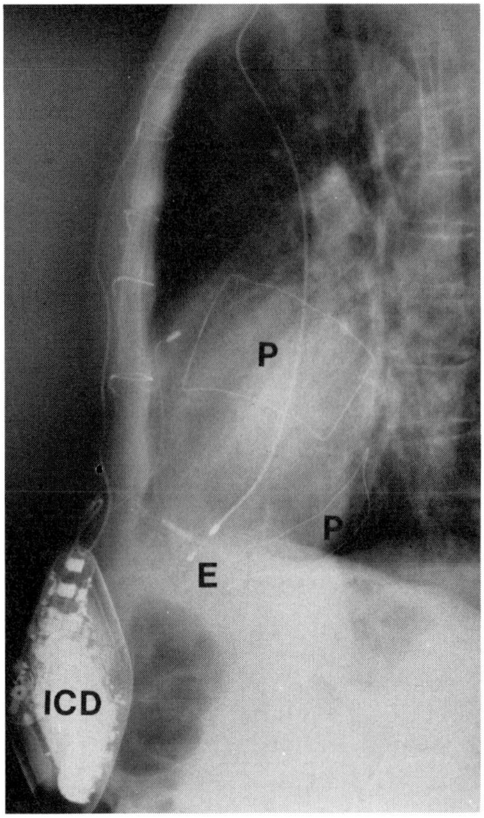

Fig. 3. *Lateral chest X-ray film showing the implantable cardioverter defibrillator system. The bipolar endocardial sensing and pacing electrode (E) extends from the right ventricular apex to the infraclavicular region and further down subcutaneously to the abdominal pocket where the defibrillator (ICD) is seen. The shock is delivered between the two patch electrodes (P). They are placed on the right ventricle anterolaterally and on the left ventricle posterobasally, respectively. The patch leads are tunnelled and connected to the defibrillator.*

Postoperative evaluation. The electrophysiologic provocation was repeated 10-14 days after the operation, using the temporary myocardial pace wires. The stimulation protocol comprised pacing down to a basic cycle length of 400 msec and up to three extra stimuli.

The implantable cardioverter defibrillator

In the two patients treated with the implantable cardioverter defibrillator, a median sternotomy was performed after implanting a bipolar sensing and pacing electrode transvenously into the right ventricular apex (Fig. 3). The two patch electrodes with a surface area of 15 cm^2 each used for cardioversion-defibrilliation were placed on the anterolateral wall of the right ventricle and the posterobasal wall of the left ventricle, respectively. The defibrillation threshold was measured (Fig. 4) and a threshold for defibrillation less than 20 joule was searched for.

The patch electrode leads were then channelled under the skin and connected to the pulse generator placed in a paraumbilical pocket. The defibrillator used was the Telectronics Guardian 4203 (weight 270 g) which also has the feature of bradycardia support. Coronary artery bypass grafting was also performed in one of the two patients.

Results

Preoperative: Sustained monomorphic VT could be induced preoperatively in 42 of the 47 patients, and VF resulted from programmed stimulation in five patients.

Peroperative: During surgery, stable monomorphic VT similar to the spontaneous VT was induced in 38 patients, in one of whom the mapping procedure could not be performed because of technical problems. In the remaining nine patients, either no arrhythmia could be provoked or VF or polymorphic VT was induced. In seven of these nine patients the area of earliest endocardial activation was estimated by pacemapping, but in the other two neither programmed stimulation nor pacemapping was successful, and an extended subendocardial resection was performed with guidance from endocardial fibrosis. A single aneurysm was found at operation in 42

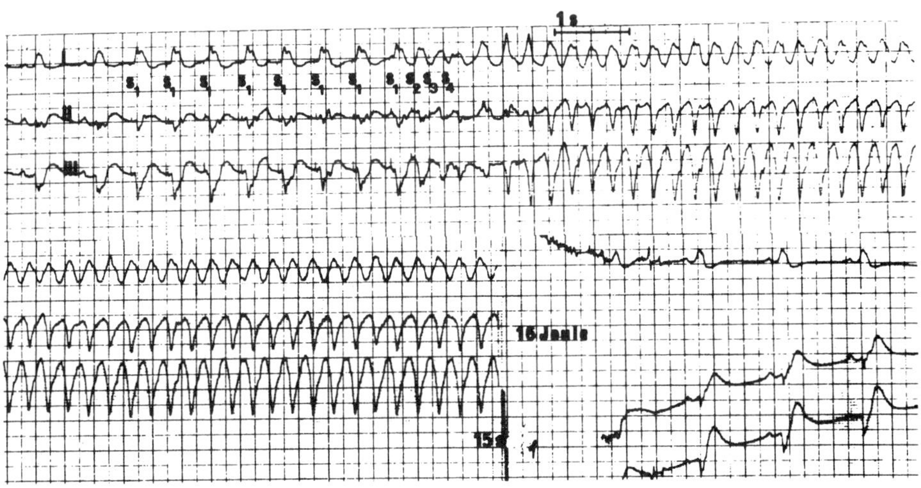

Fig. 4. *Continous recording illustrating the function of the implantable cardioverter defibrillator. Standard leads I, II and III are shown.* S_1, S_2, S_3, S_4 *are the pacestimulus artefacts. Upper left tracing shows sinus rhythm followed by programmed ventricular stimulation with a basic cycle length of* S_1-S_1 = *500 msec for eight beats after which three ventricular extrastimuli* S_2, S_3, S_4 *are introduced. This results in VT with a frequency of 220 beats/min. The VT is sensed and diagnosed by the cardioverter defibrillator. After 15 s a shock of 16 joule is delivered and sinus rhythm is restored.*

patients, while one patient had two aneurysms, giving a total of 43 aneurysmectomies. As two arrhythmogenic areas were found in the case with two aneurysms, the number of endocardial resections was also 43. Coronary artery bypass surgery was performed in 11 cases.

Postoperative: There were 4 deaths (9%) during or after surgery. One patient, preoperatively treated with Amiodarone, died in the operating room because of failed weaning from bypass. Another patient died on the first postoperative day of VF and low cardiac output, despite inotropic support and intraaortic balloon pumping. The third death occurred 2 weeks after surgery and was due to VF caused by AMI. The fourth patient died 1 month after surgery due to heart failure.

The patient with the lowest ejection fraction preoperatively (0.15) had low cardiac output after surgery and required inotropic support and intraaortic balloon pumping for 2 weeks. In two of the 12 patients who had drug-resistant heart failure before surgery, the failure persisted postoperatively, but could now be medically controlled. Spontaneous sustained VT appeared in one case on postoperative day 1 but, in contrast to the peroperative state, could now be managed with Amiodarone. Hemiparesis occurred postoperatively in one patient.

Postoperative electrophysiologic examination

Programmed electrophysiologic stimulation was repeated postoperatively in 37 of the 41 patients surviving the operation. The reasons why the other four patients were not examined were, respectively, occurrence of spontaneous VT, severe heart failure necessitating intraaortic balloon pumping for 2 weeks, hemiparesis, and withholding of consent.

VT could not be provoked in 33 of the 37 examined patients. VF resulted in two patients. Although neither patient had experienced VF before the operation, they were treated with Amiodarone postoperatively. The same VT as preoperatively could be provoked in one case. The last patient, who was inducible had had five preoperatively attacks of VF and two of VT with a cycle length of 290 msec, and the postoperative electrophysiologic provocation resulted in a slow, well tolerated VT with a cycle length of 500 msec and QRS morphology differing from the preoperative spontaneous VT. This patient was treated with disopyramide, and at electrophysiologic study a week later, VT could no longer be elicited. Thus, VT occurred spontaneously in one patient postoperatively, and VT and VF could be induced in 4 of the 37 electrophysiologically studied patients. Only in one of the four patients was the induced VT similar to the spontaneous VT.

Follow-up

The mean follow-up time was 25 (range 1-88) months. There were 8 out-of-hospital deaths. Of these 5 patients died suddenly. One of the five patients had AMI, whereas the other four patients died without AMI. Three patients died of heart failure and 2 patients experienced sudden cardiac death events with documented VF, but both patients were rescued. In total, 7 patients experienced sudden cardiaç death events and 5 of the patients died. Fig. 5 shows life table analysis of total mortality during clinical follow-up including operative mortality. Fig. 6 shows life table analysis of freedom from sudden cardiac death events during clinical follow-up.

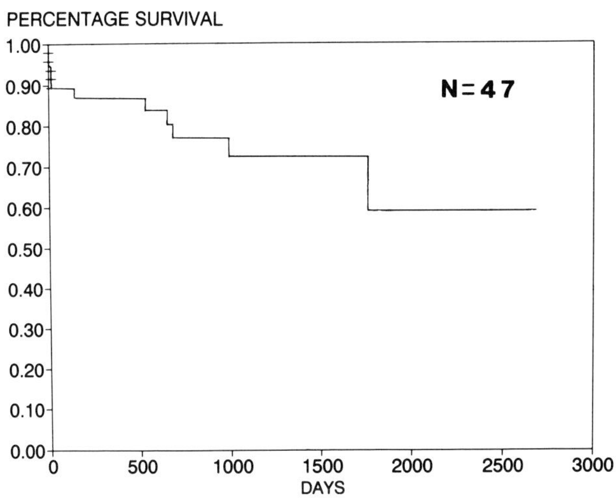

Fig. 5. *Life table analysis (Kaplan-Meier) of total mortality during clinical follow-up in 47 patients operated upon for VT/VF.*

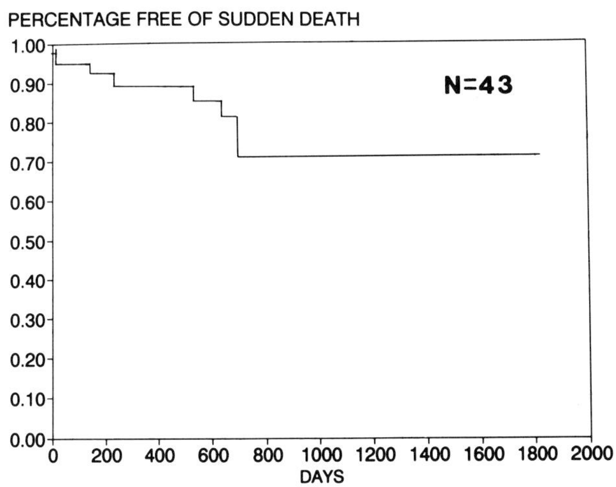

Fig. 6. *Life table analysis (Kaplan-Meier) of sudden cardiac death events during clincial follow-up in 43 patients operated upon for VT/VF. Only patients discharged from hospital are included.*

Conclusion

Various surgical approaches have been used to solve the problem of medically refractory VT/VF in patients with coronary artery disease. Coronary revascularisation alone was found by some medical investigators to have a beneficial effect on intractable VT/VF in patients with aneurysm (15), whereas others reported a high rate of late sudden death due to VT/VF (16). "Blind aneurysmectomy" alone was stated to have a 60 to 80% failure rate in such drug-resistent VT/VF (17). This is probably one of the reasons why endocardial mapping and subsequent subendocardial resection – in opposition to blind aneurysmectomy – has, for the first time allowed exclusion of areas of abnormal electrical activity located in the septum.

It must be admitted, however, that the vast majority of patients studied and operated upon had recurrent sustained VT. Too few patients with VF or non-sustained VT have been studied to allow conclusions about these substrates. In addition, aneurysmectomy for refractory malignant VT within one month after AMI has such high mortality, that it should be considered a heroic intervention (18). In the present series only one of the patients was operated within the first month of AMI.

Our experience with the implantable cardioverter defibrillator is limited to two patients. In the latest report from a world-wide register covering 3610 patients treated with the device, cumulative percentage survival from sudden cardiac death was nearly 90% after a 72 months follow-up period (7).

In conclusion, mapping-guided subendocardial resection is an effective treatment of patients with medically refractory VT/VF and left ventricular aneurysm secondary to AMI. The surgical risk appears to be acceptable in these patients with a 9% operative mortality. Clinical follow-up shows a success rate concerning sudden cardiac death events of 70%.

A realistic alternative to operation is the implantable cardioverter defibrillator. It should be mentioned, however, that both treatments are symptomatic since they are performed on patients with ischaemic heart disease. Therefore, the long-term prognosis is determined by the evolvement of the underlying heart disease.

By the time most patients die of coronary heart disease, they usually have more than one risk variable and multiple mechanisms often contribute to death. Nevertheless, non-pharmacological treatment of VT/VF can postpone death.

References

1. Horowitz LN, Josephson ME, Farshidi A, Spielman SR, Michaelson EL, Greenspan AM. Recurrent sustained ventricular tachycardia. 3. Role of the electrophysiologic study in selection of antiarrhythmic regimens. Circulation 1978; 58: 986-97.
2. Horowitz LN, Greenspan AM, Spielman SR, et al. Usefulness of electrophysiologic testing in evaluation of Amiodarone therapy for sustained ventricular tachyarrhythmias associated with coronary heart disease. Am J Cardiol 1985; 55: 367-71.
3. Josephson ME, Harken AH, Horowitz LN. Endocardial excision: A new surgical technique for the treatment of recurrent ventricular tachycardia. Circulation 1979; 60: 1430-9.
4. Horowitz LN, Harken AH, Kastor JA, Josephson ME. Ventricular resection guided by epicardial and endocardial mapping for treatment of recurrent ventricular tachycardia. N Engl J Med 1980; 302: 589-93.
5. Mirowski M, Reid PR, Mower MM, et al. Termination of malignant ventricular arrhythmias with an implanted automatic defibrillator in human beings. N Engl J Med 1980; 303: 322-4.
6. Kelly PA, Cannom DS, Garan H, et al. The automatic implantable cardioverter-defibrillator: Efficacy, complications and survival in patients with malignant ventricular arrhythmias. J Am Coll Cardiol 1988; 11: 1278-86.
7. Thomas AC, Moser SA, Smutka ML, Wilson PA. Implantable defibrillation: Eight years clincial experience. PACE 1988; 11: 2053-8.
8. Wellens HJJ, Bar FWHM, Brugada P. Ventricular tachycardia. The clinical problem. In: Josephson ME, ed. Ventricular tachycardia. Mechanism and management. New York: Future Publishing Company, 1982: 1-19.
9. Wellens HJJ, Schuilenburg RM, Durrer D. Electrical stimulation of the heart in patients with ventricular tachycardia. Circulation 1972; 46: 216-26.
10. Vandepol CJ, Farshidi A, Spielman SR, Greenspan AM, Horowitz LN, Josephson ME. Incidence and clinical significance of induced ventricular tachycardia. Am J Cardiol 1980; 45: 725-31.
11. Mason JW, Winkle RA. Accuracy of the ventricular tachycardia induction study for predicting long-term efficacy and inefficacy of antiarrhythmic drugs. N Engl J Med 1980; 303: 1073-7.
12. Ruskin JN, DiMarco JP, Garan H. Out-of hospital cardiac arrest. Electrophysiologic observations and selection of long-term antiarrhythmic therapy. N Eng J Med 1980; 303: 607-13.
13. Waller TJ, Kay HR, Spielman SR, Kutalek SP, Greenspan AM, Horowitz LN. Reduction in sudden death and total mortality by antiarrhythmic therapy evaluated by electrophysiologic drug testing: Criteria of efficacy in patients with sustained ventricular tachyarrhythmia. J Am Coll Cardiol 1987; 10: 83-9.
14. Kromann-Hansen O, Bloch Thomsen PE, Bagger H, Albrechtsen O. Surgery of ventricular tachycardia and ventricular fibrillation in patients with coronary artery disease and LV-aneurysms. Scand J Thor Cardiovasc Surg 1989; 23: 87-93.
15. Kaiser GA, Gharhamani A, Bolooki H, et al. Role of coronary artery surgery in patients surviving unexpected cardiac arrest. Surgery 1978; 78: 749-54.
16. Ricks WB, Winkle RA, Shumway NE. Surgical management of life-threatening ventricular arrhythmias in patients with coronary artery disease. Circulation 1977; 56: 38-45.
17. Harken AH, Horowitz LN, Josephson ME. Comparison of standard aneurysmectomy and aneurysmectomy with directed endocardial resection for the treatment of recurrent sustained ventricular tachycardia. J Thorac Cardiovasc Surg 1980; 80: 527-34.
18. Ostermeyer J, Borggrefe M, Breithardt G, et al. Direct operations for the management

of life-threatening ischemic ventricular tachycardia. J Thorac Cardiovasc Surg 1987; 94: 848-65.

19. Buda AJ, Stinson EB, Harrison DC. Surgery for life-threatening ventricular arrhythmias. Am J Cardiol 1979; 44: 1171-7.

25

Atrial fibrillation and the risk of embolism

JOHN GODTFREDSEN

Both stroke and atrial fibrillation (AF) are common and important clinical entities with a significant morbidity and mortality. They are also linked together through a wide variety of possible pathogenetic mechanisms. The classic theory is that in AF many, if not most, cases of ischaemic cerebral infarcts are caused by embolism originating from thrombus formation in the non-contracting left atrium.

AF can be present in any aetiological heart disease, definitely increasing with age, and AF is often associated with congestive heart failure (CHF) and high blood pressure. As the same is the case for many types of stroke, clinically and pathologically as well as in CT scan characteristics, it is not surprising that risk factors and pathogenesis of stroke in AF are presently the subject of much debate.

This review deals with these complex issues, their pathological, clinical and therapeutical features, based on recent important findings in the cardio-neurological literature. Some comprehensive review articles on the subject have been published recently (1-3). It seems reasonable to distinguish between the occurrence of stroke in AF on the one hand (the cardiologist's view) and the occurrence of AF in stroke on the other (the neurologist's view). The percentage of both total numbers of stroke in AF and total numbers of patients with AF in stroke are very similar, namely, about 15%-25% (4-6).

Pathology and pathogenesis

The pathogenetic background for thrombus formation in the atria in AF includes enlarged atria, injured mitral valve, as in rheumatic heart disease (RHD), an akinetic atrial wall, injured atrial endothelium, and stagnant and sluggish blood flow in the atria (7-9). All these mechanisms need not be present at the same time. None of them and, in particular, their interplay are completely understood; but still regarded necessary for embolism although most studies fail to find more than about 50% atrial thrombi as compared with the number of emboli (10-12). In one patho-anatomic study, however, this ratio was reversed, i.e. atrial thrombi outnumbered emboli by 2:1 (13). Thus, even though it is established that atrial thrombi are more frequent in patients with AF, and especially in patients with RHD, than in patients with sinus rhythm, this is no proof that stroke in AF is mainly of embolic origin. Although some progress seems on its way, one difficulty is the lack of a long-term animal model, as well as studies with labelled clots in the atria (14).

In two recent studies with rather strict neurological criteria for embolic stroke, the proportion of embolic origin versus localized atherothrombotic mechanisms varied between 20% and 63% (4, 15). Another important mechanism that may contribute to stroke during AF is decreased cerebral blood flow due to low cardiac output, and perhaps also to changes in coagulation factors leading to regional, localized thrombus formation (16-18). Left atrial size seems to gradually increase in the course of AF (19) and the occurrence of stroke is apparently an early event after the onset of AF (see below).

If it is maintained that increased left atrial (LA) size is an important risk factor for stroke, then the clustering of strokes early after AF-onset must be wrong or vice versa. Injured atrial endothelium in the presence of low cardiac output may of course still play an important role in thrombus formation, but only few data exist (2).

Finally, it could be that AF, in many cases of stroke, is the consequence and not the underlying cause of the acute cerebral event. Clinical evidence of such a mechanism is the very high degree of CHF in these elderly patients (4, 5), and usually larger cerebral infarcts and high mortality (2). From a cardiologist's point of view, it is no surprise that a severe cerebral disaster, whatever the cause, could precipitate overt decompensated CHF and AF in elderly, frail patients with concomitant, unstable compensated heart failure. Based on careful clinical analysis of the circumstances at the onset of AF, it was shown that in 70 of 1,212 patients (5.6%) AF was possibly precipitated by stroke, which is about 40% of the entire number of strokes in this series (5).

A recent Danish clinical and echocardiographic study of 70 patients with AF where the risk of emboli varied with the underlying aetiology points in the same direction of a very complex and varied pathogenesis of stroke in any heart disease with AF: Lone AF: primary myocardial disease: primary mitral valve disease with a ratio of 1:2:7 (20). The present situation regarding emboli as the cause of stroke in AF is thus very similar to the situation regarding the pathogenesis of AF itself: the cause is most likely multifactorial with several closely interwoven mechanisms, many of which are not yet clearly defined. Still, thrombogenesis is a common denominator, making treatment with anticoagulants attractive.

Epidemiological and clinical factors

The main sources of prospective data on stroke in AF are the Framingham Study, the British Whitehall and Regional Heart Study, and the Reykjavik Heart Study (21-23). In the Framingham Study the risk of stroke was increased 17-fold in RHD and 5.6-fold in non-valvular AF. The British Study, with its two parts, showed a relative risk of stroke in non-valvular AF of 6.9 and 2.3, respectively. In the Icelandic study the relative risk was 7.1. The incidence rate of stroke in Framingham was 5% per year as against lower figures in the British Study: 1.5% and 0.4% per year. These studies dealt with individuals in the younger age groups (30-69 years at entry) and can therefore hardly be considered representative of the much more common situation in the clinical setting, where the median age of the typical AF patient is over 70 years (5,24).

It had previously been demonstrated in a Danish study (5), and later confirmed in the Framingham Study, that the thromboembolic complications cluster shortly after the AF-onset or after the transition from paroxysmal AF (PAF) to chronic AF (CAF) (25-27). This finding, however, may be spurious, and perhaps related to the concomitant clinical presentation of AF and stroke, where AF may actually have been present before the index-stroke, or as mentioned above, the stroke may have precipitated the AF. This clustering has not been confirmed in recent, prospective studies (24). Incidence rates of thromboembolic complications in PAF and CAF are shown in a selected clinical series in Table 1 (26), and interestingly are in good accordance with the more recent epidemiological studies (21).

Table 1. *Incidence rates of thromboembolic complications in paroxysmal (PAF) and chronic (CAF) atrial fibrillation as it relates to the duration of the arrhythmia.*

	< 1 month	Up to 1 year	2-5 years
PAF (N=426)	6.8%	2%	2%
CAF (N=786)	8.2%	4%	4%

In CAF it has been shown by multifactorial Cox's analysis that a significant risk factor for stroke is the underlying aetiology, i.e. RHD, of AF, but also previous myocardial infarction (MI), hypertension, LA-enlargement and left ventricular hypertrophy seem to be relevant risk factors (8, 28, 29). Also in the British prospective study (22) in men with non-valvular AF, hypertension was a risk factor for stroke. In contrast, the patho-anatomic study from Boston (12) showed only a minor difference in the rate of systemic embolism between AF patients with RHD and those with ischaemic heart disease (IHD): 41% versus 35%. It was shown in the latest report from the Framingham Study (27) by means of multiple logistic regression analysis that age, systolic blood pressure, IHD, and CHF were also significant risk factors for stroke, though it is not entirely clear whether this analysis comprised all strokes or only those that occurred in the 59 patients with AF at entry.

Not only is there a quite high total rate of thromboembolic complications during the entire course of AF, i.e. about 17% to 50%, depending on the underlying aetiology, but also the recurrence rate and the mortality resulting from complications are both about 25% (5, 12, 15, 22, 27, 30). Thus, the important features of thromboembolic complications in AF are: (a) a definite increased risk of stroke which accounts for 60%-80% of such complications, (b) highest rate of stroke in RHD, (c) some indications that previous MI, hypertension and its followers: LA-enlargement and left ventricular hypertrophy, and perhaps CHF are associated risk factors, and (d) a recurrence rate and mortality due to complications of about 25%.

The problem of clinically silent cerebral embolism has been studied recently by means of CT scanning. In patients with CAF 48% had cortical areas of low density compared with only 28% of matched patients in sinus rhythm (31, 32). In PAF such possible cerebral infarcts were also present, but to a lesser degree and not significantly different from patients in sinus rhythm (33).

The term "lone AF" usually denotes PAF or CAF in patients without any overt underlying heart disease. In the Framingham Study of these patients (34) a 4-fold increase in the stroke rate was demonstrated compared with controls, suggesting that lone AF in this respect is not benign. However, a study from the Mayo Clinic (35) of patients with lone AF <60 days of age, 91% of whom had PAF, showed a very low incidence of thromboembolism: only 8% over 10 years of follow-up. Recent data from the same institution on older patients with lone AF showed a somewhat increased risk of transitory ischaemic attack (TIA) or stroke compared with patients with sinus rhythm (36).

Prevention of thromboembolism

Most authors agree that AF in RHD, particularly mitral stenosis, is a clear-cut indication for life-long anticoagulation treatment, as is an episode of sustained stroke in non-valvular AF patients (37). The authors of a recent retrospective study recommended prophylactic anticoagulation treatment also in non-valvular AF (38).

However, the use of anticoagulants in AF after a sustained stroke has been seriously questioned on the basis of methodological problems and as a result of evaluation of the survival rate and the recurrence of stroke in this setting as compared to patients with sinus rhythm (39).

The recently published Copenhagen AFASAK Study showed a significant reduction in thromboembolic events in out-patients with CAF after prophylactic warfarin treatment versus low-dose aspirin and placebo (24).

Presently, several randomized, prospective studies of anticoagulation treatment in non-valvular AF are underway (40). Until the results of these are known and compared with those from the Copenhagen trial, a prudent attitude seems to be an individualized evaluation in each case, and probably not to anticoagulate for more than 1-2 years, especially in older patients where this treatment carries some risk of serious side effects. The present data supporting anticoagulation treatment in PAF and in lone AF in younger patients are too sparse.

Conclusion

Non-valvular AF is definitely associated with an increased risk of stroke of about 5% per year. Prophylactic anticoagulation treatment seems to reduce this risk, and should be used in selected patients.

References

1. Cerebral embolism task force. Cardiogenic brain embolism. Arch Neurol 1986; 43: 71-84.
2. Fisher CM. Embolism in atrial fibrillation. In: Kulbertus HE, Olsson SB, Schlepper M, eds. Atrial fibrillation. Mölndal: Hässle, 1982: 192-207.
3. Alpert JS, Petersen P, Godtfredsen J. Atrial fibrillation: natural history, complications and management. Ann Rev Med 1988; 39: 41-52.
4. Britton M, Gustafsson C. Non-rheumatic atrial fibrillation as a risk factor for stroke. Stroke 1985; 16: 182-8.
5. Godtfredsen J. Atrial fibrillation. Etiology, course and prognosis. A follow-up study of 1,212 cases. Copenhagen: Munksgaard, 1975.
6. Wolf PA, Abott RD, Kannel WB. Atrial fibrillation: A major contribution to stroke in the elderly. The Framingham study. Arch Int Med 1987; 147: 1561-4.

7. Caplan LR, D'Cruz I, Hier DB, Reddy H, Shah S. Atrial size, atrial fibrillation and stroke. Ann Neurol 1986; 19: 158-61.
8. Aronow WS, Gutstein H, Hsieh FY. Risk factors for thromboembolic stroke in elderly patients with atrial fibrillation. Am J Cardiol 1989; 63: 366-7.
9. Matsuzaki M, Toma Y, Suetsugu M, et al. Analysis of blood flow velocity and thrombogenesis in left atrial appendage by transesophageal two-dimensional echocardiography. J Am Coll Cardiol 1987; 9: 212 A.
10. Åberg H. Atrial fibrillation I. A study of atrial thrombus and systemic embolism in a necropsy material. Acta Med Scand 1969; 185: 373-9.
11. Beer DT, Ghitman B. Embolization from the atria in arteriosclerotic heart disease. JAMA 1961; 177: 287-90.
12. Hinton RC, Kistler JP, Fallon JT, Friedlich AL, Fisher CM. Influence of etiology of atrial fibrillation on incidence of systemic embolism. Am J Cardiol 1977; 40: 509-13.
13. Davies MJ, Pomerance A. Pathology of atrial fibrillation in man. Br Heart J 1972; 34: 520-5.
14. Vandenberg BF, Seabold JE, Conrad GR, et al. 111-Inlabeled platelet scintigraphy and two-dimensional echocardiography for detection of left atrial appendage thrombi. Studies in a new canine model. Circulation 1988; 78: 1040-6.
15. Hart RG, Coull BM, Hart D. Early recurrent embolism associated with non-valvular atrial fibrillation: a retrospective study. Stroke 1983; 14: 688-93.
16. Gustafsson C, Blombäck M., Britton M, Hamsten A, Svensson J. Haemostatic function and the increased risk of stroke in non-valvular atrial fibrillation. Stroke 1987; 18: 25.
17. Lavy S, Stern S, Melamed E, Cooper G, Keren A, Levy P. Effect of chronic atrial fibrillation on regional cerebral blood flow. Stroke 1980; 11: 35-8.
18. Petersen P, Kastrup J, Videbæk R, Boysen G. Cerebral blood flow before and after electrical conversion of atrial fibrillation. J Cerebr Blood Flow Metab 1989; 9: 422-5.
19. Petersen P, Kastrup J, Brinch K, Godtfredsen J, Boysen G. Relation between left atrial dimension and duration of atrial fibrillation. Am J Cardiol 1987; 60: 382-4.
20. Egeblad H. Intracardiac thrombus – systemic embolism. Contribution of echocardiography. Acta Med Scand 1988; (suppl. 730): 224.
21. Wolf PA, Dawber TR, Thomas HE, Kannel WB. Epidemiologic assessment of chronic atrial fibrillation and risk of stroke: the Framingham Study. Neurology 1978; 28: 973-7.
22. Flegel KM, Shipley MJ, Rose G. Risk of stroke in non-rheumatic atrial fibrillation. Lancet 1987; 1: 526-9.
23. Önundarson PT, Thorgeirsson G, Jonmundsson E, Sigfusson N, Hardarson Th. Chronic atrial fibrillation – epidemiologic features and 14 year follow-up: a case control study. Eur Heart J 1987; 8: 521-7.
24. Petersen P, Boysen G, Godtfredsen J, Andersen ED, Andersen B. Placebo-controlled, randomised trial of warfarin and aspirin for prevention of thromboembolic complications in chronic atrial fibrillation. The Copenhagen AFASAK Study. Lancet 1989; 1: 175-9.
25. Hart RG, Easton JD, Sherman DG. Duration of non-valvular atrial fibrillation and stroke. Stroke 1987; 14: 827.
26. Petersen P, Godtfredsen J. Embolic complications in paroxysmal atrial fibrillation. Stroke 1986; 17: 622-6.
27. Wolf PA, Kannel WB, McGee DL, Meeks SL, Bharucha NE, McNamara PM. Duration of atrial fibrillation and imminence of stroke: the Framingham Study. Stroke 1983; 14: 664-7.
28. Petersen P, Godtfredsen J. Risk factors for stroke in chronic atrial fibrillation. Eur Heart J 1988; 9: 291-4.
29. Petersen P, Kastrup J, Helweg-Larsen S, Boysen G, Godtfredsen J. Risk factors for

thromboembolic complications in chronic atrial fibrillation. The Copenhagen AFASAK Study. Arch Int Med 1990 (in press)

30. Sage JI, Van Uitert RI. Risk of recurrent stroke in patients with atrial fibrillation and non-valvular heart disease. Stroke 1983; 14: 537-40.
31. Petersen P, Madsen EB, Brun B, Pedersen F, Gyldensted C, Boysen G. Silent cerebral infarction in chronic atrial fibrillation. Stroke 1987; 18: 1098-100.
32. Kempster PA, Genaty RD, Gates PC. Asymptomatic cerebral infarction in patients with chronic atrial fibrillation. Stroke 1988; 19: 955-7.
33. Petersen P, Pedersen F, Johnsen A, et al. Cerebral computed tomography in paroxysmal atrial fibrillation. Acta Neurol Scand 1989; 79: 482-6.
34. Brand FN, Abott RD, Kannel WB, Wolf PA. Characteristics and prognosis of lone atrial fibrillation. JAMA 1985; 254: 3449-53.
35. Kopecky SL, Gersh BJ, McGoon MD, et al. The natural history of lone atrial fibrillation. A population-based study over three decades. N Engl J Med 1987; 317: 669-74.
36. Kopecky SL, Gersh BJ, McGoon MD, Whisnant JP, Ilstrup DM. Lone atrial fibrillation in the elderly. A population-based long term study. Circulation 1989; 80: (suppl. II): 409.
37. Nordlander R. Anticoagulation in atrial fibrillation. In: Kulbertus HE, Olsson SB, Schlepper M, eds. Atrial Fibrillation. Mölndal: Hässle, 1982: 251-9.
38. Roy D, Marchand E, Gagné P, Chabot M, Cartier P. Usefulness of anticoagulant therapy in the prevention of embolic complications in atrial fibrillation. Am Heart J 1986; 112: 1039-43.
39. Sandercock P, Warlow C, Bamford J, Peto R, Starkey I. Is a controlled trial of long-term oral anticoagulants in patients with stroke and non-rheumatic atrial fibrillation worthwhile? Lancet 1986; 1: 788-92.
40. Walker MD. Atrial fibrillation and antithrombotic prophylaxis: A prospective meta-analysis. Lancet 1989; 1: 325-6.

26

Electrolyte disturbances and sudden cardiac death

JAN ERIK NORDREHAUG

Sudden cardiac death is most commonly associated with coronary artery disease and its consequences, which accounts for more than 80% of the cases. Other causes are left ventricular hypertrophy, myocardial disease, valvular disorders, congenital heart disease, electrophysiological abnormalities, and electrical instability related to neurohumeral and electrolyte disturbances.

Instantaneous cardiac death in patients with coronary artery disease is most commonly due to ventricular arrhythmias, especially ventricular fibrillation (VF) (1, 2). Even though the incidence of sudden death increases with advancing age, the proportion of coronary deaths that are sudden decreases with age. Thus, the problem of sudden death is important for all patients with coronary artery disease.

Experimental studies have shown that electrolyte disturbances can create electrical instability (3, 4). Potassium and magnesium have been most frequently studied clinically. These ions are of great importance for the normal cellular electrophysiology. However, chronic depletion of these and other trace metals, such as chromium, copper and selenium (5, 6), has also been suggested to result in clinical or subclinical myocardial damage. This may also predispose to arrhythmias. Although only major disturbances in extracellular calcium have been associated with arrhythmias (7, 8), intracellular calcium plays a role in mediating ischaemic cell injury (9).

Clinical studies have shown an association between low levels of potassium, magnesium and ventricular arrhythmias. The low electrolyte levels are strictly not necessarily the cause of the arrhythmias, but could be passive markers of other arrhythmogenic events. In patients with acute myocardial infarction (AMI), early agressive intravenous diuretic therapy results in a rapid decrease of potassium levels (10). These patients often also have large infarctions, and therefore a high risk of arrhythmias due to infarct size.

Furthermore, catecholamine levels are elevated early in AMI (11). Catecholamines have inherent arrhythmogenic action (2), but can also cause hypokalaemia (12) and hypomagnesaemia (13). Chronic electrolyte depletion leads to cardiomyopathy (14), and thereby increased arrhythmic potential.

On the other hand, the use of multivariate statistical analysis has identified eletrolytes, especially potassium, as independent predictors of serious ventricular arrhythmias in AMI. Such relations clearly strengthen the cause and effect concept. Sudden cardiac death has not been specifically investigated in relation to electrolyte disturbances. The link between sudden death and arrhythmias is, however, close.

Pathophysiological considerations

In spite of potassium being mainly an intracellular ion, the extracelluar fraction is very important for the cell membrane potential (3, 7). A change in potassium of 1 mmol extracellularly will change the resting membrane potential from –94 to –100 mV. The same change intracellularly of 1 mmol/l will change the membrane potential by only 0.2 mV. Hypokalaemia affects automaticity, depolarisation and repolarisation during the action potential, and is arrhythmogenic in normal hearts (3, 7, 8).

A rapid rise in extracellular potassium in the myocardium during ischaemia coincides with the occurrence of VF, but cannot solely explain this occurrence (15, 16). VF can also be initiated by ectopic currents from Purkinje fibres localised in normal myocardium close to the ischaemic border (3, 17). Such areas may reflect hypokalaemia present in the general circulation. Thus, the presence of unequal action potentials predisposes to reentry arrhythmias. Hypokalaemia may induce atrioventricular conduction blocks in experimental animal hearts, but conduction blocks grade 2 and 3 are generally only observed at serum potassium levels <2.0 mmol/l (18).

Chronic hypokalaemia is associated with myocardial damage, as reported in post-mortem studies (19). This increases the arrhythmic potential of hypokalaemia.

Magnesium is also mainly an intracellular ion. It does not directly take part in the action potential, but variations influence its amplitude, conduction and duration. The normal potassium fluxes depend on a normal magnesium concentration (20-23). Exactly how magnesium deficiency exerts antiarrhythmic action in ischaemia is not clear (24), but intracellular levels are probably more important than extracellular.

Sodium, chloride and calcium play an important role in the normal action potential. Quite extreme disturbances of these electrolytes are necessary to provoke arrhythmias experimentally (7, 8). Deficiency of trace metals such as copper, zinc, chromium and selenium have been associated with the development of cardiomyopathy and myocardial damage. This predisposes to arrhythmias.

Clinical studies – myocardial infarction

Potassium

A large number of clinical studies have shown an association between hypokalaemia and increased occurrence of ventricular arrhythmias in AMI (25-43). Recently, a few of these have identified hypokalaemia as an independent risk factor for ventricular tachycardia and VF.

The studies also indicate that hyperkalaemia confers an increased risk of serious arrhythmias. The risk is only seen at serum potassium above 7-8 mmol/l, and the hyperkalaemia has usually occurred with acidosis and in otherwise seriously ill patients with heart failure (27, 38). Therefore, it has been difficult to identify hyperkalaemia as an independent risk factor in spite of its known experimentally adverse electrophysiological actions.

There are some problems that are common to many of the potassium studies. The classification of patients into groups based on potassium values has been done in different ways. Some studies have grouped patients based on the potassium value obtained nearest in time to the particular arrhythmia under review. In this instance, patients without arrhythmias are classified according to serum potassium concentration on admission to hospital. This ensures a better temporal relationship between the serum potassium measurement and the arrhythmia, but has some major drawbacks as well. A fall in potassium concentration resulting from in-hospital diuretic treatment will only be observed in patients with arrhythmias, resulting in a falsely high incidence of hypokalaemia in such patients. Also, patients in need of diuretic treatment with a poor left ventricular function, and therefore a high risk of arrhythmias, tend to be clustered in the hypokalaemic group, resulting in a high rate of mortality and arrhythmias in this group, and making the comparison of rates of arrhythmias with the normokalaemic group difficult. Furthermore, classification into groups based on serum potassium obtained after VF and resuscitation may not be indicative of the potassium concentration before the onset of VF, since increased catecholamine levels and infusion of glucose and sodium bicarbonate during resuscitation may influence the levels of serum potassium.

Another approach has been to base the groups on potassium concentration obtained at hospital admission for all patients. This may result in a

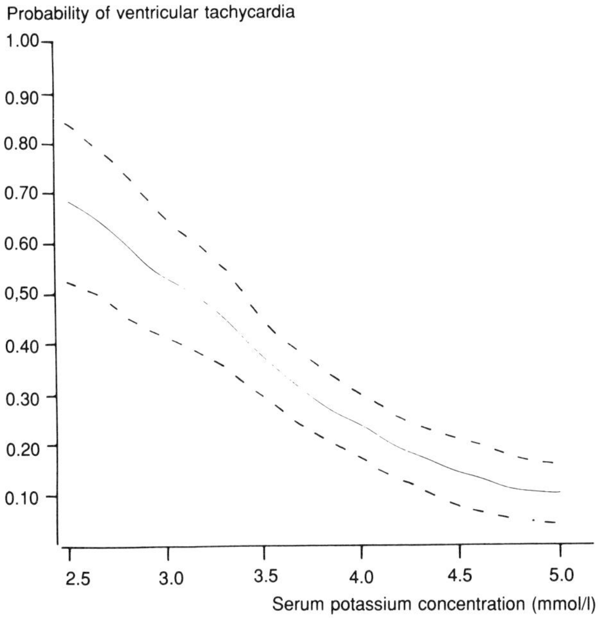

Fig. 1. *Probability of ventricular tachycardia in relation to serum potassium concentration. Dotted line denotes SD.*

loss of temporal relationship between potassium measurement and arrhythmias, but has a better chance of documenting potassium measurements at the same time of infarct evolution in the two potassium groups (37).

A closer temporal relationship between the initial serum potassium concentration and arrhythmias can be reached by detecting arrhythmia for only a short interval (26). This could also be an advantage since hypokalaemia early in AMI tends to be transient due to rapidly fluctuating catecholamine levels (11). In contrast, short-term monitoring may be inadequate for comparison of hypo- and normokalaemic groups because of the chance of spontaneous variation in the occurrence of arrhythmias. Clinical studies also generally consist of a small hypokalaemic and a large normokalaemic group, which may lead to a greater risk of detecting arrhythmias at different stages of ischaemia and infarct evolution in the two potassium groups.

Digitalis therapy may have different actions according to extracellular potassium concentrations. In the presence of normokalaemia, digitalis may prevent arrhythmias. Hypokalaemia may induce increased sensitivity to digitalis (44), which may provoke arrhythmias (45). Clinical studies (37, 40, 41) have identified hypokalaemia as a risk of arrhythmias also independent of digitalis therapy.

Most clinical studies have used conventional arrhythmia detection, this under-estimates the occurrence of arrhythmias. Prospective detection using

Holter monitoring has shown a clear association between hypokalaemia and non-sustained ventricular tachycardia (40) (Fig. 1).

Hypokalaemia is associated with diuretic therapy in most of the studies of myocardial infarction. A substantial portion of the patients with hypokalaemia have not taken diuretics. An inverse relationship between hypokalaemia and catecholamine levels early in AMI has been shown (46). This may explain the high occurrence of hypokalaemia in the absence of diuretic therapy. This hypokalaemia can be counteracted by intravenous betablockade (47).

Some main conclusions can be drawn from the clinical studies on potassium in AMI:

1. The inverse relationship between hypokalaemia and serious ventricular arrhythmias is independent of other variables usually associated with ventricular arrhythmias, such as heart failure and extensive myocardial damage. The results strongly suggest a causal role between low serum potassium levels and increased occurrence of malignant ventricular arrhythmias.
2. Hypokalaemia on admission to hospital does not confer an increased mortality during up to 33 months of follow up (38). This may be due to the finding that the arrhythmias inversely predicted by serum potassium are associated with electrical instability that is independent of a poor left ventricular function, and to the good results of resuscitation of otherwise lethal arrhythmias in the coronary care unit.
3. Hypokalaemia during the first 24 hours after hospital admission is often transient with a duration usually of 6-12 hours. There is a negative correlation between plasma adrenaline and potassium. This also indicates that patients with cornary artery disease may rapidly develop hypokalaemia and be at increased risk of ventricular arrhythmias during attacks of chest pain that provoke elevation of catecholamines. Acute hypokalaemia can be counteracted by intravenous betablockade, mediated via beta-2 receptors.

Magnesium

Hypomagnesaemia has been associated with the increased occurrence of ventricular arrhythmias in AMI (48). However, the magnesium studies suffer from the same problems as elucidated for potassium, and the problems have been solved to a lesser extent. One important problem is that intracellular magnesium levels are probably more important than extracellular levels for arrhythmias (20, 24). In one study using multivariate statistical analysis, serum potassium was a stronger predictor than serum magnesium for ventricular tachycardia (40).

Epidemiological studies have suggested an association between a low magnesium content of the diet and increased occurrence of coronary heart disease and sudden death (49). An association between low serum magnesium levels and the degree of angiographic coronary artery stenosis has also been suggested (50).

Two recent papers have shown a reduction in arrhythmias and mortality after the infusion of magnesium early in AMI (51, 52). Thus, although lacking confirmatory evidence, there is some indication that magnesium therapy has a favourable effect on arrhythmia and prognosis in AMI. Previous case reports have indicated effect of magnesium infusion also for arrhythmias and hypomagnesaemia not linked with myocardial ischaemia.

Electrolytes and hypertension

A large primary prevention trial (MRFIT) aiming at multiple risk factor intervention to reduce coronary artery disease mortality rate, suggested from retrospective analysis, a link between the use of diuretics and increased occurrence of sudden death (53). Later, several studies have reported increased occurrence of arrhythmias in diuretic-treated patients with hypertension, others have refuted this (54). Exercise-induced arrhythmias seem to be more frequent in patients who are hypokalaemic at baseline (54). No studies have so far specifically linked hypokalaemia with sudden death in hypertension.

Both potassium and magnesium therapy have favourable effects on hypertension, and a high dietary potassium is associated with a lesser incidence of mortality from stroke (55).

Conclusions

In patients with AMI, hypokalaemia on admission to hospital is associated with an increased occurrence of VF and tachycardia. Hypokalaemia may also be linked with sudden death in the prehospital phase of the infarction. Hyperkalaemia has so far only been identified as a marker of circulatory failure.

Elevated catecholamines can provoke acute hypokalaemia, this is counteracted by beta-blockers, mediated via beta-2 receptors.

There is increasing evidence for an important role of magnesium disturbances and the occurrence of arrhythmias in myocardial infarction. Increased atherosclerosis and sudden death has also been suggested to occur with low magnesium intake.

Adequate magnesium and potassium levels seem to have favourable effects on blood pressure and mortality in hypertension, a role has also been suggested for prevention of arrhythmias.

Lack of other trace metals has so far mostly been linked to the development of myocardial damage and some reduction in the left ventricular function.

Patients with pre-existing heart disease seem to be more vulnerable to the acute adverse effects of relatively small electrolyte disturbances. Based on steadily accumulating evidence, the awareness of the importance of normal electrolyte balance should be increasing, especially when caring for patients with coronary artery disease. This concerns both prophylaxis and therapy, which probably will prove to be especially important in high risk groups.

References

1. Cobb LA, Werner JA, Trobaugh GB. Sudden cardiac death. A decade's experience with out-of-hospital resuscitation. Mod Concept Cardiovasc Dis 1980; 49: 31.
2. Bigger JT, Dresdale RJ, Heissenbuttel RH, Weld FM, Wit AL. Ventricular arrhythmias in ischemic heart disease: mechanism, prevalence, significance, and management. Prog Cardiovasc Dis 1977; 19: 255.
3. Fisch C. Relation of electrolyte disturbances to cardiac arrhythmias. Circulation 1973; 47: 408-19.
4. Stanbury JB, Farah A. Effects of the magnesium on the heart and on its response to digoxin. J Pharmacol Exp Ther 1950; 100: 455.
5. Committee on biological effects of Atmosferic Pollutants. National Research Council, National Academy of Sciences. Washington DC, 1976.
6. Klevay LM, Inman L, Johnson LK, et al. Increased cholesterol in plasma in a young man during experimental copper depletion. Metabolism 1984; 33: 1112-8.
7. Zipes DP. Electrolyte derangements in the genesis of arrhythmias In: Dreyfus, Likoff, eds. Cardiac Arrhythmias. 1973: 55-69.
8. Surawicz B. Role of electrolytes in etiology and management of cardiac arrhythmias. Prog Cardiovasc Dis 1966; 49: 364-86.
9. Cheung JY, Bonventre JV, Malis CD, Leaf A. Calcium and ischemic injury. N Engl J Med 1986; 314: 1670-5.
10. Nordrehaug JE, Johannessen K-A, von der Lippe G, Sederholm M, Grøttum P, Kjekshus J. Effect of timolol on changes in serum potassium concentration during acute myocardial infarction. Br Heart J 1985; 53: 388-93.
11. Karlsberg RP, Cryer PE, Roberts R. Serial plasma catecholamine response early in the course of acute myocardial infarction: relation to infarct extent and mortality. Am Heart J 1981; 102: 24-9.
12. Brown MJ, Brown DC, Murphy MB. Hypokalaemia from beta-2-receptor stimulation by circulationg epinephrine. N Engl J Med 1983; 309: 1414-9.
13. Flink EB, Brick JE, Shane SR. Alterations of long-chain free fatty acid and magnesium content in acute myocardial infarction. Arch Int Med 1981; 141: 441-3.

14. Urbano-Marquez A, Estruch R, Navarro-Lopez F, et al. The effects of alcoholism on skeletal and cardiac muscle. N Engl J Med 1989; 320: 409-15.
15. Harris AS, Bisteni A, Russel RA, et al. Excitatory factors in ventricular tachycardia resulting from myocardial ischemia: potassium a major excitant. Science 1954; 119: 200.
16. Hill JL, Gettes LS. Effect of coronary occusion on local myocardial extracellular K+ activity in swine. Circulation 1980; 61: 768-78.
17. Janse MJ, van Capelle FJL, Morsink H, et al. Flow of "injury" current and patterns of excitation during early ventricular arrhythmias in acute regional myocardial ischemia in islolated porcine and canine hearts. Evidence for two different arrhythmogenic mechanisms. Circ Res 1980; 47: 151-64.
18. Pes de Carvalho A, Langhan WB. Influence of extracellular potassium levels on atrioventricular transmission. Am J Physiol 1963; 205: 375-81.
19. Mergner WJ, Nguyen NGA, David RG. Cardiorenal pathology in hypokalemic patients. In: Whelton, Whelton, Walker, eds. Potassium in cardiovascular and renal medicine. New York: Marcel Decker. 1986: 143-68.
20. Ebel H, Gunther T. Magnesium metabolism. A review. J Clin Chem Clin Biochem 1980; 18: 257-70.
21. Chipperfield B, Chipperfield JR. Magnesium and the heart. Am Heart J 1977; 93: 679-82.
22. Watanabe Y, Dreifus LS. Electrophysiological effects of magnesium and its interactions with potassium. Cardiovasc Res 1972; 6: 79.
23. Nayler WG. The heart cell – Some metabolic aspects of cardiac arrhythmias. Acta Med Scand 1981; (suppl 647): 17-32.
24. Dubey A, Solomon R. Magnesium, myocardial ischemia and arrhythmias. The role of magnesium in myocardial infarction. Drugs 1989; 37: 1-7.
25. Duke M. Thiazide-induced hypokalemia. Association with acute myocardial infarction and ventricular fibrillation. JAMA 1978; 239: 43-5.
26. Beck OA, Hochrein H. Initial serum potassium level in relation to cardiac arrhythmias in acute myocardial infarction. Z Kardiol 1977; 66: 187-90.
27. Dyckner T, Helmers C, Lundman T, Wester PO. Initial serum potassium level in relation to early complications and prognosis in patients with acute myocardial infarction. Acta Med Scand 1975; 197: 207-10.
28. Donelly T, Gray H, Simpson E, Rodger JC. Serum potassium in acute myocardial infarction. Scott Med J 1980: 25: 176.
29. Hulting J. In-hospital ventricular fibrillation and its relation to serum potassium. Acta Med Scand 1981; (suppl 647): 109-16.
30. Nordrehaug JE. Malignant arrhythmias in relation to serum potassium values in patients with an acute myocardial infarction. Acta Med Scand 1981; (suppl 647): 101-7.
31. Thomas RD. Ventricular fibrillation and initial plasma potassium in acute myocardial infarction. Postgrad Med J 1983; 59: 354-6.
32. Solomon RJ, Cole AG. Importance of potassium in patients with acute myocardial infarction. Acta Med Scand 1981; (suppl 647): 87-93.
33. Rolton H, Simpson E, Donnelly T, Rodger JC. Plasma potassium in acute myocardial infarction. Eur Heart J 1980; 2 (suppl 3A): 21.
34. Ramsey LE, Toner JM, Cameron HA. Diuretic use, serum potassium and ventricular fibrillation in patients with acute myocardial infarction. Proc Br Pharmacol Soc 1984; January: p. 605.
35. Johansson BW, Dziamski R. Malignant arrhythmias in acute myocardial infarction. Relationship to serum potassium and effect of selective and non-selective betablockade. Drugs 1984; 28 (suppl 1): 77-85.

36. Adams P, Murray A, Higham D, Smith AC, Julian DC, Campbell RWF. Plasma potassium and VF in acute myocardial infarction: a prospective study. Circulation 1984; 70 (suppl. II): 311.
37. Nordrehaug JE, von der Lippe G. Hypokalaemia and ventricular fibrillation in acute myocardial infarction. Br Heart J 1983; 50: 525-9.
38. Nordrehaug JE. Hypokalaemia, arrhythmias and early prognosis in acute myocardial infarction. Acta Med Scand 1985; 217: 299-306.
39. Nordrehaug JE. Malignant arrhythmias in relation to serum potassium in acute myocardial infarction. Am J Cardiol 1985; 56: 20-3.
40. Nordrehaug JE, Johannessen K-A, von der Lippe G. Serum potassium concentration as a risk factor of ventricular arrhythmias early in acute myocardial infarction. Circulation 1985; 71: 645-9.
41. Nordrehaug JE, von der Lippe G. Serum potassium concentrations are inversely related to ventricular, but not to atrial, arrhythmias in acute myocardial infarction. Eur Heart J 1986; 7: 204-9.
42. Clausen TG, Brocks K, Ibsen H. Hypokalemia and ventricular arrhythmias in acute myocardial infarction. Acta Med Scand 1988; 224: 531-7.
43. Cooper WD, Vandenburg MJ. Relationship between initial serum potassium values and cardiac arrhythmias in patients with acute myocardial infarction. In: Whelton, Whelton, Walker, eds. Potassium in renal and cardiovascular medicine. New York: Marcel Decker, 1986: 171-85.
44. Steiness E, Olesen KH. Cardiac arrhythmias induced by hypokalemia and potassium loss during maintenance digoxin therapy. Br Heart J 1976; 38: 167-72.
45. Evered DC, Chapman C. Plasma digoxin concentrations and digoxin toxicity in hospital patients. Br Heart J 1971; 33: 540-5.
46. Nordrehaug JE, Johannessen K-A, von der Lippe G, Myking OL. Circulating catecholamine and potassium concentrations early in acute myocardial infarction: Effect of intervention with timolol. Am Heart J 1985; 110: 944-8.
47. Nordrehaug JE, Johannessen K-A, von der Lippe, G, Sederholm M, Grottum P, Kjekshus J. Effect of timolol on changes in serum potassium concentration during acute myocardial infarction. Br Heart J 1985; 53: 388-93.
48. Dyckner T. Serum magnesium levels in acute myocardial infarction. Relation to arrhythmias. Acta Med Scand 1980; 207: 59-66.
49. Karppanen H, Pennanen R, Passinen L. Minerals, coronary heart disease and sudden coronary death. Adv Cardiol 1978; 25: 9-24.
50. Manthey J, Stoeppler M, Morgenstern W, et al. Magnesium and trace metals: risk factors for coronary heart disease? Associations between blood levels and angiographic findings. Circulation 1981; 64: 722-9.
51. Rasmussen HS, Norregard P, Lindeneg O, et al. Intravenous magnesium in acute myocardial infarction. Lancet 1986; 1: 872-4.
52. Abraham AS, Rosenmann D, Kramer M, et al. Magnesium in the prevention of lethal arrhythmias in acute myocardial infarction. Arch Intern Med 1987; 147: 753-5.
53. Papademetriou V. Diuretics, hypokalemia, and cardiac arrhythmias:A critical analysis. Am Heart J 1986; 111: 1217-24.
54. Holland OB, Nixon JV, Kuhnert I. Diuretic-induced ventricular ectopic activity. Am J Med 1981; 70: 762.
55. Khaw Kay-Tee, Barrett-Connor E. Dietary potassium and stroke-associated mortality. N Engl J Med 1987; 316: 235-40.

Treatment of coronary syndromes

27

Treatment of unstable coronary artery disease

LARS WALLENTIN

Background

Rapid impairment of coronary artery disease in the form of worsening angina, i.e. unstable angina, or the development of a small myocardial infarction (MI), i.e. non-Q-wave infarction, presents the patient with a severe handicap as well as much anxiety for the possible development of a larger MI (Q-wave infarction) in the near future. Several favourable treatment modes are nowadays available in the form of anti-anginal and antithrombotic medication and revascularization which can ameliorate symptoms, decrease myocardial ischaemia and reduce the risk of MI. Therefore, it is of increasing importance that persons with deterioration of coronary artery disease are immediately taken care of and given intensive pharmacological treatment and consideration given to possible revascularization.

Pathogenesis

Post mortem investigations of coronary arteries (1, 2) and observations at coronary angiography (3-5) as well as coronary angioscopy (6, 7) have resulted in general agreement on the coronary changes that cause instability in coronary artery disease. Several authors (7-9) have arrived, on the basis of these observations, at similar models describing the pathogenesis of instability in coronary artery disease (Fig. 1). The basic lesion in coronary artery disease is the slow deposition of atheromatous material leading to hardening and thickening of the arterial wall. This insidious change of the coronary artery might occur without any symptoms or with a gradual onset of stable angina pectoris. In the hard atherosclerotic arterial wall a fissure or ulceration may suddenly develop, without any warning or recognized triggering

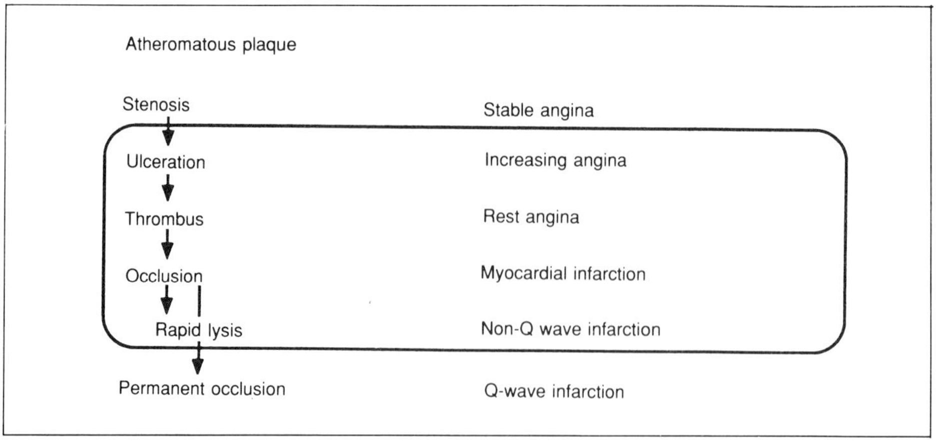

Fig. 1. *A model for the development of unstable coronary artery disease.*

factor. The lesion in the arterial wall will result in an intramural haemorrhage as well as adhesion and aggregation of platelets. The platelet plug causes a reduction in the coronary flow. A red blood clot will be formed in the stagnating blood stream due to stimulation of the coagulation process by the aggregating platelets. There is, furthermore, an increased tendency to the development of spasm of the injured arterial wall (10-13). A variable combination of a sudden lesion of the coronary vessel wall, a rapid accumulation of thrombotic material, arterial spasm and distal platelet embolization are the most likely explanations of the acute complications of coronary artery disease. The clinical consequences of this intravascular process depend on the degree and duration of the reduction of blood flow, the existence of collaterals and the myocardial oxygen demand (14). Sudden variations of coronary flow might be one reason for arrhythmias and sudden death. If the coronary blood flow is arrested over a prolonged period (hours), and if collateral blood flow is insufficient, a larger Q-wave ("transmural") MI will often develop. If the sudden coronary obstruction is of short duration or if the impediment of blood flow is subtotal and/or if there is a sufficient collateral blood flow, the clinical consequences might instead be an unstable condition – unstable coronary artery disease – with large variations in ischaemia, necrosis and functional impairment of the myocardium (14-18). In this condition the risk for the development of a Q-wave MI and death is increased until the oxygen supply to the threatened myocardium is improved either by a spontaneous healing of the arterial lesion with improvement of the blood flow past the recently formed stenosis or by the development of a sufficient collateral blood supply.

Definition and clinical presentation

Unstable coronary artery disease may be defined as the *sudden development of severe myocardial ischaemia*, usually presenting in one of the following forms:

1. unstable angina
   i.e. within the last 4 weeks, newly developed severe angina pectoris or increase in effort induced angina or onset of angina at rest
2. non-Q-wave MI (subendocardial infarction)
3. angina and/or ischaemia soon after successful thrombolysis or
4. angina and/or ischaemia soon after Q-wave MI.

Acute management

Patients with symptoms that give rise to the suspicion of unstable coronary artery disease, i.e. recent onset of severe angina, worsening effort induced angina, recent onset of angina at rest or chest pain suggesting acute MI, should always be hospitalized in a medical ward with ECG-monitoring, preferably in the CCU. It is often impossible to know whether the patient has an on-going infarction during this early phase and therefore ECG-monitoring and diagnostic laboratory tests, with serial 12-lead-ECG's and enzyme measurements, are mandatory. Repeated ECG's and serial enzyme determinations should be used liberally with recurrent episodes of severe chest pain (19).

Prognostic evaluation

The clinical presentation is useful in the evaluation of the prognosis. In the *clinical history* the existence of previous severe angina, the occurrence of repeated episodes of pain at rest and continuing episodes of chest pain during hospitalization despite medication are associated with an increased risk of serious complications. Signs of reversible ischaemia in the *ECG at rest* (transient ST-segment elevation or ST-segment depression) at time of admission or during hospitalization also carry an untoward prognostic importance (19-21).

Exercise test before discharge is of considerable value both for diagnostic and prognostic purposes in patients without obvious ischaemia at rest and in whom the pain has subsided during pharmacological treatment (21-25). There is an increased risk of developing a MI in patients with *ST-segment depression or an unexplained low exercise tolerance* at the exercise test

(21). Exercise capacity limited by chest pain as well as the occurrence of ST-segment depression or a low exercise tolerance also indicate an increased future need of revascularization because of remaining incapacitating symptoms (21). The exercise test should preferably be performed prior to discharge from hospital in order to have an optimal basis for prognostication and planning of the future treatment.

During recent years it has been shown that long-term ECG registration with tape-recorders that allow ST-segment analyses also contribute valuable prognostic information in ischaemic heart disease. The finding of ST-segment depression, despite on-going antianginal treatment, in the acute phase of unstable coronary artery disease is associated with a raised risk of future MI (26-29).

Elimination of precipitating factors

Smoking

Smokers have a well documented and generally accepted raised risk of MI and cardiac death. Smoking is associated with an increased liability of vasoconstriction and vasospasm (30), as well as a raised likelihood of thrombus formation, which can be demonstrated by a raised platelet aggregability, elevated fibrinogen concentration and impaired fibrinolysis (31-34). Immediate cessation of smoking should therefore confer some benefit on the patient by reducing symptoms and decreasing the risk of MI both in patients with unstable angina pectoris and after MI (35).

Stress and hypertension

Increased sympathetic activity raises the heart rate and the blood pressure which, in turn, increases cardiac work and myocardial oxygen demand. A reduction of psychosocial stress by a few days rest in hospital, followed by sick-leave until the symptoms have stabilized, treatment with beta-blockade and attempts at altering lifestyle may have a beneficial effect on these factors.

Pharmacological treatment

The proper comprehension of the pathogenetic basis for instability in coronary artery disease and MI is paramount for an adequate treatment. It is often impossible to determine from the clinical findings which process in the coronary arteries and which effect on the myocardium constitutes the major problem in the individual patient. Accordingly, medical treatment will often consist of a combination of different therapeutic principles whereby all known pathogenetic factors might be affected. Aggressive combined therapy will ameliorate the symptoms in most patients within a few days after which the condition frequently appears stable (36). However, the rapid symptomatic improvement does not of necessity imply that the instability of the recent coronary lesion and the threat of a large MI have subsided. Further investigations are required in the majority of patients in order to achieve a better appraisal of the risk for a MI as well as the need and timing of revascularisation.

Nitroglycerin

Sublingual nitroglycerin is an established and effective treatment, ameliorating attacks of anginal pain both in the stable and unstable phases of coronary artery disease. The effect of nitroglycerin can be prolonged and enhanced by the administration of higher doses over a prolonged period of time by an intravenous infusion (37, 38). It is, however, still not certain that intravenous nitroglycerin really is more effective than sufficient doses administered by other routes (39). Treatment can often be withdrawn after a few days of nitroglycerin infusion. Adequate effects can often be reached by the administration of high doses by other routes in patients with an increased nitroglycerin requirement following infusion (40, 41). No studies are available that demonstrate that nitroglycerin provides protection against MI or reduces mortality in unstable coronary artery disease.

Hypotension, which has been a source of worry during nitroglycerin treatment in the unstable phase of coronary artery disease, is encountered in less than 5% of the patients (40, 41). The intravenous administration has great advantages in the unstable phase of the disease as the effects are rapidly reversible and subside within 5-10 minutes after withdrawal of the infusion. Headache is a common side-effect and has been reported in 20-30% of patients in as much as they ask for simple analgetics or a reduction of the infusion rate (41). Nitroglycerin infusion should be combined with beta-blockade in unstable coronary artery disease in order to protect against reflex tachycardia which might lead to an increase in oxygen demand, which supervenes following intense vasodilation.

Beta-blockade

It has been speculated that the alpha-adrenergic dominance during beta-blockade might lead to an increased liability of coronary spasm. In the acute phase of unstable coronary artery disease, beta-blockade should preferably be combined with vasodilators – either nitroglycerin or calcium-antagonists. However, in clinical studies of unstable coronary artery disease beta-blockers reduced the risk for recurrence of angina without any indications of untoward effects (42, 43). The extensive documentation of a protective effect by beta-blockade during and after MI (44-46) should have a considerable influence on the use of beta-blockers in patients with unstable coronary artery disease. Acute intravenous beta-blockade in patients with chest pain, suspected of suffering from MI, decreases the risk of the development of MI (47, 48) and lowers mortality (44, 48). Even if there still are no randomized trials of beta-blockade, showing effects on reinfarction and mortality in unstable angina, there are hardly any reasons to believe that the effects in this situation should differ from those in patients with suspected acute MI. Therefore beta-blockers should be the drugs of first choice in patients with unstable angina.

Calcium antagonists

During treatment with calcium-antagonists (particularly nifedipine) there is a risk of a negative effect on myocardial oxygen balance, if the vasodilation leads to a rise in heart rate that increases myocardial oxygen demand (49). If calcium antagonists are used in unstable coronary artery disease, the treatment should be combined with beta-blockade or given in the form of diltiazem or verapamil which do not raise heart rate (49).

The effects of nifedipine in unstable angina pectoris have been reported in a number of studies with varying lengths of follow-up. The addition of nifedipine to beta-blockade reduces the episodes of angina and the need of revacularization because of refractory angina in all studies (42, 50, 51). However, nifedipine had a negative effect in some studies with an increased risk of MI (43, 50).

Verapamil reduces the number of episodes of pain in unstable patients with angina at rest (54-62) or with typical spasm angina of the Prinzmetal variant type (55, 56). In contrast, no favourable effects have been obtained with verapamil during or after MI (57, 58).

Diltiazem is also effective in patients with rest angina because of coronary spasm (59-61). Diltiazem conferred 40-50% reduction of angina resistant to previous treatment in non-Q-wave MI and decreased the number of reinfarctions (62, 63). In a randomized comparison of the efficacy of beta-blockade and diltiazem in a small material (64) the results of both kinds of treatment were comparable. Accordingly, diltiazem should also be

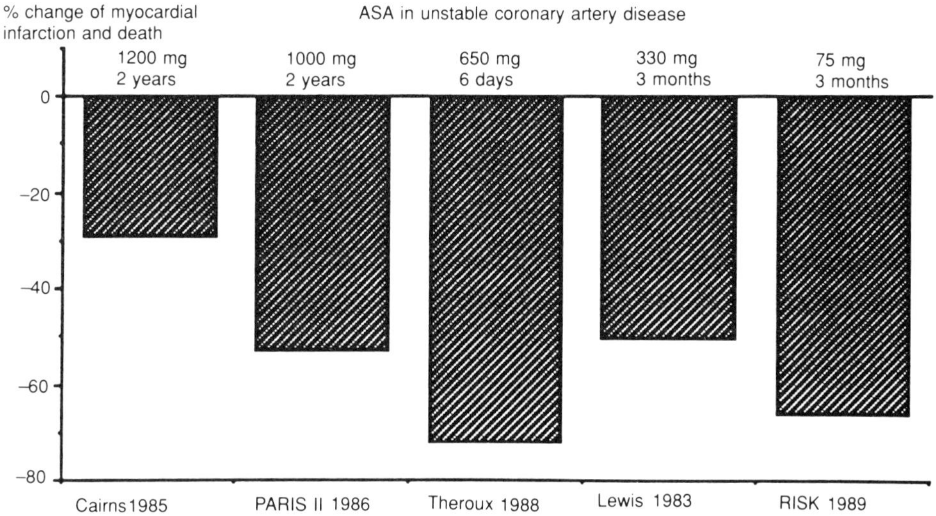

Fig. 2. *Effects of acetylsalicylic acid 75-1200 mg/day on mortality and development of myocardial infarction in unstable coronary artery disease (65-69).*

a drug of first choice in unstable coronary disease either as an addition to beta-blockade or as an alternative anti-anginal agent when beta-blockers are contraindicated.

Platelet inhibitors

Platelet inhibition reduces the risk of further thrombus formation and thereby decreases the threat of a temporary or permanent total occlusion of the coronary artery. However, platelet inhibition does not exert any immediate effect on myocardial oxygen balance as neither oxygen demand nor oxygen supply are influenced and as the permanent coronary stenosis remains unchanged for a long time. Therefore, the treatment should always be combined with conventional antianginal therapy.

During the 1980's five extensive prospective placebo controlled randomized trials (65-69) have demonstrated the efficacy of acetylsalicylic acid (ASA) 75-1200 mg/day in unstable coronary artery disease. ASA treatment reduced the rate of MI and the mortality by 30-60% during 3-24 months follow-up in all studies (Fig. 2). The efficacy of ASA treatment in these doses is well documented and should, accordingly, be routinely prescribed to all patients with unstable coronary artery disease for at least three months. As the side effects of ASA and the patient compliance are dose related, the lowest dose with proven clinical efficacy should be recommended. Treatment with ASA 75 mg daily has almost no side effects and a very high patient

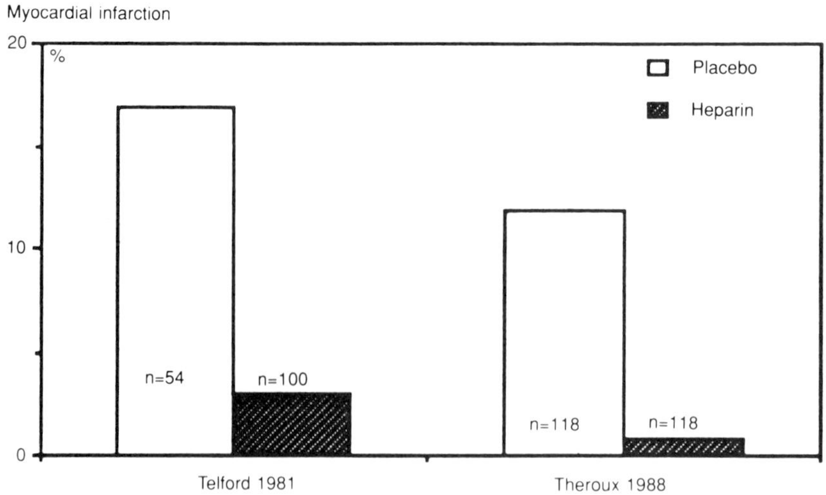

Fig. 3. *The effect of six to seven days intravenous heparin on the development of Q-wave infarction in patients with unstable coronary artery disease (68, 70).*

compliance with at least the same efficacy regarding protection against MI as higher doses (69). However, in order to obtain an immediate platelet inhibitory effect the initial dose should be at least 250 mg before continuation with the maintenance treatment of 75 mg daily.

Coagulation inhibitors

For many years heparin has commonly been employed in patients with unstable coronary artery disease, as many clinicians have found that this therapy produces favourable results. These suggestions have gained support from two clinical trials where intravenous heparin was started within the first hours after admission to hospital because of chest pain suggesting MI (Fig. 3) (68, 70). In a third study where the intravenous treatment was not started until days 1-2, the treatment was less convincing (69). However, when the intravenous heparin treatment was combined with 75 mg ASA, the intravenous treatment seemed to contribute to a further reduction in the risk of MI during ASA therapy. Thus, combined treatment with intravenous heparin and ASA should be started immediately after admission in patients with unstable coronary artery disease. The heparin treatment can often be withdrawn after a few days, provided patients continue with long term ASA therapy. The risk of side effects from a combination of intravenous heparin and 75 mg ASA is very low provided, the usual contra-indications are taken into consideration.

Thrombolysis

As a thrombotic process has pathogenetic importance in unstable coronary artery disease as well as in acute Q-wave infarction, it would seem likely that thrombolytic therapy would be beneficial. Lysis of thrombotic material at a recent coronary lesion might reduce the risk of vessel occlusion and decrease the degree of coronary stenosis. The limited number of studies of thrombolysis in unstable coronary artery disease has so far given contradictory results both regarding the effects on the coronary artery pathology and on the clinical symptoms (71-75). At present there is no scientific basis for thrombolytic treatment in unstable coronary artery disease as no beneficial effects have been demonstrated that can offset the risk for haemorrhagic complications. Future controlled studies with different forms of thrombolytic therapy will clarify the value of this mode of treatment in unstable coronary artery disease.

Revascularization

Both coronary angiography and revascularization are associated with increased risks of complications when performed as emergency procedures. Emergency interventions during the first days after admission are, however, seldom warranted in unstable coronary artery disease. The medical treatment can often be started gradually and a certain time is required for evaluation of its efficacy. With a gradual escalation of the medication around 90% of the patients can be, at least temporarily, stabilized which permits continued investigation of the remaining ischaemia and coronary angiography at a less vulnerable stage of the disease. Coronary angiography and revascularization in unstable coronary artery disease can often be performed as urgent procedures (after a day or two) rather than as an emergency procedure.

Further, the risks involved with coronary artery by-pass grafting (CABG) and percutaneous transluminal coronary angioplasty (PTCA) as urgent procedures in unstable patients are somewhat higher than with elective procedures in stable angina, but still low with an early mortality below 2% (76-87). The relief of symptoms both by CABG and PTCA is equally effective after urgent procedures in unstable angina as after elective operations in stable patients (76-87). One year after the procedure, 50% are completely free of angina and another 30-40% have obtained a considerable improvement in their symptoms. These results are considerably better than those obtained by medical treatment. Patients with remaining incapacitating symptoms during medical treatment after an episode of unstable angina should therefore be investigated by coronary arteriography and, if possible, revascularized, without delay.

Improved survival has been demonstrated in patients with left main disease and in 3-vessel disease associated with reduced left ventricular function after urgent operations in unstable coronary artery disease (86) as well as after elective operations in stable coronary artery disease (88-90). Both the European Coronary Surgery Study (89) and the American Coronary Artery Surgery Study (91) have shown that patients with ST-segment depression at exercise tests obtain an increased survival by elective CABG. It is possible that exercise tests might be similarly useful in the selection of unstable patients for surgery, but no reports on this topic are at hand as exercise tests have seldom been performed on this patient group. In all the randomized studies on by-pass surgery after stable and unstable angina pectoris, 20-30% of "medically treated" patients have been operated within 2 years because of incapacitating angina (90). Treatment costs for a regimen with prolonged attempts at medical treatment before surgery are about twice those of immediate revascularization (90). Thus, if there are signs of severe ischaemia after an episode of unstable angina pectoris, coronary angiography should be performed in order to obtain urgent revascularization.

Conclusion

Hospitalization and pharmacological treatment with a combination of anti-anginal and anti-thrombotic agents will, at least temporarily, eliminate or stabilize the symptoms in most patients with unstable coronary artery disease. However, the instability of the recent lesion in the coronary artery often remains and constitutes a continuing threat of thrombotic occlusion until it is healed. Long term treatment with ASA, which inhibits platelet function, will reduce the risk of MI by more than 50% and should be prescribed in all patients for at least three months. Urgent coronary angiography and revascularization are mandatory in patients with continuing episodes of pain at rest because of myocardial ischaemia. Patients without continuing episodes of myocardial ischaemia should be evaluated, before discharge, by an exercise test in order to identify those with a raised risk of MI and incapacitating angina during the following months. If there are signs of severe ischaemia after an episode of unstable angina pectoris, coronary angiography should be performed with the intention of urgent revascularization, also in patients without incapacitating symptoms during medical treatment.

References

1. Falk E. Unstable angina with fatal outcome: dynamic coronary thrombosis leading to infarction and/or sudden death. Circulation 1985; 71: 699-708.
2. Davies MJ, Thomas AC. Plaque fissuring – the cause of acute myocardial infarction, sudden ischaemic death, and crescendo angina. Br Heart J 1985; 53: 363-73.
3. Ambrose JA, Winters SL, Stern A, et al. Angiographic morphology and the pathogenesis of unstable angina pectoris. J Am Coll Cardiol 1985; 5: 609-16.
4. DeWood MA, Stifter WF, Carroll SS, et al. Coronary arteriographic findings soon after non-Q-wave myocardial infarction. N Engl J Med 1986; 315: 417-23.
5. Wilson RF, Holiday MD, White CW. Quantitative angiographic morphology of coronary stenoses leading to myocardial infarction or unstable angina. Circulation 1986; 73: 286-93.
6. Sherman CT, Litvack F, Grundfest W, et al. Coronary angioscopy in patients with unstable angina pectoris. N Engl J Med 1986; 315: 913-9.
7. Forrester JS, Litvack F, Grundfest W, Hickey A. A perspective of coronary artery disease seen through the arteries of living man. Circulation 1987; 75: 505-13.
8. Ambrose JA, Craig E, Hjemdahl-Monsen E, Borrico S, Gorlin R, Fuster V. Angiographic demonstration of a common link between unstable angina pectoris and non/Q/wave myocardial infarction. Am J Cardiol 1988; 61: 244-7.
9. Fuster V, Badimon L, Cohen M, Ambrose JA, Badimon JJ, Chesebro J. Insights nto the pathogenesis of acute ischemic syndromes. Circulation 1988; 77: 1213-20.
10. Maseri A, Chierchia S, Kaski J C. Mixed angina pectoris. Am J Cardiol 1985; 56: 30E-3E.
11. Plotnick GD. The pathogenesis of myocardial ischaemia in patients with unstable angina. In: Plotnick GD, ed. Unstable angina. A clinical approach. New York: Futura, 1985: 21-48.
12. Maseri A, Chierchia S, Davies G. Pathophysiology of coronary occlusion in acute infarction . Circulation 1986; 73: 233-9.
13. Hackett D, Davies G, Chierchia S, Maseri A. Intermittent coronary occlusion in acute myocardial infarction. N Engl J Med 1987; 317: 1055-9.
14. Maseri A, Chierchia S, Abbate A L. Pathogenetic mechanisms underlying the clinical events associated with atherosclerotic heart disease. Circulation 1980; 62(V): 3-13.
15. Olson HG, Lyons KP, Aronow WS, Stinson PJ, Kuperus J, Waters HJ. The high-risk angina patient. Indentification by clinical features, hospital course, electrocardiography and technetium-99m stannous pyrophosphate scintigraphy. Circulation 1981; 64: 674-84.
16. Armstrong PW, Chiong MA, Parker JO. The spectrum of unstable angina: prognostic role of serum creatine kinase determination. Am J Cardiol 1982; 65: 1849-52.
17. Nixon JW, Brown CN, Smitherman TC. Identification of transient and persistent segmental wall motion abnormalities in patients with unstable angina by two dimensional echocardiography. Circulation 1982; 65: 1497-503.
18. Thygesen K, Hørder M, Krøll L, Hyltoft Pedersen P, Haghfelt T. Creatine kinase and creatine kinase B-subunit in stable and unstable angina pectoris. Eur J Clin Invest 1986; 16: 1-4.
19. Gibson RS, Beller GA, Gheroghiade M, et al. The prevalence and clinical significance of residual myocardial ischaemia two weeks after uncomplicated non-Q-wave myocardial infarction: a prospective natural history study. Circulation 1986; 73: 1186-98.
20. Plotnick GD. Prognostic classification of the patient with rest angina. In: Plotnick GD, ed. Unstable angina. A clinical approach. New York: Futura, 1985: 191-9.

21. Swahn E, Areskog M, Berglund U, Walfridsson H, Wallentin L. Predictive importance of clinical findings and a predischarge exercise test in suspected unstable coronary artery disease. Am J Cardiol 1987; 59: 208-14.
22. Nixon JV, Hillert MC, Shapiro W, Smitherman TC. Submaximal exercise testing after unstable angina. Am Heart J 1980; 90: 772-8.
23. Vecchio C, Cobelli F, Opasich C, de Servi S, Specchia G. Exercise testing after nontransmural myocardial infarction. Cardiology 1981; 68: 218-32.
24. Butman SM, Olson HG, Gardin J, et al. Submaximal exercise testing after stabilization of unstable angina pectoris. J Am Coll Card 1984; 4: 667-73.
25. Sia TB, MacDonald PS, Horowitz JD, Goble AJ, Doyle AE. Usefulness of early exercise testing after non-Q-wave myocardial infarction in predicting prognosis. Am J Cardiol 1986; 57: 738-44.
26. Johnson SM, Mauritson DR, Winniford MD, et al. Continuous electrocardiographic monitoring in patients with unstable angina pectoris: Identification of high-risk subgroup with severe coronary disease, variant angina, and/or impaired early prognosis. Am Heart J 1982; 103: 4-12.
27. Gottlieb SO, Weisfeldt ML, Ouyang P, Mellits ED, Gerstenblith G. Silent ischaemia as a marker for early unfavorable outcomes in patients with unstable angina. N Engl J Med 1986; 314: 1214-9.
28. Nadamanee K, Intarachot V, Josephson MA, Rieders D, Mody FV, Singh BN. Prognostic significance of silent myocardial ischaemia in patients with unstable angina. J Am Coll Cardiol 1987; 10: 101-9.
29. Gottlieb SO, Weisfeldt ML, Oyang P, Mellits D, Gerstenblith G. Silent ischaemia predicts infarction and death during two year follow-up of unstable angina. J Am Coll Cardiol 1987; 10: 756-60.
30. Nadler JL, Velaco JS, Horton R. Cigarette smoking inhibits prostacyclin formation. Lancet 1983; I: 1248-50.
31. Felch JJF, McArdle BM, Burns P, Lowe GDO, Forbes CD. The effects of acute smoking on platelet behaviour, fibrinolysis and haemorrheology in habitual smokers. Thromb Haemostas 1984; 51: 6-8.
32. Rival J, Riddle JM, Stein P. Effects of chronic smoking on platelet function. Thromb Res 1987; 45: 75-85.
33. Meade TW, Imeson J, Stirling Y. Effects of changes in smoking and other characteristics on clotting factors and the risk of ischemic heart disease. Lancet 1987; II: 986-8.
34. Swahn E, Schenk HV, Wallentin L. Plasma fibrinogen in unstable coronary artery disease. Scand J Clin Lab Invest 1988; 49: 49-54.
35. Aberg A, Bergstrand R, Johansson S, et al. Cessation of smoking afte myocardial infarction. Effects of mortality after 10 years. Br Heart J 1983; 49: 416-22.
36. Mulcahy R, Awadhi AH, de Buitleor M, Tobin K, Johnson H, Contoy R. Natural history and prognosis of unstable angina. Am Heart J 1985; 109: 753-8.
37. Mikolich JR, Nicoloff NB, Robinson PH, Logue RB. Relief of refractory angina with continuous intravenous infusion of nitroglycerin. Chest 1980; 77: 375-9.
38. DePace NL, Herling IM, Kotler NM, Hakki AH, Spielman SR, Segal BL. Intravenous nitroglycerin for rest angina. Arch Intern Med 1982; 142: 1806-12.
39. Curfman DG, Heinsimer JA, Lozner EC, Fung HL. Intravenous nitroglycerin in the treatment of spontaneous angina pectoris: a prospective randomized trial. Circulation 1983; 67: 276-82.
40. Kaplan K, Davison R, Parker M, Przybylek J, Teagarden JR, Lesch M. Intravenous nitroglycerin for the treatment fo angina at rest unresponsive to standard nitrate therapy. Am J Cardiol 1983; 51: 694-7.

41. Herling IM. Intravenous nitroglycerin: clinical pharmacology and therapeutic considerations. Am Heart J 1984; 108: 141-9.
42. Muller JE, Zoltang GT, Pearle DL, et al. Nifedipine and conventional therapy for unstable angina pectoris: a randomized, double blind comparison. Circulation 1984; 69: 728-39.
43. HINT Research Group. Early treatment of unstable angina in the coronary care unit: a randomised, double blind, placebo controlled comparison of recurrent ischaemia in patients treated with nifedipin or metoprolol or both. Br Heart J 1986; 56: 400-13.
44. Hjalmarsson A, Elmfeldt D, Herlitz J, et al. Effect on mortality of metoprolol in acute myocardial infarction. Lancet 1981; II: 823-6.
45. Beta-blocker Heart Attack Trial Research Group. A randomized trial of propranolol in patients with acute myocardial infarction. I Mortality results. J Am Med Ass 1982; 247: 1707-14.
46. The International Collaborative Study Group. Reduction of infarct size with the early use of timolol in acute myocardial infarction. N Engl J Med 1984; 310: 9-15.
47. The MIAMI Trial Research Group. Development of myocardial infarction. Am J Cardiol 1985; 56: 23G-6G.
48. ISIS-1 Collaborative Group. Randomized trial of intravenous atenolol among 16027 cases of suspected actue myocardial infarction: ISIS-1. Lancet 1986; II: 57-65.
49. Braunwald MD. Mechanism of action of calcium-channel-blocking agents. N Engl J Med 1982; 307: 1618-26.
50. Muller JE, Morrison J, Stone PH, et al. Nifedipine therapy for patients with threatened and acute myocardial infarction: a randomized double blind, placebo-controlled comparison. Circulation 1984; 69: 740-7.
51. Gerstenblith G, Ouyang P, Achuff SC, et al. Nifedipine in unstable angina. N Engl J Med 1982; 306: 885-9.
52. Parodi O, Maseri A, Simonetti I. Management of unstable angina at rest by verapamil: a double blind placebo-controlled trial in CCU patients. Br Heart J 1979; 41: 167-74.
53. Mehta J, Pepine CJ, Day M, Guerrero JR, Conti CR. Short term efficacy of oral verapamil in rest angina: a doble-blind placebo controlled trial in CCU patients. Am J Med 1981; 71: 977-86.
54. Mauritson DR, Johnson SM, Winniford MD, Cary JR, Willerson JT, Hilis LD. Verapamil for unstable angina at rest: a short term randomized, double-blind study. Am Heart J 1983; 106: 652-8.
55. Johnson SM, Mauritson DR, Willerson JT, Hillis LD. A controlled trial of verapamil for Printzmetals variant angina. N Engl J Med 1981; 304: 862-6.
56. Freedman B, Dunn D R, Kelly D T. Coronary spasm during exercise: treatment with verapamil. Circulation 1981; 64: 68-75.
57. Crea F, Deanfield J, Crean P, Sharom M, Davies G, Maseri A. Effects of verapamil in preventing early postinfarction angina and reinfarction. Am J Cardiol 1985; 55: 900-4.
58. The Danish Study Group on Verapamil in Myocardial Infarction. Verapamil in acute myocardial infarction. Eur Heart J 1984; 5: 516-28.
59. Rosenthal S J, Ginsburg R, Lambe I H, et al. Efficacy of diltiazem for control of symptoms of coronary arterial spasm. Am J Cardiol 1980; 46: 1027.
60. Pepine CJ, Feldman RL, Whittle J, et al. Effect of diltiazem in patients with variant angina: a randomized double-blind trial. Am Heart J 1981; 101: 719-25.
61. Schroeder JS,Feldman RL, Giles TD, et al. Multiclinic controlled trial of diltiazem for Prinzmetals angina. Am J Med 1982; 72: 227-30.
62. Gibson RS, Boden WE, Theroux P, et al. Diltiazem and reinfarction in patients with non-Q-wave myocardial infarction. N Engl J Med 1986; 315: 423-9.

63. The Multicenter Diltiazem Postinfarction Trial Research Group. The effect of diltiazem on mortality and reinfarction after myocardial infarction. N Engl J Med 1988; 319: 385-92.
64. Waters DD, Theroux P. A comparison of the outcome of treated patients with variant angina and unstable angina. In: Hugenholtz PG, Goldman BS, eds. Unstable angina. Current concepts and management. Stuttgart-New York: Schattauer, 1985: 211-8.
65. Lewis HD, Davis JW, Archibald DG, et al. Protective effects of aspirin against acute myocardial infarction and death in men with unstable angina. N Engl J Med 1983; 309: 396-403.
66. Cairns JA, Gent M, Singer J, et al. Aspirin, sulfinpyrazone or both in unstable angina. N Engl J Med 1985; 313: 1369-75.
67. Klimt CR, Knatterud GL, Stamler J. Persantin-Aspirin Reinfarction Study. Part II. Secondary prevention with Persantine and Aspirin . J Am Coll Cardiol 1986; 7: 251-69.
68. Theroux P, Ouimet H, McCans J, et al. Aspirin, heparin or both to treat acute unstable angina. N Engl J Med 1988; 319: 1105-11.
69. Wallentin L, Andersson PO, Areskog M, et al. Risk for myocardial infarction and death during three months treatment with ASA 75 mg/day and intravenous heparin or either or neither in men with unstable coronary artery disease. Submitted 1990.
70. Telford AM, Wilson C. Trial of heparin versus atenolol in prevention of myocardial infarction in intermediate coronary syndrome. Lancet 1981; I: 1225-8.
71. Lawrence JB, Shepard JT, Bone I, Rogen AS, Fulton WFM. Fibrinolytic therapy in unstable angina pectoris / a controlled clinical trial. Thromb Res 1980; 7: 767-77.
72. Ambrose JA, Hjemdahl-Monsen C, Borrico S, et al. Quantitative and qualitative effects of intracoronary streptokinase in unstable angina and non-q-wave infarction. J Am Coll Cardiol 1987; 9: 1156-65.
73. Gold HK, Johns JA, Leinbach RC, Yasuda T. Collen D Thrombolytic therapy for unstable angina pectoris: rationale and results. J Am Coll Cardiol 1987; 10: 91B-5B.
74. Topol EJ, Nicklas JM , Kander NH, et al. Coronary revascularization after intravenous tissue plasminogen activator for unstable angina pectoris: results of a randomized double-blind placebo-controlled trial. Am J Cardiol 1988; 62: 368-71.
75. de Zwaan C, Bar FW, Janssen JHA, de Swart HB, Vermeer F, Wellens HJJ. Effects of thrombolytic therapy in unstable angina: clinical and angiographic results. J Am Coll Cardiol 1988; 12: 301-9.
76. Unstable Angina Pectoris. National Cooperative Study Group to compare medical and surgical therapy II. In hospital experience and initial follow-up results in patients with one, two and three vessel disease. Am J Cardiol 1978; 42: 839-48.
77. Rahimtoola S. Coronary bypass surgery for unstable angina. Circulation 1983; 69: 842-8.
78. de Feyter P J, Serruys P W, van den Brand M, et al. Emergency corononary angioplasty in refractory unstable angina . N Engl J Med 1985; 313: 342-6.
79. Wohlgelernter D, Cleman M, Highman HA, Zaret BL. Percutaneous transluminal angioplasty of the "culprit lesion" for management of unstable angina pectoris in patients with multivessel coronary artery disease. Am J Cardiol 1986; 58: 460-4.
80. De Feyter P, Serruys P W, Soward A, van den Brand M, Bos E, Hugenholtz P. Coronary angioplasty for early postinfarction unstable angina. Circulation 1986; 6: 1365-70.
81. Safian RD, Snyder LD, Synder BA, et al. Usefulness of percutaneous transluminal coronary angioplasty for unstable angina pectoris after non-Q-wave myocardial infarction. Am J Cardiol 1987; 59: 263-6.
82. Steffenino G, Meier B, Finci L, Rutishauser W. Follow up results of treatment of unstable angina by coronary angioplasty. Br Heart J 1987; 57: 416-9.
83. DeFeyter P, Serruys P W, van den Brand M, Soward A. Coronary angioplasty for treat-

ment of unstable angina with transient marked ST-segment elevation. Eur Heart J 1987; 8: 569-74.

84. Topol EJ, Nicklas JM, Kander N, et al. Need for definitive coronary revascularization despite intravenous tissue plasminogen activator (tPA) for unstable angina: results of a randomized placebo-controlled trial. Circulation 1987; 76 (2): 452-8.
85. De Feyter PJ, Serruys PW, Suruyapranata H, Beatt K, van den Brand M. Coronary angioplasty early after diagnosis of unstable angina. Am Heart J 1987; 114: 48-53.
86. Luchi RJ, Scott SM, Deupree R H. Comparison of medical and surgical treatment for unstable angina pectoris. Results of a Venterans Administration Cooperative Study. N Engl J Med 1987; 316: 977-84.
87. De Feyter P, Suryapranata H, Serruys PW, et al. Coronary angioplasty for unstable angina: immediate and late results in 200 consecutive patients with identification of risk factors for unfavorable early and late outcome. J Am Coll Cardiol 1988; 12: 324-33.
88. Passamani E, Davis KB, Gillespie MJ, Killip T. CASS Investigators A randomized trial of coronary artery by/pass surgery. Survival of patients witha low ejection fraction. N Engl J Med 1985; 312: 1665-71.
89. Varnauskas E. Twelve year follow up of survival in the randomized european coronary surgery study group. N Engl J Med 1988; 319: 332-7.
90. Rahimtoola S. A perspective on the three large multicenter randomized clinical trials of coronary by-pass surgery for chronic stable angina . Circulation 1985; 72: 123-35.
91. Weiner DA, Ryan TJ, McCabe C H, et al. The role of exercise testing in identifying patients with improved survival after coronary bypass surgery. J Am Coll Cardiol 1986; 8: 741-8.

28

Thrombolysis during acute myocardial infarction

ÅSMUND REIKVAM

Myocardial preservation

During the 1960's and 1970's the importance of myocardial preservation during an acute myocardial infarction (MI) attracted increased interest. Coronary occlusion will result in the death of a proportion of the myocardial cells, the ensuing deterioration of the myocardial function being dependent on the extent of loss of myocardium. Treatment was primarily aimed at factors decisive with regard to the oxygen demand of the myocardium, i.e. heart rate, left ventricle's wall tension and the contractile status of the heart. Reduction of the oxygen demand would result in salvage of myocardial cells that would otherwise die.

During the 1980's the possibility of myocardial rescuing has made substantial progress following the introduction of thrombolytic therapy.

Autopsy studies have shown a crucial role of the coronary thrombus formation for the initiation of a MI (1-3). Using coronary angiography *DeWood et al* (4) showed, in 1980, that there was thrombus material in the infarct-related artery in more than 80% of the cases of MI. Another basis is the result of animal experiments, which have shown that reperfusion of occluded coronary arteries within 3-4 hours can salvage, to a great extent, the jeopardized myocardium (5-8).

During the 1960's and 1970's streptokinase (SK) was tried in acute infarction as a long-term infusion in doses conventionally used for venous thrombosis and pulmonary embolism. These trials were so small, none involved more than 750 patients, that they yielded apparantly conflicting results. However, a recent review of their findings indicated that fibrinolytic therapy could reduce mortality by about a quarter (9).

In 1979 *Rentrop et al* (10) reported that intracoronary infusion of the infarct-related artery with SK within the first hours of the onset of chest pain resulted in reperfusion, usually within 30 minutes, in about 75% of the patients; further, that the ischaemic myocardium tolerated this reperfusion well. These findings were soon confirmed (11).

This achievement became the basis and rationale for more ambitious goals in infarct treatment. It was suggested that recanalisation of the coronary artery would provide protection against the otherwise unavoidable myocardial necrosis, and thus preserve more myocardial reserves. Hopefully, the ultimate and most important consequence would be reduced mortality and morbidity.

It was evident from the start, that intracoronary thrombolytic therapy could not be taken into routine use in most hospitals. The therapy could only be undertaken in catheterization laboratories, and this route of administration would represent a delay in the treatment of a condition where rapid and immediate therapy is critical.

Renewed interest in the intravenous route of administration showed that intravenous application in high doses over a short period, mostly 1,5 million units over 1 hour, could also give high patency rates. In general, the patency rates obtained by intravenous application seemed to be a little lower than those found by intracoronary administration, but still being in the range of 50-75% (12-15).

Thrombolytic agents

There are six thrombolytic agents currently being used or evaluated for the immediate treatment of MI:

Streptokinase (SK)
Anisoylated plasminogen-streptokinase activator complex (APSAC)
Urokinase (UK)
Recombinant prourokinase (r-pro-UK or rscu-PA)
Recombinant single-stranded tissue-plasminogen activator (rtPA, 1 chain)
Recombinant double-stranded tissue-plasminogen activator (rtPA, 2 chains)

All agents activate, directly or indirectly, plasminogen, the precursor of a native proteolytic enzyme system present in biological fluids, and which is also bound to various surfaces such as fibrin, platelets and endothelial cells. Activation of plasminogen gives rise to plasmin which has the ability to degrade fibrin and fibriogen (Fig. 1).

The thrombolytic agents are often, on the basis of their fibrin binding divided into fibrin-selective, i e., rtPA and r-pro-UK, and non-fibrin selective agents, which include SK, APSAC and UK.

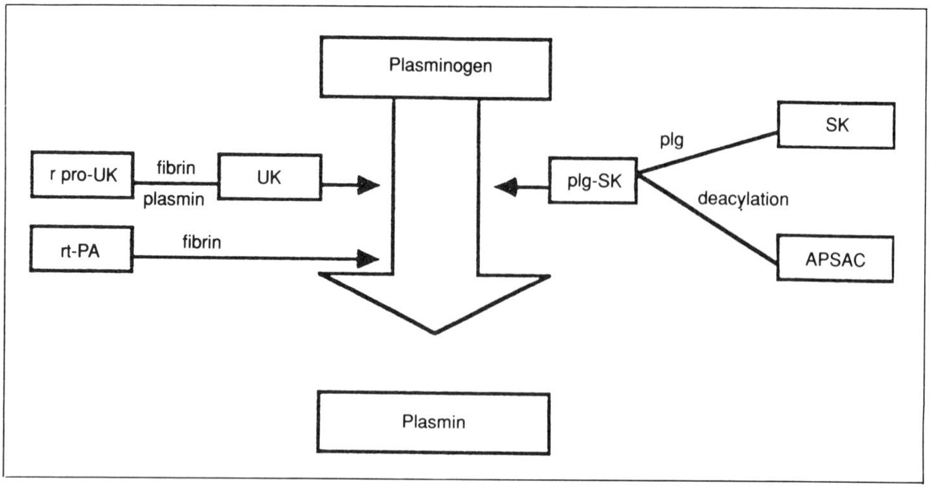

Fig. 1. *The various thrombolytic agents act through activation of plasminogen (plg) to plasmin. SK and APSAC make a plasminogen-SK activator complex. rtPA and r-pro-UK have strong fibrin binding properties. Modified after (19).*

The fibrin-selective agents were considered to have theoretical advantages over the non-fibrin selective ones. The former were supposed to attack and degrade fibrin in the thrombus and thereby have less fibrinolytic action in the circulation. However, the fibrin-selective drugs also give some reduction in the level of fibrinogen in the blood, although far less than SK and APSAC (16-18).

It should also be noted that all of the thrombolytic agents have preference for the activation of fibrin-bound plasminogen over that of plasma plasminogen.

Two aspects regarding the fibrin selectivity should be elaborated (19):

a) Fibrin-selective agents, because of their binding to fibrin independent of fibrin's binding sites for plasminogen, continue to act on fibrin even after the circulating agent has been inactivated or cleared from the plasma. Therefore they could be considered more efficient in dissolving ageing or more lysis-resistant fibrin compared with the non-selective agents.
b) There is a difference in speed and degree of plasma plasminogen activation. The non-fibrin selective drugs evoke more fibrinogenolysis and give, as a result, a more pronounced and long-lasting haemostatic defect. At first sight this seems to be an unwanted property and could be responsible for more bleeding complications. However, it is possible that this aspect of the non-selective drugs can be an advantage in thrombolytic therapy.

Reperfusion

The most important objective of the thrombolytic therapy is to reduce mortality and improve prognosis for the survivors. The proof that this can be achieved has emerged in recent years. The initial studies were, as is easily understandable, aimed at the more simple question of how efficient the actual agents could recanalize occluded coronary arteries.

If therapy is started early, within 3 hours following onset of symptoms, patency rates at the conclusion of therapy or shortly thereafter, do not appear to be much different for the various agents (20-28). Patency rates of 60-70% have usually been obtained. tPA appears to be superior to SK in some studies (29, 30). A closer evaluation attributes this advantage to a better effect on the late inclusions, i.e. more than 3-4 hours after the start of symptoms (19).

The success rates for all agents fall with increasing time from start of chest pain to fibrinolytic intervention. The fibrin selectivity of tPA can be a plausible explanation of a relatively good effect of this agent on old thrombi.

Angiographic determination of reperfusion is regarded as the gold standard for measuring the effect of thrombolytic therapy. But even this evaluation has its liminations. It does not measure flow rates. The final outcome is not known, since repetitive opening and closing of occluded vessels can occur during thrombolytic therapy and in the ensuing time. Furthermore, evaluation of flow rates by angiographic observations is subject to considerable variability.

Flow rates and flow pattern determine how fast ischaemia can be abolished, how fast toxic products are removed, and furthermore can be decisive as to whether reocclusion can represent a threat. Therefore, other factors than the simple question of patent versus occluded coronary artery, should be taken into consideration.

Viscosity changes may have some importance. SK therapy causes extensive fibrinogenolysis and is associated with a reduction in plasma and blood viscosity (31, 32). Since UK and APSAC also produce the same high degree of fibrinogenolysis, it is likely that similar viscosity changes will occur with these agents as with SK. The milder fibrinogenolysis observed with tPA was not associated with a significant reduction in blood viscosity (31).

The viscosity reduction in blood will not only increase flow rates in the coronary circulation, but could be expected to result in better flow throughout the entire circulation. Thereby, a potentially beneficial action of thrombolytic therapy could be mediated through a reduction in afterload, and by this mechanism reduce the oxygen demand of the myocardium.

These factors illustrate that a series of mechanisms during thrombolysis must be taken into consideration. A matter of patent versus occluded coronary artery may be too simple.

Mortality reduction

During recent years some large multicenter studies have been undertaken and have included such high numbers of patients that mortality could be evaluated.

The Italian GISSI study (33) included more than 11.000 patients in an open randomised comparison of SK and placebo. The hospital mortality for the SK group was 10,7% as compared to 13% for the placebo group. However, the degree of benefit was a function of time from onset of pain to infusion of SK. Significant reduction in mortality occured among patients treated within 6 hours, the reduction being 47% when treated during the first hour, 23% when treated during the first 3 hours, and 17% when treatment was started between 3 and 6 hours. There was no significant reduction in mortality when the treatment was started after 6 hours, but the number of patients in this group was rather small.

The ISIS II trial (34) randomised 17.187 patients in a double blind comparison of SK, aspirin and placebo. This trial showed a 30-40% reduction in mortality when SK therapy was initiated within 2-3 hours of onset of symptoms. The mortality reduction was less with increasing time interval, but there was a significant reduction in mortality, even in the group included 6-12 hours after start of chest pain.

It is important to note that the combination of SK and aspirin was significantly better than either agent alone. Separate effects of SK and aspirin on vascular death appeared to be additive. The group receiving SK and aspirin had about half the mortality of those given placebo for each agent if the therapy was started within 2-3 hours (Fig. 2).

The ISIS II results have, in addition to documenting the efficacy of SK, convincingly established aspirin as a key drug in the routine treatment of MI.

The AIMS study (35) included 1.004 patients in a comparison of APSAC and placebo. The one month mortality was 6,4% in the APSAC group and 12,4% in the placebo group. In this trial the percentage mortality reduction with APSAC was similar, irrespective of whether time since onset of symptoms was 0-3 hours (660 patients) or 4-6 hours (344 patients).

In the ASSET study (36) about 5.000 patients were randomised to receive tPA or placebo within 5 hours of onset of symptoms. At one month, the

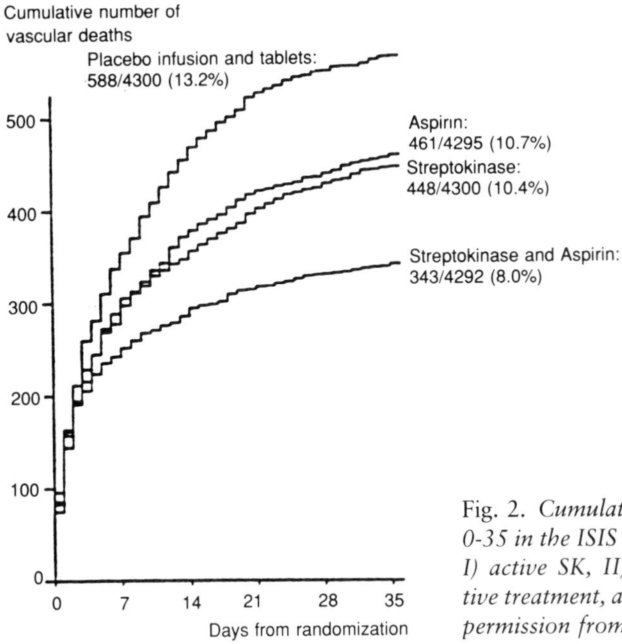

Fig. 2. *Cumulative vascular mortality in days 0-35 in the ISIS II trial (34). Patients allocated I) active SK, II) active aspirin, III) both active treatment, and IV) neither. Reprinted with permission from Lancet.*

overall case fatality rates were 7,2% in the tPA group and 9,8% in the placebo group, this being a statistically significant difference. Similar results of tPA treatment were evident in the TIMI I recanalisation trial, despite a much smaller sample size (37). Other smaller trials addressing the problem of mortality have also given indications of mortality reduction (38, 39).

Therefore, the conclusion can be drawn that thrombolytic therapy reduces the mortality of myocardial infarction.

Furthermore, ISIS II gives evidence that the benefit obtained is not lost during the first or second year of follow-up.

Left ventricular function

It is somewhat surprising that all placebo-controlled trials with thrombolytic agents have failed to show beneficial effects both on survival and on global left ventricular function (38-45). This has led to speculation that the relation between coronary reperfusion and the reduction of left ventricular dysfunction, and their effect on the improvement of both early and late survival is more complex than initially thought. Other factors that could play a beneficial part in the acute stage of an evolving MI, in addition to salvage of ischaemic myocardium, are prevention of cardial rupture and arrhythmias, and at a later stage, prevention or limitation of infarct expansion and left ventricular remodelling (46).

However, the following facts should be kept in mind. The measures available for evaluation of left ventricular function have shortcomings, and may not be good enough tools for this assessment. Secondly, the studies designed to examine the left ventricle may have had too small numbers to detect real differences.

It should be emphasized in this context that some studies, although not being of a size necessary to examine mortality reduction, have found improvement in both regional and global ventricular function after thrombolytic therapy (56, 57).

It can also be argued that when an effective thrombolytic agent is given very early in the course of an acute MI some patients with poor left ventricular function will be saved. These patients would have died if no thrombolytic therapy had been given. The low ejection fraction of these reperfused patients would mask the gain in ejection fraction obtained in other reperfused patients, and therefore distort the comparison with surviving controls (46).

Furthermore, because recovery of the mechanical function is delayed, assessment cannot be completed until relatively late after treatment, by which time loading conditions of the left ventricle, diastolic compliance of both infarct and non-infarct regions, neurohumoral stimulation of the heart, and the systolic function of the non-infarct region may change.

Bleeding complications

Fibrinolytic therapy induces a coagulation defect which carries a potential risk of internal bleeding. Fibrin-selective agents, because of their milder effect on the coagulation mechanism were expected to have a lower incidence of bleeding complications. No evidence to support this assumption has been forthcoming. Severe bleeding, i.e. requiring transfusions, has been a frequent complication of all agents, in the presence of recent invasive procedures. In the absence of the latter, the incidence has been sharply reduced, and the risk of serious spontaneous bleeding is in fact low, well below 1% (29, 30, 34, 35). Most episodes of such bleeding are related to underlying phenomena such as peptic ulcer or cerebral vascular disease.

Since haemorrhagic episodes have their origin at the sites of invasive procedures it is not surprising that the fibrin-selective agents have as high bleeding incidence as the non-fibrin selective agents. One cannot expect the drug to differentiate between protective and pathologic thrombi.

By far the most serious risk is that of intracranial bleeding. Stroke is generally thought to occur in about 1% of patients with acute MI managed conventionally. However, most strokes are ischaemic strokes, haemorrhages representing substantially fewer numbers. Although, there seems to be a slightly increased risk of cerebral bleeding related to thrombolytic therapy. This risk must be considered more than outweighed by the benefits obtained through the reduction of ischaemic strokes as clearly demonstrated in the ISIS II trial (34).

Rethrombosis

Rethrombosis after successful reperfusion is well documented. In studies using coronary angiography, reported reocclusion incidences have been stated to range from 10 to 20% (20, 22, 24, 47-49). This untoward event seems to be common to all agents, no differences have been documented between the actual agents.

Many factors influence rethrombosis during and after thrombolytic therapy. There will be an interplay between the presence of a local thrombogenic stimulus, the ability of the blood to react to the stimulus, and the dynamics of the flow. That a thrombogenic stimulus persists after thrombolytic therapy is not surprising. Lysis of the thrombus may reexpose the underlying lesion in the atheromatous plaque originally responsible for the coronary thrombosis. This may be a crack, fissure or an ulcer. Furthermore, residual thrombus, due to incomplete lysis, as is commonly present, will have thrombin bound to its surface, and serve as a stimulus for platelet aggregation and new fibrin formation.

It is preferable to have a condition of hypocoagulability, because of the threat of rethrombosis following recanalisation. tPA has a short half-life and induces a mild coagulation defect. Therefore, heparin in therapeutical doses is used for some time after tPA therapy. SK and APSAC are usually given without any intravenous heparin in the follow-up period.

However, a controversy exists as to whether and how long heparin treatment is necessary following recanalisation (50). The main focus for the therapy may be the platelets. Therefore aspirin may be the most important drug in the period after reperfusion. In ISIS II a markedly reduced incidence of reinfarction was found in the group of patients receiving aspirin in addition to SK (34).

Relation to angioplasty (PTCA)

Since thrombolytic therapy has given recanalisation in no more than 70% of the cases treated, and since a patent coronary artery was regarded as crucial, PTCA immediately or shortly after an attempt at thrombolysis became a therapeutic procedure to evaluate. In the trial of the European Cooperative Study Group (51), tPA was compared to tPA plus PTCA. Additional PCTA gave no benefit and was associated with a markedly increased frequency of bleeding.

In the trials of TAMI and TIMI, intervention with PTCA has been examined immediately after tPA treatment, after 1-2 days and after 7-10 days. Overall results showed that immediate PTCA intervention offerd no advantage (52-54).

These randomised studies have given results consistent with the simple and straightforward therapeutical regimens most commonly used. There is no reason to perform angiography as a routine with the object of undertaking PTCA or other invasive interventions. Most hospitals do not have resources for such a policy, and according to current opinion it does not offer better medical results.

An individual follow-up to select patients, who, based on clinical evaluation and eventually exercise ECG, should be subjected to angiography, seems to be the best policy to-day. The content of the quotation from *Ryan* (55) is fairly good advice: "In the absence of symptoms watchful waiting seems more sensible than a reflex response to anatomy alone".

Unsolved problems

In recent years the various pieces have begun to fall into place. Some unanswered questions are still disputed.

1. Time from onset of symptoms

The earlier the treatment starts the greater are the chances of success. Ideally, immediate thrombolytic therapy should be available.

However, the situation is that in most places, a substantial proportion of the patients will come to or be referred to hospital several hours after onset of chest pain, at a time when thrombolytic therapy is less efficient. Often a time limit of about 6 hours has been set as a prerequisite for starting fibrinolytic therapy. However, ISIS II demonstrated mortality reduction also for the late patient group, those patients whose treatment was started 6 to 24 hours after onset of symptoms (34).

More data are needed on this point and it is being addressed in ongoing trials. As has been discussed, the possible effects on the late entries may be more complex than mere salvage of the jeopardized myocardium. It should also be kept in mind, that a cumulative examination of the studies in the 60's and 70's showed a significant effect on the late entry patients (9), and was the major reason for reexamining such patients in ISIS II. With the information already present, it seems well founded to subject more late patients to this treatment which might also benefit marginal patients, especially so since it has few side-effects.

Another approach in order to get more early patients is to give the drugs to the patients before arrival in hospital. Administration of the thrombolytic drug in the ambulance can save much time and is under evaluation in some centres. Under such conditions APSAC, since it can be given as a bolus, is especially interesting and promising.

It is generally agreed that only physicians should administer the therapy. A development in the way that referring physicians can start the medication outside hospital may become a reality in the future, not least because it will be highly time-saving.

2. Relation to heparin and aspirin

Asprin has after ISIS II become a routine drug that should be given as early as possible after onset of symptoms of an acute MI. How heparin fits in relation to aspirin and in relation to the different thrombolytic agents has not been definetely settled, but this problem is also under examination in clinical trials at the present time.

3. Which agent is best?

It is still an open question as to which agent will turn out to be the best when the ultimate goals are evaluated. These goals are preservation of myocardial function, reduction of mortality and better prospects for the survivors. Time has come to undertake a direct comparison of the different agents in randomised trials with such high numbers that hard end-points can be assessed. Such studies are under way, and it will be interesting to await the results of GISSI II, ISIS III and other trials.

When more details of the medical efficacy have been determined for the different agents, other factors must be taken into consideration, such as ease of administration. SK is given over a period of one hour, tPA 3-4 hours, and at the present time followed by heparin infusion, while APSAC is especially interesting because it is given as a 5 minute bolus.

Price is another factor that may be decisive with regard to the usage of the fibrinolytic agents. SK is least expensive, APSAC is in the middle, and tPA and UK are very expensive. This picture may be adjusted or greatly changed in the coming years.

Conclusions

Thrombolytic therapy is established as a cornerstone in the treatment of acute MI. It has reduced hospital mortality substantially. These conclusions have emerged as a result of large, well-conducted, multi-centre studies. Some questions remain unanswered and will be addressed.

It will be a challenge to find out which fibrinolytic agent is the best, or if newer and more efficient drugs become available. The time limits for start of therapy have not been settled. High age was considered for a long time a contra-indication, but cannot be perceived as such any longer. The conventional contra-indications, such as previous gastrointestinal-bleeding, stroke and others, are not so absolute as they were some years ago.

This situation indicates that the whole potentiality of thrombolytic therapy has not yet been utilized, and suggests an increased and extensive usage in the coming years.

References

1. Davies MJ, Fulton WFM, Robertson WB. The relation of coronary thrombosis to ischaemic myocardial necrosis. J Pathol 1979; 172: 99-110.
2. Chapman I. The cause-effect relationship between recent coronary artery occlusion and acute myocardial infarction. Am Heart J 1974; 87: 267-71.
3. Buja LM, Willerson JT. Clinicopathologic correlates of acute ischemic heart disease syndromes. Am J Cardiol 1981; 47: 343-56.
4. DeWood MA, Spores J, Notske T, et al. Prevalence of total coronary occlusion during the early hours of transmural myocardial infarction. N Engl J Med 1980; 303: 897-902.
5. Maroko PR, Kjelkhus JK, Sobel BE, et al. Factors influencing infarct size following experimental coronary artery occlusion. Circulation 1971; 43: 67-82.
6. Reimer KA, Lowe JE, Rasmussen MM, Jennings RB. The wavefront phenomenon of ischemic cell death. Myocardial infarct size vs duration of coronary occlusion in dogs. Circulation 1977; 56: 786-93.
7. Sederholm M, Grøttum P, Erhardt L, Kjekshus J. Quantitative assessment of myocardial ischemia and necrosis by continuous vectorcardography and measurement of creatine kinase release in patients. Circulation 1983; 68: 1006-12.
8. Sonneblick EH, Ross J Jr, Braunwald E. Oxygen consumption of the heart. Newer aspects of its multifactorial determination. Am J Cardiol 1968; 22: 328.
9. Yusuf S, Collins R, Peto R, et al. Intravenous and intracoronary fibrinolytic therapy in acute myocardial infarction: overwiew of results on mortality, reinfarction and side-effects from 33 randomized controlled trials. Eur Heart J 1985; 6: 556-85.
10. Rentrop KP, Blanke H, Kostering K, Karsch KR. Acute myocardial infarction: intra-

coronary application of nitroglycerin and streptokinase in combination with transmural recanalization. Clin Cardiol 1979; 2: 354-63.

11. Mason DT, ed. Proceedings of the symposium intracoronary thrombolysis in acute myocardial infarction. Am Heart J 1981; 102: 1123-208.
12. Taylor GJ, Mikkell FL, Moses HW, et al. Intravenous versus intracoronary streptokinase therapy for acute myocardial infarction in community hospitals. Am J Cardiol 1984; 54; 256-60.
13. Rentrop KP, Feit F, Blanke H, et al. Effects of intra-coronary streptokinase and intracoronary nitroglycerin infusion on coronary angiographic patterns and mortality in patients with acute myocardial infarction. N Engl J Med 1984; 311: 1457-63.
14. Spann JF, Sherry S, Carabello BA, et al. High-dose, brief intravenous streptokinase early in acute myocardial infarction. Am Heart J 1982; 104: 939-45.
15. Kennedy JW, Ritchie JL, Davis KB, Fritz JK. Western Washington randomized trial of intracoronary streptokinase in acute myocardial infarction. N Engl J Med 1983; 309: 1477-82.
16. Owen J, Friedman KD, Grossman BA, Wilkins C, Berke AD, Powers ER. Quantitation of fragment-X formation during thrombolytic therapy with streptokinase and tissue plasminogen activator. J Clin Invest 1987; 79: 1642-7.
17. Ferres H. Preclinical pharmacological evaluation of anisoylated plasminogen streptokinase activator complex. Drugs 1987, 33 (suppl 3): 33-50.
18. Mueller HS, Rao AK, Forman SA, and the TIMI investigatiors. Thrombolysis in myocardial infarction (TIMI): comparative studies of coronary reperfusion and systemic fibrinogenolysis with two forms of recombinant tissue-type plasminogen activator. J Am Coll Cardiol 1987; 10: 470-90.
19. Sherry S. Acute myocardial infarction: Comparison of different thrombolytic agents. Current Opinion in Cardiology 1988; 3: 480-91.
20. Schrøder R, Biamino G, Enz-Rudiger L, et al. Intravenous short-term infusion of streptokinase in acute myocardial infarction. Circulation 1983; 63: 536-48.
21. Koren G, Weiss AT, Hasin Y, et al. Prevention of myocardial damage in acute myocardial ischemia by early treatment with intravenous streptokinase. N Engl J Med 1985; 313: 1384-9.
22. European Cooperative Study Group for Recombinant Tissue-Type Plasminogen Activator. Randomized trial of intra-venous recombinant tissue-type plasminogen activator versus intravenous streptokinase in acute myocardial infarction. Lancet 1985; i: 842-7.
23. Anderson JL, Marshall HW, Skins JC, et al. A randomized trial of intravenous and intracoronary streptokinase in patients with acute myocardial infarction. Circulation 1984; 70: 606-18.
24. Mathey DG, Schofer J, Sheehan FH, Becher H, Tilsner V, Dodge HT. Intravenous urokinase inacute myocardial infarction. Am J Cardiol 1985; 55: 878-82.
25. Van De Werf F, Nobuhara M, Collen D. Coronary thrombosis with human single-chain urokinase-type plasminogen activator (prourokinase) in patients with acute myocardial infarction. Ann Int Med 1986; 104: 345-8.
26. Been M, DeBono DP, Muir AL, Bouton FE, Hillis WS, Hornung R. Coronary thrombolysis with intravenous anisoylated plasminogenstreptokinase complex. BRL26921. Br Heart J 1985; 53: 253-9.
27. VanRey FJ, Bonnier HJ, Michels HR, Mamdouth IE, Hoffman J. Efficacy of BRL26921, a new fibrinolytic agent for intravenous infusion in acute myocardial infarction. In: Meyer J, Erbel R, Rupprect JH, eds. Improvement of myocardial perfusion. Thrombolysis, angioplasty, bypass surgery. Dordrecht: Martinus Nijhoff, 1985: 11-4.
28. Kasper W, Meinertz HJ. Fibrinolytic efficacy of a new acylated streptokinase-plasminogen activator complex (BRL26921) in patients with acute myocardial infarction:

comparison between intravenous and intracoronary administration (abstr). Thromb Haemost 1985; 54: P1258.

29. Chesebro JH, Knatterud G, Roberts R, et al. Thrombolysis in myocardial infarction (TIMI) trial, phase I: a comparison between intraavenous tissue plasminogen activator and intravenous streptokinase. Circulation 1987; 76: 142-54.
30. Verstraete M, Bory M, Collen D. Randomised trial of intravenous recombinant tissue-type plasminogen activator versus intravenous streptokinase in acute myocardial infarction. Lancet 1986; ii: 842-7.
31. Jan K, Reinhardt W, Chien S, et al. Altered rheological properties of blood following administrations of tissue plasminogen activator and streptokinase in patients with acute myocardial infarction. Circulation 1985, 72 (suppl. III): III-417.
32. Arntz R, Heitz J, Schäfer H, Schröder R. Hemorheology in acute myocardial infarction: effects of high dose intravenous streptokinase. Circulation 1985, 72 (suppl. III): III-417.
33. Gruppo Italiano per lo Studio della Streptochinasi nell'-infarto miocardico (GISSI). Effectiveness of intravenous thrombolytic treatment in acute myocardial infarction. Lancet 1986; i: 397-402.
34. ISIS-2 (Second International Study of Infarct Survival) Collaborative Group. Randomised trial of intravenous streptokinase, oral aspirin, both or neither among 17 183 cases of suspected acute myocardial infarction: ISIS-2. Lancet 1988; ii: 349-60.
35. AIMS Trial Study Group 1988. Effect of intravenous APSAC on mortality after acute myocardial infarction: Preliminary report of a placebo-controlled clinical trial. Lancet i: 545-9.
36. Wilcox RG, Von der Lippe G, Olsson CG, Jensen G, Skene AM, Hampton JR. For The Asset Study Group. Trial of tissue plasminogen activator for mortality reduction in acute myocardial infarction. Anglo-Scandinavian Study of Early Thrombolysis (ASSET). Lancet 1988; ii: 525-30.
37. Dalen JE, Gore JM, Braunwald E, et al. Six – and twelve-month follow-up of the phase I thrombolysis in myocardial infarction (TIMI) trial. Am J Cardiol 1988; 62: 179-85.
38. Kennedy JW, Ritchie JL, Davies KB, Stadius ML, Maynard C, Fritz JK. The Western Washington randomized trial of intracoronary streptokinase in acute myocardial infarction. A 12 month follow-up report. N Engl J Med 1985; 312: 1073-8.
39. The ISAM Study Group. A prospective trial of intravenous streptokinase in acute myocardial infarction (ISAM): Mortality, morbidity and infarct size at 21 days. N Engl J Med 1986; 314: 1465-72.
40. White HD, Norris RM, Brown MA, et al. Effect of intravenous streptokinase on left ventricular function and early survival after acute myocardial infarction. N Engl J Med 1987; 317: 850-5.
41. Guerci AD, Gerstenblith G, Brinke JA, et al. A randomized, placebo-controlled, double blind trial of intravenous plasminogen activator for acute myocardial infarction with subsequent randomization to elective coronary angioplasty. N Engl J Med 1987; 317: 1613-8.
42. O'Rourke M, Baron D, Keogh A, et al. Limitation of myocardial infarction by early infusion of recombinant tissue-type plasminogen activator. Circulation 1988; 77: 1311-5.
43. National Heart Foundation of Australia Coronary Thrombolysis Group. Coronary thrombolysis and myocardial salvage by tissue plasminogen activator given up to 4 hours after onset of myocardial infarction. Lancet 1988; i: 203-8.
44. Van de Werf F, Arnold AER. Intravenous tissue plasminogen activator and size of infarct, left ventricular function, and survival in acute myocardial infarction. Br Med J 1988; 297: 1374-9.

45. Meinertz T, Kasper W, Schumacher M, Just H. APSAC multicenter Trial Group. The German multicenter trial of anisoylated plasminogen streptokinase activator complex versus heparin for acute myocardial infarction. Am J Cardiol 1988; 62: 347-51.
46. Van de Werf F. Discrepancies between the effects of coronary reperfusion on survival and left ventricular function. Lancet 1989; 1: 1367-9.
47. Spann JF, Sherry S, Carabello BA, et al. Coronary thrombolysis by intravenous streptokinase in acute myocardial infarction: acute and follow-up studies. Am J Cardiol 1984; 53: 655-61.
48. Rogers WJ, Mantle JA, Hood WP, et al. Prospective randomized trial of intravenous and intracoronary streptokinase in acute myocardial infarction. Circulation 1983; 95: 1051-61.
49. Williams DO, Borer J, Braunwald E, et al. Intravenous recombinant tissue-type plasminogen activator in patients with acute myocardial infarction: a report from the NHLBI thrombolysis in myocardial infarction trial. Circulation 1986; 73: 338-46.
50. Kander NH, Holland KJ, Pitt B, Topol EJ. A randomized pilot trial of brief versus prolonged heparin after sucessful reperfusion of acute myocardial infarction. Circulation 1988: 78 (suppl. II): II-113 (Abstract).
51. Simoons ML, Arnold AER, Betriu A, et al. Thrombolysis with tissue plasminogen activator in acute myocardial infarction: No additional benefit from immediate percutaneous coronary angioplasty. Lancet 1988; i: 197-202.
52. Topol EJ, Califf RM, George BS, et al. A multicenter randomized trial of intravenous recombinant tissue plasminogen activator and immediate angioplasty in acute myocardial infarction. N Engl J Med 1987; 317: 581-8.
53. Passamani E, Hodges M, Herman M, et al. The thrombolysis in myocardial infarction (TIMI) phase II pilot study: Tissue plasminogen activator followed by percutaneous transluminal coronary angioplasty. J Am Coll Cardiol 1987; 10: 51B-64B.
54. The TIMI Research Group. Immediate vs delayed catheterization and angioplasty followed thrombolytic therapy for acute myocardial infarction. TIMI II A results. JAMA 1988; 260: 2849-58.
55. Ryan TJ. Letter. Thrombolysis and angioplasty in acute myocardial infarction. N Engl J Med 1988; 318: 579.
56. Armstrong P W, Baigrie R S, Daly P A, et al. Tissue plasminogen activator: Toronto (TPAT) Placebo-Controlled Randomized Trial in acute myocardial infarction. J Am Coll Cardiol 1989; 13: 1469-76.
57. Wackers F J Th, Terrin M L, Kayden D S, et al. Quantitative radionuclide assessment of regional ventricular function after thrombolytic therapy for acute myocardial infarction: Results of Phase I Thrombolysis in Myocardial Infarction (TIMI) Trial. J Am Coll Cardiol 1989; 13: 998-1005.

29

Platelet inhibitor agents in ischaemic heart disease

STEEN ELKJÆR HUSTED,
HANS KRÆMMER NIELSEN

Haemostasis is a major body defense mechanism to prevent bleeding. The so-called "haemostatic balance" is a complex interaction among the dynamics of blood flow, components of the vessel wall, blood platelets and plasma proteins. The balance between normal and abnormal haemostasis (thrombosis and haemorrhage) depends on numerous regulation factors within the platelets, the coagulation system and the fibrinolytic system. A thrombus is a mass of cellular material (red blood cells, leucocytes, platelets) bound together with fibrin strands. The relative proportion of cells and fibrin in the thrombus is determined by the rate of blood flow in the vessel and the age of the thrombus (1).

Platelets predominate in the thrombi in arteries with a high flow and shear rate, while red cells and fibrin are more important in venous thrombi, as blood flow is slow in these vessels (2). Platelets seem to be especially implicated in the thromboembolic complications of the atheromatous plaques and to have an important role in the pathogenesis of ishaemic cardiovascular disease (3).

In the 1960's a strikingly low incidence of coronary artery disease was observed among rheumatoid arthritis patients on regular acetylsalicylic acid (ASA) medication (4). Later ASA was found to have platelet inhibitory effects and an effect on thromboembolic diseases was anticipated (5). The results of 6 large clinical studies in the 1970's were, however, contradictory, and the possible antithrombotic effect of ASA as well as other platelet inhibitory agents was doubted (2). But in the 1980's a solid support for the antithrombotic efficacy of platelet inhibitors, especially ASA, has emerged and has been based on:

1. The central role of thrombosis in acute myocardial infarction (AMI)(6).
2. The central role of platelets in the pathogenesis of acute cardiac ischaemic syndromes has been demonstrated in post mortem studies (3) as well as by coronary angioscopy studies (7).
3. Newer studies have a better design, initiating the treatment with platelet inhibitors early after debute of the thromboembolic episode.

Role of platelets in thrombogenesis

Platelets are 2-3 μm nucleine free fragments of megakariocytes with an average lifetime of 7½ to 9 days. Platelets do not adhere to intact endothelium, but are activated by endothelial injury resulting in platelet aggregation. As platelets have no nucleus they cannot syntesize proteins such as enzymes etc. (8).

The haemostatic functions of platelets consist of: 1. Platelet adhesion and spreading. 2. Platelet secretion and aggregation.

Platelet adhesion and aggregation depend on platelet membrane receptors. Glycoprotein Ia binds collagen stimulating platelet adhesion to injured sites. Glycoprotein Ib are receptors for von Willebrand factor (vWF), and glycoproteins IIb and IIIa participate in adhesion and serve an important aggregating function by binding fibrinogen, fibronectin and vWF.

The platelet cytoplasma contains secretory granules, such as dense and alpha granules, lysosomes and peroxisomes. Many of the secretory products – especially ADP, serotonin, vWF and fibrinogen – are important in the platelet activation process (9). The platelet-derived growth factor is a potent mitogen and chemotactic agent for smooth muscle cells, and plays an essential role in tissue repair, and may participate in the atherosclerotic process (10, 11). Cyclic adenosine monophosphate (cAMP) plays a central role in platelet activation. cAMP reduces the intracellular Ca^{++} concentration by inhibiting the Ca^{++} mobilization from dense granules. The concentration of cAMP depends on the activity of two enzymes, adenylcyclase and phosphodiesterase. Thromboxane A_2 (TxA_2) and prostacyclin (PGI_2) as well as numerous drugs influence the activity of these enzymes.

Drugs interfering with platelet aggregation may interfere with one or more of three different steps in this process (9, 12). In *the first step* collagen, thrombin and epinephrine release Ca^{++} from the dense tubular system into the cytoplasma by the action of phospholipase on platelet membrane phophatidylinositol. The elevated free intracellular Ca^{++} activates the actin-myosin system and the platelets contract and release ADP, serotonin and

TxA_2. In *the second step* serotonin and ADP stimulate Ca^{++} release from dense granules and expose platelet binding sites of fibrinogen and vWF thus promoting platelet aggregation. Arachidonic acid released from phosphatidylcholin in the platelet membrane mediates *the third step*. Cyclooxygenase converts arachidonic acid to endoperoxides, which are transformed to TxA_2 by thromboxane synthetase. TxA_2 is a highly potent platelet aggregator and vasoconstrictor. Platelet aggregation is mediated by promoting the mobilization of intracellular Ca^{++} and facilitating the exposure of membrane receptors to fibrinogen and vWF (9).

PGI_2, which is synthetized in the endothelial cells from arachidonic acid or platelet derived endoperoxides, is a potent inhibitor of platelet aggregation by a stimulation of adenylcyclase increasing cAMP and thus reducing the Ca^{++} mobilization from dense granules (13).

An important link between the activated platelets and the coagulation system is mediated by platelet membrane lipoproteins called platelet factor III (14), which stimulates the interaction between the coagulation factors, among which thrombin is a potent platelet activator (15). The main inhibitors of thrombus formation are PGI_2, antithrombin III (ATIII), protein C and the fibrinolytic system. ATIII neutralizes activated factor II, IX, X, XI and XII, and protein C is an anticoagulant, a plasminogen activator and neutralizes the plasminogen activator inhibitor. Plasminogen in plasma is tranformed by tissue-plasminogen activator (t-PA) from endothelial cells to plasmin, which hydrolyses fibrin to soluble fragments, and degrades fibrinogen, factor II, V and VII. The fibrinolytic system is regulated by several stimulators and inhibitors (16).

Pharmacological aspects of platelet inhibitor drugs

1. Inhibitors of the arachidonic acid pathway

a. Inhibitors of cyclooxygenase

ASA and other non-steroidal anti-inflammatory drugs inhibit cyclooxygenase. ASA-acetylation of the enzyme is irreversible, and the effect persists for the life of the platelet. ASA is rapidly absorbed from the stomach and upper intestine (17), and an oral dose of 80 mg inhibits TxA_2 formation totally (18). A low dose ASA has probably the same antithrombotic effect as higher doses without toxic side-effects, and an ASA dose of 160 mg to 325 mg once daily for the prevention of arterial thromboembolic disease is currently recommended (9). ASA inhibits platelet aggregation partially as only the third step is blocked (17), and in long-term studies no tolerance to the antiaggregatory effect can be detected (19). ASA also inhibits the endothelial cyclooxygenase and production of PGI_2, but this inhibition is reversible as the endothelial cells can produce new enzymes. With low-dose ASA the platelet inhibition and low serum concentration of TxB_2 (a stable TxA_2 metabolite) can be maintained with preserved PGI_2-production. A postulated balance between PGI_2 and TxA_2 important for the thrombogenesis has not been clinically or biochemically proven and the differential effect of low-dose ASA has recently been challenged (17, 19).

Sulfinpyrazone was initially introduced as an uricosuric agent, but was shown to normalize the reduced platelet survival seen in patients with hyperuricaemia. Sulfinpyrazone is a competitive inhibitor of platelet cyclooxygenase, but it is suggested, that the drug may possess additional antiplatelet effects (17). Studies in patients with arteriovenous shunt-thrombosis indicated that at least one week of treatment was required before an effective antiplatelet activity of sulfinpyrazone was achieved (20), and this controversial "7-days rule" has made the "Anturan Reinfarction trial" difficult to interpret (21). Despite a positive effect of sulfinpyrazone in two large clinical trials on vascular events in post-AMI patients (21, 22), no effect was found in unstable angina and stroke (23, 24). Sulfinpyrazone reduces the rate of thrombotic events in patients with arteriovenous cannulas (20), and saphenous vein coronary grafts (25, 26).

Side-effects of sulfinpyrazone are hypoglycaemia when combined with sulfonylureas, precipitation of uric acid stones, exacerbation of peptic ulcer and interaction with oral anticoagulants.

b. Alteration of the platelet membrane phospholipids (fatty acids of the omega-3 series)

Atherosclerosis is apparently rare among Eskimos on a traditional diet of seal, caribou and fish, but not among those on a Western diet (27). The omega-3 fatty acids – notably eicosapentaenoic acid (20: 5 omega-3; EPA) and docosahexaenoic acid (22: 6 omega-3) – are present in high concentrations in most salt fish. These fatty acids compete with arachidonic acid for platelet and endothelial cyclooxygenase, leading to formation of TxA_3 with low biological activity and PGI_3, which has antiplatelet activity. The result is a shift in the haemostatic balance toward an antiaggregatory and vasodilatory state. A high intake of fish is also associated with some potential hazards such as increased bleeding diathesis, reduced inflammatory and immune responses and an increase in lipid peroxides because of a low concentration of vitamin E (27). In a recently published study, a daily dose of 340 mg EPA could significantly reduce mortality after AMI, but in another study 6 g daily of omega-3 fatty acids for 6 months had no effect on restenosis after coronary angioplasty (PTCA) (28).

c. Inhibition of TxA_2 synthetase

Imidazole analogues are specific thromboxane synthetase inhibitors without direct effect on the PGI_2-production, which may even increase because of an increase in platelet endoperoxides. The clinical efficacy of these drugs has been unsatisfactory, and this may be explained by the presence of the proaggregatory endoperoxides (29).

d. Blockers of thromboxane and prostaglandin endoperoxide receptors

Antagonists of the receptors for the proaggregatory and vasoconstrictor effects of endoperoxides and TxA_2 have been developed and preliminary studies have been performed in humans (30), but it remains to be demonstrated, whether these agents alone and in combination with TxA_2 synthetase inhibitors offer an advantage over ASA in clinical trials.

2. Increasing the platelet cAMP concentration.
Dipyridamole

Dipyridamole is a pyrimidopyrimidine derivative, which inhibits platelet function by several mechanisms: *1. Inhibition of the phosphodiesterase enzyme in platelets* resulting in an increase in intraplatelet cAMP, *2. Stimulation of PGI_2 release from vascular endothelium* and *3. Increasing the levels of adenosine* by inhibiting its uptake by vascular endothelium and erythrocytes (31). Adenosine enhances platelet adenylcyclase activity and has vasodilatory effects (32). Furthermore, dipyridamole seems to inhibit red cell-induced platelet activation, which may play a central role in thrombogenesis in high turbulence systems, i.e. valvular prothesis, vascular stenosis, etc. Nevertheless, after 2 decades of therapeutic use there is no firm clinical evidence for a significant antithrombotic effect of dipyridamole monotherapy in humans (31, 33).

Side-effects are headache, epigastric discomfort and nausea, but neither gastroduodenal ulcers nor bleeding tendency develop even when combined with oral anticoagulant (9).

Prostaglandin E_1 and I_2

Prostaglandin E_1 (PGE_1) and PGI_2 inhibit platelet function by an increase of platelet cAMP and in addition they are potent vasodilators. PGE_1 is used in neonates with congenital heart disease, who are dependent on the persistence of a patent ductus arteriosus until surgical correction can be done. PGI_2 induces systemic hypotension with a short duration of action of 30 minutes (9, 34). The effects on ishaemic heart disease and peripheral vascular insufficiency are controversial, but PGI_2 analogues, iloprost, carbacyclin and ciprostene, are chemically stable and have been found to be more potent in inhibiting platelet aggregation. The clinical relevance of this awaits further clinical testing (9, 35-37).

3. Inhibition of platelet agonists
Thrombin

Thrombin production is inhibited by *heparin* or *oral anticoagulants*, and thrombin activation of platelets may be attenuated. However, unfractionated heparin in vitro may stimulate ADP-induced platelet aggregation, while collagen-induced aggregation is inhibited (38). Heparin may increase the TxA_2 production, and heparin-induced paradoxical thrombosis has been described (39). Low-molecular weight heparins have a weaker effect on platelet function (40).

Heparin inhibits smooth muscle cell proliferation experimentally (41). Theoretically, this effect may be utilized to inhibit restenosis after coronary angioplasty.

The native peptide *Hirudin* has been synthesized by recombinant DNA-technology. Hirudin inhibits activation of several coagulation factors and is a powerful thrombin inhibitor, influencing platelet activation dependent on thrombin. Recently, it has been demonstrated in an animal model to be a more powerful antithrombotic agent than heparin (42).

ADP

Ticlopidine is a potent inhibitor of platelet function. It is a member of the thienopyridine family and is structurally distinct from other antiplatelet agents.

Ticlopidine appears to be a specific inhibitor of ADP-induced platelet aggregation and thereby it also attenuates collagen- and thrombin-induced platelet aggregation, which are ADP dependent (43). Optimal effect is reached after 3 days of administration and its effect lasts for several days after cessation (9).

Clinical testing of ticlopidine suggests that it is effective in patients with unstable angina for prevention of AMI and cardiovascular death (44). Ticlopidine significantly reduces the acute and late (12 months) occlusion rate after aorto-coronary bypass graft operation (45), and reduces the incidence of thrombosis after percutaneous transluminal coronary angioplasty (PTCA) (46).

Ticlopidine has been shown to reduce cardiovascular morbidity and mortality in patients with stroke and may be more effective than ASA in this respect (47). Ticlopidine has, however, frequent *side-effects* such as neutropenia and rash, and the possibility of other long-term side-effects needs to be further investigated.

4. Other possible platelet inhibitory agents

Exposure of receptors on the platelet membrane binding fibrinogen and vWF is considered to play an important role in platelet aggregation. In primates monoclonal antibodies to the platelet glycoprotein IIb/IIIa receptor abolished in vivo platelet thrombin formation in stenosed carotid artery with intimal damage and infusion of epinephrine (48). Bleeding tendency seems moderate at therapeutic dosage (48). Furthermore, intravenous infusion of arginine-glycine-aspartate-o-methyltyrosine amide, which competes with glycoprotein IIb/IIIa fibrinogen binding, effectively prevented reocclusion in canine femoral arteries with thrombi induced by electrical vascular injury and successfully recanalized by thrombolysis (49). These short-acting inhibitors of platelet aggregation seem to be promising for the prevention of arterial thrombus formation (50).

Clinical trials evaluating platelet inhibitory agents in ishaemic heart disease

Coronary atherosclerotic disease

The coronary atherosclerotic disease seems to consist of two phases: *1. A long initial asymptomatic period* with slow progression of the early non-obstructive atherosclerotic plaque during a period of 3 to 4 decades and *2. A rapid thrombotic progression* because of plaque rupture and exposure of thrombogenic material such as collagen and tissue thromboplastin from intima, promoting platelet aggregation and fibrin formation with significant occlusive or near occlusive thrombus formation (51). One of the initial factors in the development of atheromatous plaques may be platelet adhesion to areas with minor endothelial injury and the platelet release of several mitogens, i.e. platelet-derived growth factor, epidermal growth factor and others, which stimulate smooth muscle cell and fibroblast proliferation and migration from vessel wall media to intima (52).

Inhibition of platelet adhesion may therefore be beneficial in preventing atherosclerosis, but the risk of bleeding complications would hinder long-term use. Instead the slow progression of atherosclerosis must be prevented during intervention against risk factors such as hypercholesterolaemia, smoking, hypertension, hyperglycaemia etc.

In contrast, platelet function inhibitors are effective in conditions such as unstable angina, AMI and sudden ischaemic death, i.e. acute coronary syndromes, with rapid thrombogenic progression of the atherosclerotic process, because of plaque rupture and thrombus formation (53).

Primary prevention of acute myocardial infarction

The efficacy of ASA in the primary prevention of AMI has been evaluated in 2 large clinical studies. In an American study with more than 22.000 male physicians randomized to ASA 325 mg every other day or placebo for 5 years the frequency of AMI was reduced from 0.4% to 0.2%. However, a slight increase in the incidence of haemorrhagic stroke was seen in the ASA-group, and cardiovascular mortality remained unchanged (54). In a British study about 5.000 phycisians were randomized to 500 mg ASA daily or no ASA. No effect was found on the incidence of AMI, but an increase in severe strokes was registered in the ASA-treated group (55). Therefore, the general use of ASA in primary prophylaxis against AMI cannot be recommended, but in individuals with a high risk of coronary artery disease the benefits of therapy may outweigh its risk. In this respect, patients with stable angina and significant coronary atherosclerotic lesions may have a high risk of acute coronary syndromes. Ongoing studies at the Mayo clinic indicate, that platelet inhibitors reduce the incidence of AMI and prevent new lesion formation in these patients (56).

Unstable angina (Table 1)

Combined postmortem and angiographic studies have demonstrated the central role of atherosclerotic plaque rupture with thrombus formation, throm-

Table 1. *Randomized trials of platelet inhibitors for unstable angina and secondary prevention of AMI.*

References	Follow-up (months)	Number of patients	Treatment	Coronary events (%)	Cardiac deaths (%)	Deaths or MI (%)	Total deaths (%)
Unstable angina							
Lewis et al 1983 (57)	3	1216	ASA	3.5¹)	–	5.0²)	1.6
			placebo	7.8	–	10.1	3.3
Cairns et al 1985 (23)	18	555	ASA	11.5	5.0³)	–	6.6*
			Sulfinpyr.	15.0	10.0	–	10.7
			ASA+Sulf.	9.5	3.6³)	–	5.1*
			placebo	14.4	9.4	–	9.4
Théroux et al 1988 (58)	6 days	479	ASA	16.6	0	3.3³)	0
			ASA+Hepar.	11.5	0	1.6³	0
			Heparin	9.3	0	0.8³	0
			placebo	26.3	0	8.5	1.7
S.T.A.I. 1989 (44)	6	652	Ticlopidine	6.7*	–	1.9	1.9
			placebo	13.0	–	4.1	4.4
Secondsary prophylaxis							
Elwood et al 1974 (9)	12	1239	ASA	–	–	–	8.3
			placebo	–	–	–	10.9
CDPAS 1976 (9)	22	1529	ASA	8.0	4.6	9.5	5.8
			placebo	10.2	6.4	12.5	8.3
Elwood et al 1979 (9)	12	1682	ASA	14.7*	10.4	14.6	12.3
			placebo	21.2	13.5	22.4	14.8
Breddin et al 1979 (9)	24	626	ASA	7.8	1.6	12.0	8.5
			placebo	12.0	3.2	15.3	10.4
AMIS 1980 (9)	38	4524	ASA	14.1	6.0	17.1	10.8
			placebo	14.8	6.0	17.8	9.7
PARIS I 1980 (9)	44	2026	ASA	16.0	2.5	17.4	10.5
			ASA+DIP	16.8	4.0	18.6	10.7
			placebo	20.9	5.7	22.7	12.8
PARIS II 1986 (63)	23	3128	ASA+DIP	9.0*	4.9	11.6	7.1
			placebo	11.8	5.2	14.4	7.3
ART 1980 (21)	16	1558	Sulfinpyr.	–	5.5*	–	5.8
			placebo	–	7.9	–	7.9
ARIS 1982 (22)	19	727	Sulfinpyr.	9.0**	5.2	–	5.5
			placebo	15.2	5.5	–	5.8

1) $p<0.0005$, 2) $p<0.0001$, 3) $p<0.001$, ** $p<0.005$, * $p<0.05$.

bus fragmentation and peripheral embolization in patients with unstable angina (3, 7). The thrombus material is mainly aggregated platelets and the use of ASA in this condition has been very successful. In the American study ASA 324 mg daily initiated within 51 hours after debute of symptoms and with a follow-up of 12 weeks, the incidence of AMI and cardiac death was significantly reduced from 10.1% to 5.0% (57). The same risk reduction was found in a Canadian study, where ASA 1.300 mg daily was compared to placebo and sulfinpyrazone in patients with a maximum duration of symptoms of 8 days and a 2 year follow-up (23). Sulfinpyrazone was ineffective. In a recently published study of 479 patients with unstable angina, ASA (325 mg b.i.d.) was compared to intravenous heparin, the combination of both and placebo. After 6 days ASA and heparin decreased the rate of myocardial infarction by 72% and 89%, respectively. There were no significant differences between ASA, heparin and their combination (58). In an Italian study (STAI) ticlopidine 250 mg b.i.d. for 6 months reduced the incidence of AMI and mortality by >50% (44).

It can be concluded, that early ASA treatment in patients with unstable angina is highly recommended. The possible additive/synergistic effect of anticoagulants is being evaluated in ongoing studies.

Acute myocardial infarction (Table 1)

Plaque rupture and thrombus formation may completely occlude the coronary artery, resulting in non-Q wave or Q-wave AMI. A high patency rate and early peak in plasma creatine kinase suggest, that early reperfusion following spontaneous thrombolysis or resolution of vasospasm or both is important in the pathogenesis of non-Q wave infarction (59). The value of ASA administration in AMI has recently been evaluated in the large ISIS-2 study, where more than 17.000 patients with suspected AMI were randomized to ASA 160 mg daily for one month, streptokinase, both in combination or placebo. After 5 weeks vascular mortality rate was significantly reduced by 23% by ASA, 25% by streptokinase, and 42% by the combined regimen. After 2 years of follow-up the beneficial effect was still present (60). In a smaller study, 300 patients with suspected AMI and a symptom duration of median 3-4 hours were randomized to ASA 100 mg daily, 500 mg b.i.d. or placebo for 12 weeks. During the hospitalization period a significant reduction in total mortality and AMI was found in the low-dose ASA group compared with the two other groups, and a similar trend was present after 12 weeks (61). Similar results were obtained in a study of patients with less than 4 hours symptoms and electrocardiographic signs of first anterior wall AMI. All patients received streptokinase and were randomized to ASA 100 mg daily or placebo with a follow-up period of 3 months. Angiography performed within 6 weeks showed a significantly higher frequency of LAD occlusions (12 versus 1) in the placebo group (62).

Secondary prevention after myocardial infarction (Table 1)

Platelet inhibitory agents in the secondary prevention after AMI have been evaluated in several large studies with ASA monotherapy (5 studies), ASA combined with dipyridamole (2 studies) and sulfinpyrazone monotherapy (2 studies) (9). Only the last of these studies, PARIS II, with early patient inclusion showed a positive effect of the antiplatelet drugs on cardiac mortality and non-fatal AMI (63). A pooled analysis of antiplatelet therapy in these randomized studies suggests, that platelet inhibitors significantly reduce vascular mortality rate by 15%, non-fatal reinfarction rate by 30% and non-fatal stroke rate by 42% without effect on the non-vascular mortality rate. Monotherapy with sulfinpyrazone or ASA in combination with dipyridamole had no advantage compared to ASA monotherapy (33). In an open multicentre study with 2 year follow-up and inclusion within 3 weeks after the AMI, ASA 30 mg or 60 mg daily were better than 1.000 mg daily, significantly reducing reinfarction and sudden death (64).

ASA therapy in patients with AMI and for secondary prevention in survivors of AMI can be recommended and a daily dose of 150-325 mg seems suitable.

Coronary vein by-pass graft disease (Table 2)

After coronary vein by-pass about 10-15% will be occluded within 1 month postoperatively, 15-20% at 12 months and about 50% at 10 years (65). The occlusion of the vein grafts is caused by: 1. An early postoperative thrombus formation or 2. A later slow progressing atherosclerotic plaque formation with superimposed thrombotic tendency (66).

The thrombotic origin of the early vein graft occlusion often starting peroperatively with platelet deposition indicates a possible beneficial effect of peroperative administration of platelet inhibitory drugs. The slowly progressing graft atherosclerosis is not influenced by antiaggregatory drugs, but may be prevented by intervention against risk factors such as smoking, hypercholesterolaemia, etc.

The importance of an early initiation of antiplatelet treatment has been demonstrated by the fact, that no reduction in vein graft occlusion rate was obtained, when treatment started later than 48 hours postoperatively (9, 67). ASA in low-dose (100 mg daily) and ASA combined with dipyridamole

Table 2. *Randomized trials of platelet inhibitors for prevention of saphenous vein aorto-coronary by-pass occlusion.*

References	Follow-up (months)	Number of patients	Treatment	Patency rate of grafts (%)	P
Antiplatelet drugs started later than first postoperative day					
Pantely et al 1979 (67)	6	13	ASA+DIP	82	>0.05
		13	Warfarin	78	>0.05
		24	Placebo	82	
McEnamy et al 1982 (67)	21	40	ASA	80	>0.05
		34	Warfarin	84	
		37	placebo	72	
Sharma et al 1983 (67)	12	50	ASA	79	>0.05
		48	ASA+DIP	83	
		44	placebo	80	
Brooks et al 1985 (9)	12	133	ASA+DIP+AC	89	>0.05
		133	placebo+AC	87	
Limet et al 1987 (45)	12	87	Ticlopidine	84	<0.01
		86	placebo	74	
Antiplatelet drugs started within first 24 postoperative hours					
Mayer et al 1981 (67)	3-6	47	ASA+DIP	92	<0.02
		66	placebo	77	
Bauer et al 1982 (25)	7-14 days	92	Sulfinpyrazone	96	<0.02
		93	placebo	90	
Chesebro et al 1984 (69)	11-18	171	ASA+DIP	89	<0.01
		172	placebo	75	
Lorentz et al 1984 (68)	4	22	ASA	90	<0.01
		24	placebo	68	
Chevigné et al 1984 (67)	3	42	Ticlopidine	93	<0.02
		35	placebo	78	
Brown et al 1985 (2)	12	38	ASA	74	<0.05
		45	ASA+DIP	67	<0.05
		44	placebo	59	
Rajah et al 1985 (9)	6	48	ASA+DIP+AC	92	<0.01
		55	placebo+AC	75	
Goldman et al 1989 (26)	12	Totally	ASA 325 mg	93	<0.01
		555	ASA 325 tid	92	<0.01
		patients	ASA+DIP	92	<0.01
		studied	Sulfinpyrazone	90	<0.05
			placebo	85	

were shown to reduce the vein graft occlusion rate (68, 69). The low-dose ASA study was small and has been critizised, because of a higher than normal occlusion rate in the placebo group. Randomization of 555 patients to preoperative ASA 325 mg daily, ASA 325 mg t.i.d., ASA plus dipyridamole, sulfinpyrazone or placebo with angiographic assessment 6 to 60 days postoperatively showed an effect on the occlusion rate of all treatment regimens, but sulfinpyrazone was associated with transient renal failure in 5% of the patients (26). There was no additive effect of dipyridamole and no difference in the antithrombotic efficacy between the two ASA dosages. An increased bleeding tendency was seen during ASA treatment. Ticlopidine (250 mg b.i.d.) started on the 2nd postoperative day reduced the graft occlusion rate on day 10, day 180 and day 360 (45).

Treatment with ASA has been shown to be effective for at least one year, but it is not yet clear, whether ASA should be continued longer with a possible effect on rapid thrombotic progression of the atherosclerotic process.

In a recent study, 249 patients undergoing saphenous vein aortocoronary bypass surgery were assigned either to ASA (250 mg b.i.d.) plus dipyridamole (200 mg b.i.d.) or anticoagulant therapy. No difference in antithrombotic efficacy between the two groups was found (70).

It can be concluded, that ASA 100-325 mg daily initiated immediately after surgery may be recommented, while preoperative dipyridamole administration needs further clinical confirmation. Control of atherosclerotic risk factors may be an additional important measure in these patients.

Percutaneous transluminal coronary angioplasty

During PTCA stenotic lesions are dilated with fracture or splitting of the atherosclerotic vessel with the risk of acute occlusion due to intimal-medial dissection, endothelial denudation, subintimal plaque haemorrhage or vasospasms. Consequently, platelet activation and stimulation of fibrin formation leads to thrombus formation (71). Recent studies suggest that pretreatment with platelet inhibitors such as ASA (72), ASA plus dipyridamole (73) or ticlopidine (46) significantly reduces the occlusion rate and the risk of AMI.

Heparin is recommended during PTCA, although the heparin data indicating reduction of acute thrombotic complications are derived from uncontrolled studies (9).

Late restenosis after PTCA occurs with an incidence of 25-30%, and the pathogenesis seems to be multifactorial (74). An increased risk of restenosis is associated with recent onset angina, unstable angina, diabetes mellitus, dilation of multiple lesions in the same vessel, severe preangioplasty stenosis, proximal dilations and a high postangioplasty residual stenosis (9). Platelet activation, activation of the coagulation system and release of growth factors from platelets and endothelial cells inducing smooth muscle cell proliferation with intima hyperplasia may contribute to restenosis. Vasoconstrictor substances from the platelets may be an additional factor (9).

Clinical studies with antiplatelet drugs and oral anticoagulants, as well as calcium channel blockers have shown no benefit in respect of inhibition of restenosis (9).

Omega-3 fatty acids have been tested in several studies with conflicting results (9,75-77). Heparin suppresses smooth muscle cell proliferation, and may influence the tendency to restenosis (41). This is being tested in ongoing studies. Until further studies are available, ASA 325 mg daily starting at least one day before the procedure is recommended for PTCA. Heparin should be administered (100 IU/kg as a bolus followed by 150 IU/kg/hour) at the beginning and for several hours after PTCA depending on the degree of vessel wall injury and thrombotic complications during the procedure. Additional therapeutic possibilities for preventing restenosis after PTCA are badly needed.

Prosthetic valve replacement

Arterial thromboembolism is a frequent and serious complication in patients with prosthetic heart valves; the frequency is lower with bioprostheses than mechanical devices. Thromboembolic complications are more common in patients with poor left ventricular function, left atrial enlargement or atrial fibrillation. Appropriate anticoagulant therapy significantly reduces the thromboembolic complications, while platelet inhibition alone is less effective. The addition of ASA or dipyridamole augments the antithrombotic efficiency of anticoagulation, but ASA 500-1000 mg daily increases the risk of bleeding complications (78). Low-dose ASA combined with anticoagulants has not been studied.

Life-long anticoagulation therapy is recommended in patients with mechanical devices starting in the immediate postoperative period after valve replacement. Treatment with dipyridamole may be added in high risk patients or patients with prior embolism. Patients with bioprostheses should be anticoagulated for at least 3 months postoperatively, although life-long in high risk patients or prior embolism.

Summary

The central role of platelets in thrombogenesis of the coronary arteries and especially in the pathogenesis of acute cardiac syndromes has been documented.

Platelet inhibitory agents are highly effective against cardiac morbidity and mortality in patients with unstable angina, AMI and in secondary prevention after AMI, with ASA 150-325 mg daily as the best documented therapy.

An alternative is combined treatment regimens with fatty acids of the omega-3 series, ticlopidine, platelet glycoprotein IIb/IIIa receptor antibodies or antagonists although these need further documentation, but they seem especially promising in coronary vein by-pass graft disease and after PTCA, where ASA alone or in combination with dipyridamole is not sufficiently effective.

ASA therapy in the primary prevention of AMI in healthy people cannot be recommended, while stable angina seems to be a future indication.

References

1. Mustard JF, Packham MA, Kinlough-Rathbone RL. Mechanisms in thrombosis. In: Colman RW, Hirsh J, Marder VJ, Salzman EW, eds. Hemostasis and thrombosis. Philadelphia: Lippincott 1987: 618-50.
2. Harker LA. Clinical trials evaluating platelet-modifying drugs in patients with atherosclerotic cardiovascular disease and thrombosis. Circulation 1986; 73: 206-23.
3. Falk E. Thrombosis in unstable angina: Pathologic aspects. Cardiovasc Clin 1987; 18: 137-49.
4. Cobb S, Anderson F, Bauer W. Length of life and cause of death in rheumatoid arthritis. N Engl J Med 1953; 249: 553-6.
5. O'Brian JR. Effects of salicylates on human platelets. Lancet 1968;i: 779-83.
6. DeWood MA, Spores J, Notske R, et al. Prevalence of total coronary occlusion during the early hours of transmural myocardial infarction. N Engl J Med 1980; 303: 897-902.
7. Sherman CT, Litvack F, Grundfest W, et al. Coronary angioscopy in patients with unstable angina pectoris. N Engl J Med 1986; 315: 913-9.
8. Schmidt K Gjerløff. Trombocytter. Christensen BE, Jøhnsson V, eds. Hæmatologi. FADL's Forlag 1988: 33-40.
9. Stein B, Fuster V, Israel DH, et al. Platelet inhibitor agents in cardiovascular disease: An update. J AM Coll Cardiol 1989; 14: 813-36.
10. Ross R, Raines EW, Bowen-Pope DF. The biology of platelet-derived growth factor. Cell 1986; 46: 155-69.
11. Westermark B, Heldin C-H. Platelet-derived growth factor: structural and functional aspects. J Int Med 1989; 225: 55-8.
12. Vargaftig BB, Chignard M, Le Couedic JP, Benveniste J. One, two, three or more pathways for platelet aggregation. Acta Med Scand 1980; (suppl 642): 23-9.
13. Oates JA, FitzGerald GA, Branch RA, Jackson EK, Knapp HR, Roberts LJ. Clinical implications of prostaglandin and thromboxane A_2 formation. N Engl J Med 1988; 319: 689-98 and 761-7.
14. Hawiger J. Formation and regulation of platelet and fibrin hemostatic plug. Human Pathol 1987; 18: 111-22.
15. Walsh PN, Schmaier AH. Platelet-coagulation protein interaction. Colman RW, Hirsh J, Marder VJ, Salzman EW, eds. Hemostasis and thrombosis. Philadelphia: Lippincott 1987: 689-709.

16. Jespersen J. Pathophysiology and clinical aspects of fibrinolysis and inhibition of coagulation. Lægeforeningens Forlag, 1987. (Thesis).
17. Pedersen AK, FitzGerald GA. The human pharmacology of platelet inhibition: pharmacokinetics relevant to drug action. Circulation 1985; 72: 1164-76.
18. Jakubowski JA, Stampfer MJ, Vaillancourt R, Deykins D. Cumulative antiplatelet effect of low-dose enteric coated aspirin. Br J Hematol 1985; 60: 635-42.
19. Bochner F, Lloyd J. Is there an optimal dose and formulation of aspirin to prevent arterial thrombo-embolism in man? Clin Sci 1986; 71: 625-31.
20. Kaegi A, Pineo GF, Shimizu A, Trivedi H, Hirsh J, Gent M. Arteriovenous shunt thrombosis: Prevention by sulfinpyrazone. N Engl J Med 1974; 290: 304-6.
21. The anturane reinfarction trial research group: Sulfinpyrazone in the prevention of sudden death after myocardial infarction. N Engl J Med 1980; 302: 250-6.
22. Report from the anturane reinfarction Italian study. Sulfinpyrazone in post myocardial infarction. Lancet 1982; i: 237-42.
23. Cairns JA, Gent M, Singer J, et al. Asprin, sulfinpyrazone or both in unstable angina. Results of a Canadian multicenter trial. N Engl J Med 1985; 313: 1369-75.
24. The Canadian Cooperative Study Group. A randomized trial of aspirin and sulfinpyrazone in threatened stroke. N Engl J Med 1978; 299: 53-9.
25. Bauer HR, van Tassel RA, Pierach CA, Gobel RL. Effects of sulfinpyrazone on early graft closure after myocardial revascularization. Am J Cardiol 1982; 49: 420-4.
26. Goldman S, Copeland J, Moritz T et al. Saphenous vein graft patency 1 year after coronary artery bypass surgery and effects of antiplatelet therapy. Results of Veterans Administration Cooperative Study. Circulation 1989; 80: 1190-7.
27. Zhu B-Q, Parmley WW. Modification of experimental and clinical atherosclerosis by dietary fish oil. Am Heart J 1990; 119: 168-78.
28. Burr ML. Effects of changes in fat, fish and fibre intakes on death and myocardial reinfarction: diet and reinfarction trial (dart). Lancet 1989; ii: 757-61.
29. FitzGerald GA, Reilly LA, Pedersen AK. The biochemical pharmacology of thromboxane synthetase inhibition in man. Circulation 1985; 72: 1194-201.
30. Saussy DL Jr, Mais DE, Knapp DR, Halushka PV. Thromboxane A_2 and prostaglandin endoperoxide receptors in platelets and vascular smooth muscle. Circulation 1985; 72: 1202-7.
31. FitzGerald GA. Dipyridamole. N Engl J Med 1987; 316: 1247-57.
32. Saniabadi AR, Tomiak RHH, Lowe GDO, Barbenel JC, Forbes CD. Dipyridamole inhibits red cell-induced platelet activation. Atherosclerosis 1989; 76: 149-54.
33. Antiplatelet trialists' collaboration. Secondary prevention of vascular disease by prolonged antiplatelet treatment. Br Med J 1988; 296: 320-31.
34. Vane JR. Prostaglandins and the cardiovascular system. Br Heart J 1983; 49: 405-9.
35. Whrittle BJR, Moncada S. Platelet actions of stable carbocyclic analogues of prostacyclin. Circulation 1985; 72: 1219-25.
36. Fisher CA, Kappa JR, Sinka AK, Cottrell ED, Reiser HJ, Addonizio VP. Comparison of equimolar concentrations of iloprost, prostacyclin and prostaglandin E_1 on human platelet function. J Lab Clin Med 1987; 109: 184-90.
37. Raizner A, Hollman J, Demke D, Wakefield L. Beneficial effects of ciprostene in PTCA: a multicenter, randomized, controlled trial (abstr) Circulation 1988; 78 (suppl II): II-290.
38. O'Brien JR, Shoobridge SM, Finch WJ. Comparison of the effect of heparin and citrat on platelet aggregation. J Clin Path 1969; 22: 28-31.
39. Arthur CK, Isbister JP, Aspery EM. The heparin induced thrombosis – thrombocytopenia syndrome (H.I.T.T.S.): a review. Pathology 1985; 17: 82-8.
40. Huisse M-G, Guillin M-C, Bezeaud A, Toulemonde F, Kitzis M, Andreassian B. Heparin-

associated thrombocytopenia. In vitro effects of different molecular weight heparin fractions. Thromb Res 1982; 27: 485-90.
41. Reilly CF, Fritze LMS, Rosenberg RD. Heparin inhibition of smooth muscle cell proliferation: a cellular site of action. J Cell Physiol 1986; 129: 11-9.
42. Heras M, Chesebro JH, Penny WJ, Bailey KR, Badimon L, Fuster V. Effects of thrombin inhibition on the development of acute platelet-thrombus deposition during angioplasty in pigs. Circulation 1989; 79: 657-65.
43. Maffrand J-P, Defreyn G, Bernat A, Delebassee D, Tissinier A-M. Reviewed pharmacology of ticlopidine. Act Méd Int – Angiologie 1988; (suppl 77): 6-13.
44. Violi F, Scrutinio D, Cimminiello C, et al. S.T.A.I. (Study of Ticlopidine in Unstable Angina) (Abstr) J Am Coll Cardiol 1989; 13 (suppl A): 238A.
45. Limet R, David JL, Magotteaux P, Larock MP, Rigo P. Prevention of aorta-coronary bypass graft occlusion. J Thorac Cardiovasc Surg 1987; 94: 773-83.
46. White CW, Chaitman B, Lassar TA, et al. Antiplatelet agents are effective in reducing the immediate complications of PTCA: results from the ticlopidine multicenter trial (abstr). Circulation 1987; 76 (suppl IV): IV-400.
47. Gent M, Blakely JA, Easton JD, et al. The Canadian American ticlopidine study (CATS) in thromboembolic stroke. Lancet 1989; i: 1215-20.
48. Coller BS, Folts JD, Smith SR, Scudder LE, Jordan R. Abolition of in vivo platelet thrombus formation in primates with monoclonal antibodies to the platelet GPIIb/IIIa receptor. Correlation with bleeding time, platelet aggregation, and blockade of GPIIb/IIIa receptors. Circulation 1989; 80: 1766-74.
49. Haskel EJ, Adams SP, Feigen LP, et al. Prevention of reoccluding platelet rich thrombi in canine femoral arteries with a novel peptide antagonist of platelet glycoprotein IIb/IIIa receptors. Circulation 1989; 80: 1775-82.
50. Fitzgerald DJ. Platelet inhibition with an antibody to glycoprotein IIb/IIIa. Circulation 1989; 80: 1918-9.
51. Fuster V, Steele PM, Chesebro JH. Role of platelet and thrombosis in coronary atherosclerotic disease and sudden death. J Am Coll Cardiol 1985; 5: 175B-84B.
52. Ross R. The pathogenesis of atherosclerosis - an update. N Engl J Med 1986; 314: 488-500.
53. Falk E. Unstable angina with fatal outcome, dynamic coronary thrombosis leading to infarction and/or sudden death. Autopsy evidence of recurrent mural thrombosis with peripheral embolization culminating in total vascular occlusion. Circulation 1985; 71: 699-708.
54. The steering committee of the physicians' health study research group. Final report on the aspirin component of the ongoing physicians' health study. N Engl J Med 1989; 321: 129-35.
55. Peto R, Gray R, Collins R, et al. A randomised trial of the effects of prophylactic daily aspirin among male British doctors. Brit Med J 1988; 296: 313-6.
56. Chesebro JH, Webster MWI, Smith HC, et al. Antiplatelet therapy in coronary disease progression: reduced infarction and new lesion formation (abstr). Circulation 1990 (in press).
57. Lewis HD, Davis JW, Archibald DG, et al. Protective effects of aspirin against acute myocardial infarction and death in men with unstable angina. Results of a veterans administration cooperative study. N Engl J Med 1983; 309: 396-403.
58. Théroux P, Ouimet H, McCans J, et al. Aspirin, heparin, or both to treat acute unstable angina. N Engl J Med 1988; 319: 1105-11.
59. DeWood M, Stifter WF, Simpson CS, et al. Coronary angiographic findings soon after non-Q wave myocardial infarction. N Engl J Med 1986; 315: 417-23.
60. ISIS-2 (second international study of infarct survival) collaborative group. Randomized

trial of intravenous streptokinase, oral aspirin, both, or neither among 17.187 cases of suspected acute myocardial infarction: ISIS-2. Lancet 1988; ii: 349-60.
61. Husted SE, Nielsen H Kræmmer, Krusell LR, Færgeman O. Acetylsalicylic acid 100 mg and 1000 mg daily in acute myocardial infarction suspects: a placebo-controlled trial. J Intern Med 1989; 226: 303-10.
62. Verheugt FWA, Küpper AJF, Galema TW, Roos JP. Low dose aspirin after early thrombolysis in acute myocardial infarction. Am J Cardiol 1988; 61: 904-6.
63. Klimt CR, Knatterud GL, Stampler J, Meier P. Persantine-aspirin reinfartion study. Part II. Secondary coronary prevention with persantine and aspirin. J Am Coll Cardiol 1986; 7: 251-69.
64. Hoffmann W, Förster W. Two years follow-up cottbus reinfarction study with 30 and 60 mg acetylsalicylic acid. Prostaglandins Clin Res 1987; 393-7.
65. Fuster V, Chesebro JH. Role of platelets and platelet inhibitors in aorto- coronary artery vein-graft disease. Circulation 1986; 73: 227-32.
66. Bulkley BH, Hutchins GM. Accelerated "atherosclerosis": a morphologic study of 97 saphenous vein coronary artery bypass grafts. Circulation 1977; 55: 163-9.
67. Verstraete M, Brown BG, Chesebro JH, et al. Evaluation of antiplatelet agents in the prevention of aorto-coronary bypass occlusion. Eur Heart J 1986; 7: 4-13.
68. Lorenz RL, Schacky CV, Weber M, et al. Improved aortocoronary bypass patency by low-dose aspirin (100mg daily): effects on platelet aggregation and thromboxane formation. Lancet 1984; i: 1261-4.
69. Chesebro JH, Fuster V, Elveback LR, et al. Effect of dipyridamole and aspirin an late vein-graft patency after coronary bypass operations. N Engl J Med 1984; 310: 209-14.
70. Pfisterer M, Burkart F, Jockers G, et al. Trial of low-dose aspirin plus dipyridamole versus anticoagulants for prevention of aortocoronary vein graft occlusion. Lancet 1989; ii: 1-7.
71. Waller BF. "Crackers, breakers, stretchers, drillers, scrapers, shavers burners, welders and melters": the future treatment of atherosclerotic coronary artery disease? A clinical-morfologic assessment. J Am Coll Cardiol 1989; 13: 969-87.
72. Barnathan ES, Schwartz JS, Taylor L, et al. Aspirin and dipyridamole in the prevention of acute coronary thrombosis complicating coronary angioplasty. Circulation 1987; 76: 125-34.
73. Schwartz L, Bourasse MG, Lesperance J, et al. Aspirin and dipyridamole in the prevention of restenosis after percutaneous transluminal coronary angioplasty. N Engl J Med 1988; 318: 1714-9.
74. McBride W, Lange RA, Hillis LD. Restenosis after successful coronary angioplasty. Pathophysiology and prevention. N Engl J Med 1988; 318: 1734-7.
75. Dehmer GJ, Popma JJ, van den Berg EK, et al. Reduction in the rate of early restenosis after coronary angioplasty by a diet supplemented with n-3 fatty acids. N Engl J Med 1988; 319: 733-40.
76. Milner MR, Gallino RA, Leffingwell A, et al. Usefulness of fish oil supplements in preventing clinical evidence of restenosis after percutaneous transluminal coronary angioplasty. Am J Cardiol 1989; 64: 294-9.
77. Reis GJ, Boucher TM, Sipperly ME, et al. Randomised trial of fish oil for prevention of restenosis after coronary angioplasty. Lancet 1989 ii: 177-81.
78. Chesebro JH, Ezekowitz M, Badimore L, Fuster V. Intracardiac thrombi and systemic thromboembolism detection, incidence and treatment. Am Rev Med 1985; 36: 579-605.

30

Mural thrombi in acute myocardial infarction

KARL-ARNE JOHANNESSEN

Thromboembolism is a clinically important complication in patients with acute myocardial infarction (MI). Peripheral emboli to the arterial circulation is known to occur in 2-5% of the patients with acute infarcts, and an association between intraventricular mural thrombi located at the infarcted myocardium and peripheral arterial embolization has been known for many decades. This complication has been intensively examined the last 10 years with non-invasive techniques that have made it possible to study this problem without any hazards to the patients. Whereas studies performed until a decade ago addressed this issue in all patients with acute MI, recent results have defined subgroups of patients that have the largest risk of such complications, with the potential to improve the risk-benefit ratio of future interventions.

The diagnosis of left ventricular thrombi

Until recently, the accurate diagnosis of left ventricular (LV) thrombi was possible only at the time of autopsy. Several autopsy series reported a similar incidence of left ventricular thrombi following MI; 32-48% of patients who died within the first 3 months had a mural thrombus at autopsy (1-6).

The current diagnostic techniques for detecting LV thrombi are listed in Table 1. The radionuclide technique with 111-Indium labelled platelets reflects the thrombus activity which also seems to indicate their embolic potential; a positive scan being associated with the highest risk for embolization (7). The radionuclide angiography and contrast angiography detect a space-occupying lesion seen as absence of contrast within the left ventricle, whereas both X-ray computed tomographic (CT) scanning and resonance imaging may generate images of the thrombi (8). However, the accuracy of

Table 1. *Diagnostic techniques for detecting left ventricular thrombi.*

Diagnostic technique	Sensitivity, %	Specificity, %
Indium 111 platelet imaging	70	100
Radionuclide angiography	31-62	92-100
Contrast angiography	31-62	75-100
X-ray computed tomography		
Magnetic resonance imaging		
Two-dimensional echocardiography	77-95	88-100

these two techniques has not been studied in detail. Furthermore, they are expensive and not generally available, and their usefulness for diagnosing thrombi in large groups of patients may therefore be limited.

In contrast to the other techniques, two-dimensional echocardiography gives information about both the anatomic location, the size, and the morphologic features of thrombi. Being an inexpensive and widely available technique that may be performed on even critically ill patients, it has gained preeminence for the detection of thrombi in patients with acute MI. However, although it has a sensitivity of about 85% and specificity of 95% (9-12), it has several limitations. Approximately 5-10% of studies are technically poor and cannot exclude or prove the presence of a thrombus. Furthermore, anatomical structures such as trabeculations, papillary muscles, abberrant bands and tumors may be mistaken for thrombi. Artefacts due to noise or limited technical resolution (reverberations) may also cause problems (13-15). However, when these limitations are controlled, the technique is probably more suitable than any other for the study of LV thrombi in acute MI.

Incidence of left ventricular thrombi in acute myocardial infarction

Since the first prospective echocardiographic study of left ventricular thrombi in acute MI was reported in 1981 (16), several other studies using two-dimensional echocardiography have reported on the incidence of LV thrombi in acute MI. As seen in Table 2, most studies have found an incidence of 30-40% thrombi in anterior MI, in contrast to almost none in patients with other infarct locations (17-23). The overall pooled incidence in anterior MI may be about 34%.

A constant finding in patients with thrombi is apical akinesia or dyskinesia. This seems to be a prerequisite for thrombus development. Using colour Doppler flow imaging, the blood stasis and the flow pattern in the presence of apical akinesia has been described (24, 25). It has also been

Table 2. *Incidence of LV thrombus in anterior MI.*

	N	LVT	(%)
Asinger 1981	35	12	(34)
Friedman 1982	49	11	(22)
Keating 1983	54	17	(32)
Visser 1983	96	18	(19)
Johannessen 1984	53	15	(28)
Nordrehaug 1985	27	7	(26)
Eigler 1985	10	7	(70)
Johannessen 1988	150	55	(37)
Weinreich 1984	130	44	(34)
Domenicucci 1988	109	59	(54)
Kupper 1989	92	30	(33)
Turpie 1989	88	28	(32)
Overall	893	303	(34)

N=Number of patients, LVT=Number of patients with ventricular thrombus.

Table 3. *Risk of systemic embolization if LV thrombus present in AMI.*

	LVT	Antic.	PE	(%)
Asinger 1981	12	7	0/12	(0)
Friedman 1982	11	9	2/11	(18)
Keating 1983	17	10	6/17	(35)
Haugland 1984	31	NA	9/31	(29)
Johannessen 1984	15	15	4/15	(27)
Visser 1984	22	22	1/22	(4)
Weinreich 1984	43	18	7/43	(16)
Spirito 1985	24	0	1/24	(4)
Tramarin 1986	34	17	1/34	(3)
Domenicucci 1988	59	0	5/59	(8)
Johannessen 1988	55	55	15/55	(27)
Turpie 1989	33	8	3/33	(9)
Overall	402	161	66/402	(16)

established that large and transmural anterior infarcts have the highest risk of thrombus development, and this is probably due to more extensive wall motion abnormalities seen with increasing infarct size. One study that reported increased occurrence of LV thrombi in patients receiving betablocker treatment in the acute phase of an anterior MI, found the higher thrombus incidence to be associated with more extensive apical hypokinesia and akinesia with betablocker treatment (26). Similar findings were later reported in a larger study (27).

There may be several reasons why LV thrombi are mainly seen with anterior MI. Anterior infarcts are larger than infarcts with other locations, which predispose to increased release of substances that promote local thrombus formation. Moreover, although an inferior infarct may cause inferior or lateral wall motion abnormalities, the blood coming through the mitral annulus is moving passively along the inferior wall. Thus, even in the presence of inferior wall akinesia, blood stasis may not be present to the same extent as with apical akinesia.

Time of development of left ventricular thrombi

The time of thrombus development after the acute MI has been described in several studies in which serial echocardiograms have been performed (16, 19, 28-31). Only about 15% of thrombi develop in the first 24 hours, whereas 45-55% of thrombi may be present within the first 48 hours. Within 8-10 days of the infarction, 85-100% of thrombi have developed. In one study, 12% formed later than two weeks (29). Thus, echocardiograms done within the first 3-4 days after the infarction cannot exclude the possibility of later thrombus development, if apical akinesia is present. Since the risk of thrombus formation seems to decline with improved wall motion, patients with hypokinesia or normal wall motion in the apical region probably do not need further echocardiograms with respect to thrombus development.

Embolic risk of LV thrombi

Although the incidence of arterial emboli in a large group of patients with acute MI is invariably between 2-5% (32-34), the reported incidence of embolic events in studies of patients with echocardiographically detected thrombi has varied between 0 and 35% (Table 3). Although most large studies have shown a substantial embolic risk – and the risk pooled from all studies is about 16% – agreement has not been uniform that LV thrombi are associated with such an increased embolic risk. A recent report even claimed that LV thrombi may be of benefit to the patient (35), which markedly contrasts to other reports (17, 22, 23).

These apparent discrepancies are difficult to reconcile, but may be due in part to differing clinical and anticoagulant routines, differing diagnostic criteria for thrombus and embolus, and baseline differences among patient groups. Some studies may have used echocardiographic criteria for a thrombus with high "sensitivity" but of low specificity, thus including false positive "thrombi" without embolic risk.

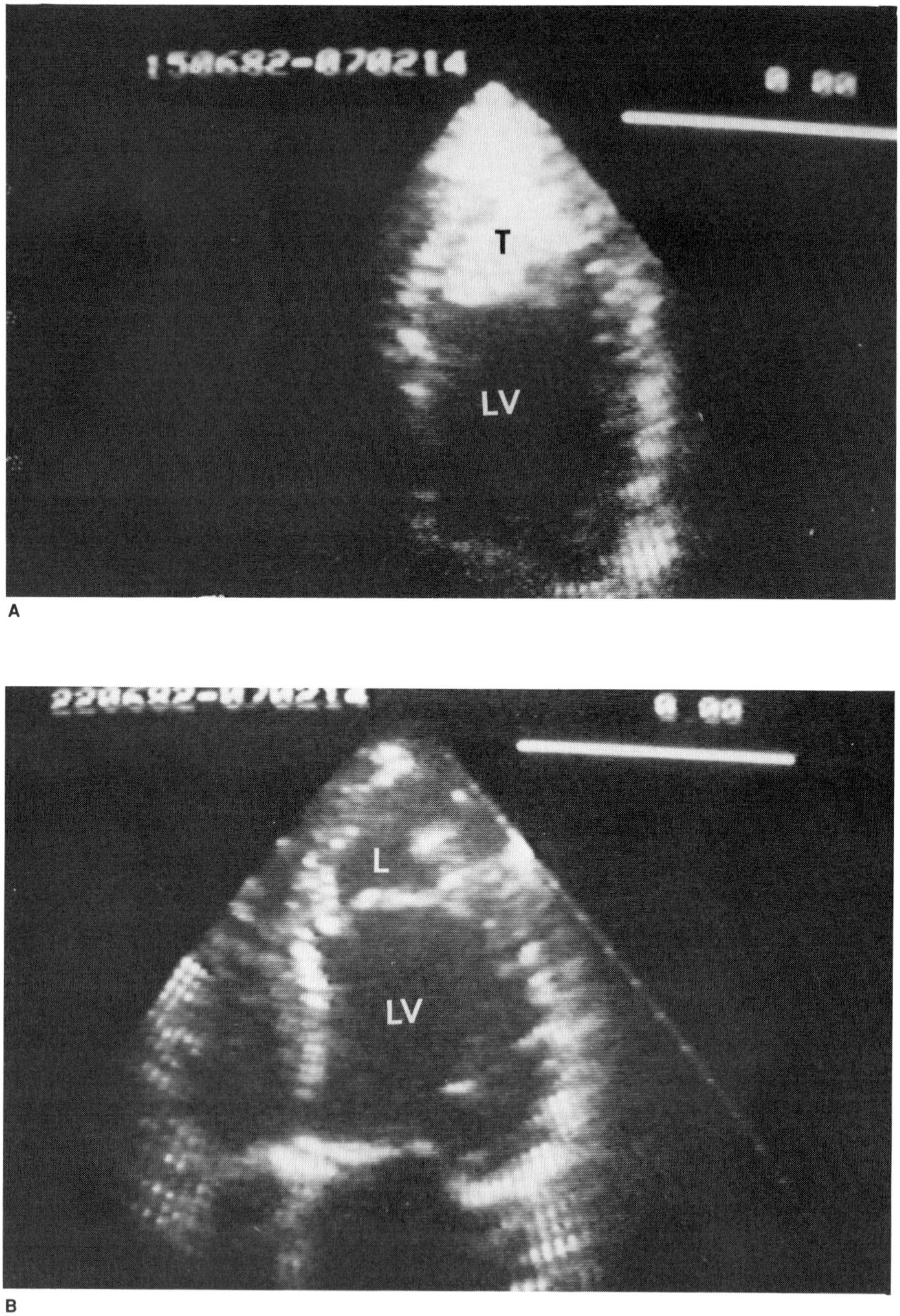

Fig. 1. A) *Thrombus* (T) *in the apex of the left ventricle* (LV). B) *Weeks later the thrombus has developed central lysis* (L) *or echolucency.* C) *A thrombus consisting of two separate clots located in the apical region.*

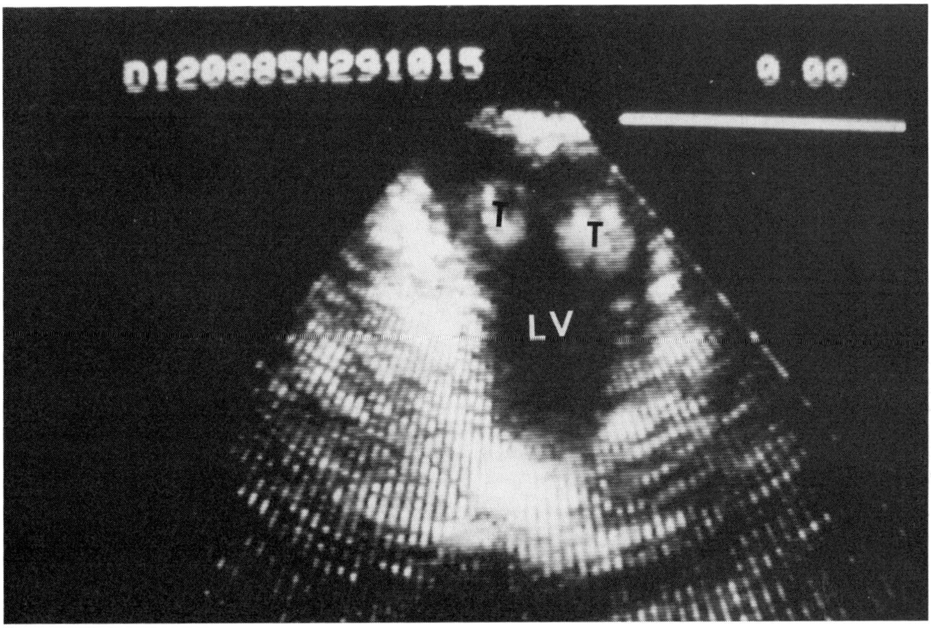

c

The distribution of emboli

The distribution of clinically detected emboli is approximately 75% to the cerebral and 25% to the peripheral circulation. Whether this reflects a true relation of emboli is unclear. Most cerebral emboli are symptomatic and therefore clinically detected, whereas emboli in the kidneys, spleen or other locations may frequently be silent and therefore remain undetected. The reported incidence of emboli is therefore probably a minimum number.

The time of occurrence of emboli

In most studies that have reported emboli from LV thrombi, they have mainly occurred within the first 3 months after the acute MI. However, thrombi from remote infarcts may also embolize, in particular thrombi that have a positive Indium scan (7, 36). Late occurrence and recurrence of thrombi (up to 6 months post MI) has also been reported (37). Since fresh thrombi seem to have higher embolic risk than old, organized and endothelialized thrombi, the late development of thrombi may be of importance. Interventions to reduce embolization therefore must be initiated within the first weeks of thrombus formation.

Predictors of embolization from left ventricular thrombi

No clinical features strongly predict embolization in a patient with a LV thrombus. Several echocardiographic features, however, have been reported to be useful (23, 38-40). Thrombus protrusion into the ventricular lumen and thrombus mobility may be of some use for predicting embolization. Of all thrombi, approximately 50% protrude into the ventricular cavity and 30-55% embolize as compared to only 10-15% of flat thrombi. Some thrombi develop central echolucency, which possibly represents central lysis. Such thrombus remains may have vigorous movements during the cardiac contractions and theoretically imply a high risk of embolization. Thrombus mobility, defined as movement of the thrombus or part of it independent of the underlying myocardium, occurs in 15-30% of all clots, and between 35 and 83% of mobile thrombi seem to embolize.

Anticoagulation treatment and LV thrombi

In addition to the possible effectiveness of acute anticoagulation for reducing venous thromboembolism, substantial evidence suggests that early anticoagulation reduces the risk of stroke. In three large old randomized trials of anticoagulation in acute MI, a total of 3562 patients in whom the presence or absence of left ventricular thrombi was unknown were studied (32-34). Approximately 2% to 5% of patients in these control groups had embolic events as compared to 1% to 2% in the anticoagulated groups. The autopsy prevalence of LV thrombi in 112 patients was 49% in non-anticoagulated patients as compared to 19% of patients who received anticoagulation treatment (32, 34).

These studies were hampered by the fact that many patients were given anticoagulants when there was no need for such treatment. The bleeding risk was 5% to 13% in the treatment groups and only 1% to 5% in the control groups. Thus, anticoagulation of all patients with acute MI may probably reduce peripheral emboli, but exposes some patients with a low embolic risk to possible bleeding complications. With our current knowledge that ventricular thrombi mainly develop in patients with anterior infarcts, therapy can be targeted at this high-risk group.

Recent studies using echocardiographic detection of thrombi as the endpoint have reported conflicting results (27, 30, 31, 41-43) (Table 4). These trials differ markedly in the heparin dose and the treatment, if any, of the control group, and most studies have been small. The largest study, performed by *Turpie et al*, randomized 221 patients to receive either low dose

Table 4. *Randomized trials of anticoagulation treatment to prevent LV thrombi in acute MI.*

	N	Hours to start of treatment	AC regimen	Control regimen	% LV treated	Thrombi control	P-val
Nordrehaug 1985	53	4.6+2.5	H+W	Placebo	0	21	<0.05
Davis 1986	52	<12	H+W	Low-doseH	56	56	ns
Gueret 1986	46	5.2+4.6	H	No therapy	38	52	ns
Arvan 1987	30	6.5+3.3	H+W	No therapy	31	35	ns
Turpie 1989	221	<36	H 12000	H 5000 bid	9	31	<0.01

N=Number of patients in study. AC=Anticoagulation treatment. H=Heparin. W=Warfarin.

Table 5. *Systemic emboli in patients with diagnosed LV thrombi after anterior MI: The role of anticoagulation (AC) treatment.*

	Duration of follow up (months)	Full dose AC	No full dose AC
Asinger 1981	7	0/5 (0)	0/7 (0)
Friedman 1982	11	1/9 (11)	1/2 (50)
Keating 1983	11	0/10 (0)	6/7 (86)
Weinreich 1984	15	0/25 (0)	7/18 (39)
Davis 1986	<1	0/14 (0)	1/15 (7)
Gueret 1986	0.6-1.7	1/8 (12)	1/13 (8)
Tramarin 1986................................	12	1/17 (6)	0/17 (0)
Johannessen 1987	3	12/40 (30)	3/12 (25)
Arvan 1987...................................	<1	1/4 (25)	1/6 (17)
Turpie 1989	<1	1/8 (12)	3/25 (12)
Overall		17/140 (12)	23/122 (19)

(5,000 units b.i.d.) heparin or high dose (12,500 units b.i.d.) heparin, and found a significantly lower incidence of thrombi in the high-dose group. It seems that short time from onset of infarction to start of treatment, and high dose intravenous treatment with monitoring of the treatment effect may reduce the thrombus incidence, whereas standard or low-dose anticoagulation does not. A small trial suggested that if anticoagulation treatment is discontinued one month after the MI, thrombi may develop in a substantial number of patients during the next 2 months (37).

There are relatively few and conflicting data concerning the efficacy of early anticoagulation in reducing the risk of systemic embolism in patients with diagnosed LV thrombi (Table 5). Whereas some studies have claimed that anticoagulants are beneficial in respect of embolization from thrombi, other studies have concluded negative in this respect. However, many studies have been retrospective, not designed to address the issue properly, and treatments has been left to the discretion of the individual physician. Nevertheless, at present it seems that treatment, initiated after LV thrombi have formed, is of limited value.

Platelet inhibitors and LV thrombi

Two studies using aspirin and dipyridamole reported a thrombus incidence similar to placebo or no treatment at all (44, 45). This is probably what would be expected, considering the fact that LV thrombi are probably "red" or "venous thrombi" despite their "arterial" location.

Fibrinolytic treatment and left ventricular thrombi

Only a few and rather small studies have been reported about this topic and their conclusions are conflicting (46-50) (Table 6). An effect of such treatment on LV thrombi, if any, might probably be due mainly to an improvement in wall motion, since the effect on the coagulation system is too short to be of significance for a complication that may develop as late as 10 days after the acute MI. Whether fibrinolytic agents may be used for the lysis of LV thrombi after they have formed is unclear, but a small trial using urokinase reported promising results (51).

Summary

LV thrombi occur in 30-35% of patients with acute anterior myocardial infarctions and rarely in patients with other infarct locations. Patients with the largest infarcts and apical akinesia have the highest risk of thrombus formation, and 90-100% of thrombi develop during the first 10 days after the acute infarct. Arterial embolization has been reported in up to 30% of patients with ventricular thrombi, and embolization has an overall incidence of 15-20% in this patient group as compared to only 2-5% in patients without thrombi. Early, high dose anticoagulation therapy (24,000-26,000 IU Heparin/day or the equivalent) initiated <4-6 hours after the onset of infarction in patients with large anterior infarcts may reduce or prevent thrombus formation and anticoagulation therapy should be continued for

Table 6. *Incidence of LV thrombi with fibrinolytic treatment in anterior MI.*

	n	LVT	(%)
Eigler 1984 SK iv	12	1	(8)
Sharma 1985 SK ic	30	8	(27)
Stratton 1985 SK ic	42	5	(12)
Held 1988 SK/TPA	65	9	(14)
Lupi 1989 SK iv	19	4	(21)
Overall	168	27	(16)

at least 3-6 months following the acute infarct. Fibrinolytic treatment in the acute phase of the infarction may possibly reduce the incidence of LV thrombi, but further studies on this issue are needed.

References

1. Parkinson J, Bedford DE. Cardiac infarction and coronary thrombosis. Lancet 1928; 1: 4-11.
2. Garvin CF. Mural thrombi in the heart. Am Heart J 1941; 21: 713-20 .
3. Bean WB. Infarction of the heart: III. Clinical course and morphological findings. Ann Intern Med 1943; 12: 71-94.
4. Ford AG. Embolism and thrombosis in coronary heart disease. JAMA 1948; 138: 1009-12.
5. Jordan RA, Miller RD, Edwards JE, et al. Thromboembolism in acute and healed myocardial infarction: Intracardiac mural thrombosis. Circulation 1952; 6: 1-6.
6. Miller RD, Jordan RA, Parker RL, et al. Thromboembolism in acute and healed myocardial infarction: Systemic and arterial occlusions. Circulation 1952; 6: 7-15.
7. Stratton JR, Ritchie JL. Positive Indium-111 platelet scans for left ventricular thrombi predict increased embolic risk. J Am Coll Cardiol 1988; 11: 214A.
8. Goldstein JA, Schiller NB, Lipton MJ, et al. Evaluation of left ventricular thrombi by contrast-enhanced computed tomography and two-dimensional echocardiography. Am J Cardiol 1986; 57: 757-60.
9. Lupi G, Chiarella F, Bellotti P, et al. Left ventricular thrombosis: A two-dimensional echocardiographic and anatomic study. G Ital Cardiol 1987; 17: 134-8. (Engl Abstr)
10. Ezekowitz MD, Wilson DA, Smith EO, et al. Comparison of Indium-111 platelet scintigraphy and two-dimensional echocardiography in the diagnosis of left ventricular thrombi. N Engl J Med 1982; 306: 1509-13.
11. Stratton JR, Lighty GW, Pearlman AS, Ritchie JL. Detection of left ventricular thrombus by two-dimensional echocardiography: sensitivity, specificity, and causes of uncertainty. Circulation 1982; 66: 156-66.
12. Visser CA, Kan G, David GK, Lie KI, Durrer D. Two-dimensional echocardiography in the diagnosis of left ventricular thrombus: a prospective study of 67 patients with anatomic validation. Chest 1983; 228-32.
13. Keren A, Billingham ME, Popp RL, et al. Echocardiographic recognition and implications of ventricular hypertrophic trabeculations and abberrant bands. Circulation 1984; 70: 836-42.
14. Mikell FL, Asinger RW, Elsperger KJ, Anderson WR, Hodges M. Regional stasis of blood in the dysfunction of left ventricle: echocardiographic detection and differentiation from early thrombus. Circulation 1982; 66: 755-61.
15. Mikell FL, Asinger RW, Elsperger KJ, Hodges M. Tissue acoustic properties of fresh left ventricular thrombi and visualization by two-dimensional echocardiography: Experimental observations. Am J Cardiol 1982; 49: 1157-65.
16. Asinger RW, Mikell FL, Elsperger J, Hodges M. Incidence of left ventricular thrombosis after acute transmural myocardial infarction. N Engl J Med 1981; 306: 297-302.
17. Keating EC, Gross SA, Schlamowitz RA, et al. Mural thrombi in myocardial infarctions. Am J Med 1982; 74: 989-95.
18. Friedman M, Carlson K, Marcus FI, Woolfenden JM. Clinical correlations in patients with acute myocardial infarction and left ventricular thrombus detected by two-dimensional echocardiography. Am J Med 1982; 72: 894-8.

19. Visser CA, Kan G, Lie KI, Durrer D. Left ventricular thrombus following acute myocardial infarction: A prospective serial echocardiographic study of 96 patients. Eur Heart J 1983; 4: 333-7.
20. Benichou M, Aubry J, Larbi MB. Detection of left ventricular thrombi in the acute phase of myocardial infarction by two-dimensional echocardiography: A series of 103 cases (Fren). Arch. Mal. Coeur Vaiss. 1983; 76/9: 1012-9.
21. Johannessen KA. Nordrehaug JE, von der Lippe G. Left ventricular thrombosis and cerebral vascular accident in acute myocardial infarction. Br Heart J 1984; 51: 553-6.
22. Weinreich DJ, Burke JF, Pauletto FJ. Left ventricular mural thrombi complicating acute myocardial infarction. Ann Intern Med 1984; 100: 789-94.
23. Johannessen KA, Nordrehaug JE, von der Lippe G. Risk factors for embolisation in patients with left ventricular thrombi and acute myocardial infarction. Br Heart J 1988; 60: 104-10.
24. Delemarre BJ, Visser CA, Bot H, et al. Apical flow pattern and thrombus formation after acute myocardial infarction. Circulation 1987; 76 (suppl. IV): IV-227.
25. Maze SS, Kotler MN, Parry WR. Flow characteristics in the dilated ventricle with thrombus: qualitative and quantitative doppler analysis. J Am Coll Cardiol 1989; 13: 873-81.
26. Johannessen KA, Nordrehaug JE, von der Lippe G. Increased occurrence of left ventricular thrombi during early treatment with timolol in acute myocardial infarction. Circulation 1987; 75: 151-5.
27. Turpie AGG, Robinson JG, Doyle DJ, et al. Comparison of high-dose with low-dose subcutaneous heparin to prevent left ventricular mural thrombosis in patients with acute transmural anterior myocardial infarction. N Engl J Med 1989; 320: 352-7.
28. Spirito P, Bellotti P, Chiarella F, et al. Prognostic significance and natural history of left ventricular thrombi in patients with acute anterior myocardial infarction: A two-dimensional echocardiographic study. Circulation 1985; 72: 774-80.
29. Domenicucci S, Bellotti P, Chiarella F, et al. Spontaneous morphologic changes in left ventricular thrombi: A prospective two-dimensional echocardiographic study. Circulation 1987; 75: 737-43.
30. Gueret P, Dubourg O, Ferrier A, et al. Effects of full-dose heparin anticoagulation on the development of left ventricular thrombosis in acute transmural myocardial infarction. J Am Coll Cardiol 1986; 8:419-26.
31. Davis MJE, Ireland MA. Effect of early anticoagulation on the frequency of left ventricular thrombi after anterior wall myocardial infarction. Am J Cardiol 1986; 57: 1244-7.
32. Veterans Administration Hospital Investigators. Anticoagulants in acute myocardial infarction. JAMA 1973; 225: 724-9.
33. Report of the Working Party on Anticoagulant Therapy in Coronary Thrombosis to the Medical Research Council. Assessment of short-term anticoagulant administration after cardiac infarction. Br Med J 1969; 1: 335-42.
34. Drapkin A, Merskey C. Anticoagulant therapy after acute myocardial infarction: relation of therapeutic benefit to patients age, sex, and severity of infarction. JAMA 1972; 222: 541-8.
35. Nihoyannopolous P, Smith GC, Maseri A, et al. The natural history of left ventricular thrombus in myocardial infarction: A rational in support of masterly inactivity. J Am Coll Cardiol 1989; 14: 903-11.
36. Stratton JR, Nemanich JW, Johannessen KA, et al. Fate of left ventricular thrombi in patients with remote myocardial infarction or idiopathic cardiomyopathy. Circulation 1988: 78: 1388-93.
37. Johannessen K-A, Nordrehaug JE, von der Lippe G. Left ventricular thrombi after short time high dose anticoagulants in acute myocardial infarction. Eur Heart J 1987; 8: 975-8.

38. Haugland JM, Asinger RW, Mikell FL, Elsperger KJ, Hodges M. Embolic potential of left ventricular thrombus detected by two-dimensional echocardiography. Circulation 1984, 70: 588-98.
39. Visser CA, Kan G, Meltzer RS, et al. Embolic potential of left ventricular thrombus after myocardial infarction: A two-dimensional echocardiographic study of 119 patients. J Am Coll Cardiol 1985; 5: 1276-80.
40. Meltzer RS, Visser CA, Kan G, et al. Two-dimensional echocardiographic appearance of left ventricular thrombi with systemic emboli after myocardial infarction. Am J Cardiol 1984; 53: 1511-3.
41. Nordrehaug JE, Johannessen KA, von der Lippe G. Usefulness of high dose anticoagulants in preventing left ventricular thrombus in acute myocardial infarction. Am J Cardiol 1985; 55: 1491-3.
42. Arvan S, Boscha K. Prophylactic anticoagulation for left ventricular thrombi after acute myocardial infarction: A prospective randomized trial. Am Heart J 1987; 113: 688-93.
43. Tramarin R, Pozzoli M, Febo O, et al. Two-dimensional echocardiographic assessment of anticoagulation therapy in left ventricular thrombosis early after acute myocardial infarction. Eur Heart J 1986; 7: 482-92.
44. Johannessen KA, Stratton JR, Taulow E, et al. Usefulness of aspirin plus dipyridamole in reducing left ventricular thrombus formation in anterior wall acute myocardial infarction. Am J Cardiol 1989; 63: 101-2.
45. Funke Kupper AJ, Verheugt FWA, Peels CH, et al. Effect of low dose acetyl-salicylic acid on the frequency and hematologic activity of left ventricular thrombus in anterior wall acute myocardial infarction. Am J Cardiol 1989; 63: 917-20.
46. Eigler N, Maurer G, Shah P. Effect of early systemic thrombolytic therapy on left ventricular mural thrombus formation in acute myocardial infarction. Am J Cardiol 1984; 54: 261-3.
47. Sharma B, Carvalho A, Wyeth R, et al. Left ventricular thrombi diagnosed by echocardiography in patients with acute myocardial infarction treated with intracoronary streptokinase followed by intravenous heparin. Am J Cardiol 1985; 56: 422-5
48. Stratton JR, Speck SM, Caldwell JH, et al. Late effects of intracoronary streptokinase on regional wall motion, ventricular wall aneurysm and left ventricular thrombus in myocardial infarction: Results from the Western Washington Randomized Trial. J Am Coll Cardiol 1985; 5: 1023-8.
49. Held AC, Gore JM, Paraskos J, et al. Impact of thrombolytic therapy on left ventricular mural thrombi in acute myocardial infarction. Am J Cardiol 1988; 62: 310-1.
50. Lupi G, Domenicucci S, Chiarella F, et al. Influence of thrombolytic treatment followed by full dose anticoagulation on the frequency of left ventricular thrombi in acute myocardial infarction. Am J Cardiol 1989; 64: 588-90.
51. Kremer P, Fiebig R, Tilsner V, et al. Lysis of left ventricular thrombi with urokinase. Circulation 1985; 72: 112-8.

31

The importance of alpha-blockade during acute ischaemia

KETIL GRONG,
JØRGEN WESTBY

Introduction

There is an increase in the sympathetic activity in acute myocardial ischaemia (1-4). Increased sympathetic drive has a positive inotrophic and chronotrophic effect mainly mediated by cardiac β-adrenergic receptor stimulation. The altered demands for oxygen and perfusion in the myocardium associated with sympathetic activation, further worsen the insufficient ratio between oxygen delivery and demand in acute myocardial ischaemia (5). These notions form the theoretical and experimental background for the beneficial effects of β-adrenergic blockers observed in acute myocardial infarction in man (6, 7).

The importance of sympathetic α-adrenergic receptor stimulation in acute myocardial ischaemia is less clear. In the following, the theorethical aspects of α-adrenergic receptor blockade and the experimental knowledge with relation to myocardial ischaemia will be reviewed, with special emphasis on myocardial blood flow regulation.

Alfa-receptors – classification

In 1948 *Ahlquist* described two types of adrenergic receptors, the α- and the β-receptor (8). This model explained many of the observed effects of catecholamines, by the use of pharmacological substances selectively stimulating these receptors. Stimulation of vascular α-adrenergic receptors mediates vasoconstriction, whereas β-adrenergic receptors mediates vasodilatation. Administration of epinephrine raises blood pressure, whereas a pressure reduction is observed if epinephrine is administered after α-adrenergic blockade. *Lands* described in 1967 two types of β-adrenergic receptors, the β_1-receptor with relation to the myocardium and the β_2-receptor with relation to vessels and other tissues (9). It is now clear that both β-receptors coexist in blood vessels, although the relative distribution between β_1 and β_2-receptors varies in the vascular beds of different tissues and species.

With the development of new selective adrenergic antagonists and agonists it became clear that α-adrenergic receptors did not solely influence the effector organ, for instance smooth muscle cells in blood vessels, but also affect the release of neuro-transmitters following stimulation of adrenergic nerves. *Langer* described in 1974 two types of α-adrenergic receptors associated with the adrenergic neuro-muscular junction in vessels (10). The postsynaptic or postjunctional receptor, named α_1, causes contraction in smooth muscle cells by norepinephrine released from the nerve terminal, and thus vasoconstriction. The prejunctional receptors, called α_2, inhibit by negative "feed-back" further release of norepinephrine from the vesicles in the nerve terminal, thus modulating the responce to adrenergic nervous stimulation. Although some experimental studies indicate that prejunctional α_1-receptors also exist and exert such inhibitory effects (11, 12), the prejunctional α_2-adrenergic receptor is the most important receptor for modulation of norepinephrine release (13).

However, a postjunctional α-receptor mediated response not sensitive to selective α_1-blockade was described (14). Postjunctional α_2-adrenergic receptors also mediate vascular smooth muscle contraction and thereby vasoconstriction (15, 16). One among other new pharmacological substances, SK&F 104078, is claimed to be a relative selective postjunctional α_2-receptor antagonist with low affinity for presynaptic α_2-receptors (17-20). This indicates structural and biochemical differences between pre- and postjunctional α_2-adrenergic receptors. From current knowledge, the subtypes of α-adrenergic receptors are classified in respect of the pharmacological substances that selectively block or stimulate the receptor rather than according to their anatomical localization.

It was originally suggested that the α_1- was independent whereas α_2-mediated contraction was dependent on extracellular calcium influx. These conclusions were based on experiments demonstrating that α_2-, and not α_1-mediated contraction, was inhibited by calcium channel blockers (21-23). However, there are experiments suggesting that α_1-mediated contraction also depends on the influx of extracellular calcium (24-27).

Alpha-receptors – myocardial and vascular effects

Phenylephrine (an α-agonist with relative selectivity for α_1-receptors) increases inotrophy in the myocardium, this effect is blocked by the selective

α_1-antagonist prazosin (29). Furthermore, in the normal non-ischaemic myocardium α-adrenergic stimulation has an antiarrhythmic effect by increasing the duration of the plateau phase and duration of the action potential and prolonging the refractory period (30). In myocardial ischaemia, α-adrenergic stimulation seems to provoke arrhythmia, especially in situations with myocardial reperfusion. Several experimental studies have demonstrated that α-adrenergic blockers decrease the incidence of ventricular fibrillation and tachycardia in acute myocardial infarction and reduce reperfusion arrhythmias (31, 32). The reason for this reversed α-receptor effect during ischaemia is not clear, but could be related to an increase in the number of α-receptors in the ischaemic myocardium (33).

Both postjunctional α_1- and α_2-adrenergic receptors elicit vasoconstriction in the pheripheral vascular bed. This has been demonstrated both *in vitro* and *in vivo* in experimental models and also in humans (14, 15, 34-37). Studies indicate that α_1-receptors dominate on the arterial side whereas both α_1 – and α_2-receptors act on the venous side.

We have studied the effects of repeated test doses of 0.05 μg/kg norepinephrine on diastolic blood pressure in anaesthetized cats with atrial pacing and previous non-selective β-adrenergic blockade with propranolol (Fig. 1). Whereas a test dose of norepinephrine increased diastolic blood pressure by an average of 19.9% in the control situation, the blood pressure increase was 9.2% after additional selective α_1-adrenergic blockade with doxazosin, and a further reduction occurred to 3.4% after the postsynaptic α_1-blocker SK&F 104078 was added (Fig. 1). This demonstrates that in the cat both subtypes of postjunctional α-adrenergic receptors are important for regulation of blood pressure and total vascular resistance.

Both postjunctional α_1 – and α_2-receptors are present in coronary vessels, and experimental data indicate that vasoconstriction in large coronary arteries is mediated by α_1-receptor stimulation, whereas vasoconstriction in small resistance arteries is mediated both by α_1- and α_2-receptor stimulation (36-39).

When studying the effects of adrenergic blockers on myocardial blood flow, concomitant changes in heart rate, contractility, left ventricular systolic and end-diastolic pressure will change the demands and conditions for myocardial perfusion. The interpretation of the results with regard to direct vascular effects in the coronary circulation can thus only be done in experimental settings where these haemodynamic variables are kept relatively unaltered. Furthermore, interaction between the different adrenergic receptor effects must also be considered. For instance, a vasodilatatory effect observed for an α-blocker could either result from blockade of α-

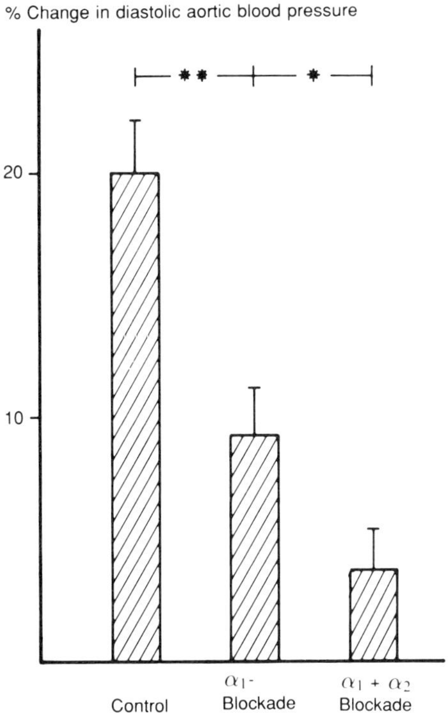

Fig. 1. *% Change in diastolic aortic blood pressure induced by i.v. bolus injection of norepinephrine (0.05 µg/kg) in ten cats pretreated with propranolol (1mg/kg) with subsequent administration of doxazosin (200 µg/kg) and SK&F (2mg/kg). Analysis of variance for repeated measurements (ANOVA) with Newman-Keuls multiple range tests.*
*** $P<0.001$, * $P<0.03$.*

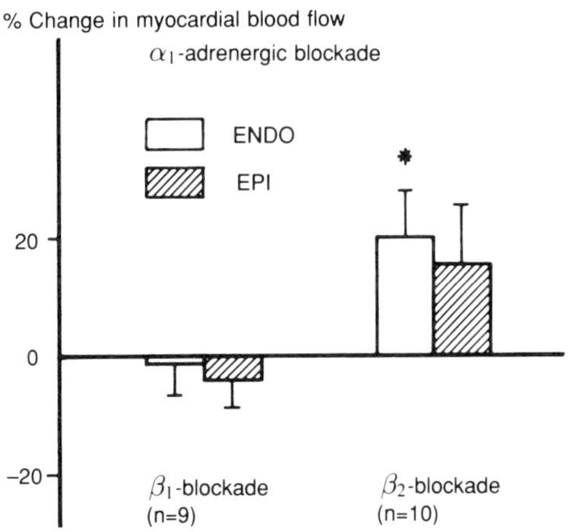

Fig. 2. *% Change in blood flow in well-perfused myocardium following α_1-adrenergic antagonism with doxazosin in two groups of LAD-occluded cats pretreated with either β_1- (atenolol) or β_2-adrenergic blockade (ICI 118.551).*
** Denotes significant difference from unity by Student's t-test ($P<0.05$).Data adapted from (Westby et al (40) and Kvitting et al (41)).*

receptor mediated constriction, from unopposed β-mediated vasodilatation, or both. This is illustrated from our data presented in Fig. 2. In two studies in LAD-occluded hearts, heart rate, left ventricular systolic pressure, mean aortic pressure, and left ventricular end-diastolic pressure were kept constant (40, 41). Heterogenity in blood flow response was observed following α_1-antagonism with doxazosin in animals pretreated with either selective β_1 (atenolol)- or β_2 (ICI 118.155)-adrenergic blockade (Fig. 2). The increase in blood flow in a well-perfused myocardium following doxazosin in the β_2-blocked group is probably due to unopposed β_1-receptor mediated vasodilatation. These findings demonstrate that non-selective β-antagonism with for instance propranolol should be preferred when the proper cardiovascular effects of α-adrenergic antagonism is studied.

Early studies addressing the α-adrenergic effects on the coronary circulation were often undertaken with the use of antagonists that influenced both α-adrenergic subtypes pre- and postjunctionally. More recent studies have focused on the two subtypes of postjunctional α-adrenergic receptors and there are rather diverging conclusions concerning the importance of these receptors in the coronary circulation. Some authors conclude that α_1-adrenergic receptors are mainly responsible for mediating coronary vasoconstriction (42, 43), but most studies conclude that both types or mainly postjunctional α_2-adrenoceptors mediate this response to both neural and humoral sympatethic stimulation (37, 44-50). It has also been demonstrated that α-adrenergic vasoconstriction is mainly localized in the epicardium and this transmural heterogenity has been claimed to be benefical in terms of governing blood flow towards the more vulnerable endocardium and is referred to as the "anti-steal" mechanism (51). The influence of α-adrenergic activity on the autoregulative capabilities in hypoperfused, nonoccluded segments of the coronary circulation, is the experimental approach with the most exciting clinical relevance. The significance of a coronary α-adrenergic vasoconstriction has also been demonstrated in such experimental models, although the importance and degree of this vasoconstriction has been disputed (52-57).

Studies in our laboratory on cats have demonstrated that mainly postjunctial α_2-receptors are responsible for the adrenergic coronary vasoconstriction observed in non-ischaemic control hearts with established β-adrenergic blockade (propranolol 1mg/kg) (Fig. 3). In non-ligated hearts *(controls)* both endocardial and epicardial blood flow were unaltered after postjunctional α_1-adrenergic blockade with doxazosin (200 μg/kg) (58, 59), but increased following additional postjunctional α_2-adrenergic blockade with SK&F 104078 (2 mg/kg). A remarkable finding is the lack of effect on blood flow in the well-perfused myocardium after combined α-adrenergic blockade in hearts with coronary occlusion. No effects could be demonstrated in the ischaemic zone, probably due to the very low coronary collateral circulation in the feline heart. Both experimental groups were paced at a constant heart rate, and mean aortic blood pressure was kept stable with an aortic balloon. This finding suggests that the metabolic vasodilatation in well-perfused myocardium in hearts with an ischaemic region is not restrained

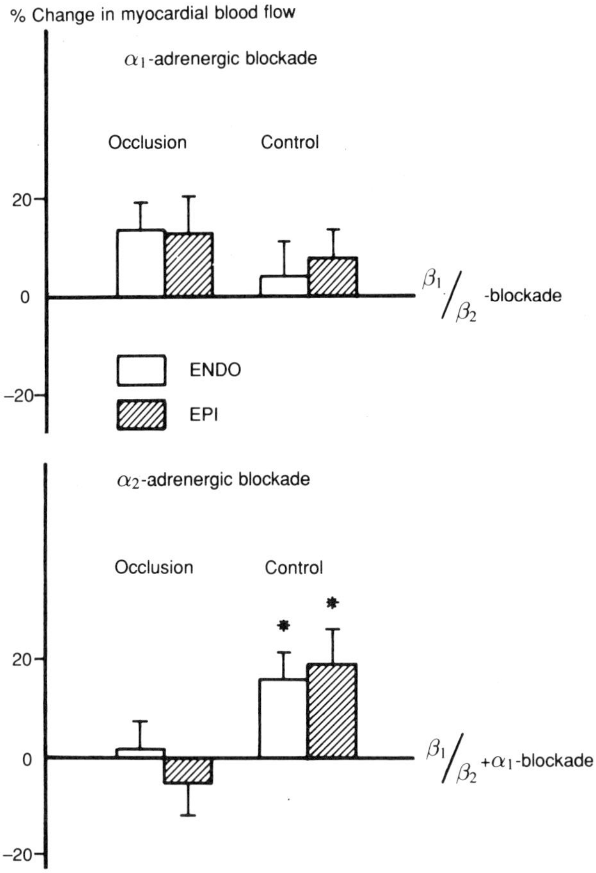

Fig. 3. *% Change in blood flow in well-perfused myocardium following α_1- (doxazosin 200μg/kg) (upper panel) and subsequent α_2-adrenergic (SK&F 104078 2 mg/kg) (lower panel) antagonism in LAD occluded cats (n=10) and controls (n=10) pretreated with propranolol.*
** Significant difference from unity by Student's t-test (P<0.03).*

by any α-adrenergic vasoconstriction. The influence of myocardial metabolic stress on the remaining well-perfused myocardium due to cardiac pacing, and the fact that the study was performed on anaestethized animals, could explain this lack of superimposed α-adrenergic vasoconstriction in the LAD occluded hearts. The significance of α-adrenergic coronary vasoconstriction in conscious animals with acute myocardial ischaemia or sympathetic activation is, however, well documented (44, 50, 60-62). Our data confirm and extend the line of evidence that postjunctional α_2-antagonists should be addressed more specifically in further investigations aimed at possible beneficial effects of α-adrenergic antagonism in acute myocardial ischaemia.

Clinical experience with alpha-blockers

In spite of these theoretically interesting aspects of α-adrenergic blockade during acute ischaemia, the use of these drugs has been limited in clinical practice. Systemic blood pressure reduction will obviously cause a reduction of coronary perfusion pressure also, and could thereby result in a critical reduction of myocardial perfusion. Furthermore, blood pressure reduction is followed by secondary tachycardia thereby increasing the metabolic demands for oxygen and perfusion.

The introduction of labetalol, an adrenergic blocker acting both as α_1- and non-selective β-blocker, initiated experimental studies with regard to reduction of infarct size. With its unique receptor affinity profile, this drug has the same beneficial effects on myocardial oxygen consumtion as β-blockers, but could in addition prevent coronary vasoconstriction caused by unopposed α-receptor stimulation. In the rat myocardium labetalol is superior to the non-selective β-blocker propranolol in reducing infarct size (63). However, a clinical trial involving 166 patients with suspected acute myocardial infarction randomized to either conventional treatment or additional labetalol administration could not demonstrate any favourable effect of labetalol (64). In fact, labetalol treatment resulted in a significantly increased release of the enzyme marker for myocardial damage, CK-MB. Although not statistically significant, more patients died during admission in the labetalol treated group, and more patients had heart failure on discharge or later. Large clinical studies parallel to the β-blocker trials are lacking.

In clinical practice α-adrenergic blockers have been used in coping with systemic hypertension associated with acute myocardial infarction. Reduction of cardiac afterload in this situation will reduce the myocardial demands for oxygen and perfusion (65), and probably reduce the incidence of further complications (66, 67). Both the non-selective α-receptor blocker phentolamine (68), and the combined β- and α_1-blocker labetalol have been used (69). Both these regimes effectively reduced blood pressure. However, phentholamine was best when the cardiac index was reduced. In acute myocardial infarction complicated with cardiac failure, systemic vasodilatatory therapy has been found usefull. Reducing preload is favourable both with regard to perfusion of the myocardium, especially the endocardium, and improves cardiac function. Furthermore, reduction of afterload in this situation can be beneficial in order to reduce cardiac work, α-adrenergic blockers have been used for this purpose (70). Whether this therapy is more or less usefull than for instance nitrates or calcium antagonists with regard to important parameters like mortality or infarct size, is not known. However, nitrates and other vasodilators are preferred in clinical practice (71, 72).

The concept of myocardial reperfusion therapy with thrombolysis with streptokinase, urokinase, plasminogen activators, PTCA, or even surgery paved the way for a new and interesting use of α-adrenergic blockers. Arrhythmias associated with myocardial reperfusion are very frequently observed. The striking antiarrhythmic effect of α-adrenergic blockers found in experimental myocardial reperfusion studies (31, 32), led to some clinical use of α-adrenergic blockers in connection with reperfusion procedures. However, reperfusion arrhythmias are rather benign, and can be successfully treated with conventional antiarrhythmic agents.

Conclusion

Although experimental results have revealed interesting aspects of α-adrenergic blockers in the treatment of acute myocardial ischaemia, this group of pharmacologic agents is not frequently applied in clinical medicine due to lack of evidence of superiority to other therapeutic regimens. A recent review of clinical trials of agents (other than β-blockers) that potentially limit myocardial infarct size does not include any studies on α-adrenergic antagonists (73). However, further development of new specific postsynaptic α_2-antagonists which seem to reduce resistance in small coronary arteries/arterioles in particular and thereby improve blood flow in sympathetic stimulated hearts, could actualize the use of α-adrenergic antagonists in acute myocardial ischaemia.

References

1. Videbaek J, Juel Christensen N, Sterndorff B. Serial determination of plasma catecholamins in myocardial infarction. Circulation 1972; 46: 846-55.
2. Goldstein DS. Plasma norepinephrine as an indicator of sympathetic neural activity in clinical cardiology. Am J Cardiol 1981; 48: 1147-54.
3. Honda T, Ninomiya I. Changes in AdSNA and arterial catecholamines to coronary occlusion in cats. Am J Physiol 1988; 255: H704-10.
4. Schömig A. Adrenergic mechanisms in myocardial infarction. Cardiac and systemic catecholamine release. J Cardiovasc Pharmacol 1988; 12 (suppl 1): S1-S7.
5. Maroko PR, Kjekshus JK, Sobel BE, et al. Factors influencing infarct size following experimental coronary artery occlusions. Circulation 1971; 43: 67-82.
6. Yusuf S, Peto R, Lewis J, Collins R, Sleight P. Beta blockade during and after myocardial infarction: an overview of the randomized trials. Progr Cardiovasc Dis 1982; 247: 1707-14.
7. Hjalmarson Å. International beta-blocker review in acute and postmyocardial infarction. Am J Cardiol 1988; 61: 26B-9B.
8. Ahlquist RP. A Study of the adrenotropic receptors. Am J Physiol 1948; 153: 586-600.
9. Lands AM, Arnold A, McAuliff JP, Ludvena FP, Brown RG Jr. Differentiation of receptor systems activated by sympathomimetic amines. Nature 1967; 214: 597-8.
10. Langer SZ. Presynaptic regulation of catecholamine release. Biochem Pharmacol 1974; 23: 1793-800.
11. Docherty JR. An investigation of presynaptic α-adrenoceptor subtypes in the pithed rat heart and in the isolated vas deferens. Br J Pharmacol 1984; 82: 15-23.

12. Uchida W, Kimura T, Satoh S. Presence of presynaptic inhibitory adrenoceptors in the cardiac symphathetic nerves of the dog: effects of prazosin and yohimbine on sympathetic neurotransmission to the heart. Eur J Pharmacol 1984; 103: 51-6.
13. Jie K, van Brummelen P, Vermey P, Timmermans PBMWM, van Zwieten PA. Modulation of noradrenalin release by pheriperal presynaptic α_2-adrenoceptors in humans. J Cardiovasc Pharmacol 1987; 9: 407-13.
14. Drew GM, Whiting SB. Evidence for two distinct types of postsynaptic α-adrenoceptor in vascular smooth muscle in vivo. Br J Pharmacol 1979; 67: 207-15.
15. Timmermans PBMWM, van Zwieten PA. The postsynaptic α_2-adrenoceptor. J Autonom Pharmacol 1981; 1: 171-83.
16. McGrath JC. Evidence for more than one type of postjunctional α-adrenoceptor. Biochem Pharmacol 1982; 31: 467-84.
17. Hieble JP, Sulpizio AC, Nichols AJ, et al. Pharmacologic differentiation of pre- and post-junctional alpha$_2$-adrenoceptors. Hypertension 1986; 4 (suppl 6): S189-92.
18. Ruffolo RR Jr, Sulpizio AC, Nichols AJ, Demarinis RM, Hieble JP. Pharmacologic differentiation between pre- and postjunctional α_2-adrenoceptors by SK&F 104078. Naunyn-Schmiedeberg's Arch Pharmacol 1987; 336: 415-8.
19. Daly RN, Sulpizio AC, Levitt B, et al. Evidence for heterogenity between pre- and postjunctional alpha-$_2$ adrenoceptors using 9-substituted 3-benzazepines. J Pharmacol Exp Ther 1988; 247: 122-7.
20. Hieble JP, Sulpizio AC, Nichols AJ, Willette RN, Ruffolo RR Jr. Pharmacologic characterization of SK&F 104078, a novel alpha-$_2$-adrenoceptor antagonist which discriminates between pre- and postjunctional alpha2-adrenoceptors. J Pharmacol Exp 1988; 247: 645-52.
21. Van Meel JAC, de Zoeten K, Timmermans PBMWM, van Zwieten PA. Impairment by nifedipine of vasopressor responses to stimulation of postsynaptic α_2-adrenoceptors in ganglion-blocked rabbits. Further evidence for the selective inhibition of the postsynaptic α-adrenoceptor-induced pressor responses by calsium entry blockade. J Auton Pharmacol 1982; 2: 13-20.
22. Cavero I, Shepperson NB, LeFèvre-Borg F, Langer SZ. Differential inhibition of vascular smooth muscle responses to and α_2-adrenoceptor agonists by dilitazem and verapamil. Circ Res 1983; 52 (suppl I): I-69-76.
23. Llenas J, Massingham R. A comparison of the effects of verapamil and cinnarizine upon responses elicted by selective α_1- and α_2-adrenoceptor agonists in the autoperfused canine hindlimb. Eur J Pharmacol 1983; 87: 53-9.
24. Cauvin C, Loutzenhiser R, van Breemen C. Mechanisms of calsium antagonist-induced vasodilatation. Ann Rev Pharmacol Toxicol 1983; 23; 373-96.
25. Holck MI, Jones CHM, Haeusler G. Differential interactions of clonidine and methoxamine with the post-synaptic alpha adrenoceptor of rabbit main pulmonary artery. J Cardiovasc Pharmacol 1983; 5: 240-8.
26. Janssens W, Verhaeghe R. Sources of calcium used during alpha$_1$ and alpha$_2$-adrenergic contractions in canine saphenous veins. J Physiol 1984; 347: 525-32.
27. Knight DR, Vatner SF. Calcium channel blockers induce preferential coronary vasodilation by an α_1- mechanism. Am J Physiol 1987; 253: H604-13.
28. Wynsen JC, Gross GJ, Brooks HL, Warltier DC. Changes in adrenergic pressor responses by calcium channel modulation in conscious dogs. Am J Physiol 1987; 253: H531-9.
29. Skomedal T, Osnes JB, Øye I. Competitive blockade of α-adrenergic receptors in rat heart by prazosin. Acta Pharmacol Toxicol 1980; 47: 217-22.
30. Benfey BG. Function of myocardial α-adrenoceptors. Life Sci 1982; 31: 101-12.
31. Sheridan DJ, Penkoske PA, Sobbel E, Corr PB. Alpha adrenergic contribution to dys-

rythmia during myocardial ischemia and reperfusion in cats. J Clin Invest 1980; 65: 161-71.
32. Aubry ML, Davey MJ, Petch B. Cardioprotective and antidysrhythmic effects of α_2-adrenoceptor blockade during myocardial ischaemia and reperfusion in the dog. J Cardiovasc Pharmacol 1985; 7 (suppl. 6): S93-S102.
33. Corr PB, Shayman JA, Kramer JB, Kipnis RJ. Increased renergic receptors in ischaemic cat myocardium. J Clin Invest 1981; 67: 1232-6.
34. de Mey J, Vanhoutte PM. Uneven distribution of postjunctional $alpha_1$- and $alpha_2$-like adrenoceptors in canine arterial and venous smooth muscle. Circ Res 1981; 48: 875-83.
35. Weinstein JS, Grossman W, Weintraub RM, Thurer RL, Johnson RG, Morgan KG. Differences in α-adrenergic responsiveness between human internal mammary arteries and saphenous veins. Circulation 1989; 79: 1264-70.
36. Rimele TJ, Rooke TW, Aarhus LL, Vanhoutte PM. Alpha-1 adrenoceptors and calcium in isolated canine coronary arteries. J Pharmacol Exp Ther 1983; 226: 668-72.
37. Heusch G, Deussen A, Schipke J, Thämer V. α_1- and α_2-adrenoceptor-mediated vasoconstriction of large and small canine coronary arteries in vivo. J Cardiovasc Pharmacol 1984; 6: 961-8.
38. Young MA, Vatner SF. Regulation of large coronary arteries. Circ Res 1986; 59: 579-96.
39. Woodman OL, Vatner SF. Coronary vasoconstriction mediated by α_1- and α_2-adrenoceptors in conscious dogs. Am J Physiol (Heart Circ Physiol 22) 1987; 253: H388-93.
40. Westby J, Kvitting P, Birkeland S, Grong K, Lekven J. Does α_1-adrenergic blockade influence regional blood flow regulation in hearts with coronary artery occlusion? Clin Physiol 1989; 9: 107-20.
41. Kvitting P, Westby J, Birkeland S, Lekven J, Grong K. Regional perfusion in hearts with acute coronary artery occlusion and subsequent β_2- and α_1-adrenergic blockade. Clin Physiol 1990 (in press).
42. Liang IYS, Jones CE. α_1-adrenegic blockade increases coronary blood flow during coronary hypoperfusion. Am J Physiol 1985; 249: H1070-7.
43. Dai XZ, Sublett E, Lindstrom P, Schwartz JS, Homans DC, Bache RJ. Coronary flow during exercise after selective α_1- and α_2-adrenergixc blockade. Am J Physiol 1989; 256:H1148-55.
44. Gwirtz PA, Overn SP, Mass HJ, Jones CE. α_1-Adrenergic constriction limits coronary flow and cardiac function in running dogs. Am J Physiol 1986; 250: H1117-26.
45. Holtz J, Saeed M, Sommer O, Bassenge E. Norepinephrine constricts the canine coronary bed via postsynaptic α_2-adrenoceptors. Eur J Pharmacol 1982; 82: 199-202.
46. Heusch G, Deussen A. The effects of cardiac sympathetic nerve stimulation on perfusion of stenotic coronary arteries in the dog. Circ Res 1983; 53: 8-15.
47. Deussen A, Heusch G, Thaemer V. α_2-adrenoceptor-mediated coronary vasoconstriction persists after exhaustion of coronary dilator reserve. Eur J Pharmacol 1985; 115: 147-53.
48. Saeed M, Holtz J, Elsner D, Bassenge E. Sympathetic control of myocardial oxygen balance in dogs mediated by activation of coronary vascular α_2-adrenoceptors. J Cardiovasc Pharm 1985; 7: 167-73.
49. Kopia GA, Kopaciewics LJ, Ruffolo RR Jr. Alpha adrenoceptor regulation of coronary artery blood flow in normal and stenotic canine coronary arteries. J Pharmacol Exp Ther 1986; 239: 641-7.
50. Woodman OL. The role of α_1- and α_1-adrenoceptors in the coronary vasoconstrictor responses to neuronally released and exogenous noradrenalin in the dog. Arch Pharmacol 1987; 336: 161-8.
51. Chiariello M, Ribeiro LGT, Davis MA, Maroko PR. "Reverse coronary steal" induced by coronary vasoconstriction following coronary artery occlusion in dogs. Circulation 1977; 56: 809-15.

52. Gewirtz H, Most AS, Williams DO. The effect of generalized alpha-receptor stimulation on regional myocardial blood flow distal to a severe coronary artery stenosis. Circulation 1982; 65: 1329-36.
53. Jones CE, Farrell TA, Ator R. Evidence that a coronary α-adrenergic tone limits myocardial blood flow and oxygenation in acute hemorrhagic hypotension. Circ Shock 1983; 11: 329-40.
54. Nathan HJ, Feigl O. Adrenergic vasoconstriction lessens transmural steal during coronary hypoperfusion. Am J Physiol 1986; 250: H645-53.
55. Dole WP. Autoregulation of the coronary circulation. Exhaustion of coronary dilator reserve. Progr Cardiovasc Dis 1987; 29: 293-323.
56. Young MA, Knight DR, Vatner SF. Autonomic control of large coronary arteries and resistance vessels. Progr Cardiovas Dis 1987; 30: 211-34.
57. Chilian W, Ackell PH. Transmural differences in sympathetic coronary constriction during exercise in the presence of coronary stenosis. Circ Res 1988; 62: 216-25.
58. Vincent J, Elliot HL, Meredith PA, Reid JL. Doxazosin, an α_1-adrenoceptor antagonist: pharmacokinetics and concentration-effect relationship in man. Br J Clin Pharmacol 1983; 15: 719-25.
59. Young RA, Brogden RN. Doxazosin. A review of its pharmacokinetic properities, and therapeutic efficacy in mild and moderate hypertension. Drugs 1988; 35: 525-41.
60. Heyndrickx GR, Muylaert P, Pannier JL. α-adrenergic control of oxygen delivery to myocardium during exercise in conscious dogs. Am J Physiol 1982; 242: H805-9.
61. Huang AH, Feigl EO. Adrenergic vasoconstriction helps maintain uniform transmural blood flow distribution during exercise. Circ Res 1988; 62: 286-98.
62. Seitelberger R, Guth BD, Heusch G, Lee JD, Katayama K, Ross J Jr. Intracoronary α_2-adrenergic receptor blockade attenuates ischemia in conscious dogs during exercise. Circ Res 1988; 62: 436-42.
63. Chiariello M, Brevetti G, de Rosa G, et al. Protective effects of simultaneous alpha and beta adrenergic receptor blockade on myocardial cell necrosis after coronary artery occlusion in rats. Am J Cardiol 1980; 46: 249-54.
64. Heber ME, Rosenthal E, Thomas N, et al. Effect of labetalol on indices of myocardial necrosis in patients with suspected acute infarction. Eur Heart J 1987; 8: 11-18.
65. Braunwald E. Control of myocardial oxygen consumption. Am J Cardiol 1971; 27: 416-32.
66. Fox KM, Tomlinson IW, Portal RW, Aber CP. Prognostic significance of acute systolic hypertension after myocardial infarction. Br Med J 1975; 3: 128-30.
67. Christensen DJ, Ford M, Reading J, Castle CH. Effect of hypertension on myocardial rupture after myocardial infarction. Chest 1977; 72: 618-22.
68. Kelly DT, Delgado CE, Taylor DR, Pitt B, Ross RS. Use of phentolamine in acute myocardial infarction associated with hypertension and left ventricular failure. Circulation 1973; 47: 729-35.
69. Renard M, Jacobs P, Liebens I, Abou Hamdam B, Bernard R. A comparison of the effects of combined or separate alpha- and beta-blockade in the treatment of hypertension in the acute stage of myocardial infarction. Int J Cardiol 1986; 10: 149-58.
70. Majid PA, Sharma B, Taylor SH. Phentolamine for vasodilator treatment of severe heart-failure. Lancet 1971; 2: 719-24.
71. Hockings BEF, Cope GD, Clarke GM, Taylor RR. Randomised controlled trial of vasodilator therapy after myocardial infarction. Am J Cardiol 1981; 48: 345-52.
72. Verma SP, Silke B, Hussain M, et al. First-line treatment of left ventricular failure complicating acute myocardial infarction: a randomised evaluation of immediate effects of diuretic, venodilator, arteriodilator, and positive inotropic drugs on left ventricular function. J Cardiovasc Pharmacol 1987; 10: 38-46.

73. Yusuf S. An overview of the clinical trials of agents (other than β-blockers) that potentially limit myocardial infarct size. J Cardiovasc Pharmacol 1988; 12 (suppl 1): S48-S55.

32

Percutaneous transluminal coronary angioplasty

PER HENNINGSEN

Atherosclerosis of the coronary arteries is a progressive and incurable disease, and prevention has not been able to demonstrate any worth-while results regarding a reduction in the incidence and for this reason there is considerable necessity for palliative treatment. The latter has also demonstrated especially good results.

Since the Swiss radiologist *Andreas Grüntzig* reported in 1978 (1) his first successful percutaneous transluminal coronary angioplastis (PTCA), this method for the palliative treatment of atherosclerotic stenosis of the coronary arteries has become wide-spread in those countries where the incidence of ischaemic heart disease is high, for example in the USA and Western Europe.

In the USA, a central registry for PTCA was established shortly after the publication of Grüntzig's report, under the auspecies of the National Heart, Lung and Blood Institute (NHLBI). This register was able to report on the first 600 PTCA carried out in the USA and Europe in a total of 34 centres in 1982 (2). Since then, the development has almost run riot. In 1989 almost 300,000 PTCA were carried out in the USA and almost 200,000 in Western Europe. It is noteworthy, that the number of coronary by-pass operations (CABG) within the same period has risen to similar heights, thus, roughly 1 million patients per year are given invasive treatment for their ischaemic heart disease; about one half employing CABG and the other half PTCA. The Scandinavian countries have been somewhat behind in this respect, and first began PTCA treatment in 1983-84. While the PTCA frequency in the USA is now more than 1,000 per 1 million inhabitants per year, there are considerable differences in Europe, ranging from 600 PTCA per million inhabitants in Holland to roughly 50 per million in Denmark.

The explanation of this extensive expansion is mainly that we now have, for the treatment of the main manifestation of ischaemic heart disease, angina pectoris, a method that is effective, reasonably simple to carry out and does not subject the patient to greater stress. However, part of the explanation is that the indications for the procedure have been extended and with this the number of patients liable to benefit from the procedure.

Indication for PTCA

There are two aspects with regard to the indication: 1) the clinical, i.e., the patient's symptoms (frequently classified according to the Canadian Cardiovascular Society's 4 classes), which indicate angiography and 2) the pathoanatomy of the coronary arteries, upon which the technical evaluation of whether PTCA is possible and reasonable, with acceptable risks.

In the first report from the NHLBI registry, 97% of the patients were in CCS class 2-4 (60% in class 3 and 4), and 80% had one vessel disease with a short, proximal, discrete, non-calcified stenosis and good left ventricular function (3).

ISFC/WHO Task Force.

Class I: Accepted indications
Chronic stable angina unresponsive to medical therapy or unstable angina:

1. Preferably with objective evidence of myocardial ischaemia
2. With good left ventricular function
3. With a single significant coronary stenosis suitable for PTCA

Class II: Evolving indications

1. Chronic stable angina or unstable angina in patients with multivessel disease
2. Angina in patients with recent coronary occlusion (less than three months)
3. No angina or mild angina following medical therapy with a strongly positive exercise stress test
4. Documented variant angina with significant fixed lesions
5. Acute myocardial infarction
6. Angina after coronary by-pass surgery
7. Angina in inoperable/high-risk patients
8. Angina in elderly patients ($\geq$75 years)

Class III: Relative contra-indications

1. No angina or mild angina without evidence of myocardial ischaemia
2. Severe left ventricular dysfunction (ejection fraction <25%)
3. Significant left main coronary artery stenosis
4. Patients in whom the only lesions are chronic coronary occlusions (older than three months)

Recently, two official reports were published on "Task Forces on Coronary Angioplasty". One report by the International Society and Federation of Cardiology, in cooperation with the World Health Organisation (4) which divide the indications into 3 classes.

These indications include patients without angina pectoris, but with a positive exercise test, all patients with acute myocardial infarction (AMI), irrespective of whether they have angina pectoris or not, and all patients above the age of 75 years with angina pectoris.

The other report, from the American College of Cardiology/American Heart Association Task Force, goes even further, and in actual fact, lays most emphasis on contra-indications, so that patients who have been subjected to angiography must be subjected to angioplasty if this is technically possible and the risk acceptable. A complicated table has been compiled, where the indications depend on the symptoms, degree of ischaemia, the coronary pathoanatomy and the expectations regarding sucess and/or complications to PTCA.

The absolute contra-indications are:

1. No significant obstruction
2. Multi vessel disease with severe, diffuse atherosclerosis
3. Left main branch lesion (unless protected by a graft)
4. No surgical back-up

Seven relative contra-indications are also given, of which the following are worthy of mention: blood coagulation disorders, no evidence of ischaemia, the dilatated vessel supplying more than 40% of the myocardium, variant angina with stenosis less than 60%. In addition, some more technical contra-indication are mentioned. It can be clearly seen that the indications from being very restrictive have gone over to being consideration as to the technical possibility of carrying out the procedure against the risks involved. In order to determine whether this widening of the indications is justified, one has to look at the risks incured, i.e., complications to the procedure itself, results, both immediate and long-term, as well as special indications, i.e., unstable angina pectoris, post-AMI treatment, and graft dilatation etc.

A not inconsiderable percentage of the increase in the number of PTCA results from the improvement in technical equipment: smaller balloons, coated balloons, thinner catheters, better guide-wires etc., which has meant that more and narrower stenoses can be dilatated, and that even occluded vessels can be re-opened. These technical aspects of the procedure will not be discussed here – or only very briefly.

Success and complications

The immediate success rate and frequency of complications have been the object of considerable improvement from the first data supplied by the NHLBI registry, where 63% of the attempts at PTCA were successful with a 9.2% more serious complication rate (AMI, acute CABG or death) (3) to a few very routined, American centres with a success rate of 95% with 2-3% serious complications (6). This results partly from the greater routine of the cardiologists who carry out the procedure and partly from selection of patients (7).

In the larger European centres, dilatation is successful in 76-91%, with serious complications in 6.8-10% and a mortality of less than 0.5% (8, 9).

An analysis was attempted of 400 PTCA in order to find predictors of acute complications, the most important being acute occlusion of the dilatated vessel (10). Clinically, women had acute closure twice as often as men, while age, diabetes, smoking, hyperlipidaemia, unstable angina pectoris and re-PTCA were of no importance. There were, in contrast, several angiographic variables which were of predictive value in respect of complications: stenoses where the vessel bent or branched, long stenoses, eccentric stenoses as well as two and three vessel disease and thromboses.

Two and three vessel disease

The indications have been widened, in step with the improved results, from mainly applying to patients with atherosclerosis in one vessel to two and three vessel disease. The same success rate can be achieved (90%) by careful selection of these patients and with only a slight increase in the frequency of complications (11%) as compared to one vessel disease (11). The mortality with PTCA is, however, higher for patients with two or three vessel disease (1-2%) than for patients with one vessel disease, and in some studies higher than with CABG (12). Part of the explanation of this is that a number of patients subjeceted to PTCA having two or three vessel disease are inoperable in respect of CABG, and therefore cannot be subjected to acute coronary surgery if the dilatated vessel should close during the procedure. Acute CABG occurs in 4-6% and is accompanied by myocardial infarction in approx. 50%. This complication has, however, been reduced considerably following the introduction of the perfusion catheter, which ensures circulation during the waiting time for surgery. The surgeons, as a rule, are unable to employ the internal mammary artery in acute cases. The procedure of PTCA in cases of two or three vessel disease has frequently to be carried out in several sessions and is therefore relatively expensive.

Stenosis of the left main branch has been considered a contra-indication to PTCA, as it is related to serious risk (i.e., the patient's death if the main branch should close acutely) unless the main branch is protected by a graft to at least one of the two left-sided arteries (13) or a good collateral circulation is present from the non-stenosed right coronary artery.

Long-term results with one vessel disease

The long-term results in patients with one vessel disease are favourable. One thousand patients in the NHLBI registry from 13 laboratories were followed for 5 years (14). Sixtythree per cent of the patients were in functional class 3 or 4 at the time of treatment. Five years later, 65% were free from symptoms and 31% in group 1 or 2. Thirteen per cent had been subjected to re-angioplasty. The annual mortality was approx. 1%, and there were 1.6% non-fatal AMI per year. However, it has been demonstrated that patients with one vessel disease, who are given medical or surgical treatment also have a good prognosis (15). The advantage thus lies in the fact that PTCA patients have fewer symptoms than those under medical treatment, and that PTCA treatment is cheaper and less traumatic than CABG. However, randomized studies of whether the one method of treatment is most advantageous, partly from the patient's point of view and partly from a financial point of view, are lacking.

Long-term results with two or three vessel disease

Sufficiently re-vascularised two or three vessel disease has a good prognosis also, but the follow-up time has often only been a couple of years. Seventyfour per cent of the patients are symptom-free, 16% in functional class 1. Thirty per cent have been subjected to re-PTCA (11). Insufficiently re-vascularised patients (i.e., where one or more stenoses of more than 70% reduction in diameter still remain) were more frequently subjected to secondary by-pass operation and more cases of death, AMI, angina pectoris were reported than in completely re-vascularised patients. The picture is, however, somewhat confusing, inasmuch as the results depend to a great extent on the condition of the coronary vessels prior to PTCA (2 or 3 vessel disease, one or more stenoses in each vessel, occluded vessels, previous AMI, left ventricular function, duration of angina pectoris, etc.) (16, 17). It is, in addition, remarkable that the level of activity is similar for the successful and non-succesful PTCA patients with two or three vessel disease in the NHLBI registry (18). The indications for treating patients with two or three vessel disease are therefore very complicated and technical, (5) and will not be discussed further here. However, it can be said, in general, that the more stenoses that are dilatated the greater the risk of complications and re-stenosis. Until a clinically controlled study of two or three vessel, several stenoses PTCA versus CABG has been carried out, the majority of patients with two or three vessel disease will be candidates for by-pass surgery.

Occluded vessels

It is often possible to re-open occluded vessels with a special guide-wire, provided that occlusion is not too old (less than 4-6 months) or is not too long (less than 1.5 cm); it is worth trying, especially if the myocardium peripheral to the occlusion functions well. The success rate is about 67%. Sixty per cent of the patients become symptom-free and 50% of the vessels remain open.

Re-stenosis

It was reported very early in the history of balloon dilatation that in approx. 30-40% of the successfully dilatated vessels, the stenosis was re-formed within 5-6 months. Re-stenosis occurs most frequently in those with the most severe stenosis prior to dilatation, and if remains of a stenosis were present at the time of dilatation. Eccentric stenoses, long stenoses and stenoses at the site of bending or branching of the vessel more often re-stenose. Patients with duration of angina of less than 2 months, unstable angina, a positive spasm test or diabetes run a greater risk of developing re-stenosis.

Re-formation of the arteriosclerotic plaque has occurred in a few cases, but most frequently the re-stenosis has been caused by particularly strong growth of the intimal hyperplasia which always takes place at the site of dilatation following PTCA. Re-stenosis takes place within 2-4 months after the dilatation (6) and is, in about 2/3rds of the cases, accompanied by clinical recurrence. Clinical recurrence of angina pectoris occurring later will often be the result of progression of the arteriosclerotic disease (20). About 5% of PTCA patients develop clinical recurrence without showing angiographic re-stenosis.

However, there are some quite difficult problems in defining angiographic re-stenosis and relating this to the functional reduction in the coronary flow (21).

Considerable efforts have been made to reduce the frequency of re-stenosis (22). Acetylsalicylic acid appears to reduce the frequency of re-stenosis in patients with angina pectoris of more than 6 months duration. Eicosapentaenic acid treatment or a reduction in the level of cholesterol have shown some effect in a few studies, but not in others. Calcium antagonists seem to have no effect. Certain of the procedures during dilatation (long dilatation time, high ballon pressure) have no effect. The problem must presumably be solved by drug therapy, perhaps by the inhibition of certain growth factors (19).

The treatment of re-stenosis is re-dilatation, unless the coronary pathoanatomy indicates that the patient should be directly referred to CABG, or perhaps to drug treatment only. Re-dilatation should first be carried out 5 months after the initial dilatation. The frequency of secondary re-stenosis can be reduced in this manner from 40 to 20% (23).

PTCA after CABG

CABG is carried out in increasing numbers, despite the fact that surgeons feared the opposite at the time PTCA made its appearance. Five to ten per cent annually of the patients subjected to by-pass operation develop recurrent angina pectoris, which results either from a poor graft, progression of the atherosclerosis or incomplete re-vascularisation. The technique of re-operation is difficult, involves an increased risk and is only successful in about 2/3rds of the cases. The possibilities presented by angioplasty in this patient group have been discussed in a number of studies (24). Dilatation is successful in 80-94% of the cases attempted. The rate of complications (4-6%) is lower following graft dilatation than with PTCA of the cononary vessels. On average, re-stenosis occurs in about 48%, varying from 19% after dilatation of distal graft anastomoses to 56% with dilatation of the graft itself. Grafts of the internal mammary artery can be successfully dilatated (25). Patients subjected to by-pass operation who develop recurrent angina pectoris should therefore be subjected to angiography with the object of performing PTCA.

Patients above 70 years of age

PTCA has been found to be just as effective in patients above 70 years of age as in younger patients, and there is no higher frequency of complications nor re-stenosis. The long-term results are similarly good, corresponding to age (26).

Unstable angina pectoris

Unstable angina pectoris is a clinical syndrome, which is difficult to define. In many American studies the term unstable angina and recently occurring angina pectoris are employed synonymously, thus up to 67% of patients in an angina pectoris population are termed unstable. The reason is that many consider angina pectoris unstable until it has been stable for 2-3 months. In Europe the requirement for the diagnosis is that prolonged periods of pain at rest have to be present with electrocardiographic signs of ischaemia and no increase in enzymes, however, accelerating angina triggered by exercise is termed unstable. The angiographic picture is a severe stenosis (>90%) with one, two or three vessel disease. Coronary angioscopy (27) and autopsy (28) have demonstrated plaque-fissure and thrombus formation in the majority of these patients. The risk is of developing AMI and sudden death.

The treatment has been intensive drug therapy or, if this fails, CABG. Seveval studies, also larger series, describe good results of PTCA (29, 30), some with higher frequencies of complications and more re-stenoses than following PTCA in cases of stable angina pectoris, others without. Thus, *Plokker et al* (31) treated 469 patients having unstable, drug intractable angina pectoris with PTCA successfully in 88-90% and with a mortality of 1%. The actuarial survival was 94% at 5 years with 79% having no angina pectoris, AMI, re-PTCA, CABG or death. The results correspond to those achieved with stable angina pectoris, although there was no control group. Some have given treatment with thrombolytic agents and have been able, in this manner, to eliminate the angina pectoris, but there were 25% with bleeding complications (32). *Mayo et al* found that the complications were halved provided one waited 2 weeks after the onset of symptoms before carrying out PTCA (33). In patients with multiple vessel disease, it is only necessary to dilate the "unstable" stenosis.

The conclusion is that patients with unstable angina pectoris should be subjected to angiography and invasive PTCA or CABG, if they do not rapidly become symptom-free following medical treatment, and in actual fact, all patients with unstable angina pectoris should be subjected to angiography prior to deciding the continued treatment. However, controlled studies comparing the three types of treatment are lacking.

PTCA after acute myocardial infarction

Thrombolytic treatment has, in later years, become the standard treatment of patients with AMI, if the treatment can be commenced within the first

6 hours after the onset of symptoms. Thrombolytic treatment does not, however, remove the causative stenosis with or without plaque rupture. It is therefore natural to supplement thrombolytic treatment with angioplasty. This could present two advantages: 1, reduce the frequency of re-occlusion and re-infarction and, 2, re-establish full perfusion of the myocardium and with this the function of the left ventricle.

These aspects have been studied in several different set-ups. The European Cooperative Study Group (34) randomized 367 patients treated with thrombolysis to conservative treatment or angiography and angioplasty; the later was carried out on average 42 minutes after commencing the treatment with a thrombolytic agent. PTCA reduced the extent of the stenosis and increased perfusion in the infarct related artery, but the price was a high frequency of re-occlusion, a considerably higher incidence of episodes of ischaemia, hypotension, ventricular fibrillation and bleeding complications. The mortality in the invasive group was more than twice as high as in the conservative group. There was no difference in left ventricular function between the two groups. The study group concluded that there was no advantage to be gained from immediate PTCA of patients with AMI.

A group under the National Institute of Health (The Thrombolyses and Angioplasty in Myocardial Infarction (TAMI) Trial) also found an increased mortality and increased number of by-pass operated patients in those treated with PTCA. The same TAMI group, found that one third of the dilatated arteries re-occluded, and that no improvement was seen in left ventricular function, and therefore the treatment could not be recommended (35).

The TAMI group (36) found, by comparing acute and late (7-10 days) PTCA treated AMI patients, that there was a similar incidence of re-occlusion and similar ventricular ejection fraction on discharge in the two groups. In addition, the mortality and frequency of by-pass surgery were higher in the acute group. Neither have smaller studies of acute PTCA versus thrombolysis shown any significant differences in the mortality, or the left ventricular function, but, a lower degree of stenosis in the PTCA treated patients (37). Neither could this be seen even when the thrombolytic agent was given intracoronarily (38). This acute treatment strategy was feared by many cardiologists because it would have entailed considerable expense and added duty time for the cardiological laboratories, the numbers of which should be increased considerably in order to comply with these demands. However, the results provided the basis for many cardiologists, especially those in the USA, who would prefer to send their patients home with "open vessels", in other words, that all AMI patients are PTCA treated when the most acute phase has passed. The question then remains, is this justifiable?

The second study of the Thrombolyses In Myocardial Infarction (TIMI) included 3262 AMI patients treated with thrombolysis, randomized to PTCA – if possible – after 18-48 hours, or conservative treatment, i.e., PTCA in only patients who showed spontaneous or exercise induced ischaemia. Fiftyseven per cent in the first group were subjected to PTCA, 16% in the conservative group. There was no difference in the incidence of re-infarction or death, neither was there any difference in the ejection fraction within 42 days between the two groups. This also applied to the 3-year follow-up between smaller randomized groups in respect of the morbidity and mortality between PTCA treated and conservatively treated patients (40). The prophylactic value of PTCA after AMI is thus not demonstrated, and the TIMI group suggest a "watchfull waiting" strategy after thrombolysis, i.e., angiography and PTCA with symptoms or positive exercise ECG.

However, not all the European centres will term this strategy as conservative. We do not know whether drug therapy is just as good as invasive treatment in this patient group. *Holt et al* (41) found a high frequency of acute CABG and other cardiac events about 2 years after AMI in patients treated with PTCA. There was no control group, and one does not know the spontaneous course in corresponding patients. A controlled study of invasive treatment (PTCA or CABG) versus drug therapy after AMI in patients with angina pectoris or a positive exercise ECG has been planned in Denmark (DANAMI). Patients will be followed for 1 and 5 years.

A small group of AMI patients with cardiogenic shock appears to gain advantage from rapid (a few hours) PTCA treatment. Both the mortality and the long-term results are improved dramatically (42).

PTCA and left ventricular function

There are contradictory reports as to whether PTCA can improve left ventricular function. There is, however, no doubt that "stunned" myocardium with reduced or absent wall movement, but with post extrasystolic improvement of contractility and the uptake of thalliunm 201 in the affected areas, can be brought to function normally following dilatation of the stenosis in the related vessels (43). The diastolic function of the left ventricle can also be improved (44).

PTCA in patients with no or very little angina pectoris

Asymptomatic patients or those with minimal symptoms, with or without "silent ischaemia", will often be subjected to coronary arteriography and be found suitable for PTCA treatment. It is, however, an unanswered question as to whether this treatment should be carried out even though the centre in question has good results and few complications. It is known from among other sources, the CASS studies, that patients with one and two vessel disease and good ventricular function – who comprise the majority of this group of PTCA candidates – have a good prognosis when on drug therapy (45). Patients with the best improvement in prognosis – three vessel disease and poor left ventricular function – following invasive treatment (CABG) are rarely suitable for PTCA. In addition, the initial PTCA will often, of necessity, be followed by re-PTCA or CABG (46), and thus it will be necessary to look at the costs. The problem will hardly be solved before the results of a randomized, controlled clinical investigation are available, for example those of the Veterans Administration ACME study.

Costs and advantages of PTCA versus CABG

One of the arguments for PTCA, since the start of the PTCA era, has been that it is the cheaper of the two. In respect of one vessel disease, *Reeder et al* (47) found that PTCA was 15% cheaper than CABG, when measured over the first year. *Black et al* (48) found a considerable spreading of the costs with regard to multiple vessel PTCA (mean: 9,138 $, range: 4,820-33,820) versus CABG (mean: 22,771 $ range: 15,601-66,322). It is not clear whether the costs of surgical stand by have been included. There is agreement that treatment of re-stenosis after PTCA, either re-PTCA or CABG, increases the costs of this procedure considerably.

The advantages of PTCA rather than CABG include shorter hospitalization, shorter convalescence and a less traumatic procedure. The CASS study showed that almost all were working prior to CABG, but that the number fell by about 20% over the next 5 years (49). Several studies have shown that 84-100% of PTCA patients return to work (50), and that several factors play a role: age above 50 years, whether or not the patient was working prior to treatment and the presence or absence of angina pectoris. It appears that the patient's own attitude to the problem is more important than medical factors (51). The problem is accentuated in countries where there is a long waiting time. In particular, this can be up to one year for surgery, while for PTCA it is often merely a question of a few weeks or months. Patients with a waiting time of more than 3 months after the decision to carry out invasive treatment has been made and until treatment has been concluded, rarely work again.

Similar to after CABG, patients treated with PTCA have a higher quality of life – in other words, less pain, greater physical capacity and less drug consumption – than patients given medical treatment. Which of the two invasive methods is best suited to which patients must await the results of clinical controlled investigations, partly under the control of NHLBI, By-pass, Angioplasty, Re-vascularisation, Intervention (BARI) and partly at the Emory University in Atlanta, Emory Angioplasty or Surgery Trial (EAST) as well as an English study: The Randomized Intervention Treatment of Angina (RITA) Trial (52), a French (CABRI) and a German study.

The future and development

Angioplasty has during its short existence established itself as an invasive, palliative treatment of angina pectoris. There are, however, still a number of unsolved problems in several respects. Just how are the results when compared to drug therapy of patients with slight angina pectoris? – How are they for multiple vessel disease as compared to CABG? – Which post-AMI patients should be treated invasively, and who should be given drug therapy? Current randomized, clinically controlled studies will hopefully provide an answer to these questions.

Another problem is re-stenosis, which still runs at 30-35%. Several technical innovations are being tested in order to make dilatation more effective, both in the short and long term. Laser beams, partly as sources of warmth, partly "naked" (Excimer Laser (53)) have been tried on patients and have shown promising results. Special units for percutaneous, transluminal, intracoronary arterectomy (Simpson's atherocath.) are being tested clinically; as is a diamond drill, which rotates at a speed of 50,000 RPM (Rotablator). All of these methods for the removal of arteriosclerotic plaques must, as a rule, be followed by balloon dilatation.

In order to reduce the rate of re-stenosis, both acute and chronic, *Sigwart* has been working with intravascular stents (54), which unfortunately present a number of problems. In all probability the problem of re-stenosis will be solved medically; a number appear to be the result of spasms (55).

One must conclude that at present we have not yet seen "the end of the line" in respect of PTCA treatment. However, we must still remember that it is a palliative treatment of a chronic, progressive disease, and that in many patients, one of the most important effects of PTCA treatment will be to delay by-pass operation for up to 5-10 years. Both invasive methods await effective drug prophylaxis and therapeutic methods, which are not available today.

References

1. Grüntzig AR. Transluminal dilatation of coronary artery stenosis. Lancet 1978; 1: 263.
2. Kent MK, Bentivoglio LG, Block PC, et al. Percutaneous Transluminal Coronary Angioplasty. Report from the Registry of the National Heart, Lung and Blood Institute. Am J Cardiol 1982; 49: 2011-20.
3. Dorros G, Cowley MJ, Simpson J, et al. Percutaneous Transluminal Coronary Angioplasty. Report of complications from the National Heart, Lung and Blood Institute, PTCA Registry. Circulation 1983; 67: 723-30.
4. Bourassa MG, Alderman EL, Bertram DM, et al. Report of the Joint ISFC/WHO Task Force on Coronary Angioplasty. Circulation 1988; 78: 780-9.
5. Fisch C, Desanctis RW, Dodge HT, Reeves TJ, Weinberg SL. Guidelines for Percutaneous Transluminal Coronary Angioplasty. Circulation 1988; 78: 486-502.
6. Anderson HV, Roubin GS, Leimgruber PP, Douglas JS Jr, King III SB, Grüntzig AR. Primary angiographic success rate of Percutaneous Transluminal Coronary Angioplasty. Am J Cardiol 1985; 56: 712-7.
7. Hamad N, Pechard AK, Lyle HRP, Lindsay J. Results of Percutaneous Transluminal Coronary Angioplasty by multiple, relatively low frequency operators 1986-87 experience. Am J Cardiol 1988; 61: 1229-31.
8. Ellis SG, Roubin GS, King III SB, et al. Angiographic and clinical predictors of acute closure after native vessel coronary angioplasty. Circulation 1988; 77: 372-9.
9. Steffenino G, Meier B, Finci L, et al. Acute complications of elective coronary angioplasty: a review of 500 consecutive procedures. Br Heart J 1988; 59: 151-8.
10. Sowton E, Timis AD, Crick JCP, et al. Early results after Percutaneous Transluminal Coronary Angioplasty in 400 patients. Br Heart J 1986; 56: 115-20.
11. Disciascio G, Cowley MJ, Vetrovec GW, Kelly KM, Lewis SA. Triple vessel coronary angioplasty: Acute outcome and long-term results. J Am Coll Cardiol 1988; 12: 42-8.
12. Detre K, Holubkov R, Kelsey S, et al. Percutaneous Transluminal Coronary Angioplasty in 1985-86 and 1977-88. N Engl J Med 1988; 318: 265-70.
13. O'Keefe JH, Hartzler GO, Rutherford BD, et al. Left main coronary angioplasty early and late results of 127 acute and elective procedures. Am J Cardiol 1989; 64: 144-7.
14. Kent KM, Cowley MJ, Kelsey CF, et al. Long term follow-up of the NHLBI-PTCA Registry. Circulation 1986; 74 (suppl 2): II 280.
15. Danchin N, Brengard A, Ethevenot G, et al. Ten year follow-up of patients with single vessel disease that was suitable for Percutaneous Transluminal Coronary Angioplasty. Br Heart J 1988; 59: 275.
16. Reeder GS, Holmes DR, Detre K, Costigan T, Kelsley SF. Degree of revascularization in patients with multivessel coronary disease: a report from the NHLBI PTCA Registry. Circulation 1988; 77: 638-44.
17. Deligonul U, Vandormael MG, Kern MJ, Zelman R, Galan K, Chaitman BR. Coronary Angioplasty: A therapeutic option for symtomatic patients with two and three vessel coronary disease. J Am Coll Cardiol 1988; 11: 1173-9.
18. Detre K, Holubkov R, Kelsey S, et al. One year follow-up results of the 1985-86 NHLBI's PTCA Registry. Circulation 1989; 80: 421-8.
19. Liu MW, Roubin GS, King III SB. Restenosis after coronary angioplasty. Circulation 1989; 79: 1374-87.
20. Cequir A, Bonan R, Crépeau J, et al. Restenosis and progression of coronary atherosclerosis after coronary angioplasty. J Am Coll Cardiol 1988; 12: 49-55.
21. Serruys PW, Luijten HE, Beatt J, et al. Incidence of restenosis after successfull coronary angioplasty: a timerelated phenomenon. J Am Coll Cardiol 1989; 77: 361-71.

22. Blackshear JL, O'Callaghan WG, Califf RM. Medical approaches to prevention of restenoses after coronary angioplasty. J Am Coll Cardiol 1987; 9: 834-48.
23. Black AJR, Anderson HV, Roubin GS, Powelson SW, Douglas JS, King III SB. Repeat coronary angioplasty: correlate of a second restenosis. J Am Coll Cardiol 1988; 11: 714-8.
24. Chokshi SK, Meyers S, Abi-Mansour P. Percutaneous Transluminal Coronary Angioplasty: ten years experience. Progr Cardiovasc Dis 1987; 30: 147- 210.
25. Simshak TM, Giorgi LV, Johnson WL, et al. Application of Percutaneous Transluminal Coronary Angioplasty to the internal mammary artery graft. J Am Coll Cardiol 1988; 12: 1205-14.
26. Simpendorfer C, Raymond R, Schraider J, et al. Early and long-term results of Percutaneous Transluminal Coronary Angioplasty in patients 70 years of age and older with angina pectoris. Am J Cardiol 1988; 62: 959-61.
27. Sherman CT, Litvak F, Grundfest W, et al. Coronary angioscopy in patients with unstable angina pectoris. N Engl J Med 1986; 315: 913-9.
28. Falk E. Unstable angina with fatal outcome: dynamic coronary thrombosis leading to infarction and/or sudden death. Circulation 1985; 71: 699-708.
29. Defeyter PJ, Serruys PW, Van den Brand M, et al. Emergency coronary angioplasty in refractory unstable angina. N Engl J Med 1985; 313: 342-6.
30. Halon DA, Merdler A, Shefer A, Flugelman MY, Lewes BS. Indentifying patients at high risk for restenosis after Percutaneous Transluminal Coronary Angioplasty for unstable angina pectoris. Am J Cardiol 1989; 64: 289-93.
31. Plokker HWT, Ernst MPG, Bal ET, et al. Percutaneous Transluminal Coronary Angioplasty with unstable angina pectoris refractory to medical therapy long-term clinical and angiographic results. Cath Cardiovasc Diag 1988; 14: 15-8.
32. Topol EJ, Nicklas JM, Kander NH, et al. Coronary revascularization after intravenous tissue plasminogen activator for unstable angina pectoris: results of a randomized double-blind, placebo-controlled trial. Am J Cardiol 1988; 62: 368-71.
33. Mayo J, Myler RK, Webb J, Shae RE, Stertzen SH, Ryan C. Is timing after coronary angioplasty (PTCA) important for early and late outcome in unstable angina pectoris. Circulation 1989; 80-II: 172.
34. Simoons ML, Arnold A, Betriu A, et al. Thrombolyses with tissue plasminogen activator in acute myocardial infarction: no additional benefit from immediate Percutaneous Coronary Angioplasty. Lancet 1988; I: 197-202.
35. Califf RM, Topol EJ, George BS, et al, and the TAMI Study Group. Characteristics and outcome of patients in whom reperfusion with intravenous tissue – type plasminogen activator fails: results of the thrombolysis and angioplasty in myocardial infarction (TAMI) I trial. Circulation 1988; 77: 1090-9.
36. Topol EJ, Califf RM, George BS, et al. A randomized trial of immediate versus delayed elective angioplasty after intravenous tissue plasminogen activator in acute myocardial infarction. N Engl J Med 1987; 317: 581-8.
37. DeWood MA, Fisher MJ, for the Spokane Heart Research Group. Direct Percutaneous Transluminal Coronary Angioplasty versus intravenous r-t PA in acute myocardial infarction. Preliminary results. Circulation 1989; 80: II-418.
38. O'Neill W, Timmis GC, Bourdillon PD, et al. A prospective randomiced clinical trial of intracoronary streptokinase versus coronary angioplasty for AMI. N Engl J Med 1986; 314: 812-8.
39. The TIMI Study Group. Comparison of invasive and conservative strategies after treatment with intravenous tissue plasminogen activator in acute myocardial infarction. N Engl J Med 1989; 320: 618-27.
40. Erbel R, Pop T, Diefenbach C, Meyer J. Long-term results of thrombylytic therapy with

and without Percutaneous Transluminal Coronary Angioplasty. J Am Coll Cardiol 1989; 14: 276-85.

41. Holt GW, Gersh BJ, Holmes DR, et al. Results of Percutaneous Transluminal Coronary Angioplasty for angina pectoris early after acute myocardial infarction. Am J Cardiol 1988; 61: 1238-42.
42. Verna E, Repetto S, Boscarini M, Ghezzi I, Binachi G. Emergency Coronary Angioplasty in patient with severe left ventricular dysfunction or cardiogenic shock after acute myocardial infarction. Eur Heart J 1989; 10: 958-66.
43. Cohen M, Charney R, Hersman T, Fuster V, Gorlin T, Francis X. Reversal of chronic ischemic myocardial dysfunction after transluminal coronary angioplasty. J Am Coll Cardiol 1988; 12: 1193-8.
44. Mizuno K, Arakawa K, Shibuya T, et al. Improved regional and global diastolic performance in patients with coronary artery disease after Percutaneous Transluminal Coronary Angioplasty. Am Heart J 1988; 115: 302-6.
45. Mock MB, Ringquist I, Fisher L, et al. Survival of medically treated patients in the coronary artery surgery study (CASS) Registry. Circulation 1982; 66: 562-8.
46. Snydeer LD, Baim DS, McCabe CH, et al. Should patients with mildly symptomatic angina pectoris be managed with Percutaneous Transluminal Coronary Angioplasty. Circulation 1986; 74-II: 281.
47. Reeder GS, Krishan I, Nobrega FT, et al. Is Percutaneous Transluminal Coronary Angioplasty les expensive than bypass surgery? N Eng J Med 1984; 311: 1157-62.
48. Black AJR, Roubin GS, Sutor C, et al. Comparative costs of Percutaneous Transluminal Coronary Angioplasty and coronary artery bypass grafting in multivessel coronary artery disease. Am J Cardiol 1988; 62: 809-11.
49. Coronary Artery Surgery Study (CASS). Quality of life in patientes randomly assigned to treatment groups. Circulation 1983; 68: 951-60.
50. Lairo-Meeter K, Erdman RAM, van Domburg R, et al. Probability of a return to work after either coronary ballon dialtation or coronary bypass surgery. Eur Heart J 1989; 10: 917-22.
51. Fitzgerald ST, Becker DM, Celentano DD, Swank R, Brinker J. Return to work after Percutaneous Transluminal Coronary Angioplasty. Am J Cardiol 1989; 64: 1108-12.
52. Henderson RA. The randomized intervention treatment of angina (RITA) trial protocol: a long term study of coronary angioplasty and coronary artery bypass surgery in patients with angina. Br Heart J 1989; 62: 411-4.
53. Karsch KR, Haase KK, Maiser M, et al. Percutaneous coronary excimer laser angioplasty: initial clinical results. Lancet 1989; II: 647-50.
54. Sigwart U, Puel J, Mirkovitch V, Joffre F, Kappenberger L. Intravascular stents to prevent occlusion and restenosis after transluminal angioplasty. N Engl J Med 1987; 316: 701-6.
55. Bertrand ME, Lablanche JM, Fourrier JL, Traisnel G. Percutaneous Transluminal Coronary Angioplasty in patients with spasm superimposed on atherosclerotic narrowing. Br Heart J 1987; 58: 469-72.

33

Coronary artery bypass grafting

EDVARDAS VARNAUSKAS

Introduction

It was selective coronary angiography (1) that provided the indispensible basis for the pioneering efforts of *Favaloro* (2) which resulted in the first surgical procedure able to reliably and reproducibly improve blood perfusion of ischaemic myocardium in coronary artery disease.

Coronary artery bypass grafting (CABG) marks a new milestone of therapy: revascularization of the myocardium is a realistic alternative to traditional drug-induced suppression of myocardial oxygen demand in the treatment of the clinical consequences of myocardial ischaemia.

Spectacular relief of angina pectoris following operation contributed decisively to a rapid spreading of the new procedure. Meanwhile, a claim that CABG also prevents myocardial infarction and cardiac death provoked turbulent discussions and animated debate. Eventually, many clinicians questioned the therapeutic role of CABG in treating patients with coronary artery disease.

Controlled studies appeared to be badly needed to establish the principles of the new treatment.

Clinical trials supplemented by numerous non-randomized investigations confirmed the initial clinical impression that CABG works and helped to explain why it works. Moreover, they provided guidelines for a proper timing of operation, at least in some categories of patients with coronary artery disease.

Principal effects of coronary artery bypass grafting

Practical implications of clinical trials. During the 1970s CABG was on trial in a number of studies. Our present knowledge about the principal effects of surgery is provided, to a considerable extent, by the three large trials: Veterans Administration Study (VA) (3), European Coronary Surgery Study (European) (4) and Coronary Artery Surgery Study (CASS) (5).

The advantages and limitations of design largely define the implications of these trials.

The trials were designed to compare a group of patients randomized to medical treatment with a group randomized to early surgery. For statistical comparisons, all patients alloted to medical treatment who subsequently received surgery because of worsening symptoms and all those randomized to surgery who refused operation are retained in their original randomization groups. Consequently, the trials answer an important pragmatic and practical question: Would an "aggressive" policy of immediate surgery prove superior in terms of prognosis to "conventional" treatment with medical therapy in the first place, reserving surgery for those whose symptoms demand it?

All three studies included a substantial number of patients alloted to medical treatment who subsequently received surgery and a few "surgical" patients who refused operation. It is generally recognized that "cross-overs" from experimental to conventional treatment may dilute potential benefits of the experimental treatment (6). Although study protocols stipulated criteria as the basis for making use of surgery in patients alloted to medical treatment, the final decision as to whether or not to operate was highly influenced by the physicians' interpretation of symptoms and their attitude towards emerging reports on survival benefits of surgery. Thus, a lack of positive effect of surgery in these trials may be real, or due to a significant dilution effect that may remain undetected.

On the other hand, a result favouring CABG would clearly indicate that a supposed dilution effect was insufficient to completely obscure the real potential of surgical treatment; the benefits of early surgery appeared not because of "cross-overs" but rather inspite of them.

The next question is to what extent possible differences between patient populations of the three trials may affect the results?

Principally, the trial populations consisted of male patients, younger than 66 with significant coronary artery disease and chronic angina pectoris, not sufficiently severe to warrant instant surgery. On average, however, the VA patients had distinctly more advanced symptoms and some of them had impaired left ventricular function (3); the European patients had moderate angina and good left ventricular function (4); the CASS patients constituted the most heterogeneous population – they had mild or no angina at all and two relatively small groups of them had recent myocardial infarction and

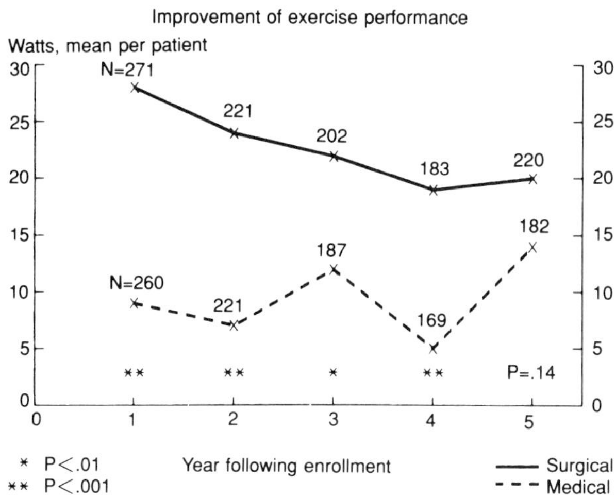

Fig. 1. *Improvement of exercise performance between 1 and 5 years after randomization as compared to baseline values. Variations of improvement among the patients alloted to the medical treatment depend to some extent on those who received surgery because of symptomatic deterioration. (European Study, 1982).*

lower than normal left ventricular ejection fraction, respectively (7). Consequently, one may suppose that the results of the two treatments would vary between the studies both with regard to total populations and to different subgroups. These differences between the patient populations and conceivable variability in results do not preclude a possibility that the three studies are complementary and that the emerging conclusions are thus applicable to a large proportion of patients with chronic coronary artery disease.

Great caution is mandatory in applying the conclusions of the trials to other categories of coronary patients.

The benefits and drawbacks of coronary surgery

CABG improves symptoms related to myocardial ischaemia. The improvement is spectacular especially in patients with refractory angina.

During the first postoperative year, *angina pectoris* ceases in 60-80% of patients and significantly decreases in an additional 10-20%. The demand for *antianginal drugs* diminishes markedly. *Physical performance* increases permiting higher levels of daily activities, Fig. 1. Although some observational studies (8) suggest an increased *return to work*, the controlled trials do not confirm this observation (9).

Later on, the initially improved "quality of life" gradually decreases with time. Annual recurrence of symptoms amounts to approximately 4% between 1 and 12 years after operation among surviving patients (10).

Surgery improves long-term survival. The policy of early surgery is superior to the policy of conventional treatment reserving surgery for those

Table 1. *Late Mortality.*

	No. of Pts.					
	M	S	M	S	M	S
European Study			*At 5 yr.*		*At 10 yr.*	
All Patients	373	394	17	8*)	30	24*)
3-VD	188	219	18	6*)	32	22*)
Markedly positive exercise ECG-test	150	159	24	8*)	38	25*)
CASS			*At 5 yr.*		*At 10 yr.*	
All Patients	390	390	8	5	21	18
3-VD	135	123	10	7	25	24
Impaired LVF	82	78	17	8	39	21*)
VA Study			*At 7 yr.*		*At 10 yr.*	
Total	354	332	30	23*)	43	42
3-VD	156	135	37	25	50	44
Impaired LVF	175	150	37	26*)	51	47

M = medical group, S = surgical group, VD = vessel disease, LVF = left ventricular function. Markedly positive Exercise ECG-test = ST deviation and/or ischaemic symptoms at a relatively low maximal workload and maximal heart rate achieved.
*) significant M-S difference.

patients whose symptoms demand it, Table 1. The survival improvement is almost exclusively due to a decreased incidence of sudden and non-sudden cardiac deaths.

As could be expected, the greatest survival benefits are observed in patients who have a relatively poor prognosis defined by older age and pathophysiologic consequences of disease – advanced myocardial ischaemia at rest and/or on exercise, impaired left ventricular function and signs of generalised atherosclerosis. The prognostically important anatomical counterparts of these clinical predictors are characterized by significant obstructions in either the main left coronary artery or the three major coronary branches (3-vessel disease). A significant stenosis in the proximal segment of the left anterior descending artery as a component of 3- or 2-vessel disease further augments the risk (11). Moreover, left ventricular ejection fraction less than 0.5 is also an independent prognostic predictor (3, 5).

An intriguing observation of the European study suggests that a history of arterial hypertension, although associated with relatively poor prognosis, predicts no survival benefits after surgery, Fig. 2. (11). This observation has not been confirmed by other studies and may be real or a random finding.

Nevertheless, a plausible explanation for this finding could be that CABG is unable to fully restore the limited coronary reserve of hypertrophied hypertensive myocardium thereby sustaining a tendency to myocardial ischaemia and increased risk of lethal complication (12, 13). On the other

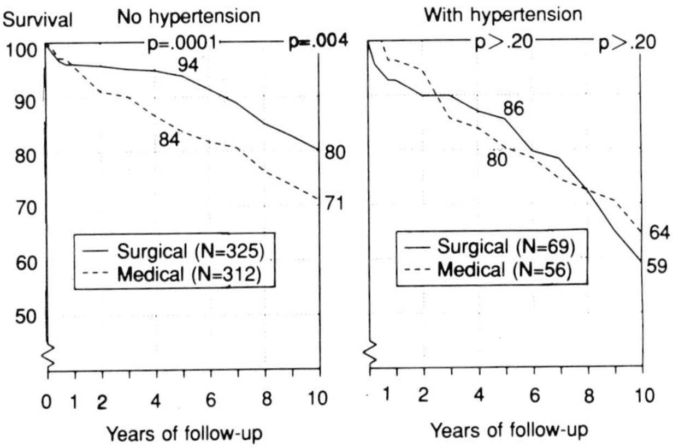

Fig. 2. *Long-term survival in per cent for the patients randomized to the medical or surgical treatment subdivided into those who have (right) or who have not (left) a history of arterial hypertension. P-values are given for the survival differences for 5 and 10 year follow-up, respectively. (European Study, 1988).*

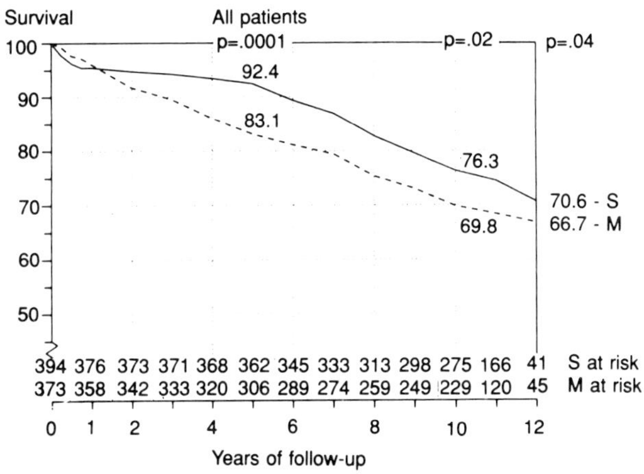

Fig. 3. *Long-term survival in per cent for all patients randomized to medical or surgical treatment. M=medical and S=surgical treatment groups. P-values are given for 5, 10 and 12 year follow-up, respectively. (European Study, 1988).*

hand, other mechanisms unrelated to surgery may just as well be responsible for an increased rate of graft occlusions and cardiac mortality in hypertensive patients.

An extraordinary study of a large number of surgically treated patients demonstrated that significant independent predictors of poorer long-term survival include cardiomegaly, use of IABP and postoperative kidney failure (15).

The most marked difference in survival between the two treatment policies appears 5-7 years after surgery. The gain in survival that can be attributed to surgery may vary between 30% and 60% at five years depending on the risk level. This gain in survival gradually diminishes during the subsequent years. The significant difference between the two treatments may still be present at 10-12 years, as indicated by the European Study, (Fig. 3) (11) or may be absent as in VA patients with more advanced disease (3) and rather heterogeneous CASS populations (14). The decrease in survival difference is due to accelerated late mortality among the patients alloted to early surgery. The most marked acceleration of mortality occures between 5 and 10 years in the subgroup of hypertensive patients (Fig. 2) followed by the subgroup of patients with left main disease (11).

It is equally important to note that no significant survival benefits of early surgery are seen in patients with a relatively good prognosis – young men without significant ECG changes at rest and/or exercise and with good left ventricular function. However, this does not preclude that surgery might save life in individual low risk patients.

It is interesting to note, that the contribution of CABG to the decline in coronary heart disease mortality in the USA was nil in 1970. From 1971 to 1984, the percentage contribution increased from 0.19% to 13.21%, respectively (15).

A new nonfatal myocardial infarction is not prevented by surgery (9, 16, 17), although some observational studies claim the opposite. On the other hand, a significantly decreased postoperative incidence of sudden and non-sudden cardiac deaths strongly suggests that fatal infarction is prevented. It is generally recognized that the assessment of per- and postoperative infarction incidence is a difficult task due to usual diagnostic uncertanties and the variability of diagnostic criteria employed by different studies. It is quite likely that the rate of infarction is frequently underestimated. This restriction applies to both medically and surgically treated patients.

Patency of grafts and native vessels is essential for good long-term results. Patent and well functioning grafts are generally accompanied by total or partial relief of myocardial ischaemia as demonstrated frequently, although not invariably, by postoperatively improved results of electrocardiographic, radionuclear and haemodynamic investigations.

Graft patency is also important for the maintenance of clinical improvement. A significantly larger proportion of patients with at least one patent graft improved angina and survival over a period of 12 years as compared to those without patent graft. On the other hand, a few patients with no patent grafts may have partial or total relief of angina, suggesting that other mechanisms, whether related to the surgery or not (scarring after an infarction, periarterial coronary denervation or placebo) may play an important role in such cases (10, 18).

After the initial drop in graft patency by approximately 20% during the first year, the annual rate of graft closure is roughly 1% between 1 and 5 years and as much as 4-5% between 6 and 11 years after operation. Moreover, more than 50% of the patent grafts are significantly narrowed at 10 years (18).

Graft occlusion is usually caused by thrombosis during the first year after operation, frequently associated with focal narrowing due to inappropriate surgical techniques and/or intimal hyperplasia, while late occlusions are associated with changes attributed to atheroslerosis.

The natural history of atherosclerosis in native coronary vessels is another important factor for the late outcome. Lesions present preoperatively may show significant progression at 10-12 years in 66% of arteries, while new significant stenoses seem to appear in 7% of ungrafted arteries and in 14% of grafted arteries (10).

Thus, the advance of atherosclerotic disease in grafts and native arteries, which may lead to recurrent myocardial ischaemia and new infarction, appears to be the major mechanism responsible for the late symptomatic deterioration and accelerated cardiac mortality after surgery.

The need to repeat surgery arises when symptoms and signs related to myocardial ischaemia recur.

Angina which recurs in the first two months after surgery is most often due to graft failure. When syptoms recur later on, the majority of reoperated patients show disease progression or have new lesions in their native coronary arteries and/or grafts (19, 20).

Nearly a third of patients appear to have lost previously normal left ventricular function during the period between the two operations.

The baseline characteristics of patients receiving repeat surgery include young age, women, those with less extensive coronary disease, less left ventricular impairment, no internal mammary artery graft, incomplete revascularization (20).

Reoperation carries a markedly increased operative mortality, on average of 12.6% (15) while morbidity appears to be the same as with the initial operation. This is one of the good reasons for avoiding, if possible, surgery at a too early date

The annual incidence of reoperation increases as the length of follow-up increases, being 0,9% and 2,7% at five and ten years. The cumulative percentage of repeat surgery is 19% at 12 years.

Improvement of surgical and medical care over time

To what extent are the results of medical and surgical treatment performed in the 1970s applicable to current clinical decision making?

A study from the Duke Databank for Cardiovascular Diseases attempted to answer this question by investigating 2-year survival probability in both medically and surgically treated patients over the time period between 1970 and 1984 (21). The study showed that survival over time improved with both treatment modalities. However, the improvement in survival benefits of CABG appeared at a more rapid rate than with medical therapy in all categories of coronary artery disease. The authors concluded that the improvement in medical patients was due to less sick patients being treated, while that observed in surgical patients was due to refinements in care. The refinements in care of surgical patients have been manifold (22). Advanced myocardial preservation, more complete coronary revascularization, better intraoperative support, refined operative technique are the means primarily aimed at improving in-hospital morbidity and mortality (22).

Furthermore, increased use of antiplatelet drugs and internal mammary artery grafting, and adoption of more efficient risk factor modification programmes may have resulted in decreased progression of atherosclerosis in grafts and native vessels accompanied by increased long-term survival (23-26).

The Duke study supports the notion that conclusions emerging from the three trials are principally valid even today. However, a fitting remark is that results from the 1970s may need to be modified when selecting the approach that is most appropriate for current clinical decision making (21).

Approach to current clinical decision making

The results of trials and vast clinical experience convincingly demonstrate that CABG can be utilized with great success to relieve unacceptable angina pectoris and/or to prevent cardiac death even when angina is adequately controlled by medical therapy.

Stable angina pectoris not yielding to medical therapy causes no great problems in clinical decision making. Coronary angiography is done without delay to establish whether coronary anatomy is suitable for intervention and whether CABG or angioplasty is to be preferred.

While angioplasty is nowadays generally used in patients with single vessel disease, the majority of patients with multivessel disease usually need surgery for adequate revascularization. On the other hand, the possibility of internal mammary artery grafting makes the use of CABG attractive, also in patients with single vessel lesions, especially if a large area of myocardium is at jeopardy, implying a high risk of premature death. The risk for repeat surgery seems to have decreased due to the superior patency of the internal mammary artery, this may favourably affect survival. Meanwhile, angioplasty, in contract to CABG, is not yet established as an equally successful method for preventing cardiac death.

Prevention of cardiac death even when angina is controlled by medical treatment requires first of all reasonably reliable information as to the relative odds of continued medical therapy and early surgery. This is obtained by risk stratification, using clinical variables predictive of impaired prognosis and significantly improved survival with surgery. The clinical predictors established by the trials are: (i) middle age or older, (ii) resting-ECG changes reflecting myocardial ischaemia and/or old infarction, (iii) markedly positive exercise ECG (ST deviation >1.5mm on low work level), (iv) impaired left ventricular function (confirmed by radionuclear ventriculography, if necessary).

Moreover, history and signs of peripheral artery disease and absence of a history of treated hypertension appears to favour surgery. An ejection fraction lower than 0.25 carries an unreasonably high operative mortality and poor long-term survival.

Two or more of the established clinical prognostic predictors indicate a "high risk" profile while less than two predictors suggest a "low risk" profile.

The next step in patients at high risk of premature cardiac death is to perform coronary angiography, in order to confirm that the clinical evidence of increased risk has its counterpart in coronary and ventricular anatomy: 50% or greater stenoses in (i) the left main artery or (ii) two or more major coronary branches, one of which is the proximal segment of the left descending artery and/or (iii) left ventricular ejection fraction of 0.25-0.5. Moreover, angiographic findings determine the feasibility of surgery.

Bearing in mind the fact that surgery can improve long-term prognosis by 30-60% in high risk patients who have anyone of the above anatomical risk factors, CABG should be performed without delay.

There is no urgent indication for surgery in patients with mild angina who have no apparent evidence of a high risk of premature death. The initial treatment approach in these patients is a comprehensive medical therapy and thorough monitoring for possibly evolving clinical risk factors. This noninvasive management can be continued as long as the hazard involved is less than that of early operation. As soon as clinical evidence of increased risk appears, coronary angiography and subsequent surgery are strongly indicated, even if a simultaneous worsening of the angina does not occur. The patient is to be regarded and taken care of as a high risk patient.

This treatment approach actually represents a modified policy of early surgery tested in clinical trials. The modification implies utililization of the advantages of noninvasive treatment before making use of preventive surgery.

We can call for the sake of convenience, this treatment approach the *strategy of elective early surgery*.

Although the strategy of elective early surgery would principally apply only to patients who meet the characteristics of those with stable chronic angina included in the trials, it is reasonable to suppose that the basic concept of *this strategy may also apply to other categories of coronary patients in a stabilized clinical condition.*

Unstable angina. The initially much apprecciated emergency revascularization of patients with unstable angina has lost ground, as the efficiency of medical therapy to "cool" and stabilize the condition increased and no convincing survival benefits could be demonstrated of CABG (27, 28). However, the strategy of elective early revascularization seems applicable, if used after the stabilization of angina (29).

Acute myocardial infarction. CABG has been advocated in acute myocardial infarction (sometimes also defined as impending or evolving infarction) to preserve myocardial contractility, decrease infarction size and favourably affect survival (30, 31). Although it has been shown that emergency surgery can be performed with as low an operative mortality rate as 2.3% in selected patient categories (30), the achievement of these goals has not been reliably documented. Emergency surgery is presently not acceptable as the treatment of choice in patients with uncomplicated acute myocardial infarction.

After thrombolytic treatment of acute myocardial infarction revascularization is indicated to relieve persistent or recurrent symptomatic or asymptomatic myocardial ischaemia. Prophylactic revascularization immediately after thrombolysis with no ischaemic symptoms and signs offers no advantages in terms of reduced mortality or prevention of new infarction over the strategy of elective early intervention (32).

It has not been determined as yet whether surgery or angioplasty is the most beneficial method of revascularization in order to improve the prognosis in this phase of disease.

Early postinfarction period. Although coronary revascularization early after acute myocardial infarction is considered feasible and relieves angina in the majority of patients, its role in preventing or postponing postinfarction death remains obscure.

Following acute infarction several prognostic indices have been developed which can identify high and low risk patients. A low risk group of patients has a mortality not greatly different from that of the general population, while the high risk group can have a first year mortality as high as 27% (33). One cannot say that surgery is the treatment of choice due to heterogeneity of the patient population, except when angina is poorly controlled by medical means or there is evidence of increased risk of premature cardiac death (34). Coronary angiography does not appear to be indicated in all postinfarction patients, although it is practiced in many hospitals. The need of it is preferably defined by symptoms and clinical risk stratification. Evidently, the strategy of elective early surgery appears applicable.

Left ventricular failure. The two trials (3, 5) which included patients with decreased left ventricular ejection fraction suggest that surgery is indicated to relieve angina and/or to improve prognosis in these high risk patients.

No clinical trials evaluated survival benefits of CABG in patients with far advanced left ventricular dysfunction. Observational studies demonstrate that operative mortality is markedly increased (2-25%) and long-term survival is rather low in these patients with an ejection fraction below 0.30. CABG may relieve their angina, but it is unable to improve the failing ventricle (35). Consequently, if surgery may be rightly considered as being hazardous and questionable to relieve angina, then it is definetely not indicated to improve cardiac function and prognosis in patients with an ejection fraction less than 0.30-0.20.

Silent myocardial ischaemia. A generally recognized urgent need to prevent myocardial infarction and sudden death in apparently normal people has focussed great attention on silent ischaemia as it is detected by ECG during exercise test or Holter monitoring. Prophylactic revascularization has been considered and to a limited extent used in these individuals in whom coronary angiography disclosed significant coronary artery disease.

One of the most systematic studies of this subject (36) suggests that silent ischaemia has characteristics of clinically and angiographically highly progressive disease, eventually requiring surgery because of evolving angina, although the annual rate of sudden death is less than 1% over a period of 8-10 years. Significantly lower baseline maximal heart rate during exercise test as well as lower work performance were identified as clinical predictors of disease progression. This observation may be of help in considering coronary angiography and revascularization in individuals who have professions involving public safety, such as air pilots.

However, the knowledge about the natural history of silent ischaemia and the effect of intervention are as yet too limited to provide medically sound and psychologically acceptable guidelines for prophylactic revascularization in apparently normal individuals. Population screening for silent ischaemia seems justified only for the purpose of research. The strategy of elective early surgery aimed at preventing sudden cardiac death is applicable if and when ischaemic symptoms appear.

Conclusions

The primary objective of coronary artery bypass grafting is either to *relieve* refractory angina pectoris or to *prevent* premature cardiac death in high risk patients.

The most dramatic improvement of symptoms is seen in patients with the most incapacitating angina and the greatest survival benefits are recorded in patients with markedly increased mortality risk defined by clinical and angiographic prognostic predictors which also forecast the outcome of surgery.

A strategy of elective early surgery is adopted: progressive high-level medical care is expanded by cardiac catheterization as soon as angina becomes unacceptable or clinical risk predictors evolve. Surgery, if anatomically feasible, is performed without delay. This strategy appears applicable to all patients in the *stable phase* of symptomatic coronary artery disease.

Surgery has *no* established position in the treatment of sequels of coronary artery disease without associated symptoms and signs of myocardial ischaemia, for instance congestive heart failure.

Extensive clinical *research is still needed* to define the exact role of prophylactic revascularization in silent ischaemia.

References

1. Sones FM Jr, Shirey EK. Cine coronary arteriography. Mod Concepts Cardiovasc Dis 1962; 31: 735-8.
2. Favaloro RG. Saphenous vein aorto-graft replacement of severe sequential coronary artery occlusion: operativetechnique. Ann Thorac Surg 1968; 5: 334-9.
3. The Veterans Administration Coronary Artery Bypass Surgery Cooperative Study Group. Eleven-year survival in the Veterans Administration randomized trial of coronary bypass surgery for stable angina.N Engl J Med 1984; 311: 1333-9.
4. European Coronary Surgery Study Group. Long-term results of prospective randomised study of coronary artery bypass surgery in stable angina pectoris. Lancet 1982; 2: 1173-80.
5. Killip T, Passamani E, Davis K, CASS Principal Invistigators and Their Associates. Coronary Artery Surgery Study (CASS): a randomized trial of coronary bypass surgery: eight years follow-up and survival in patients with reduced ejection fraction. Circulation 1985; 72 (suppl. V): V102-9.
6. May GS, Chir B, DeMets DL, Friedman LM, Furberg C, Passamani E. The randomized clinical trial: bias in analysis. Circulation 1981; 64: 669-73.
7. CASS Principal Investigators and Their Associates. Coronary Artery Surgery Study (CASS): a randomized trial of coronary artery bypass surgery: survival data. Circulation 1983; 68: 939-50.
8. Walter PJ, ed. Return to work after coronary artery bypass surgery – psychosocial and economic aspects. Berlin Springer Verlag, 1985.
9. Varnauskas E. European Coronary Surgery Study Group. Survival, myocardial infarction, and employment status in a prospective randomized study of coronary bypass surgery. Circulation 1985; 72 (suppl. V): V90-V101.

10. Campeau L, Bourassa MG, Enjalbert M, Lesperance J. Improvement of angina and survival 1 to 12 years after aortocoronary bypass surgery: correlations with changes in grafts and in the native coronary circulation. Heart Transplant 1984; 3: 220-3.
11. Varnauskas E and the European Coronary Surgery Study Group. Twelve-year follow-up of survival in the randomized European Coronary Surgery Study.N Engl J Med 1988; 319: 332-7.
12. Stauer B-E. Ventricular function and coronary hemodynamics in hypertensive heart disease. Am J Cardiol 1979; 44: 999-1006.
13. Marcus ML, Harrison DG, Chilian WM, et al. Alterations in the coronary circulation in hypertrophied ventricles. Circulation 1987; 75 (suppl. I): I19-I25.
14. Alderman EL, Bourassa MG, Cohen LS, et al. Ten year follow-up of Coronary Artery Surgery Study (CASS) randomized patients. Circulation 1988; 78 (suppl. II): II-636.
15. Doliszny KM. Coronary artery graft surgery from 1970 through 1984 in the Seven-County Twin Cities Metropolitan area. 1989 (Thesis).
16. CASS Principal Investigators and Their Associates. Myocardial infarction and mortality in the Coronary Artery Surgery Study (CASS) randomized trial. N Engl J Med 1984; 310: 750-8.
17. Murphy ML, Meadows WR, Thomsen J, et al. The effect of coronary artery bypass surgery on the incidence of myocardial infarction and hospitalization. Progr Cardiovasc Dis 1986; 28: 309-17.
18. Bourassa MG, Fisher LD, Campeau L, Gillespie MJ, McConney M, Lespérance J. Long-term fate of bypass grafts: the Coronary Artery Surgery Study (CASS) and Montreal Heart Institute experiences. Circulation 1985; 72 (suppl. V): V71-V78.
19. Loop FD, Lytle BW, Gill CC, Golding LAR, Cosgrove DM, Taylor PC. Trends in selection and results of coronary artery reoperations. Ann Thorac Surg 1983; 35: 380-8.
20. Loop FD, Cosgrove DM. Repeat coronary bypass surgery: selection of cases, surgical risks, and long-term outlook. Mod Concepts Cardiovasc Dis 1986; 55: 31-6.
21. Pryor DB, Harrel FE, Rankin JS, et al. The changing survival benefits of coronary revascularization over time. Circulation 1987; 76 (suppl. V): V13-V21.
22. Wheatley DJ, ed. Surgery of Coronary Artery Disease. London: Chapman and Hall, 1986.
23. Fuster V, Chesebro JJ. Aortocoronary artery vein-graft disease: experimental and clinical approach for the understanding of the role of platelets and platelet inhibitors. Circulation 1985; 72 (suppl. V): V65-70.
24. Cameron A, Kemp HG, Green GE. Bypass surgery with the internal mammary artery graft: 15 year follow-up. Circulation 1986; 74 (suppl. III): III30-6.
25. Loop FD, Lytle BW, Cosgrove DM, et al. Influence of the internal-mammary-artery graft on 10-year survival and other cardiac events.N Engl J Med 1986; 314: 1-6.
26. Blakenhorn DH, Nessim SA, Johnson RL, et al. Beneficial effects of combined Colestipol-Niacin therapy on coronary atherosclerosis and coronary venous bypass grafts. JAMA 1987; 257: 3233-40.
27. Russell RO, Moraski RE, Kouchoukos N, et al. Unstable angina pectoris: National Cooperative Study Group to compare surgical and medical therapy. II. In-hospital experience and initial follow-up results in patients with one-, two-, and three-vessel disease. Am J Cardiol 1978; 42: 839-48.
28. Rahimtoola SH, Nunley D, Grunkemeier G, et al. Ten-year survival after coronary bypass surgery for unstable angina. N Engl J Med 1983; 308: 676-81.
29. Cohn LH, Alpert J. Koster K, et al. Changing indications for the surgical treatment of unstable angina. Arch Surg 1978; 113: 1312-6.

30. Berg R, Selinger SL, Leonard JJ, et al. Surgical management of acute myocardial infarction. Cardiovasc Clin 1982; 12: 61-74.
31. Phillips SJ, Zeft RH, Kongtahworu C, et al. Surgery for evolving myocardial infarction. JAMA 1982; 248: 1325-8.
32. The TIMI Study Group. Comparison of invasive and conservative strategies after treatment with intravenous tissue plasminogen activator in acute myocardial infarction. N Engl J Med 1989; 320: 618-27.
33. Theroux P, Waters DD, Halphen C, et al. Prognostic value of exercise testing soon after myocardial infarction. N Engl J Med 1979: 301-41.
34. The European Postinfarction Coronary Surgery Study. Unpublished 1990.
35. Alderman EL, Fisher LD, Litwin P, et al. Results of coronary artery surgery in patients with poor left ventricular function (CASS). Circulation 1983; 68: 785-95.
36. Erikssen J, Thaulow E. Follow-up of patients with asymptomatic myocardial ischemia. In: Rutishauser W, Roskamm H, eds. Silent myocardial ischemia. Berlin: Springer Verlag, 1984: 156-64.

Late management, risk stratification and prognosis

34

Prognosis after acute myocardial infarction

ERLING BIRK MADSEN

Decline in mortality after myocardial infarction

The prognosis after acute myocardial infarction (MI) has shown considerable improvement over the last 3 decades. This improved survival for patients with MI is one of the major explanations of the significant declining mortality trend in coronary heart disease (1).

Short-term prognosis: Before introduction of coronary care units acute mortality in hospital was above 30% (2). After the first 10 years of coronary care with intensive treatment of life-threatening ventricular arrhythmias, mortality in hospital was still around 25% in 1970 (3) (Table 1). Better prehospital care and attendance to anti-ischaemic therapy after admission caused a further reduction in mortality to 15% in 1980 (4). The introduction in recent years of thrombolytic therapy has been a major break through, with 8% reported mortality after 5 weeks among treated patients (5). The acute mortality for patients with MI will probably settle around 5% in the nineties. Therefore, in the last 20 years we have seen acute mortality after MI diminished in the order of 80% to 1/5 of the original mortality.

Long-term prognosis: Mortality in the first year after MI and in the following years has also been declining, although not at the same rate as compared to the reduction in acute mortality (Table 1). In 1970 the one-year mortality for patients discharged after MI was around 15% (6). Ten years later in 1980 the mortality had decreased to 10% (7), probably due to more emphasis on post-MI treatment, with beta-blocking agents and better secondary prevention. The current one-year mortality is approximately 5% (5) due to more intensive acute treatment with thrombolysis and better evaluation before discharge. In the last 20 years one-year mortality has decreased in the order of 66% to 1/3 of the original mortality.

Table 1. *Declining mortality after acute myocardial infarction in 20 years.*

	Mortality	
	Hospitalization	One-year
1970	25%	15%
1980	15%	10%
1990	5%	5%

Prognostic evaluation

Risk related to therapy: The prognosis after MI can be evaluated by identifying important factors related to increased mortality, early and late, after MI. An abundance of prognostic studies have described many different prognostic patient characteristics in various patient populations. The basic mortality for the patient population has a strong influence on the prognostic conclusions. Therefore a very pertinent point for evaluation of prognostic studies is the time period for the study (Table 1). In addition, the optimal prognostic study should take more objective quantitative techniques into account for patient evaluation. Finally, multivariate statistical analytic techniques are essential for identifying the most important independent risk factors (8).

The ultimate goal of the prognostic work-up is to identify the individual patients in various risk groups according to the characteristics of the particular patient. The incidence of selected prognostic variables will identify low- and high-risk groups with a high grade of accuracy. The prognostic classification of patients has been best for high-risk patients with 90% of the deaths correctly classified into the predicted high-risk group (8). The actual mortality among patients predicted to be at low risk has been very low, at 1-2%.

The prognostic evaluation has important therapeutic implications both for patients with low predicted mortality (i.e. early discharge) and for patients with high predicted mortality (i.e. more aggressive treatment). The available prognostic information today allows precise prognostic evaluation early on admission to hospital, later during hospitalization and at the time of discharge.

Prognosis on admission to hospital

History: Age is a very important prognostic factor with markedly increased hospital mortality even in patients in their mid-sixties (16%) and very high mortality (32%) in patients 75 years or more (9). Patients above 60-65 years carry a more grave prognosis from the start and require proper therapeutic management according to their quality of life.

The presence of previous MI implies at least a two-fold increase in mortality even if the previous MI was not recognized by the patient (10). Hospital mortality is very high in patients with diabetes mellitus, around 30% due to more serious coronary disease and larger infarctions (11). Patients with previous congestive heart failure and chronic obstructive pulmonary disease also have higher mortality during the acute phase.

Electrocardiogram: Patients with anterior MI have two to four times higher hospital mortality as compared to patients with inferior MI (12). The acute mortality among patients with non-Q wave MI is approximately one half the mortality in patients with Q wave MI (12, 13). Non-Q wave infarctions tend to be smaller with lower enzyme levels and better ventricular function. A non-Q wave MI is rarely caused by total occlusion of the infarct-related vessel. However, non-Q wave infarctions denote an unstable long-term condition with progression to Q wave infarctions in 21% of the patients during 9 months follow-up (14). The prognosis is particularly serious if infarct extension occurs during hospitalization (15) and if large perfusion abnormalities can be demonstrated on thallium scintigrams (16). A subgroup of patients with non-Q wave MI with no localisable repolarisation abnormalities appears to have a more favourable outcome (17).

Infarct size: The myocardial damage with impaired ventricular function is directly related to infarct size. Peak creatine kinase level can provide an estimate of infarct size directly related to prognosis (18, 19). The extent of myocardial injury estimated from the electrocardiographic leads with ST-elevation is directly correlated to mortality and efficacy of thrombolytic therapy (20). Long-term follow-up patients with small infarctions and low peak creatine kinase levels seem to be more unstable with a higher incidence of angina and later death (21).

Prognosis during hospitalization

Heart failure: Evidence of compromised left ventricular function is the most important prognostic factor. Acute mortality among patients with moderate left ventricular failure evaluated by clinical or radiologic pulmonary congestion is approximately 15% (18, 22). Mortality in patients with pulmonary oedema is 30% (18) and the presence of cardiogenic shock, even with the most aggressive treatment, carries a 65% acute mortality (23).

Ischaemia: Ongoing myocardial ischaemia with persistent episodes of pain during hospitalization indicates an unstable condition (24). Ischaemia is often caused by coronary spasm when ST-segment depression occurs in the same area where Q waves are located and prognosis is relatively benign (25). The persistence of ST-segment changes in leads with no Q waves denotes distant ischaemia with a more dubious prognosis (26). Ongoing ischaemia can lead to infarct extension with a significantly increased risk of progression to cardiogenic shock (23) and death (15). Restoration of anterograde coronary flow by thrombolysis or coronary angioplasty to relieve ischaemia is essential for improving the prognosis in patients with ongoing ischaemia (27).

Arrhythmia: Early ventricular fibrillation occurring during the first two days of hospitalization increases the hospital mortality to 25% but has no deleterious effects on the long-term prognosis (28,29). Very early primary ventricular fibrillation during the first few hours in patients with no symptoms of left ventricular failure does not appear to increase the risk of death later during hospitalization (30).

Ventricular tachycardia during the first 24 hours is often transient and benign. Ventricular tachycardia presenting later is often associated with left ventricular dysfunction with increased mortality (31). Ventricular premature beats during the acute phase are not related to hospitalization prognosis. Even complex warning arrhythmias (frequent or multiform premature beats, beats with early coupling and couplets or salvos) are not harbingers of ventricular fibrillation or death (32). Sinus tachycardia and atrial fibrillation often signify left heart failure or ongoing ischaemic injury (33) and the independent prognostic value is limited.

Third-degree atrioventricular block complicating anterior MI is often caused by extensive septal necrosis with concomitant severe left ventricular failure and high mortality (34). Patients with inferior MI complicated by complete atrioventricular block usually demonstrate less myocardial necrosis and an only slightly increased risk of death. Development of intraventricular block indicates a two- to three-fold increase in acute mortality (35). Bifascicular block is associated, in particular, with extensive myocardial necrosis and high hospital mortality approaching 50% (36).

Prognosis on discharge from hospital

Early discharge: Patients with a low risk of complications and death can leave hospital after 5 to 7 days (37, 38). Discharge even after only 3 days in hospital has also been reported in selected patients with uncomplicated MI treated by thrombolysis, angioplasty, or both (39). The low-risk group feasible for early discharge comprises patients below 70 years of age, patients with no previous MI, patients without persistent chest pain or infarct extension and patients with no signs of congestive heart failure or severe arrhythmias (37). The risk of death, cardiac arrest and development of shock after early discharge in selected patients is very low, at 1-2% (37).

Left ventricular dysfunction: The most important independent long-term prognostic characteristic is depressed left ventricular function (22, 40), quantitated by left ventricular ejection fraction (LVEF). Patients with LVEF below 0.40 have a 30% one-year mortality (22, 30). With LVEF below 0.20 the mortality increases to 50%. The predictive value of a low LVEF is greatest in the first year after discharge, since the presence of severe coronary lesions appears to contain more prognostic power later (41).

LVEF is directly measured by radionuclide ventriculography or estimated by echocardiography. LVEF can be roughly estimated from an abnormal chest radiograph (42) or the peak creatine kinase level (43). The presence of clinical or radiographic signs of congestive heart failure can augment the predictive value of a depressed LVEF (44). Left ventricular wall motion abnormalities are also good predictors of later death (45).

Exercise testing: Evaluation of functional capacity and detection of exercise-induced ischaemia and arrhythmias in patients without any symptoms at rest is essential for long-term prognostic assessment and therapeutic management. Exercise testing can be performed safely to a submaximal level before early discharge and to maximal stress soon after discharge (46). Inability to perform exercise testing due to advanced age, congestive heart failure, or impaired medical condition is in itself a stong predictor for later death (47, 48).

Low functional capacity is related to left ventricular function and implies a higher long-term mortality (48). Patients with low functional capacity (multiples of resting oxygen consumption [MET] below 4) have a cardiac event rate in one year follow-up of 18% (death, new MI) compared to a 2% event rate among patients with higher functional capacity (47).

Exercise-induced ischaemic ST-segment abnormalities are related to the magnitude of coronary disease and multiple vessel disease can be identified (49). Significant ST-segment depression of more than 1 mm is related to higher long-term mortality (50). The development of these ischaemic changes at low work loads increases the predictive value for multi-vessel disease (46). Ischaemic ST-changes can enhance the predictive value of signs of pulmonary congestion during the acute phase and a low LVEF (51). Other adverse exercise test prognostic factors are the development of angina (46, 52) and inadequate blood pressure response (50).

Silent asymptomatic ischaemia during exercise seems to have identical prognostic value as compared to symptomatic ischaemia (53), particularly for the subsequent development of angina and reinfarction (54). Utilization of thallium imaging and radionuclide ventriculography during exercise testing can further identify severe multi-vessel coronary lesions associated with increased long-term risk (55, 56).

The predictive value of exercise test variables is influenced by aggressive modern revascularization procedures and secondary prevention with beta-blockers. Recent studies indicate that exercise-induced angina and ST-segment depression in the modern therapeutic setting could have relative limited predictive value for later death and reinfarction during four years follow-up (57). The recently reported limited value of exercise testing in 141 patients with uncomplicated non-Q wave MI needs confirmation in larger patient populations (58).

Ambulatory monitoring: Ambulatory Holter-monitoring before discharge can disclose the presence of ventricular premature beats. Frequent and complex premature beats are associated with left ventricular dysfunction and multi-vessel disease and increase the risk of later death (59). More than ten ventricular premature beats per hour have been identified as the most important predictor for death in the MILIS study of 533 patients followed 18 months (30). In the parallel Multicenter Postinfarction Research Group study of 866 patients the same variable from 24-hour ambulatory monitoring ranked second to LVEF and congestive heart failure for prediction of death during two years follow-up (22).

For prognostic purposes it appears that depressed left ventricular function, indicated by low LVEF, has a higher predictive value for later outcome than the presence of increased ventricular activity from ambulatory monitoring. Complex ventricular arrhythmias seem to carry more independent prognostic information not related to LVEF among patients with non-Q wave MI (60). Silent ischaemic ST-segment changes detected during ambulatory monitoring are also predictive of later death (53) but the definitive value of this variable in the prognostic work-up needs more clarification.

Coronary angiography: Detection of extent of coronary artery disease by coronary angiography is necessary before later prospective revascularization with bypass surgery or angioplasty. Coronary artery abnormalities also demonstrate predictive value for later survival. The presence of significant three-vessel disease is related to 22% mortality during two years follow-up (61). Other studies have emphasized the long-term prognostic value of the number of diseased vessels (62, 63), and a special coronary artery jeopardy score (64). In these invasive studies evaluation of compromised left ven-

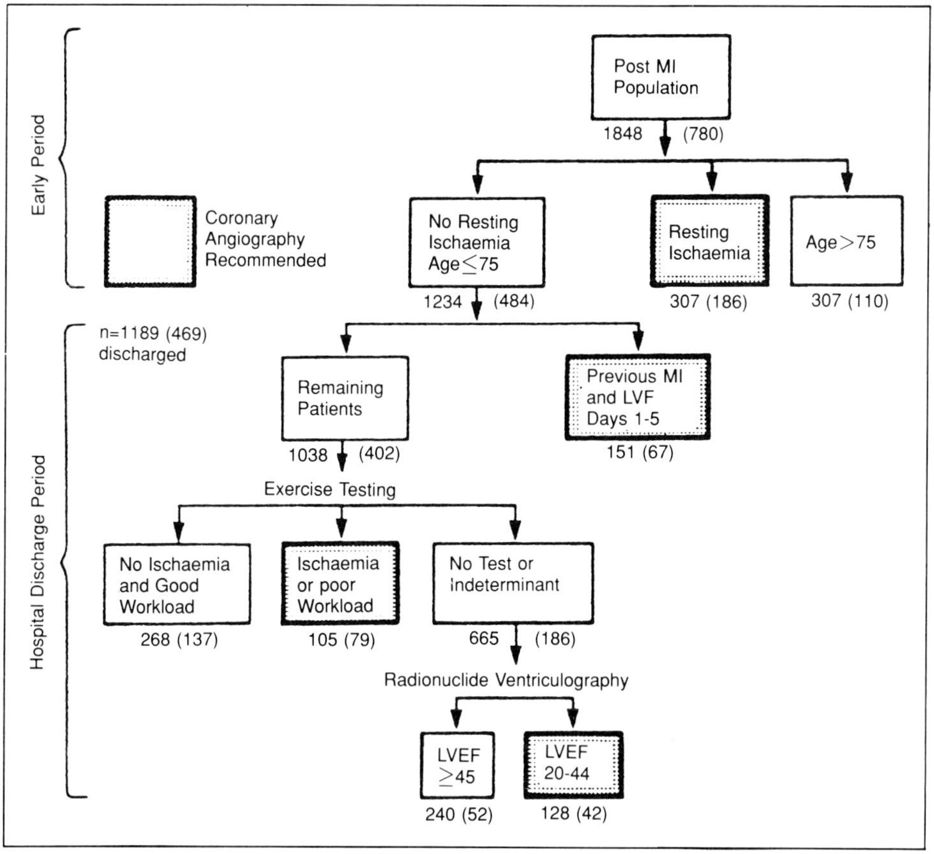

Fig. 1. *Stratification scheme for selection of patients for coronary angiography. Early period: For patients surviving the first 5 days. Later stratification is for patients discharged from hospital. Coronary angiography is recommended for selected groups (stippled boxes). Numbers under boxes show the distribution of patients in the original population and a validation sample (in parentheses).*
MI: myocardial infarction. LVF: left ventricular failure. LVEF: left ventricular ejection fraction. (Reprinted with permission from Ross et al. [69]).

tricular function with LVEF contained more prognostic information than coronary artery abnormalities.

Survival in some sub-groups of patients after MI can be improved by invasive intervention with surgery or angioplasty after the acute phase. Patients with high-grade stenosis of the left main coronary artery and patients with three-vessel disease combined with left ventricular dysfunction can benefit from surgery (65,66). Coronary angiography should be performed on patients with a high likelihood of these severe lesions contributing to increased mortality after MI.

The presence of left ventricular dysfunction or exercise-induced ischaemia can be applied for classification of patients into a high-risk group. Various criteria for selection of patients to coronary angiography have been presented (24, 67, 68). Fig. 1 shows a stratification scheme obtained from analysis of a large group of 1,848 patients with further validation in 780 patients (69). Coronary angiography is recommended in the following subgroups of high-risk patients:

1. Patients with persisting ischaemic pain beyond first 24 hours with 31% one-year mortality.
2. Patients with previous MI and left ventricular failure during the first five days in hospital with 25% mortality.
3. Patients with depressed LVEF between 0.20 and 0.44 with 19% mortality.
4. Patients with exercise-induced ischaemia (at least 2 mm ST-segment depression) or poor workload (below 4 METS) with 11% mortality.

Coronary angiography is neither feasible in patients above 75 years of age (31% mortality) nor in patients with LVEF of less than 0.20 (33% mortality). Invasive interventions in these high-risk subgroups will not improve survival. One-year mortality is low (3%) in patients with normal exercise tests with good workload without ischaemia. Patients with normal LVEF above 0.45 also demonstrate fairly low mortality (5%). Coronary angiography is not advisable in these large low-risk groups of patients since only a few patients will display high-risk coronary lesions amendable to invasive intervention (69). Coronary angiography is suggested in 43% of patients surviving the first five days of hospitalization.

Summary

With the introduction of intensive coronary care and thrombolysis survival both in hospital and later has been significantly improved over the last three decades. With up-to-date prognostic characteristics, patients with MI can be classified into various risk groups directing to specified therapeutic implications. On admission to hospital important prognostic variables are data from history (age, previous MI), from electrocardiogram (anterior MI, non-Q wave MI) and infarct size (peak enzyme level). Prominent variables from hospitalization are signs of congestive heart failure, of ongoing myocardial ischaemia and severe ventricular arrhythmias. At time of discharge remarkable variables are evidence of left ventricular dysfunction (LVEF) and data from exercise testing (ischaemia or low functional capacity). Coronary angiography is advisable in selected high-risk patients leading to improved survival from invasive revascularization procedures.

References

1. Stern MP. The recent decline in ischemic heart disease mortality. Ann Intern Med 1979; 91: 630-40.
2. Hughes WL, Kalbfleisch JM, Brandt ENJr, Costiloe JP. Myocardial infarction prognosis by discriminant analysis. Arch Intern Med 1963; 111: 338-45.
3. Birk Madsen E, Rasmussen S, Lysbo Svendsen T. Short-term prognostic index in acute myocardial infarction. Multivariate analysis by Cox model. Eur J Cardiol 1979; 10: 359-68.
4. Gillum RF, Folsom A, Luepker RV, et al. Sudden death and acute myocardial infarction in a metropolitan area, 1970-1980. The Minnesota Heart Survey. N Engl J Med 1983; 309: 1353-8.
5. ISIS-2 (Second international study of infarct survival) Collaborative Group. Randomised trial of intravenous streptokinase, oral aspirin, both, or neither among 17.187 cases of suspected acute myocardial infarction: ISIS-2. Lancet 1988; II: 349-60.
6. Birk Madsen E, Gilpin E, Henning H. Evaluation of prognosis one year after myocardial infarction. J Am Coll Cardiol 1983; 1: 985-93.
7. Gilpin EA, Koziol JA, Madsen EB, Henning H, Ross JJr. Periods of differing mortality distribution during the first year after acute myocardial infarction. Am J Cardiol 1983; 52: 240-4.
8. Birk Madsen E, Gilpin E, Henning H. Short-term prognosis in acute myocardial infarction: Evaluation by different prediction methods. Am Heart J 1984; 107: 1241-51.
9. Goldberg RJ, Gore JM, Gurwitz JH, et al. The impact of age on the incidence and prognosis of initial acute myocardial infarction: the Worcester Heart Attack Study. Am Heart J 1989; 117: 543-9.
10. Kannel WB, Abbott RD. Incidence and prognosis of unrecognized myocardial infarction. An update on the Framingham study. N Engl J Med 1984; 311: 1144-7.
11. Smith JW, Marcus FI, Serokman R. Prognosis of patients with diabetes mellitus after acute myocardial infarction. Am J Cardiol 1984; 54: 718-21.
12. Stone PH, Raabe DS, Jaffe AS, et al. Prognostic significance of location and type of myocardial infarction: Independent adverse outcome associated with anterior location. J Am Coll Cardiol 1988; 11: 453-63.
13. Nicholson MR, Roubin GS, Bernstein L, Harris PJ, Kelly DT. Prognosis after an initial non-Q wave myocardial infarction related to coronary arterial anatomy. Am J Cardiol 1983; 52: 462-5.
14. Hutter AMJr, DeSanctis RW, Flynn T, Yeatman LA. Nontransmural myocardial infarction: A comparison of hospital and late clinical course of patients with that of matched patients with transmural anterior and transmural inferior myocardial infarction. Am J Cardiol 1981; 48: 595-602.
15. Maisel AS, Ahnve S, Gilpin E, et al. Prognosis after extension of myocardial infarct: the role of Q wave or non-Q wave infarction. Circulation 1985; 71: 211-7.
16. Gibson RS, Beller GA, Gheorghiade M, et al. The prevalence and clinical significance of residual myocardial ischemia two weeks after uncomplicated non-Q wave infarction: A progressive natural history study. Circulation 1986; 73: 1186-98.
17. Boden WE, Kleiger RE, Gibson RS, et al. Favourable long-term prognosis in patients with non-Q wave acute myocardial infarction not associated with specific electrocardiographic changes. Diltiazem Reinfarction Study. Br Heart J 1989; 61: 396-402.

18. Henning H, Gilpin E, Covell JW, Swan EA, O'Rourke RA, Ross JJr. Prognosis after acute myocardial infarction: A multivariate analysis of mortality and survival. Circulation 1979; 59: 1124-36.
19. Geltman EM, Ehsani AA, Campbell MK, Schechtman K, Roberts R, Sobel BE. The influence of location and extent of myocardial infarction on long-term ventricular dysrhythmia and mortality. Circulation 1979; 60: 805-14.
20. Mauri F, Gasparini M, Barbonaglia L, et al. Prognostic significance of the extent of myocardial injury in acute myocardial infarction treated by streptokinase (the GISSI trial). Am J Cardiol 1989; 63: 1291-5.
21. Pi'erard LA, Dubois C, Albert A, Chapelle JP, Carlier J, Kulbertus HE. Prognostic significance of a low peak serum creatine kinase level in acute myocardial infarction. Am J Cardiol 1989; 63: 792-6.
22. The Multicenter Postinfarction Research Group. Risk stratification and survival after myocardial infarction. N Engl J Med 1983; 309: 331-6.
23. Hands ME, Rutherford JD, Muller JE, et al. The in-hospital development of cardiogenic shock after myocardial infarction: incidence, predictors of occurrence, outcome and prognostic factors. The MILIS Study Group. J Am Coll Cardiol 1989; 14: 40-6.
24. Epstein SE, Palmeri ST, Patterson RE. Evaluation of patients after acute myocardial infarction: Indications for cardiac catheterization and surgical intervention. N Engl J Med 1982; 307: 1487-92.
25. Moran TJ, French WJ, Abrams HF, Criley JM. Postmyocardial infarction angina and coronary spasm. Am J Cardiol 1982; 50: 197-202.
26. Schuster EH, Bulkley BH. Early post-infarction angina. N Engl J Med 1981; 305: 1101-5.
27. Cigarroa RG, Lange RA, Hillis LD. Prognosis after acute myocardial infarction in patients with and without residual anterograde coronary blood flow. Am J Cardiol 1989; 64: 155-60.
28. Nicod P, Gilpin E, Dittrich H, et al. Late clinical outcome in patients with early ventricular fibrillation after myocardial infarction. J Am Coll Cardiol 1988; 11: 464-70.
29. Volpi A, Cavalli A, Franzosi MG, et al. One-year prognosis of primary ventricular fibrillation complicating acute myocardial infarction. Am J Cardiol 1989; 63: 1174-8.
30. Mukharji J, Rude RE, Poole WK, et al. Risk factors for sudden death after acute myocardial infarction: two-year follow-up. Am J Cardiol 1984; 54: 31-6.
31. Bigger JT, Weld FM, Rolnitsky LM. Prevalence, characteristics and significance of ventricular tachycardia (three or more complexes) detected with ambulatory electrocardiographic recording in the late hospital phase of acute myocardial infarction. Am J Cardiol 1981; 48: 815-23.
32. Lie KJ, Wellens HJJ, Dorsnar E, Durrer D. Observations on patients with primary ventricular fibrillation complicating acute myocardial infarction. Circulation 1975; 52: 755-9.
33. Hod H, Lew AS, Keltai M, et al. Early atrial fibrillation during evolving myocardial infarction: a consequence of impaired left atrial perfusion. Circulation 1987; 75: 146-50.
34. Biddle TL, Ehrich DA, Yu PN, Hodges M. Relation of heart block and left ventricular dysfunction in acute myocardial infarction. Am J Cardiol 1977; 39: 961-6.
35. Hindman MC, Wagner GS, Jaro M, et al. The clinical significance of bundle branch block complicating acute myocardial infarction. 1. Clinical characteristics, hospital mortality and one-year follow-up. Circulation 1978; 58: 679-88.
36. Godman MJ, Lassers BW, Julian DG. Complete bundle-branch block complicating acute myocardial infarction. N Engl J Med 1970; 282: 237-40.

37. Birk Madsen E, Hougaard P, Gilpin E, Pedersen A. The length of the hospitalization in acute myocardial infarction determined by risk calculation. Circulation 1983; 68: 9-16.
38. McNeer JF, Wagner GS, Ginsburg PB, et al. Hospital discharge one week after acute myocardial infarction. N Engl J Med 1978; 298: 229-32.
39. Topol EJ, Burek K, O'Neill WW, et al. A randomized controlled trial of hospital discharge three days after myocardial infarction in the era of reperfusion. N Engl J Med 1988; 318: 1083-8.
40. Bigger JT, Fleiss JL, Kleiger R, Miller JP, Rolnitzky LM. The relationships among ventricular arrhythmias, left ventricular dysfunction and mortality in the two years after myocardial infarction. Circulation 1984; 69: 250-8.
41. De Cock CC, Visser FC, van Eenige MJ, Roos JP. Short-term and long-term prognosis after myocardial infarction: prognostic value of coronary anatomy and left ventriculography. Int J Cardiol 1989; 24: 197-209.
42. Birk Madsen E, Gilpin E, Slutsky RA, Ahnve S, Henning H, Ross JJr. Usefulness of the chest x-ray for predicting abnormal left ventricular function after acute myocardial infarction. Am Heart J 1984; 108: 1431-6.
43. Dewhurst NG, Muir AL. Comparative prognostic value of radionuclide ventriculography at rest and during exercise in 100 patients after first myocardial infarction. Br Heart J 1983; 49: 111-21.
44. Nicod P, Gilpin E, Dittrich H, et al. Influence on prognosis and morbidity of left ventricular ejection fraction with and without signs of left ventricular failure after acute myocardial infarction. Am J Cardiol 1988; 61: 1165-71.
45. Pièrard LA, Albert A, Chapelle JP, Carlier J, Kulbertus HE. Relative prognostic value of clinical, biochemical, echocardiographic and haemodynamic variables in predicting in-hospital and one-year cardiac mortality after acute myocardial infarction. Eur Heart J 1989; 10: 24-31.
46. Starling MR, Crawford MH, Kennedy GT, O'Rourke RA. Treadmill exercise tests predischarge and six weeks post-myocardial infarction to detect abnormalities of known prognostic value. Ann Intern Med 1981; 94: 721-7.
47. Birk Madsen E, Gilpin E, Ahnve S, Henning H, Ross JJr. Prediction of functional capacity and use of exercise testing for predicting risk after acute myocardial infarction. Am J Cardiol 1985; 56: 839-45.
48. Fioretti P, Brower RW, Simoons ML, et al. Prediction of hospital survivors of myocardial infarction. Comparison of predischarge exercise testing and radionuclide ventriculography at rest. Br Heart J 1984; 52: 292-8.
49. Akhas F, Upward J, Keates J, Jackson G. Early exercise testing and elective coronary artery bypass surgery after uncomplicated myocardial infarction. Effect on morbidity and mortality. Br Heart J 1984; 52: 413-7.
50. Waters DD, Bosch X, Bouchard A, et al. Comparison of clinical variables and variables derived from a limited predischarge exercise test as predictors of early and late mortality after myocardial infarction. J Am Coll Cardiol 1985; 5:1-8.
51. Dwyer EMJr, Greenberg HM, Steinberg G. Clinical characteristics and natural history of survivors of pulmonary congestion during acute myocardial infarction. The Multicenter Postinfarction Research Group. Am J Cardiol 1989; 63: 1423-8.
52. Peart I, Odemuyiwa O, Albers C, Hall A, Kelly C, Hall RJ. Exercise testing soon after myocardial infarction: its relation to course and outcome at one year in patients aged less than 55 years. Br Heart J 1989; 61: 231-7.
53. Ouyang P, Shapiro EP, Chandra NC, Gottlieb SH, Chew PH, Gottlieb SO. An angiographic and functional comparison of patients with silent and symptomatic treadmill ischemia early after myocardial infarction. Am J Cardiol 1987; 59: 730-4.
54. Fox JP, Beattie JM, Salih MM, Davies MK, Littler WA, Murray RG. Silent ischemia

following myocardial infarction: frequency, characteristics and prognosis. Eur Heart J 1988; 9 (suppl N): 108-13.
55. Hung J, Goris ML, Nash E, et al. Comparative value of maximal treadmill testing, exercise thallium myocardial perfusion scintigraphy and exercise radionuclide ventriculography for distinguishing high- and low-risk patients soon after acute myocardial infarction. Am J Cardiol 1984; 53: 1221-7.
56. Hakki A, Nestico PF, Heo J, Unwala AA, Iskandrian AS. Relative prognostic value of rest thallium-201 imaging, radionuclide ventriculography and 24 hour ambulatory electrocardiographic monitoring after acute myocardial infarction. J Am Coll Cardiol 1987; 10: 25-32.
57. Fioretti P, Deckers JW, Salm E, Baardman T, Roelandt JR. Four-year prognostic value of exercise-induced angina and painless ST-segment depression early after myocardial infarction. Eur Heart J 1988; 9 (suppl N): 123-7.
58. Krone RJ, Dwyer EMJr, Greenberg H, Miller JP, Gillespie JA. Risk stratification in patients with first non-Q wave infarction: limited value of the early low level exercise test after uncomplicated infarcts. The Multicenter Post-Infarction Research Group. J Am Coll Cardiol 1989; 14: 31-7.
59. Taylor GJ, Humphries JO, Mellits ED, et al. Predictors of clinical course, coronary anatomy and left ventricular function after recovery from acute myocardial infarction. Circulation 1980; 62: 960-70.
60. Maisel AS, Scott N, Gilpin E, et al. Complex ventricular arrhythmias in patients with Q wave versus non-Q wave myocardial infarction. Circulation 1985; 72: 963-70.
61. De Feyter PJ, van Eenige MJ, Dighton DH, Visser FC, de Jong J, Roos JP. Prognostic value of exercise testing, coronary angiography and left ventriculography 6-8 weeks after myocardial infarction. Circulation 1982; 66: 527-36.
62. Sanz G, Castaner A, Betriu A, et al. Determinants of prognosis in survivors of myocardial infarctions: A prospective clinical angiographic study. N Engl J Med 1982; 306: 1065-70.
63. Schulman SP, Achuff SC, Griffith LS, et al. Prognostic cardiac catheterization variables in survivors of acute myocardial infarction: A five year prospective study. J Am Coll Cardiol 1988; 11: 1164-72.
64. Califf RM, Phillips HR, Hindman MC, et al. Prognostic value of a coronary artery jeopardy score. J Am Coll Cardiol 1985; 5:1055-63.
65. Breyer RH, Engelman RM, Rousou JA, Lemeshow S. Postinfarction angina: An expanding subset of patients undergoing coronary artery bypass. J Thorac Cardiovasc Surg 1985; 90: 532-40.
66. Pigott JD, Kochoukos NT, Oberman A, Cutler GR. Late results of surgical and medical therapy for patients with coronary artery disease and depressed left ventricular function. J Am Coll Cardiol 1985; 5:1036-45.
67. Ross JJr, Brandenberg RO, Dinsmore RE, et al. Guidelines for coronary angiography: Report of the Joint American College of Cardiology/American Heart Association Task Force on Assessment of Cardiovascular Procedures. J Am Coll Cardiol 1987; 10: 935-50.
68. DeBusk RF, Blomqvist CG, Kochoukos NT, et al. Identification and treatment of low-risk patients after acute myocardial infarction and coronary-artery bypass graft surgery. N Engl J Med 1986; 314: 161-6.
69. Ross JJr, Gilpin EA, Madsen EB, et al. A decision scheme for coronary angiography after acute myocardial infarction. Circulation 1989; 79: 292-303.

35

Identification of high-risk patients after recovery from acute myocardial infarction. The role of exercise testing

KARI I. SAUNAMÄKI

After acute myocardial infarction (AMI) the survival of the patients is closely related to the extent of the myocardial damage, to the number of obstructed coronary arteries and to the occurrence of ventricular arrhythmias (1-3). Thrombolytic therapy has improved the prognosis after AMI (4). The effect seems to be mediated both through established patency of the infarct related artery and by myocardial salvage (5-7).

A recent large scale trial has indicated that a routine coronary angiography followed by percutaneous coronary angioplasty in suitable cases does not improve the clinical outcome after thrombolysis for AMI (8). However, there is a widespread acceptance that coronary angiography is indicated in selected high-risk patients (7, 8). So far there is only partial agreement as to which criteria should be used for further invasive investigations of post AMI patients (9). Exercise testing during early recovery from AMI has become an important method in the evaluation of these patients (9, 10). The role of exercise testing in this connection is still undergoing development and the topic of this review is to examine the present experience for the most appropriate use of exercise testing in post AMI patients.

The relative prognostic significance of left venticular function and coronary artery disease after myocardial infarction

Tables 1 and 2 present data from 3 post AMI angiographic studies. The patients were investigated before discharge (11), 4 weeks after AMI (1) and 6-8 weeks after AMI (2), respectively.

Table 1. *Post AMI mortality in relation left ventricular ejection fraction.*

Author	Follow up time (years)	Cardiac mortality(%) Ejection fraction(%)				
		≤20	<30	≥30	21-49	≥50
Taylor et al (11)	2.5	–	86	14	–	4
Sanz et al (1)	1.0	42	–	–	8	2
DeFeyter et al (2)	1.0	–	16	1	–	–
	2.0	–	26	4	–	–
	3.0	–	36	9	–	–

Table 2. *Post AMI mortality in relation to extent of coronary artery disease.*

Author	No. of patients	Follow up time (years)	Cardiac mortality (%) No. of diseased vessels		
			1-2	3	Total
Taylor et al (11)	106	2.5	4	27	12
Sanz et al (1)	259	1.0	4	18	7
DeFeyter et al (2)	179	1.0	3	4	
		2.0	5	20	
		3.0	9	36	6

A low left ventricular ejection fraction (LVEF) was associated with high mortality, especially during the first year after AMI (1, 2, 11), but the risk of dying also remained increased during the subsequent years (2, 11) (Table 1).

The significance of the extent of the coronary artery disease (CAD) in the above mentioned 3 studies (1, 2, 11) is shown in table 2. One- and 2-vessel disease was associated with relatively low mortality, but the risk of dying was considerably increased in patients with 3-vessel disease. One-year mortality was relatively low in patients with 3-vessel disease in the study by *DeFeyter et al* but it was increased markedly during the subsequent years (2). Angiography was performed 2-4 weeks later after AMI in this study than it was done in the two other series.

Sanz et al analyzed the combined effect of LVEF and CAD in their patients (1). They found that 1-year mortality was unaffected by the number of diseased coronary arteries with LVEF ≤20% or ≥50%. In the intermediate group (LVEF=21-49%) patients with 3-vessel disease had higher mortality than those with 1-2 vessel CAD (20% vs.4%). This group constituted one half of the total population.

Reperfusion therapy has further modified the factors which determine the survival of the patients. The prognosis of patients with patent infarct related artery has improved more than what could be expected on the basis of myocardial salvage (5-7).

Multivariate analysis in a series of thrombolyzed patients by *Stadius et al* showed that adequate perfusion of the infarcted myocardial region was more closely related to improved survival than LVEF (5).

The goal of the post-AMI non-invasive evaluation of the patients is thus to identify those who might benefit from invasive revascularisation, including: 1) Relief of symptoms; 2) Improvement of prognosis by a) trying to establish adequate perfusion and sustained patency of infarct related artery in patients with occlusion or restenosis after thrombolysis, b) treating other critical coronary artery narrowings.

Early post-myocardial exercise testing in the identification of high risk patients

Exercise testing after AMI gives information on the most important factors that determine the prognosis of the patients. ST-segment depression, exercise indexes of left ventricular function and exercise induced arrhythmias reflect myocardial ischaemia, cardiac pump function and electrical instability which are major determinants of subsequent survival (3, 9, 10).

1. Exercise induced ST-segment depression

Table 3 shows the 1-year mortality in relation to the presence or absence of exercise induced ST-segment depression (≥0.1 mV) in 8 post-AMI series

Table 3. *Significance of ST-segment depression during exercise testing early after AMI.*

Reference	Number of patients (deaths) (%)	Pct. with ST-depr.	Mortality (%) (1 year) ST-depression Yes	No	Sensitivity
(12)	210 (9.5)	30	27	2	85%*
(13)	225 (9.3)	31	17	6	57%*
(14)	103 (8.7)	30	10	8	33%
(15)	205 (5.8)	43	3	7	25%
(16)	222 (7.2)	23	12	6	38%
(17)	667 (4.9)	25	4	2	21%
(ST-0.2 mV)	– –	9	5	5	9%
(18)	300 (6.7)	42	6	8	35%
(19)	338 (7.1)	42	8	7	46%

One-year mortality after myocardial infarction in relation to occurrence of ST-segment depression (≥0.1 mV) during predischarge exercise testing.(For ref.17 the significance of 0.2 mV ST-depression is also indicated)(* = significant difference in mortality between patients with ST-depression and those without)

Table 4. *Significance of ST-segment depression during predischarge post AMI exercise testing in relation to AMI type.*

AMI-type	Number of patients (deaths) (%)	Pct. with ST-depr.	Mortality (%) (2 year) ST-depression Yes	No	Sensi-tivity
Q-wave	138 (10.9)	33	11	11	33%
(ST-0.2mV)	– –	15	19	9	27%
Non-Q-wave	55 (20)	31	53	5	82% *

Two-year mortality after myocardial infarction in relation to occurrence of ST-segment depression (≥0.1 mV) during pre-discharge exercise testing in Q-wave and non-Q-wave infartion, respectively. (Significance of 0.2 mV ST-depression in Q-wave AMI is also indicated) From Klein et al (20) (* = significant difference in mortality between patients with ST-depression and those without).

with a total of 2270 patients (12-19). ST-depression was able to discriminate significantly between dead and living patients in 2 studies only (12, 13). A more pronounced ST-depression (≥0.2 mV) was not helpfull either (17). Further, the sensitivity of ST-depression for identifying high-risk patients was unacceptably low in all but one series (12).

2. Q-wave vs. non-Q-wave infarction

Klein et al compared the prognostic value of ST-depression in Q-wave and in non-Q-wave infarction (20) (Table 4). They found that ST-depression had no prognostic significance in patients with Q-wave infarction, irrespective of it's magnitude. In patients with non-Q-wave infarction the ST-depression was highly predictive of mortality and had also very high sensitivity. Other investigators have found ST-depression to be predictive of mortality, other cardiac events and of critical CAD in patients with non-Q-infarction (21, 22).

Thus, in a general AMI-population, exercise induced ST-depression is of no value as a prognostic predictor unless there is a considerable number of patients with a non-Q infarction in the population. This probably explains the variable results in the series shown in Table 3.

3. Angina pectoris during exercise

Angina pectoris during exercise testing indicates myocardial ischaemia but it has not been predictive of mortality in general post-AMI populations (16, 20). The presence of angina has increased the sensitivity of the test in patients with non-Q-infarction (without reducing specificity too much) for detection of subsequent death or recurring AMI (21) and of critical coronary artery lesions (22).

4. Exercise indexes of left ventricular function

Exercise indexes of left ventricular function include exercise capacity with systolic blood pressure and heart rate responses. In 6 post-AMI exercise series with a total 1975 patients the following exercise LV-function indexes were used: maximal systolic blood pressure (17, 23), change of systolic blood pressure (14, 16, 18) or of pressure-rate-product (24) from rest to maximal exercise. A low value of these variables was in all series associated with significantly increased 1-year mortality ranging from 12% to 32% versus 3%-7% in patients with corresponding high values. The high-risk variables were present in 8%-41% of the patients. The sensitivities for identification of high-risk patients ranged from 32% to 70%.

An adequate diagnostic test should allow identification of a high-risk group which consists of less than a half of the population and contains most of the end-points. In the above mentioned series the LV-function indexes fulfilled the first criterion in all cases and the second one in all except two (17, 23).

5. Exercise induced ventricular arrhythmias

Occurrence of ventricular arrhythmias during predischarge Holter monitoring has been associated with increased subsequent mortality independent of the LV function (3, 25). Ventricular arrhythmias occurring during post-AMI exercise testing have also been independent predictors of mortality (13, 17, 23, 24). *Saunamäki and Andersen* confirmed the prognostic significance of the exercise induced ventricular arrhythmias in two subsequent post-AMI patient series (24). *Henry et al* found that exercise associated ventricular arrhythmias were better predictors of mortality than arrhythmias detected during ambulatory Holter monitoring (26). The increased risk of dying has especially been associated with increasing frequency of single ventricular premature beats (VPB) and to the occurrence of repetitive VPBs (23, 24).

The post-AMI risk assessement can be improved by combining relevant exercise variables. By using an exercise index of LV function and occurrence of ventricular arrhythmias in a series of 455 patients, *Saunamäki and Andersen* identified a low risk group of 185 patients with 1-year mortality of 3% vs. 16% in the remaining high-risk group which thus contained 90% of all deaths (19).

Concluding remarks

About 10-15% of post AMI patients have very poor LV function with LVEF <30% and hence high subsequent mortality (3, 25). These patients can be identified non-invasively by means of 2-dimensional echocardiography (27). The role of exercise testing in this sub-population is not yet clarified. However, exercise testing has been useful in identifying low-risk subjects (1-year mortality=zero) in a clinical high-risk population with a 1-year mortality of 20% (19).

Exercise testing is a valuable and cost-effective method for risk stratification in the great majority of post AMI patients. The present evidence indicates that in subjects with a Q-wave infarction exercise indexes of LV function and exercise induced ventricular arrhythmias should be used as risk variables.

Angina pectoris indicates a need for possible symptomatic revascularisation. The risk stratification in patients with non-Q-infarction can be based on the occurrence of ST-depression during exercise and probably also on the occurrence of angina pectoris.

References

1. Sanz G, Castaner A, Betriu A, et al. Determinants of prognosis in survivors of myocardial infarction. A Prospective angiographic study. N Eng J Med 1982; 306: 1065-70.
2. DeFeyter PJ, v.Eenige MJ, Dighton DH, et al. Prognostic value of exercise testing, coronary angiography and left ventriculography 6-8 weeks after myocardial infarction. Circulation 1982; 66: 527-36.
3. (The)Multicenter Postinfarction Research Group. Risk Stratification and survival after myocardial infarction. N Eng J Med 1983; 309: 331-6.
4. ISIS-2 Collaborative Group. Randomized trial of intravenous streptokinase, oral aspirin, both or neither among 17187 cases of suspected acute myocardial infarction: ISIS-2. Lancet 1988; II: 349-60.
5. Stadius ML, Davis K, Maynard C, Ritchie JL, Kennedy JW. Risk stratification for 1 year survival based on charateristics identified in the early hours of acute myocardial infarction. Circulation 1986; 74: 703-11.
6. Stack RS, Califf RM, Hinohara T, et al. Survival and cardiac event rates in the first year after emergency coronary angioplasty for acute myocardial infarction. J Am Coll Cardiol 1988; 11: 1141-9.
7. Califf RM, Topol EJ, Gersh BJ. From myocardial salvage to patient salvage in acute myocardial infarction: The role of reperfusion therapy. J Am Coll Cardiol 1989; 14: 1382-8.
8. TIMI Study Group. Comparison of invasive and conservative strategies after treatment with intravenous tissue plasminogen activator in acute myocardial infarction. N Eng J Med 1989; 320: 618-27.
9. Ross Jr J, Gilpin EA, Madsen E, et al. A decision scheme for coronary angiography after acute myocardial infarction. Circulation 1989; 79: 292-303.

10. Saunamäki KI. Early post-myocardial infarction exercise testing. Exercise response and clinical value. Dan Med Bull 1988; 35: 549-64.
11. Taylor GJ, Humphries JO, Mellits ED, et al. Predictors of clinical course, coronary anatomy and left ventricular function after recovery from acute myocardial infarction. Circulation 1980; 62: 960-9.
12. Theroux P, Waters DD, Halphen C, Debaisieux JD, Mizgala HF. Prognostic value of exercise test soon after myocardial infarction. N Eng J Med 1979; 301: 341-5.
13. Waters DD, Bosch X, Bouchard A, et al. Comparison of clinical variables and variables derived from a limited predischarge exercise test as predictors of early and late mortality after myocardial infarction. J Am Coll Cardiol 1985; 5: 1-8.
14. Jennings K, Reid DS, Hawkins T, Julian DJ. Role of exercise testing early after myocardial infarction in identifying candidates for coronary surgery. Br Med J 1984; 288: 185-7.
15. Williams WL, Nair RC, Higginson LAJ, et al. Comparison of clinical and treadmill variables for the prediction of outcome after myocardial infarction. J Am Coll Cardiol 1984; 4: 477-86.
16. Handler CE. Submaximal predischarge exercise testing after myocardial infarction: prognostic value and limitations. Eur Heart J 1985; 6: 510-7.
17. Krone RJ, Gillespie JA, Weld FM, et al. Low-level exercise test after myocardial infarction: usefulness in enhancing clinical risk stratification. Circulation 1985; 71: 80-9.
18. Fioretti P, Brower RW, Simoons ML, et al. Prediction of mortality during the first year after acute myocardial infarction from clinical variables and stress test at hospital discharge. Am J Cardiol 1985; 55: 1313-8.
19. Saunamäki KI, Andersen JD. Clinical significance of the ST-segment response and other early exercise test variables in uncomplicated vs. complicated myocardial infarction. Eur Heart J 1987; 8: 603-10.
20. Klein J, Froelicher VF, Detrano R, Dubach P, Ray Y. Does the rest electrocardiogram after myocardial infarction determine the predictive value of exercise-induced ST-depression? A 2 year follow-up study in a Veteran population. J Am Coll Cardiol 1989; 14: 305-11.
21. Swahn E, Areskog M, Wallentin L. Prognostic importance of early exercise testing in men with suspected unstable coronary artery disease. Eur Heart J 1987; 8: 861-9.
22. Sia B, MacDonald PS, Horowittz JD, Goble AJ, Doyle AE. Usefulness of early exercise testing after non-Q-wave myocardial infarction in predicting prognosis. Am J Cardiol 1986; 57: 738-44.
23. Weld MF, Chu KL, Bigger Jr JT, Rolnitzky LM. Risk stratification with low-level exercise testing 2 weeks after acute myocardial infarction. Circulation 1981; 64: 306-14.
24. Saunamäki KI, Andersen JD. Post-myocardial infarction exercise testing: clinical significance of a left ventricular function index and ventricular arrhythmias. Acta Med Scand 1985; 218: 271-8.
25. Bigger Jr JT, Fleiss JL, Kleiger R, Miller JP, Rolnitzky LM, Multicenter Post-Infarction Research Group. The relationships among ventricular arrhythmias, left ventricular dysfunction and mortality in the 2 years after myocardial infarction. Circulation 1984; 69: 250-8.
26. Henry RL, Kennedy GT, Crawford MH. Prognostic value of exercise-induced ventricular ectopic activity for mortality after acute myocardial infarction.Am J Cardiol 1987; 59: 1251-5.
27. Erbel R, Schweizer P, Krebs W, Meyer J, Effert S. Sensitivity and specificity of two-dimensional echocardiography in detection of impaired left ventricular function. Eur Heart J 1984; 5: 477-89.

36

The tip of the J-curve

JOHN KJEKSHUS

Hypertension is strongly associated with the occurence of coronary heart disease. It is therefore disappointing that prevention of coronary events has generally not been found in most treatment trials when blood pressure is reduced (1, 2). The mechanism that links hypertension to coronary disease is not clearly defined. Obviously the relationship is not a direct one since the importance of hypertension as a risk factor is different between men and women. Roughly, the coronary heart disease risk among men corresponds to the risk for women with 50 mmHg higher systolic blood pressure (3). This contrasts a comparable incidence of stroke between males and females. Furthermore, hypertension does not seem to affect the atherosclerosis in human arteries to the same extent. The coronary arteries are severly affected while the adjacent mammary arteries are usually spared. These differences clearly point to other important mechanisms than solely the hydraulic effect of blood pressure.

The lack of prevention has been attributed to an unfavorable effect of the intervention and also to excessive reduction of blood pressure. Although of small, and as yet of hypothetical importance, antihypertensive drugs may cause an unfavorable effect on the lipid profile, which is suggested to compensate for a favorable effect of reducing blood pressure (4).

The J-curve

Recently, it has been pointed out that the association between blood pressure and coronary mortality is J-formed, suggesting that a systolic blood pressure below 115 mmHg or diastolic below 90 mmHg (5-8) is associated with an increased risk of myocardial infarction (MI).

Retrospective analysis of large intervention studies of hypertension have also shown J-shaped relation between diastolic blood pressure during treatment and MI (1, 8, 9). The lowest point (the J-point) was at a diastolic blood pressure between 85 and 90 mmHg. It has been claimed to be independent of the choice of treatment (9). The non-linear relationship was mainly observed among patients with ischaemic heart disease, while in non-ischaemic patients (defined as those with no previous MI, no angina and no ischaemic ECG changes and no intermittent claudication) the relationship between treated diastolic blood pressure and coronary death was positive and linear. A hypothesis has therefore been suggested that hypertensive patients with myocardial hypertrophy and severe coronary stenosis have a poor coronary reserve which makes the myocardium vulnerable to reduction of coronary perfusion pressure (10, 11). The defenders of the hypothesis claim that it is unlikely that the results can be caused by poor left ventricular function. However, no determination of left ventricular function has been made which can convincingly prove or disprove this hypothesis. The physiological basis underlying the hypothesis is suggested to be abolition of autoregulation ultimately resulting in myocardial ischaemia when blood pressure is reduced (12).

Coronary perfusion pressure and coronary autoregulation

Obviously, the hypothesis is true, if there is a primary reduction in coronary perfusion pressure with unchanged loading conditions and oxygen requirement of the left ventricle. During coronary constriction, the coronary autoregulation compensates for the drop in coronary perfusion pressure by arteriolar vasodilatation until a coronary perfusion pressure of 60 mmHg is attained (13). The autoregulation is effected by a myogenic mechanism sensitive to a reduction of coronary arteriolar transmural pressure and by a metabolic autoregulation effected by the release of adenosine (14, 15). Further constriction causes a rapid reduction of flow (Fig. 1). Oxygen extraction from the coronary flow is almost complete at rest. Lowering of coronary perfusion pressure below the point of autoregulation is followed by proportional reduction of coronary flow and an immediate ischaemic myocardial response causing ventricular dilatation and evidence of myocardial ischaemic injury (16). In the hypertrophic myocardium and especially during an increase in left ventricular filling pressure or during tachycardia, the autoregulation of the coronary resistance is completely exhausted at higher coronary perfusion pressures than during resting conditions (13) (Fig. 1). This may explain the larger infarctions and poorer prognosis following acute coronary occlusion among patients with myocardial hypertrophy and tachycardia (17). This condition is different from when the perfusion pres-

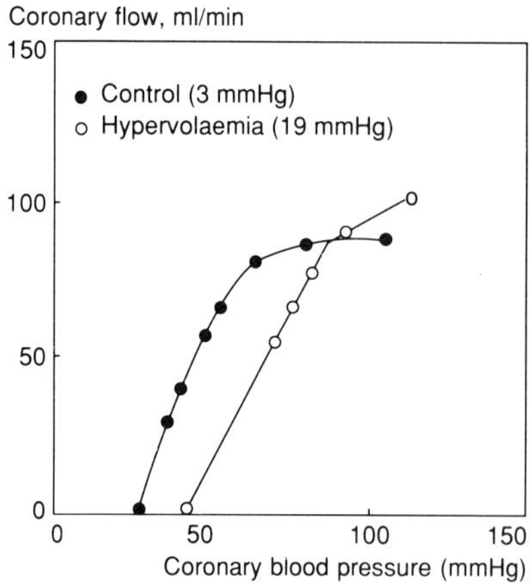

Fig. 1. Coronary pressure-flow relationship before and during elevation of left ventricular end-diastolic pressure. Coronary blood pressure was measured distal to an occlusion on the coronary artery. Coronary flow was measured by an electromagnetic flowmeter on the same artery.

sure is reduced secondary to a reduction of systemic arterial blood pressure, which reduces both myocardial oxygen requirement and coronary perfusion pressure in parallel.

Systemic blood pressure and coronary autoregulation

Animal experiments have demonstrated that when blood pressure was reduced by the arteriolar vasodilator trimethaphan comphor sulfonate, myocardial oxygen consumption and flow were reduced in proportion to the reduction in mean arterial pressure, without evidence of disturbed ventricular contractile pattern, and calculated coronary resistance remained unchanged or increased (18). This was in contrast to haemorrhagic hypotension alone in which coronary resistance decreased reflecting reduced coronary reserve (Fig. 2). However, when blood pressure was lowered by haemorrhage during beta-receptor blockade, coronary resistance increased. The J-curve concept depends entirely on a reduction of the myocardial supply demand ratio during pressure reduction. *Maroko et al* (19) found that haemorrhagic hypotension in animals with acute occlusion of the left descending coronary artery increased epicardial ST segment elevation. These animals had a reflex tachycardia and inotropic stimulation which increased myocardial oxygen demand in a heart with a fixed coronary occlusion.

Provided myocardial contractility and wall tension and consequently myocardial oxygen consumption are decreased in proportion to the reduction of systemic blood pressure without any reflex tachycardia, coronary reserve may remain intact because of preserved metabolic autoregulation.

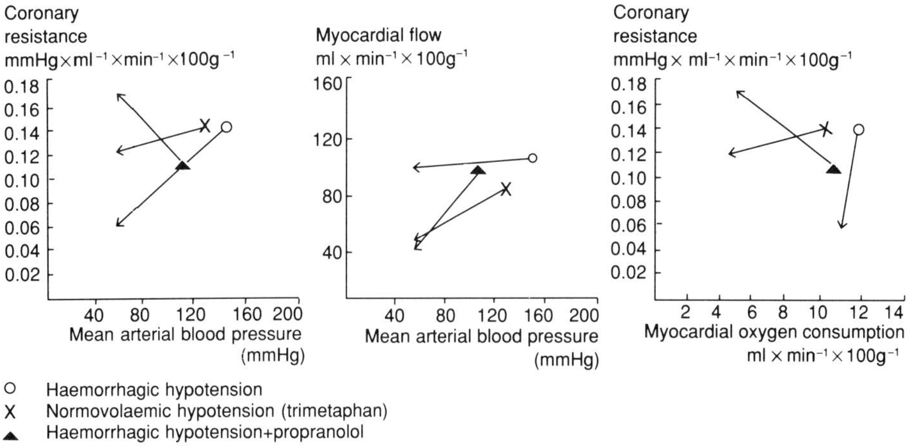

Fig. 2. *The different effects on coronary resistance of reducing systemic blood pressure by haemorrhagic hypotension, normovolaemic hypotension (trimetaphan) and haemorrhagic hypotension with propranolol. Reduction of blood pressure during haemorrhage alone is not associated with a reduction in coronary flow or myocardial oxygen consumption. Accordingly coronary resistance is decreased. Reduction of blood pressure by trimetaphan or haemorrhage during beta blockade was associated with a proportional reduction in coronary flow and myocardial oxygen consumption with no change or an increase in coronary resistance (Ref. 18).*

Reduction of blood pressure and mortality

A low blood pressure may reflect a subset of high risk patients due to myocardial dysfunction and severe coronary artery disease. According to the J-curve hypothesis these patients would be at increased cardiac risk during further reduction of blood pressure. An alternate hypothesis is that reduction of blood pressure may unload the dilated left ventricle and reduce oxygen demand more than the reduction of oxygen supply.

The effect of lowering of blood pressure on mortality has been examined in high risk patients with severe myocardial dysfunction in the Cooperative North Scandinavian Enalapril Survival Study (CONSENSUS) (20).

The CONSENSUS study included 253 patients in severe congestive heart failure (NYHA class IV) from 35 hospitals in Norway, Sweden and Finland. The patients were randomized to enalapril or indentical placebo in a blinded randomized fashion. Details of inclusion procedure and results have been presented elsewhere (20). The mean age was 70 years, (range 36-91), coronary heart disease was the cause of congestive heart failure in 73%. All patients were on diuretics and 94% on digitalis, while 50% received vasodilators other than ACE inhibitors. The treatment dose of enalapril was

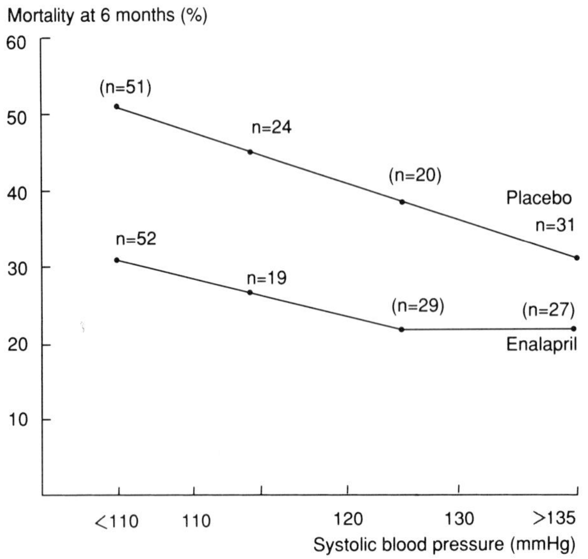

Fig. 3. *Relationship between systolic blood pressure at baseline and mortality at 6 months after treatment with enalapril or placebo (Ref. 26).*

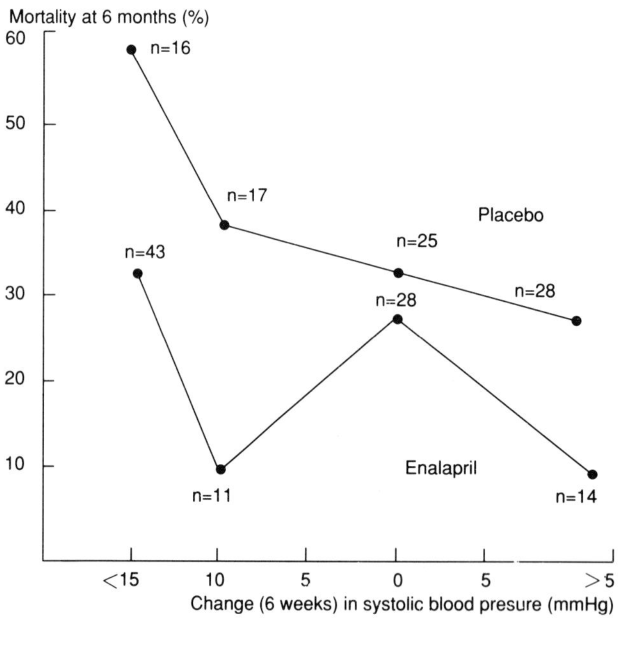

Fig. 4. *Relationship between change in systolic blood pressure from baseline to 6 weeks and mortality at 6 months among patients treated with enalapril or placebo (Ref. 26).*

2.5-40 mg daily. The mortality calculated from life table analysis was 48% at six months, which was the primary objective in the placebo group and reduced by 40% to 29% in the enalapril group. Enalapril reduced average systolic blood pressure by 10 mmHg, compared to 4 mmHg with placebo. Heart rate was reduced respectively 5 and 1 beats/min (21). Thus, there was a significant reduction in the pressure rate product in the enalapril group, which is a major determinant of myocardial oxygen consumption. There was also a reduction of circulating catecholamines which may have further reduced the myocardial oxygen requirement (24).

A trend in both treatment groups could be demonstrated of increasing mortality rates as the baseline systolic blood pressure decreased (Fig. 3). For example, the crude six month mortality rates for patients with systolic blood pressure of 110 mmHg or less at baseline was 51% in the placebo group contrasting 31% in the enalapril group, while the rates for patients with systolic blood pressure higher than 135 mmHg were 32% and 22%, respectively. Enalapril reduced the mortality for any given blood pressure at baseline. Fortythree patients in the enalapril group reduced systolic blood pressure by more than 15 mmHg compared to only 16 patients in the placebo group. Yet the mortality was 33% in the enalapril group as compared to 56% in the placebo group (Fig. 4). A similar trend was observed for diastolic blood pressure changes. Thus, a clear reduction in mortality for any change in blood pressure was observed, meaning that no excess mortality was observed, despite a major reduction in systolic blood pressure with enalapril. This suggests that although a low blood pressure identifies patients with a poor myocardial risk and high six months mortality, further reduction of blood pressure by enalapril conferred long-term protection compared to patients with similar blood pressure at baseline treated with placebo.

All patients in the CONSENSUS trial had major myocardial dysfunction and were in functional class IV (NYHA). The finding of a negative relationship between blood pressure and six months mortality suggests that the CONSENSUS population is at the tip of the J-curve and that their severe prognosis is determined by poor myocardial function. Autopsy findings of the patients showed a mixture of diffuse coronary artery disease, extensive old myocardial infarction, and myocardial hypertrophy in the remaining myocardium

Progression of congestive heart failure was the most frequently observed cause of death in the CONSENSUS trial, which may result from a permanent overloaded myocardial condition (22). The effect of enalapril was also shown to be caused by reduction of death caused by progression of congestive heart failure (20, 21) and no unfavorable effect could be demonstrated on documented MI. Unloading of the myocardium by reducing preload and afterload may therefore be the most likely explanation of the improvement of patient symptoms and survival. Enalapril treatment was associated with a clear reduction in heart size (20) and improvement in systolic time intervals (23) as well as a reduction of neuro-hormones (24). The treatment-induced fall in blood pressure was well tolerated and did not increase the number of coronary events or episodes of symptomatic myocardial ischaemia (21). However, the effects of lowering the blood pressure were associated with more frequent observations of dizziness, when compared to the placebo group (21). This may be anticipated when perfusion pressure is reduced to the brain while its metabolic demand remains unchanged.

In a previous study in which captopril and enalapril were given in higher than therapeutic doses, frequent hypotensive reactions from the central nervous and renal systems were observed yet no myocardial ischaemic events were reported (25). Thus, hypoperfusion symptoms are more likely to occur in organs with fixed oxygen requirement which is independent of the reduction in blood pressure than in the heart when the oxygen requirement is reduced in proportion to the reduction in systemic arterial pressure.

The CONSENSUS study refutes the hypothesis that a moderate reduction of blood pressure impairs myocardial supply among patients with low coronary flow reserve. The prevailing data suggest that the brain and the kidney may be more sensitive than the heart to reduction in systemic blood pressure. The explanation in some epidemiological and interventional studies of a non-linear relationship between MI and systemic blood pressure is that the relationship is a consequence rather than a cause of poor left ventricular function. In hypertensive men after MI, mortality and infarct size are largest among those with the largest fall in blood pressure, and this relationship is independent of drug treatment, as observed in the CONSENSUS trial. The J-point therefore describes a population of high risk patients rather than consequenses of blood pressure lowering intervention.

There is an obvious danger in over emphasizing the importance of the J-curve, when this will lead to inadequate dosing of ACE inhibitors and consequently less reduction of mortality compared to a more aggressive approach.

The CONSENSUS trial clearly demonstrates the importance of prospective randomized studies in defining mortality effects among high risk patients.

Conclusion

Among patients with severe congestive heart failure, there is a negative relationship between blood pressure and mortality. However, further reduction of systemic blood pressure by enalapril improved survival and reduced mortality from progressive congestive heart failure, irrespective of blood pressure at baseline. The reduction of arterial blood pressure did not seem to jeopardize the myocardium of patients in severe heart failure.

A proportional reduction of systemic arterial blood pressure and myocardial oxygen requirement may explain the myocardial tolerance to the reduction in perfusion pressure and refutes the J-curve hypothesis.

References

1. Wilhelmsen L, Berglund G, Elmfeld D, et al. On behalf of the Heart Attack Primary Prevention in Hypertension Trial Research Group. Beta-blockers versus diuretics in hypertensive men: main results from the HAPPHY trial. J Hypertension 1987; 5(5): 561-72.
2. Medical Research Council Working Party. MRC trial of treatment of mild hypertension: principal results. Br Med J 1985; 291: 97-104.
3. Holme I, Waaler HT. Five-year mortality in the city of Bergen, Norway, according to age, sex and blood pressure. Acta Med Scand 1976; 200: 229-39.
4. Ames RP. Negative effects of diuretic drugs on metabolic risk factors for coronary heart disease, possible alternative drug therapies. Am J Cardiol 1983; 51: 632-8.
5. Anderson TW. Re-examination of some of the Framingham blood pressure data. Lancet 1978; ii: 1139-41.
6. Stewart IMcDG. Relation of reduction in pressure to first myocardial infarction in patients receiving treatment for severe hypertension. Lancet 1979; i: 861-5.
7. Cruickshank JM, Thorp JM, Zacharias FJ. Benefits and potential harm of lowering high blood pressure. Lancet; 1987; i: 581-4.
8. Samuelsson O, Wilhelmsen L, Andersson OK, Pennert K, Berglund G. Cardiovascular morbidity in relation to change in blood pressure and serum cholesterol levels in treated hypertension. Results from the Primary Preventin Trial in Goteborg, Sweden. JAMA 1987; 258: 1768-76.
9. Cruickshank JM, Pennert K, Sorman AE, Thorp JM, Zacharias FM, Zacharias FJ. Low mortality from all causes, including myocardial infarction, in well-controlled hypertensives treated with a beta-blocker plus other antihypertensives. J Hypertension 1987; 5: 489-98.
10. Stewart IMcDG. Relation of reduction in pressure to first myocardial infarction in patients receiving treatment for severe hypertension. Lancet 1987; i: 581-4
11. Cruickshank JM. Coronary flow reserve and the J curve relation between diastolic blood-pressure and myocardial infarction. Br Med J 1988; 297: 1227-30.
12. Strandgaard S, Haunsø S. Why does antihypertensive treatment prevent stroke but not myocardial infarction? Lancet 1987; ii: 658-61.
13. Kjekshus J. Mechanism for flow distribution in normal and ischemic myocardium during increased ventricular preload in the dog. Circ Res 1973; 33: 489-99.
14. Belardinelli L, Linden S, Berne J M. The cardiac effects of adenosine. Progr Cardiol Dis 1989; 32: 73-97
15. Klocke FJ. Control of coronary blood flow. An Rev Med 1980; 31: 489-508.
16. Lekven J, Mjøs OD, Kjekshus JK. Compensatory mechanisms during graded myocardial ischemia. Am J Cardiol 1973; 31: 467-73.
17. Kjekshus JK. Importance of heart rate in determining betablocker efficacy in acute and long-term myocardial intervention trials. Am J Cardiol 1986; 51: 437-97.
18. Bugge-Asperheim B, Kjekshus J. Effects of prolonged hypotension on myocardial function in dogs. Scand J Clin Lab Invest 1968; 21: 145-56.
19. Maroko PR, Kjekshus JK, Sobel BE, et al. Factors influencing infarct size following experimental coronary artery oclusions. Circulation 1971; 18: 67-82.

20. The Consensus Trial Study group. Effects of enalapril on mortality in severe congestive heart failure. N Engl J Med 1987; 316: 1429-35.
21. Kjekshus J, Swedberg K. For The Consensus Trial Study Group. Enalapril for congestive heart failure. Am J Cardiol 1989; 63: 26D-32D
22. Katz AM. Cardiomyopathy of overload : a major determinant of prognosis in congestive heart failure. N Engl J Med 1990; 322: 100-10.
23. Eriksson SV, Offstad J, Kjekshus J. M-Mode echocardiography in patients with severe congestive heart failure. A subgroup analysis in the Cooperative North Scandinavian Enalapril Survival Study (CONSENSUS) Drugs 1990.
24. Swedberg K, Eneroth P, Kjekshus J, Wilhelmsen L. For the CONSENSUS Trial Study Group. Hormones regulating cardiovascular function in patients with severe congestive heart failure and the relation to mortality. Circulation (in press).
25. Packer M, Hung Lee W, Yurshak M, Medina N. Comparison of captopril and enalapril in patients with severe chronic heart failure. N Engl J Med 1986; 315: 847-53.
26. Kjekshus J, Swedberg K. Consensus Study and beyond. In Cardiac and renal failure: An expanding role for ACE inhibitors. In: Dollery CT, Sherwood LM, eds. Philadelphia: Hanley and Belfus, Inc. 1989: 210-21.

Late management, therapeutic approach

37

Strategy for therapy after myocardial infarction

TERJE R. PEDERSEN

Patients surviving an acute myocardial infarction (MI) face a relatively high risk of suffering new manifestations of coronary heart disease. The strategy for secondary prevention of these manifestations must incorporate intervention on several pathological processes. The most important are 1) sudden, unexpected heart arrest, mostly due to primary ventricular fibrillation (VF), 2) recurrent coronary thrombosis leading to a new MI, 3) developement of pump failure due to damage of large areas of the myocardium, 4) ischaemia of the remaining myocardium due to multiple coronary stenoses, coronary artery spasm and raised end-diastolic intraventricular pressure which leads to postinfarction angina, 5) symptomatic cardiac arrhythmias and 6) endocardial thrombus formation leading to cerebral and periferal embolia. The risk of each of these complications varies between patients according to size and location of the infarction and the extent of coronary atheromatosis. As methods are being developed to assess the risks, it has to some extent become possible to tailor the secondary preventive therapy to each individual victim of acute MI. Such therapy should always be adjusted to the patient's psychological, social and physical status and should be planned as part of the rehabilitation process.

The different strategies of secondary prevention may be classified according to the pathophysiology that are targets of intervention. One of these is the jeopardized metabolism of the ischaemic myocardium giving rise to dangerous arrhythmias as well as deteriorated contractility. A second target is the formation of thrombus by activation of platelet aggregation as well as fibrin formation. A third is the progress of coronary atheromatosis, probably facilitated by the same factors that initiated it. Several specific remedies and interventions have been tested to cope with these processes, the most important are listed in Table 1. The formal requirement for accepting a new

Table 1. *Strategies for secondary prevention.*

	Proven benefit on survival
Beta-adrenergic blocking agents	+
Calcium antagonists	−
Nitrates	−
ACE inhibitors (in heart failure)	+
Antiarrhythmic agents	−
Antiplatelet agents	+
Intervention on primary risk factors	−
Anticoagulation	+
Surgical revascularization	(+) *)
Physical training	−

*) Benefit proven only in trials with patients with and without infarction.

therapy is that it has been of proven value in randomized, controlled clinical trials of adequate size and design. In the following, the most promising strategies will be delt with in detail.

Long-term beta-adrenergic blockade

At present, beta-adrenergic blockade is the therapy with the most convincing documentation of protective effects against sudden cardiac death following infarction. This stragey also rests on extensive evidence from experimental research showing the deleterious effects of sympathetic stimulation during myocardial ischaemia. Increased activation of beta-adrenergic receptors is a fundamental part of myocardial ischaemia (1). Such activation leads to increased oxygen consumption which in turn leads to increased myocardial damage as the oxygen demand cannot be met (2, 3). At the same time adrenergic activation lowers the threshold for VF (4).

Studies of animals with experimentally induced coronary artery occlusion have shown that treatment with beta-adrenergic blocking agents, particularily when given prior to occlusion, reduces infarct size up to 50% compared to control animals (3, 5, 6) and reduces the risk of VF (7). Pretreatment with beta-adrenergic blocking drugs increases the threshold of VF induced by electrophysiological stimulation in dogs with and without ischaemia (8, 9).

Eighteen randomized placebo controlled clinical trials have been published since 1972, on the use of beta-adrenergic blocking drugs following acute MI (10-27). These trials have included more than 19,000 patients. Most of the studies failed to demonstrate significant reductions in mortality and reinfarction due to insufficient sample size or inclusion of patients with relatively low risk of sudden death and reinfarction or both. The trend in favour of therapy was, however, present in most trials. The three studies that succeeded in demonstrating a significant reduction in mortality through therapy were designed to avoid the errors made in the non-conclusive studies.

The Norwegian multicentre study with timolol was the first to demonstrate convincingly that overall mortality could be reduced (19). Among 3,647 consecutive survivors of acute MI 1,884 (52%) could be included in the study. Those who were excluded from participation were patients with accepted contra-indications to beta-adrenergic blockade (18%), other serious diseases (7%) or logistic and administrative reasons precluding participation (23%). Life-table cumulative total mortality was 21.9% in the placebo-group (152 deaths among 939 patients) against only 13.3% in the timolol group (98 deaths among 945), (p=0.0003) during the follow-up period of 12-33 months (Fig. 1). This trial also showed a reduced incidence of non-fatal reinfarction, 16.4 % in the placebo-group against 11.8% in the timolol group (p=0.001) (28).

In the Beta-blocker Heart Attack Trial (BHAT) which was carried out in the USA using propranolol, only 23 % of all patients considered were included in the study. Life-table total mortality was 13.3 % in the placebo-

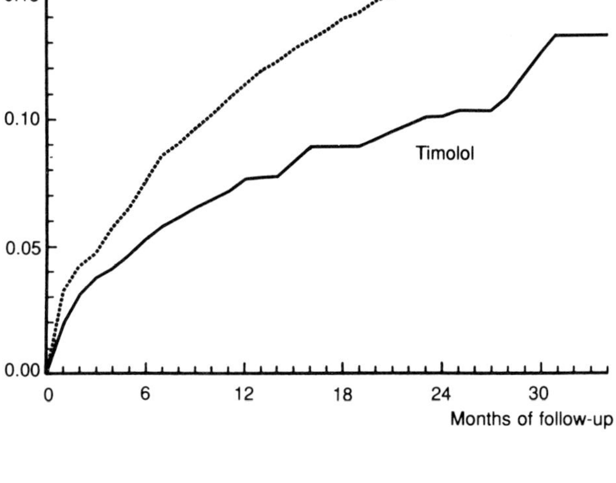

Fig. 1. *Life table cumulative probability of total death, including deaths after withdrawal (intention-to-treat) in the Norwegian Multicentre Study on Timolol in Secondary Prevention after Infarction (from 28).*

group (188 deaths among 1,921 patients) against 10.3 % in the propranolol group (138 deaths among 1,916) during the follow-up period of up to 36 months ($p < 0.01$).

In a study from Gothenborg using metoprolol, randomization was carried out upon arrival in hospital, starting with intravenous administration of placebo or metoprolol and continuing with peroral treatment for 3 months. The study comprised a large proportion of high-risk patients and only 47% of admitted patients were excluded from randomization. Mortality was reduced from 8.9% in the placebo-group (62 deaths among 697 patients) to 5.7% in the metoprolol group (40 deaths among 698) ($p=0.024$).

Mechanism of action

The reasons for the success of beta-adrenergic blockade following acute MI are still being discussed (29). In the Norwegian timolol-study, 76 patients in the placebo group had a definite or probable primary heart arrest against only 26 in the timolol group (28). In the metoprolol study from Gothenborg 18 placebo-treated patients had VF during hospitalization against only 6 in the metoprolol group (30). In the study by *Hansteen*, the number of instantaneous deaths plus patients found dead was 20 in the placebo-group and 10 in the propranolol group (14). Prevention of primary VF therefore seems to be the major mechanism of action and is in accordance with results from animal experiments (8, 9).

In addition to the timolol-study, trials using sotalol (18) and metoprolol (13) demonstrated significant reductions in non-fatal reinfarction. Timolol has no clinically important effect on platelet aggregation (31). The preventive effect therefore must be due to other steps in the reinfarction process. *Maroko and coworkers* gradually reduced coronary blood flow in dogs during simultaneous infusion of isoproterenol (32). After pretreatment with propranolol, blood flow could be reduced more than during control conditions before signs of myocardial damage became evident. This was presumed to be due to conservation of ATP and mitochondrial function during hypoxia (33).

Beta-adrenergic blockade attenuates lipolysis caused by adrenergic stimulation. The myocardial tissue thus reduces the uptake of free fatty acids and increases the uptake of glucose (34, 35). This might explain some of the reduced demand for high-energy phosphates in ischaemic conditions. Collateral blood flow during a critical stenosis or occlusion of coronary arteries might be sufficient to avoid or at least minimize necrosis when the demand for high energy phosphates is reduced.

A central aspect of the process of acute MI and unstable angina is the rupture of an atherosclerotic plaque with subsequent thrombus formation. Beta-adrenergic blocking agents reduce heart rate and contractility. If mechanical forces acting upon the sclerotic plaque during each heart beat are important in producing plaque fissures, beta-adrenergic blockade might possibly decrease the tendency of "material fatigue" by reducing motion and streching-bending forces on the coronary artery. This hypothesis remains to be tested.

Candidates for beta-adrenergic blocking treatment

Results from the timolol-study indicate that 75-80% of all patients aged 75 years or less might start therapy before discharge from hospital, or they are already receiving such treatment on admission. Although patients with small infarctions will also benefit from therapy, the risk of sudden cardiac death in such patients is small and prevention of reinfarction is probably as effective with treatments giving less side effects such as aspirin or warfarin. Patients with small infarctions are candidates for beta-blockade, especially if they have post-infarction angina or evidence of myocardial ischaemia as judged from an exercise test during convalecense. In patients with large and complicated infarctions, beta-adrenergic blockade should be started as soon as the patient is haemodynamically stable. Aggresive therapy with diuretics, digitalis and vasodilatators should be attempted in patients with clinical signs of congestive heart failure before beta-adrenergic therapy is started. Such patients have the highest risk of VF and consequently the highest relative benefit of therapy with beta-adrenergic blocking agents, if they are tolerated. Patients with hypotension (i.e. systolic blood pressure of 105 mmHg or less) tolerate beta-blockade poorly and should be excluded from therapy. Bradycardia during therapy is mostly well tolerated, even with heart rates down to 40 beats per minute.

Starting and terminating treatment

The advantages of starting therapy very early in the course of the infarction have been less convincing, although several investigations indicate reduction of infarct size through intravenous administration on admission to hospital (36-40). In large scale trials of selected patients, only modest benefits have been observed in short-term follow-up (41, 42). In trials showing substantial long-term benefit, treatment was started after the patients had been clinically stable for some days.

During the first year after the infarction a large number of the patients will develop angina pectoris making cessation of therapy less practical among those who tolerate beta-adrenergic blockade well. Since the risk of VF is greatest during the first year after the infarction, therapy should be continued for at least that period in patients at high risk, even if minor side effects are present. Concern has been raised that treatment with beta-adrenergic blocking agents over several years might have an unfavourable effect on progression of atheromatosis through the effect on plasma lipids (43). However, during an extended follow-up of the patients in the timolol study, there was no sign of a diminished effect on survival in patients continuing on therapy for up to six years (44).

Choice of drug and dosage

When comparing results from different trials it is not possible to draw any conclusions about preference for one beta-adrenergic blocking agent over the others because of the difference in selection of study patients in the various trials. One exception seems to be that trials using drugs with intrinsic sympathomimetic activity tend to yield less benefit than trials with drugs devoid of such an effect. The last published study using a high dose of oxprenolol was interrupted prematurely after including 1,700 patients as the difference in mortality between the placebo and the treated group showed a trend in disfavour of oxprenolol (17). *Raeder at al* investigated the effect of several beta-adrenergic blocking agents on the threshold of inducable VF in dogs (45). In accordance with the findings by *Anderson et al* (8) the authors found an increased threshold for all types of drugs. The effect of pindolol, however, having strong instrinsic sympathomimetic activity, was quickly attenuated in comparison with other drugs. The optimal dosage has not yet been determined. *Anderson et al* showed increasing effects on the threshold of VF when dosage was increased. A relatively high dosage was necessary with most beta-adrenergic blocking agents to achieve maximal protection. In the timolol study, the dosage choosen produced a mean heart rate reduction of as much as 18 beats per minute.

If the main effect of therapy is to protect from casual catecholamin-induced lowering of the VF threshold, a continuing protection throughout the day and night as well as a good patient compliance seems as important as a high dosage. Until more data become available to document the mechanisms of action of therapy, dosages used in the clinical trials should be used in clinical practice.

Clinical guidelines

Long-term therapy with beta-adrenergic blocking agents is clearly indicated in patients with moderate or large infarct size and therapy should start as soon as the patient is clinically stable. Drugs without intrinsic sympathomimetic activity should be chosen. Standard therapy would be timolol 10 mg b.i.d, propranolol 60-80 mg t.i.d or metoprolol 100 mg b.i.d. Treatment should be continued for at least 1-2 years. In patients with very high risk or with angina, treatment should be continued for the rest of their life. In patients with small infarctions and a low risk of sudden death, beta-adrenergic therapy represents an option to prevent reinfarction.

Other strategies

Calcium antagonists

Calcium antagonists have been as extensively studied in secondary prevention following infarction as beta-adrenergic blocking agents. In contrast to the latter, such therapy has not been shown to influence survival (46). In one trial using diltiazem, the risk of reinfarction was reduced if therapy was given to patients with non-Q-infarction (47). Preliminary results of a recent trial using verapamil also showed that the risk of reinfarction was reduced, compared to placebo, when therapy was started 1-3 weeks following the onset of infarction (48). Trials with nifedipine have indicated, if anything, a possible deleterious effect on infarct size, when used in the acute stage (46). Diltiazem and verapamil might have a place in the treatment of angina following non-Q-wave and smaller infarctions if beta-adrenergic blocking agents are contra-indicated. Other calcium-antagonists so far seem to have no place in secondary prevention regimens.

Nitrates

Isosorbide dinitrate in combination with hydralazine reduced mortality in patients with severe congestive heart failure in one trial (49). The difference compared to placebo was of borderline statistical significance. Approximately 40% of the patients had previous MI. However, at present no randomized controlled clinical trial has demonstrated secondary preventive effects of nitrates per se. Therefore, such therapy is only indicated as symptomatic therapy when beta-blocking agents are contra-indicated or have insufficient antianginal effect.

Angiotensin converting enzyme inhibitors

So far, ACE inhibitors have only been tested in randomized clinical trials in patients with severe congestive heart failure. In the CONSENSUS trial, the majority of patients had severe congestive heart failure because of MI (50). This trial demonstrated marked improvement in survival in the group using enalapril compared to the placebo-treated group. Whether patients with less extensive myocardial damage will benefit from such therapy remains to be proven.

Antiarrhythmic drugs

Several clinical trials have been performed with various antiarrhythmic drugs of Class I and Class III, but none have shown beneficial effects on fatal arrhythmias (51). On the contrary, trials using encainide and flecaninide have indicated a deleterious effect of such therapy, proably due to a proarrhythmic effect (52). Such therapy is therefore contra-indicated in patients with ischaemic heart disease, with the exception of patients with invalidizing arrhythmia.

Antiplatelet agents

An overview of all clinical trials with antiplatelet therapy in secondary prevention of vascular disease (53), as well as the ISIS-2 using aspirin with and without the combination with streptokinase (54) showed reduced mortality with use of such therapy following infarction. Dosages ranging from 160-1500 mg aspirin daily have been used in these trials. Addition of dipyridamole or sulphinpyrazone have not contributed with an increase of effect. In a recent Swedish trial using 75 mg aspirin, benefits of the same magnitude were indicated as seen with larger dosages, whereas side-effects were not observed with the lower dose (55). Low-dose aspirin therefore seems indicated to reduce the risk of fatal and non-fatal reinfarction.

Intervention on primary risk factors

Leren showed that lipid-lowering diet after acute MI reduced the incidence of reinfarction, however, the study was too small to demonstrate any effect on mortality (56). Trials using lipid-lowering drugs have also failed to demonstrate an improvement in overall survival, possibly due to a relatively modest efficiency of the drugs being used. More effective modern drugs are currently being tested in clinical trials. Randomized trials on the effect of cessation of smoking following infarction have not been carried out. However, in the Oslo Study Diet and Antismoking Trial, healthy men at high risk of coronary heart disease had significantly lower incidence of a first infarction and sudden death when subjected to an antismoking and diet intervention programme (57). In an extended follow-up, overall mortality was also reduced compared to the control group, although the difference was of borderline statistical significance (58). Since such advice involves little or no expense and since epidemiological and other experience indicate a relationship between smoking and coronary thrombosis, all smokers should be advised to quit.

Anticoagulants, revascularization and physical training

Anticoagulants, revascularization and organized physical training are important elements in the rehabilitation and secondary prevention of post-infarction complications. The effects of these interventions will be discussed in the following chapters.

References

1. Raab W, Van Lith P, Lepeschkin E, Herrlich HC, Louis DA. Catecholamine-induced myocardial hypoxia in the presence of impaired coronary dilatability independent of external cardiac work. Am J Cardiol 1962; 9: 455-70.
2. Katz L, Williams FL, Laurent D, Bolene-Williams C, Feinberg H. Effects of l-norepinephrine and l-epinephrine on coronary flow and oxygen consumption of the intact open chest dog. Fed Proc 1956; 15: 106-7.
3. Maroko PR, Kjekshus JK, Sobel BE, et al. Factors influencing infarct size following experimental coronary artery occlusion. Circulation 1971; 43: 67-82.
4. Corr PB, Witkowsky FX, Sobel BE. Increased adrenergic tone in ischemic myocardium undergoing ventricular fibrillation. Clin Res 1977; 25: 454A.
5. Singh BN, Miura M, Thomas R, Ganz W, Shell WE. Effects of propranolol on gross anatomic infarctsize following experimental coronary artery occlusion. In: Hjalmarson Å, Wilhelmsen L, eds. Acute and longterm medical management of myocardial ischemia. Göteborg: Hässle 1978: 238-46.
6. Smith FF, Schmuck GA, Carrwo BA, Lefer AM. Infarct size restriction in cats by the beta-adrenergic blocker timolol. Eur J Pharmacol 1982; 77: 153-8.
7. Kahn MI, Hamilton JT, Manning GW. Protective effect of beta-adrenergic blockade in experimental coronary occlusion in conscious dogs. Am J Cardiol 1972; 30: 832-7.
8. Anderson JL, Rodier HE, Green LS. Comparative effects of beta-adrenergic blocking drugs on experimental ventricular fibrillation threshold. Am J Cardiol 1983; 51: 1196-202.
9. Gang ES, Bigger JT, Uhl EW. Effects of timolol and propranolol on induceable sustained ventricular tachyarrhythmias in dogs with subacute myocardial infarction. Am J Cardiol 1984; 53: 275-81.

10. Wilhelmsson C, Vedin AJ, Wilhelmsen L, Tibblin G, Werkö L. Reduction of sudden deaths after myocardial infarction by treatment with aprenolol: preliminary results. Lancet 1974; 2: 1157-60.
11. Manger Cats V, van Capelle FJL, Lie KI, Durrer D. Effect of treatment with 2X100 mg metoprolol on mortality in a single-center study with low placebo mortality-rate after infarction. Circulation 1983; 68 (suppl III): III-8.
12. Baber NS, Evans DW, Howitt G, et al. Multicentre post-infarction trial of propranolol in 49 hospitals in the United Kingdom, Italy and Yugoslavia. Br Heart J 1980; 44: 96-100.
13. Olsson G. Effects of chronic metoprolol treatment after acute myocardial infarction. Stockholm, 1984. (Thesis).
14. Hansteen V, Möinichen E, Lorentsen E, et al. One year's treatment with propranolol after myocardial infarction: preliminary report of Norwegian multicentre trial. Br Med J 1982; 284: 155-60.
15. Australian and Swedish Pindolol Study Group. The effect of pindolol on two years mortality after complicated myocardial infarction. Eur Heart J 1983; 4: 367-75.
16. European Infarction Study Group. European infarction study (E.I.S.). A secondary prevention study with slow release oxprenolol after myocardial infarction: morbidity and mortality. Eur Heart J 1984; 5: 189-202.
17. Taylor SH, Silke B, Ebutt A, Sutton GC, Prout BJ, Burley DM. A long-term prevention study with oxprenolol in coronary heart disease. N Engl J Med 1982; 307: 1293-301.
18. Julian DG, Prescott RJ, Jackson FS, Szekely P. Controlled trial of sotalol for one year after myocardial infarction. Lancet 1982; i: 1142-7.
19. Multicentre International Study. Supplementary Report. Reduction in mortality after myocardial infarction with long-term beta-adrenoceptor blockade. Br Med J 1977; 2: 419-21.
20. Norwegian Multicenter Study Group. Timolol-induced reduction in mortality and reinfarction in patients surviving acute myocardial infarction. N Engl J Med 1981; 304: 801-7.
21. Beta-blocker Heart Attack Trial Research Group. A randomized trial of propranolol in patients with acute myocardial infarction. I. Mortality results. JAMA 1982; 247: 1707-14.
22. Reynolds JL, Whitlock RML. Effect of beta-adrenrgic receptor blocker in myocardial infarction treated for one year from onset. Br Heart J 1972; 34: 252-9.
23. McIlmoyle L, Evans A, Boyle D McC, et al. Early intervention in myocardial ischaemia. Proc Br Cardiac Soc. December 1981: 3-4.
24. Wilcox R, Roland JM, Banks DC, Hampton JR, Mitchell JRA. Randomized trial comparing propranolol with atenolol in immediate treatment of suspected myocardial infarction. Br Med J 1980; 280: 885-8.
25. Barber JM, Boyle D McC, Chatuverdi NC, Singh N, Walsh MJ. Practolol in acute myocardial infarction. Acta Med Scand 1976; (suppl 587): 213-9.
26. Hjalmarson Å, Elmfeldt D, Herlitz J, et al. Effect on mortality of metoprolol in acute myocardial infarction: a double-blind randomized trial. Lancet 1981; ii: 823-7.
27. Andersen MP, Bechsgaard P, Frederiksen J, et al. Effect of alprenolol on mortality among patients with definite or suspected acute myocardial infarction: preliminary results. Lancet 1979; ii: 865-8.
28. Pedersen TR, The Norwegian Multicenter Study Group. A multicenter study on timolol in secondary prevention after myocardial infarction. Acta Med Scand 1983; 214 (suppl 674): 1-129.
29. Fitzgerald JD. By what means might beta blockers prolong life after actue myocardial infarction? Eur Heart J 1987; 8: 945-51.
30. Rydén L, Arniego R, Arnman K, et al. A double-blind trial of metoprolol in acute

myocardial infarction: effects on ventricular tachyarrhythmias. N Engl J Med 1983; 308: 614-8.
31. Thaulow E, Kjekshus J, Eriksen J. Effect of timolol on platelet aggregation in coronary heart disease. Acta Med Scand 1981; (suppl 651): 101-9.
32. Maroko PR, Libby P, Braunwald E. Effect of pharmacologic agents on the function of the ischemic heart. Am J Cardiol 1973; 32: 930-6.
33. Braunwald E, Muller JE, Kloner Ra, Maroko PR. Role of beta-adrenergic blockade in the therapy of patients with myocardial infarction. Am J Med 1983; 74: 113-23.
34. Marchetti G, Merlo L, Neseda V. Myocardial uptake of free fatty acids and carbohydrates after beta adrenergic blockade. Am J Cardiol 1968; 22: 370-4.
35. Opie LH, Thomas M. Propranolol and experimental myocardial infarction: substrate effect. Postgrad Med J 1976; 52 (suppl. 4): 124-32.
36. Norris RM, Clarke ED, Sammel NL, Smith WM, Williams B. Protective effect of propranolol in threatened myocardial infarction. Lancet 1978; ii: 907-9.
37. Yusuf S, Ramsdale D, Peto R. Early intravenous atenolol in suspected acute myocardial infarction. Preliminiary report of a randomized trial. Lancet 1980; ii : 273-6.
38. Jürgensen HJ, Fredriksen J, Hansen DA, Pedersen-Bjergaard D. Limitation of myocardial infarct size in patients less than 66 years treated with alprenolol. Br Heart J 1981; 45: 583-8.
39. Herlitz J, Elmfeldt D, Hjalmarson Å, et al. Effect of metoprolol on indirect signs of the size and severity of acute myocardial infarction. Am J Cardiol 1983; 51: 1282-8.
40. International Collaborative Study Group. Reduction of infarct size with the early use of timolol in acute myocardial infarction. N Engl J Med 1984; 310: 9-15.
41. The MIAMI Trial Research Group: Metoprolol In Acute Myocardial Infarction (MIAMI). A randomized placebo-controlled international trial. Eur Heart J 1985; 6: 199.
42. ISIS-1 (First International Study of Infarct Survial) Collaborative Group: Randomized trial of intravenous atenolol among 16,027 cases of suspected acute myocardial infarction: ISIS-I. Lancet 1986; ii: 57.
43. Schulman RS, Herbert PN, Capone RJ, et al. Effects of propranolol on blood lipids and lipoproteins in myocardial infarction. Circulation 1983; 67 (suppl. I): I19-21.
44. Pedersen TR, for The Norwegian Multicenter Study Group. Six-year follow-up of the Norwegian Multicenter Study on Trimolol after acute myocardial infarction. N Engl J Med 1985; 313: 1055-8.
45. Raeder EA, Verrier RL, Lown B. Intrisic symptahomimetic activity and the effects of beta-adrenergic blocking drugs on vulnerability to ventricular fibrillation. J Am Coll Cardiol 1983; 16: 1442-6.
46. Held PH, Yusuf S, Furberg CD. Calcium channel blockers in acute myocardial infarction and unstable angina: an overview. Br Med J 1989; 299: 1187-92.
47. Gibson RS, Boden WE, Theroux P, et al. Diltiazem and reinfarction in patients with non-Q wave infarction. N Engl J Med 1986; 315: 423-9.
48. Fischer Hansen J. Effect of verapamil on mortality and reinfarction after acute myocardial infarction. Presented at American College of Cardiology, 39th annual scientific session, New Orleans, Lousiana, March 18-22, 1990.
49. Cohn JN, Archibald DG, Ziesche S, et al. Effect of vasodilator therapy on mortality in chronic congestive heart failure: results of a Veterans Administration Cooperative Study. N Engl J Med 1986; 314: 1547-52.
50. The CONSENSUS Trial Study Group. Effects of enalapril on mortality in severe congestive heart failure. Results of the Cooperative North Scandinavian Enalapril Survival Study (CONSENSUS). N Engl J Med 1987; 316: 1429-35.
51. Hine LK, Laird NM, Hewitt P, Chalmers TC. Meta-analysis of empirical long-term antiarrhythmic therapy after myocardial infarction. JAMA 1989; 262: 3037-40.

52. Cardiac Arrhythmias Suppression Trial. Preliminary report: effect of encainide and flecainide on mortality in a randomized trial of arrhythmia supression after myocardial infarction. N Engl J Med 1989; 321: 406-12.
53. Hennekens CH, Buring JE, Sandercock P, Collins R, Peto R. Aspirin and other antiplatelet agents in the secondary and primary prevention of cardiovascular disease. Circulation 1989; 80: 749-56.
54. ISIS-2 (Second International Study of Infarct Survival) Collaborative Study Group. Randomized trial of intravenous streptokinase, oral aspirin, both or neither among 17,187 cases of suspected acute myocardial infarction. Lancet 1988; ii: 349-60.
55. Wallentin L. ASA 75 mg and/or heparin after an episode of unstable coronary artery disease - risk for myocardial infarct death in a randomized placebo-controlled study. Eur Heart J 1989; 10: II-49.
56. Leren P. The Oslo diet-heart study. Eleven-year report. Circulation 1970; 17: 935-42.
57. Hjermann I, Byre KV, Holme I, Leren P. Effect of diet and smoking intervention on the incidence of coronary heart disease. Report from the Oslo Study Group of a randomised trial in healthy men. Lancet 1981; ii: 1303-10.
58. Hjermann I, Holme I, Leren P. Oslo Study Diet and Antismoking Trial: Results after 102 months. Am J Med 1986; 80 (2A): 7-11.

38

Anticoagulation after myocardial infarction

PÅL SMITH,
HARALD ARNESEN

Background

Thrombus formation on a ruptured atheromatous plaque in the infarct-related artery is a frequent finding at autopsy after acute myocardial infarction (AMI) (1-3). Moreover, epidemiological research has pinpointed the relation of clotting factor VII and fibrinogen with subsequent increased risk of cardiovascular death and morbidity in putatively healthy subjects (5-7), and angiographic studies in the early phase of AMI have clearly demonstrated the association of thrombus with the clinical event (8, 9). The effects of thrombolysis as depicted angiographically (10) and clinically (11-13) have provided additional support to the concept of a causal relationship between coronary thrombus and AMI.

Once recovered from a AMI, a patient faces a 15-20 per cent risk of a recurrence, a 4-5 per cent risk of having a stroke, and a 15-20 per cent risk of succumbing to cardiovascular disease within the next 2-5 years (14, 15). Moreover, increased levels of the rapid inhibitor of tissue plasminogen activator, PAI-1, are associated with increased risk of recurrency in younger patients with AMI (16). The theoretical rationale for the use of anticoagulant therapy after AMI is to prevent cardiac chamber thrombus and coronary thrombus formation.

Despite the rationale for antithrombotic prevention, clinical trials have as yet not been able to produce conclusive evidence of a benefit of anticoagulant therapy after AMI (17). This chapter reviews the role of anticoagulants after AMI with particular reference to data from the Warfarin Re-Infarction Study (WARIS), the latest study in this field (18).

History

Few topics have engendered as much controversy in cardiological practice as the use of anticoagulants after AMI. In 1948, *Wright et al* (19) reported less mortality with the use of heparin and dicoumarol in the first six weeks after AMI. Although the conclusions were challenged because of inadequate randomization of the patients, they opened an era of enthusiastic clinical trials during the fifties and sixties. However, while most of the early trials are considered deficient by modern study design criteria, a series of more pessimistic studies from the 60's were also seriously flawed (20). Furthermore, few of those studies which failed to find a benefit, did achieve an intensity of hypocoagulation regarded as adequate by todays standards (21).

In 1969, *Gifford and Feinstein* criticized the accumulated literature in a paper that became very influential. They stated that only two of 32 clinical studies had satisfied more than half of the criteria of adequate trial design, and that methodological short-comings had been especially serious in those studies claiming benefit from anticoagulation (22).

Neither later clinical studies, most of which reported that long-term anticoagulation therapy was indeed effective, nor a comprehensive review article which concluded that combined analysis of six randomized trials revealed a reduction in mortality by anticoagulants by 21 per cent (23), could stop the decline in enthusiasm.

The Sixty Plus trial revived the debate when published in 1980 (24). It was a large study, including 878 patients with an average age of 67.6 years. The desired range of anticoagulant therapy was 5-10 per cent Thrombotest (4.8 to 2.8 INR) (25), which was subsequently achieved in about 70 per cent of the prothrombin time determinations. The average follow-up was 2 years. When analyzed for total mortality on intention-to-treat basis the difference just failed to attain statistical significance ($p=0.07$), whereas an analysis based on protocol adherents yielded a statistically significant difference ($p=0.017$). Analyzing the endpoint reinfarction, there was an unequivocal reduction by oral anticoagulants: $p=0.0005$ on intention-to-treat basis and $p=0.0001$ considering only those who were actually taking the test medication at the time of event. However, as those entered into this study had already been treated with oral anticoagulants for an average of more than six years, it was argued that the study tested the danger of stopping anticoagulant treatment, not the benefit of starting it (17, 26). Thus, the anticoagulant problem was still not solved, and the need for a conclusive trial was discussed both in the national (27) and in international medical journals (17).

The WARIS trial

Design and methods: The Warfarin Re-Infarction Study (WARIS) (18) was designed as a randomized, placebo-controlled and double blind trial. The major goal of this study was to assess safety and efficacy of anticoagulant therapy after AMI. Treatment allocation was stratified for chronic beta-blockade, to ensure even distribution of subjects on such drugs in the two study groups.

Patients of either sex aged 75 or less were eligible at discharge from hospital after a documented AMI (28) if they exhibited no specific contra-indication to treatment with oral anticoagulants, lived in the study area, had anticipated acceptable compliance and gave their informed consent. They were recruited from five cardiological centres serving the Oslo area with 570.000 inhabitants.

Prothrombin time measurements were performed with Thrombotest (Nycomed, Oslo) with a target range of 2.8-4.8 INR (International Normalized Ratio) (25). An INR between 2.5 and 4.8 has been proposed as being suitable for preventing arterial thrombosis (21).

Blood was drawn from all patients at the follow-up visits which, after initial stabilization of the prothrombin time, were scheduled every 4-6 weeks. In the placebo group the dosage was changed according to preset criteria.

Inclusion, treatment and endpoints: During the accrual period from January 10, 1983 through March 24, 1986, 1,918 eligible patients were identified of whom 1,214 (63 per cent) were entered into the study. Apart from total cholesterol being higher in the warfarin group ($p<0.001$), the patients' characteristics were well balanced across the treatment groups. Overall duration on test medication averaged 37 months (range, 24 to 63 months). An analysis of the adequacy of treatment after termination of the study, showed that two thirds of the patients had a prothrombin time within the desired range at any given time. Mortality and reinfarction were primary endpoints, stroke a secondary endpoint. Endpoints were taken to have occurred on treatment if occurring within 28 days after stopping test medication. For the intention-to-treat analysis all events after randomization were counted.

Results: Data on reduction in mortality, total reinfarction and stroke are summarized in Table 1. Non-fatal reinfarction on treatment occurred in 75 patients in the placebo group compared with 38 in the warfarin group, a reduction by 49 per cent.

Bleeding complications: Five patients in the warfarin group suffered an intracranial haemorrhage while on treatment, three of which were fatal (0.16 fatal events per 100 patients per year). Major extracranial bleeding

Table 1. *Results of anticoagulant treatment after myocardial infarction. Per cent risk in placebo (PL) versus warfarin group (W).*

	PL (n=607)	W (n=607)	p
Intention-to-treat			
Mortality	20.2	15.4	0.0267
Reinfarction	20.4	13.5	0.0007
Stroke	7.2	3.2	0.0015
On treatment			
Mortality	15.1	9.8	0.0050
Reinfarction	20.0	11.5	0.0001
Stroke	6.7	2.6	0.0003

occurred in 8 patients Thus, the combined incidence of major bleeding was 0.6 per 100 patients per year. Minor bleeding, requiring dose adjustment, was observed in 69 patients of whom 25 were in the placebo group. In 7 of the patients with major extracranial bleeding, this was associated with peptic ulcer, cancer or illegitimate intake of antiplatelet drugs.

Anticoagulants after thrombolysis?

After termination of patient accrual in the WARIS study, thrombolysis became established as effective therapy for improving survival and preserving left ventricular function after AMI (11-13). Data from the ISIS-2 trial, involving 17,187 patients, showed that both aspirin and streptokinase were superior to placebo when considered alone, reducing the mortality at 5 weeks by 23-25 per cent (12). The combination of streptokinase with aspirin 160 mg/day reduced the risk of death more than each of the two treatments alone. Reinfarction was 15 per cent higher in the SK group, while this was reversed to a reduction by 37 per cent by adding aspirin to the treatment. Presently no data are available from randomized trials on warfarin after thrombolysis. However, the Italian SCATI group, which compared the efficacy of calcium heparin 12,500 Units daily with placebo, demonstrated a significantly lower mortality both in the overall groups and in the subgroups receiving streptokinase by heparin (29). Thus, antithrombotic therapy with anticoagulants seems worthwhile, also after thrombolysis. A randomized comparison of warfarin with aspirin in this setting has not yet been performed.

Warfarin versus aspirin

Two studies have compared aspirin and oral anticoagulants in one and the same trial (30, 31). The German-Austrian trial randomized 946 patients to treatment with either phenprocoumon (320 patients), aspirin (317 patients) or placebo (309 patients) and reported that aspirin was numerically more effective against reinfarction and death than placebo or phenprocoumon (30). The French EPSIM study (31), which randomized 1,303 patients to anticoagulant therapy or aspirin, found 65 deaths in the former group and 72 in the latter. The number of reinfarctions were also higher in the aspirin group: 33 versus 20. None of the differences in the two studies were statistically significant.

The benefit of aspirin and anticoagulants has recently been evaluated by meta-analyses, concluding that aspirin seemed to reduce mortality by approximately 13 per cent and non-fatal reinfarction by 31 per cent (32). Taken separately, however, no aspirin study has so far yielded a statistically significant reduction in mortality alone. In comparison, aggregated data from a recent review on the effect of oral anticoagulants, suggest a reduction in mortality by 40 per cent and a reduction in the reinfarction rate by two thirds in studies applying adequate anticoagulation (33). Only a randomized comparison of the two treatments can, however, definitely indicate if one treatment is superior to the other.

Clinical implications

The WARIS study has unequivocally shown that long-term treatment with warfarin after AMI brings about a substantial reduction in the risk of subsequent death, reinfarction and thromboembolic stroke. The slightly increased risk of adverse effects is clearly counter-balanced by the benefits. Thus, if considering an antithrombotic prevention after AMI, oral anticoagulants should be recommended. The efficacy of oral anticoagulants versus aspirin, which has also proved effective in this setting, has not yet been established. Considering the accumulated data on efficacy, the risk reduction by aspirin seems less pronounced than that by oral anticoagulants (32, 33). Furthermore, aspirin seems less likely to reduce the risk of cardiogenic emboli (33). As the 60+ Study (34) showed that stopping anticoagulation after many years has a deleterious effect, anticoagulant treatment should probably be continued indefinitely, provided the patient complies with the treatment regimen. Otherwise, this treatment should be discontinued.

References

1. Blumgart HL, Schlesinger MJ, Davis D. Studies on the relation of the clinical manifestations of angina pectoris, coronary thrombosis, and myocardial infarction to the pathologic findings. Am Heart J 1940; 19: 1-91.
2. Davies MJ, Woolf N, Robertson WB. Pathology of acute myocardial infarction with particular reference to occlusive coronary thrombi. Br Heart J 1976; 38: 659-64.
3. Falk E. Plaque rupture with severe pre-existing stenosis precipitating coronary thrombosis. Br Heart J 1983; 50: 127-34.
4. Falk E. Unstable angina with fatal outcome: dynamic coronary thrombosis leading to infarction and/or sudden death. Circulation 1985; 71: 699-708.
5. Meade TW, North WRS, Chakrabarti R, et al. Haemostatic function and cardiovascular death: early results of a prospective study. Lancet 1980; 1: 1050-4.
6. Wilhelmsen L, Svärdsudd K, Korsan-Bengtsen K, Larsson B, Welin L, Tiblin G. Fibrinogen as a risk factor for stroke and myocardial infarction. N Engl J Med 1984; 311: 501-5.
7. Dalaker K, Hjermann I, Prydz H. A novel form of factor VII in plasma from men at risk for cardiovascular disease. Br J Haematol 1985; 61: 315-22.
8. DeWood MA, Spores J, Notske R, et al. Prevalence of total coronary occlusion during the early hours of transmural myocardial infarction. N Engl J Med 1980; 303: 897-902.
9. Vetrovec GW, Cowley MJ, Overton H, Richardson DW. Intracoronary thrombus in syndromes of unstable myocardial ischemia. Am Heart J 1981; 102: 1202-8.
10. Rentrop P, Blanke H, Karsch KR, Kaiser H, Kostering H, Leitz K. Selective intracoronary thrombolysis in acute myocardial infarction and unstable angina pectoris. Circulation 1981; 63: 307-17.
11. Gruppo Italiano Per Lo Studio Della Streptochinasi Nell Infarto Miocardico. Long-term effects of intravenous thrombolysis in acute myocardial infarction: Final report of the Gissi Study. Lancet 1987; 2: 871-4.
12. ISIS-2 (Second International Study of Infarct Survival) Collaborative Group. Randomized trial of intravenous streptokinase, oral aspirin, both or neither among 17,187 cases of suspected acute myocardial infarction. ISIS-2. Lancet 1988; 2: 349-60.
13. Wilcox RG, Olsson CG, Skene AM, Von der Lippe G, Jensen G, Hampton JR. Trial of tissue plasminogen activator for mortality reduction in acute myocardial infarction. Lancet 1988; 2: 525-30.
14. Helmers C, Lundman T, Maaring R, Wester PO. Mortality pattern among initial survivors of acute myocardial infarction using a life-table technique. Acta Med Scand 1976; 200: 469-73.
15. The Norwegian Multicenter Study Group. Timolol-induced reduction in mortality and reinfarction in patients surviving acute myocardial infarction. N Engl J Med 1981; 304: 801-7.
16. Hamsten A, Walldius G, Szamosi A, et al. Plasminogen activator inhibitor in plasma: risk factor for recurrent myocardial infarction. Lancet 1987; 2: 3-9.
17. Mitchell JRA. Anticoagulants in coronary heart disease retrospect and prospect. Lancet 1981; 1: 257-62.
18. Smith P, Arnesen H, Holme I. The effect of warfarin on mortality and reinfarction after myocardial infarction. N Engl J Med (in press).
19. Wright IS, Marple CD, Back DF. Report of the committeee for the evaluation in the treatment of coronary thrombosis with myocardial infarction; a progress report on the statistical analysis of the first 800 cases by this committee. Am Heart J 1948; 36: 801-15.
20. Bertelé V, Salzman EW. Antithrombotic therapy in coronary artery disease. Arteriosclerosis 1985; 5: 119-34.

21. Loeliger EA. Laboratory control, optimal therapeutic ranges and therapeutic quality control of oral anticoagulation. Acta Haemat 1985; 74: 125-31.
22. Gifford RH, Feinstein AR. A critique of methodology in studies of anticoagulation for acute myocardial infarction. N Engl J Med 1969; 280: 351-7.
23. Chalmers TC, Matta RJ, Smith H, Kunzler A. Evidence favoring the use of anticoagulants in the hospital phase of acute myocardial infarction. N Engl J Med 1977; 297: 1091-6.
24. The Sixty Plus Reinfarction Study Research Group. A double-blind trial to assess long-term oral anticoagulant therapy in elderly patients after myocardial infarction. Lancet 1980; 2: 989-93.
25. Loeliger EA, Poller L, Samama M, et al. Questions and answers on prothrombin time standardisation in oral anticoagulant control. Thrombos Haemostas 1985; 54: 515-7.
26. Graham I, Mulcahy R, Hickey N. Anticoagulants after myocardial infarction. Lancet 1981; 1: 223.
27. Abildgaard U. Antikoagulasjon etter hjerteinfarkt. Tidsskr Nor Lægeforen 1981; 101: 1346.
28. Nomenclature and criteria for diagnosis of ischemic heart disease. Report of the Joint International Society and Federation of Cardiology/World Health Organization task force on standardization of clinical nomenclature. Circulation 1979; 59: 607-9.
29. The SCATI Group. Randomised controlled trial of subcutaneous calcium-heparin in acute myocardial infarction. Lancet 1989; 2: 182-6.
30. Breddin K, Loew D, Lechner K, Ueberla K, Walter E. Secondary prevention of myocardial reinfarction a comparison of acetylsalicylic acid, placebo and phenprocoumon. Haemostasis 1980; 9: 325-44.
31. The E.P.S.I.M. Research Group. A controlled comparison of aspirin and oral anticoagulants in prevention of death after myocardial infarction. N Engl J Med 1982; 307: 701-8.
32. Yusuf S, Wittes J, Friedman L. Overiew of results of randomized clinical trials in heart disease. JAMA 1988; 260: 2088-93.
33. Loeliger EA. Oral anticoagulation in patients surviving myocardial infarction. A new approach to old data. Eur J Clin Pharmacol 1984; 26: 137-9.
34. Petersen P, Godtfredsen J, Boysen G, Andersen ED, Andersen B. Placebo-controlled randomised trial of warfarin and aspirin for prevention of thromboembolic complications in chronic atrial fibrillation. Lancet 1989; 1: 175-9.

39

Myocardial remodelling after myocardial infarction

KARL SWEDBERG

The syndrome of congestive heart failure (CHF) develops when the pumping (systolic) function of the heart can no longer perfuse vital organs satisfactorily. The underlying mechanism is a disturbance of myocardial function caused by disease or damage. In most cases the cause is an underlying coronary artery disease which has resulted in a myocardial infarction (MI). It is obvious that if this damage is very extensive there is not enough myocardium left to produce energy that will be able to generate an adequate cardiac output and perfusion pressure. However, in many situations the acute damage to the myocardium is not that extensive and yet there is development of left ventricular dysfunction leading to CHF. It is the intention of the present review to discuss the mechanisms that may create this myocardial dysfunction and potential interventions that may counteract that process.

Animal experiments

Several studies have looked into the dynamics of the healing process early after the onset of a MI (1-3). *Bulkley and coworkers* have named the early effects of the healing process infarct expansion, that is disproportionate thinning and dilation of acutely infarcted myocardium. They have also demonstrated in a rat model after ligation of the left anterior descending artery that infarct expansion was not dependent on infarct size but seems to be related to the age of the infarct (4). The hearts were examined on days 1, 2 and 3 after ligation. The extent of expansion increased markedly for each day. Expansion is thus a very early finding during the healing process. Another important observation was that significant wall thinning and increased regional radius of the curvature were also seen in adjacent and remote regions of the hearts with expansion. This observation indicates the effects upon the non-infarcted myocardium during the early phase.

Interstitial tissue has been shown to be very sensitive to ischaemia. Collagen fibres are also sensitive to increased stress. *Weber and coworkers* have shown that the collagen volume fraction is increased following coronary embolization (5). The fibres were markedly changed in structure the result of ischaemia and/or stress may be infarct expansion.

Also in a rat model *Pfeffer et al* demonstrated that infarct size after LAD-ligation predicted survival (6). They also found that treatment with the angiotensin-converting enzyme (ACE-) inhibitor captopril improved survival. Similar observations have been reported by *Sweet et al* using enalapril (7).

Human studies

It is obviously more difficult to interpret clinical studies in the context of myocardial remodelling. We have very limited information as regards myocardial structural changes. Measurements of left ventricular function have to be limited in numbers and the available techniques also limit the interpretation of the information.

Considerable left ventricular dilation may occur within the first days of an acute MI. One obvious explantion is that the remaining non-infarcted myocardium undergoes diastolic lengthening by the Frank-Starling mechanism. However, there are observations supporting the concept of expansion of the infarcted area in causing ventricular dilation (8, 9). The early (within <3 days) expansion has also been studied by the same group. In 27 patients with acute anterior infarctions it was observed that the early ventricular dilation was due to the dilation of the infarcted segment. A recent report (10) from *Behrenbeck et al* at the Mayo Clinic using ultrafast CT-scanning, found a dilation of the infarcted segment that occurred from one to six weeks.

Studies of the fate of the non-infarcted myocardium in man have been limited. *Wynne et al* found that the regional ejection fraction in non-infarcted segments was abnormal in 69% of patients with anterior infarction and in 30% posterior infarctions (11). The changes within two weeks after successful thrombolysis were studied by *McKay et al* (12). A left ventricular angiogram was performed within 10 hours from onset of symptoms in patients with a first infarction. Thereafter thrombolytic therapy was administered. In 30 patients where vessel opening was achieved, a repeat investigation was performed after 14 days (9-18 days). During this period both left ventricular end-diastolic and end-systolic diameter had increased. In those patients where the increase was at least 20% (26 patients) serial endocardial perimeter measurements were performed. There was a mean increase of 13% in the perimeter length of the infarcted segments and a 19% increase in the non-infarcted segments. The magnitude of the remodelling process was proportional to the infarct size in contrast to the observations in the experimental situation referred above.

In a long-term follow-up *Pfeffer and collaborators* compared left ventricular volume changes in patients after a first anterior MI between three weeks and one year post-infarct in 59 patients (13). They observed that there was a significant left ventricular dilation, in particular in patients with large akinetic areas. However, the dilation was due to a lengthening of non-infarcted segments.

Remodelling

The entire left ventricle is exposed to a change early after a MI. This remodelling also seems to be significant in non-infarcted areas. It involves an immediate change in diastolic function, initially by increased distensibility. An increased stiffness occurs as the healing process evolves. This will increase the filling pressure and shift the pressure-volume relation upwards. The result will be increased wall stress.

The formation of a scar will reduce distensibility and further increase wall stress. Increased stress may provide the stimulus for myocardial hypertrophy and the combination of fibre elongation and wall thickening will return wall stress towards normal. It is also possible that dilation of the left ventricle may vary in different areas depending on the time from infarction. In the early healing period (<one week) the expansion of the infarcted area is the most important. Later in this process (<3-4 weeks) a remodelling of the non-infarcted segments may be of greater importance. A schematic presentation of this process is seen in Fig. 1.

Factors that may affect the remodelling include hypertension and activation of neuroendocrine mechanisms. Hypertension will increase wall stress and thus hasten expansion. Neuroendocrine activation of the sympathetic and renin-angiotension systems will result in an increase in peripheral resistance and thus increase systolic blood pressure which also increases wall stress.

There are, in addition, potential direct effects upon the myocardium from this hormonal activation. It has been demonstrated in animals and believed to be important in man, that long term increase in sympathetic activity will

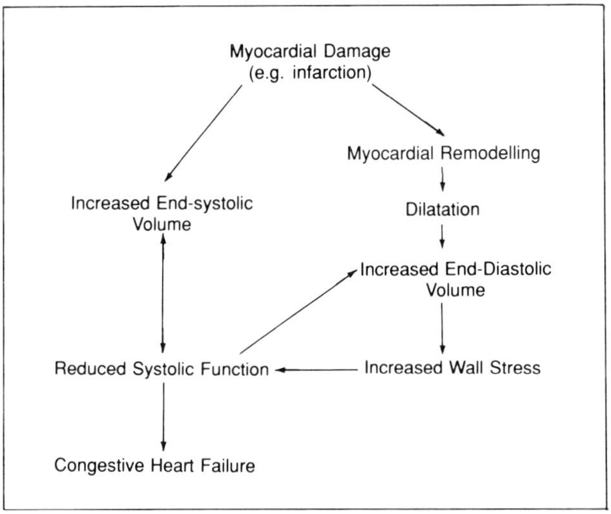

Fig. 1. *Schematic presentation of the pathogenetic development of congestive heart failure.*

adversely affect the myocardium (14). Furthermore, angiotensin II stimulates cellular growth (15). It also has deleterious effects upon the myocardial cell and interstitial tissue (16).

Treatment

Interventions aimed at reducing the remodelling and thus decreasing the risk of development of CHF are limited so far. Therapy should probably affect unloading of the left ventricle as well as myocardial protection. Different approaches would be the use of nitroglycerin, betablockers and ACE-inhibitors. Early administration of intravenous nitroglycerin has been demonstrated to have a beneficial influence upon infarct size both in animals (17) and humans (18). These effects could be achieved primarily through unloading of the heart. The direct myocardial effects from nitroglycerin are unclear. Long-term effects from prophylactic therapy is unclear. A pooled analysis from nitroglycerin trials indicates a beneficial effect (19).

Early intervention with betablockers seems to limit infarct size and has been demonstrated to improve survival after two weeks as well after three months (20, 21). It is not clear whether the incidence of CHF is reduced during these periods. It has not been shown that betablockers affect myocardial remodelling post-infarction.

Administration of ACE-inhibitors has been shown to limit infarct size and reverse infarct expansion in animal studies (4-6). In humans the progressive left ventricular dilation is reduced during the first week after early addition of captopril to successful thrombolysis (22). The long-term dilation of left ventricular volumes post-infarction has also been shown to be reduced by captopril (13, 23). It is not known if these effects may be translated into improved morbidity or survival. These questions will be addressed in a large multicentre trial in Denmark, Finland, Norway and Sweden called CONSENSUS II. The answers will hopefully be available in 1992. Other trials studying this issue are also planed.

Summary

After an acute MI there is a progressive dilation of both infarcted and non-infarcted myocardium, starting within the first couple of days. This process is probably important for the long-term prognosis. There are indications that deterioration in myocardial function may be counteracted by ACE-inhibitors. There are ongoing trials that will answer the question of whether survival is improved by prophylactic ACE-inhibitor therapy post-MI.

References

1. Eaton LW. Bulkley BH. Expansion of acute myocardial infarction: its relationsship to infarct morphology in canine model. Circ Res 1981; 49: 80-8.
2. Hocman JS, Bulkley BH. Expansion of acute myocardial infarction: Am experimental study. Circulation. 1982; 65: 1446-50.
3. Eaton LW, Weiss JL, Bulkley BH, Garrison JB, Weisfeldt ML. Regional cardiac dilation after acute myocardial infarction. Recognition by two-dimensional echocardiography. N Engl J Med 1979; 300: 57-62.
4. Weisman HF, Bush DE, Mannisi JA, Bulkley BH. Global cardiac remodeling after acute myocardial infarction: A study in the Rat Model. J Am Coll Cardiol 1985; 5: 1355-62.
5. Caroll E, Janicki JS, Pick R, Weber KT. Myocardial stiffness and reparative fibrosis following coronary embolization in the rat. J Am Coll Cardiol 1989; 13: 1A
6. Pfeffer MA, Pfeffer JM, Steinberg C, Finn P. Survival after an experimental myocardial infarction: Beneficial effects of long-term therapy with captopril. Circulation. 1985; 72: 406-12.
7. Sweet CS, Emmert SE, Stabilito II, Ribeiro LGT. Increased survival in rats with congestive heart failure trated with enalapril. J Cardiovasc Pharmacol 1987; 10: 636-42.
8. Eaton LW, Weiss JL, Bulkley BH, Garrison JB, Weisfeldt ML. Regional cardiac dilation after acute myocardial infarction. Recognition by two-dimensional echocardiography. N Engl J Med 1979; 300: 57-62.
9. Erlebacher JA, Weiss JL, Eaton LW, Kallman C, Weisfeldt ML, Bulkley BH. Late effects of acute cardiac dilation on heart size: A two dimensional echocardiographic study. Am J Cardiol 1982; 49: 1120-6.
10. Behrenbeck T, Ramberger JA, Gersh BJ, et al. Effect of infarct size on left ventricular remodeling after a first myocardial infarction. Circulation 1989; 80 (suppl II): II 589.
11. Wynne J, Sayres M, Maddox DE, et al. Regional left ventricular function in acute myocardial infarction: Evaluation with quantitative radionuclide ventriculography. Am J Cardiol 1980; 45: 203-9.

12. McKay RG, Pfeffer MA, Pasternak RC, et al. Left ventricular remodeling after myocardial infarction: A corollary to infarct expansion. Circulation 1986; 74: 693-702.
13. Pfeffer MA, Vaughn DE, Parisi AF, Braunwald E. Effect of captopril of progressive ventricular dilation after anterior myocardial infarction. N Engl J Med 1988; 319: 80.
14. Swedberg K. Neurohormonal activation is deleterious to the long-term outcome in patients with congestive heart failure. Protagonists's viewpoint. J Am Coll Cardiol 1988; 12: 550-4.
15. Dzau VJ. Implications of local angiotensin production in cardiovascular physiology and pharmacology. Am J Cardiol 1987; 59: 59A-65A.
16. Tan L-B, Jalil JE, Janicki JS, Weber KT, Clark WA. Cardiotoxic effects of angiotensin II. J Am Coll Card 1989; 13 (suppl A):2A.
17. McGregor M. Pathogenesis of angina pectoris and role of nitrates in relief of myocardial ischemia. Am J Med 1983; 74 (suppl): 21-7.
18. Jugdutt BI, Warnica JW. Intravenous nitroglycerin therapy to limit myocardial infarct size, expansion, and complications. Effect of timing, dosage, and infarct location. Circulation 1988; 78: 906-19.
19. Yusuf S, Collins R, MacMahon S, Peto R. Effect of intravenous nitrates on mortality in acute myocardial infarction: an overview of the randomized trials. Lancet 1988; i: 1088-92.
20. Hjalmarsson Å, Elmfeldt D, Herlitz J, et al. Effect on mortality of metoprolol in acute myocardial infarction. Lancet 1981; 2: 823-827.
21. The Miami Trial Group. Metoprolol in acute myocardial infarction (MIAMI). A randomised placebo-controlled trial. Eur Heart J 1985; 6: 199-226.
22. Nabel EG, Topal EJ, Galeana A, et al. A Randomized, Double-Blind, Placebo controlled, pilot trial of combined early intravenous captopril and tPA therapy in acute myocardial infarction. Circulation 1989; 80: (suppl II): II 112.
23. Sharpe N, Murphy J, Smith H, Hannan S. Treatment of patients with symptomless left ventricular dysfunction after myocardial infarction. Lancet 1988; i: 225-59.

40

Antiatherosclerotic therapy in secondary prevention after myocardial infarction

OLE FÆRGEMAN,
IB CHRISTIAN KLAUSEN

Early after myocardial infarction (MI), prognosis is largely determined by the extent and location of myocardial damage, residual ischaemia and the risk of thrombotic reocclusion of the infarct related artery. With time, however, progression of the slow, underlying atherosclerotic process reassumes its importance as a determinant of prognosis. Analogously, the long-term prognosis for the patient with angina pectoris and the patient treated by coronary by-pass surgery or coronary angioplasty is also determined by the progression of atherosclerosis.

Any treatment that interrupts the long chain of events leading to atherosclerosis could theoretically inhibit further progression and possibly induce regression. Some animal studies have suggested that betablockers may retard formation of atheromatous plaques (1). This concept is not supported by the only human angiographic study published to date (2), although the beneficial effects of betablocker therapy on clinical events in secondary prevention are well established. According to a preliminary report, combined treatment with acetylsalicylic acid and dipyridamole inhibits formation of new lesions but not the further progression of older lesions in human coronary arteries (3). The effects of antiplatelet drug therapy are discussed in another chapter of this book. Although extensively employed, the possible clinical benefits of chelation therapy with EDTA have not been documented by publication of a well designed study. A trial of this kind with mainly nonangiographic end-points relating to intermittent claudication is in progress in Denmark and scheduled for termination in 1990 (*Rolf Jelnes,* personal communication).

Trials of dietary and pharmacological lipid reduction and treatment with calcium antagonists have been performed in humans with angiographic evaluation. In this chapter we briefly review the effects of calcium antagonists and lipid reduction in patients with coronary and, in some trials, femoral atherosclerosis. The focus will be on angiographic studies.

Angiography

In humans, the effect of intervention can be studied by the controlled clinical trial with MI and cardiac death as end-points. Secondary preventive trials of this kind require fewer patient-years of observation than do the trials of primary prevention, because event rates are higher once the diasease is present.

Most economical in terms of patient numbers are the angiographic trials, in which most of the patients contribute end-point data after only a few years of observation. The angiographic studies, on the other hand, are invasive, and they pose high demands on techniques of execution and interpretation. Moreover, arteriograms provide information about the lumen of the artery but not about the pathology of lumenal narrowing or dilation. Stenosis may for example be atherosclerotic, thrombotic, or due to spasm or arteritis. Methods of quantitation of stenoses vary in the trials published to date. Some trials have relied on visual, semiquantitative assessment, whereas others have employed caliper or vernier measurements or some form of computer assisted evaluation (4, 5). In all the studies cited in this chapter, the arteriograms have been evaluated without knowledge of the treatment group.

Calcium antagonists

Animal studies of the possible antiatherogenic effect of calcium antagonists have provided conflicting results (6). Nevertheless, a limited number of studies has been performed to test the hypothesis in humans. In a retrospective study of 17 control patients and 26 patients treated with verapamil, *Kober et al* (7) reported that verapamil caused less progression and significant regression of severe stenoses as visualised in coronary angiograms slightly more than a year apart. The authors have initiated a much larger angiographic prospective study of verapamil.

Loaldi et al (2) allocated 113 patients with coronary heart disease to treatment with nifedipine (n = 39), propranolol (n = 36) or isosorbide dinitrate (n = 38) for 2 years. Quantitative coronary angiograms showed significantly less progression and significantly more regression in arterial segments in the nifedipine group than in the 2 other groups. Also, significantly fewer nifedipine patients experienced progression. Nifedipine did not affect risk factors including lipids, whereas propranolol typically raised triglycerides and lowered high density lipoproteins (HDL).

In a preliminary communication, *Waters et al* (8) reported no effect of nicardipine on progression or regression of coronary lesions in 383 patients as evaluated by computer assisted angiography 2 years apart. A subgroup analysis, however, did suggest inhibition of progression of lesions less than 20% diameter stenosis. In another preliminary publication, *Gottlieb et al* (9) reported the development of fewer lesions in coronary bypass grafts in patients treated with nifedipine than in placebo treated controls. Another nifedipine study, the International Nifedipine Trial on Antiatherosclerotic Therapy (INTACT), has not yet been published (see addendum p. 487).

The use of calcium antagonists as a class of drugs in secondary prevention has not been clarified. Extensive experience with nifedipine indicates little or no clinical benefit, and some trials have actually demonstrated harmful effects (10). In contrast, diltiazem trials suggest benefit in survivors of non-Q myocardial infarction, and the Danish verapamil study provided subgroup data suggesting benefit in patients given verapamil 2 to 3 weeks after infarction (11). A later study by the same authors has shown that verapamil started 2 weeks after infarction significantly reduces reinfarction and the combined incidence of reinfarction and total mortality (*Jørgen Fischer Hansen,* personal communication).

Lipid reduction

In several (12-15) but not all studies (16), progression of atheroslcerosis has been shown to be correlated to low levels of HDL and to high levels of low density lipoproteins (LDL) in serum. Atherosclerosis can in several animal species, including non-human primates, be induced and regressed by respectively increasing and decreasing serum cholesterol (17). The methodological problems involved in this kind of animal work have been reviewed by *Malinow* (18).

Angiographic studies

A number of studies of lipid intervention without adequate control groups have reported the inhibition of further progression of coronary or femoral atherosclerosis.

In an early study without a control group, *Kuo et al* provided angiographic data suggestive of inhibition of progression in hypercholesterolaemic patients treated with colestipol (19).

Nikkilä et al (12) treated 26 men and 2 women with diet, clofibrate and in some cases nicotinic acid for 7 years and compared the developments in the coronary arteries with those of 20 non-randomized control men. The treated group experienced significantly less development of angina and significantly fewer deaths (annual mortality rates 1.5% vs. 7.0%). Angiographic changes were assessed visually. As in most of the studies described here, results were given for each patient and for segments of the coronary arteries. No regression was observed, but lesions progressed in all but one of the surviving 13 control subjects vs. 19 of the 28 treated subjects. Two year angiographic findings were used in 4 treated subjects not surviving 7 years. The authors considered their results suggestive of benefit of the intervention employed.

Nash et al (20) performed coronary angiography before and after 2 years of colestipol treatment of 24 men and 1 woman previosly shown to respond to colestipol with at least 15% reduction in serum cholesterol. The non-randomized control group was composed of 13 male and 4 female non-responders to colestipol. Visual assessment of the arteriograms indicated significantly less progression in drug treated subjects (3/25) than in controls (8/17). Inadequate data were given concerning 19 patients who did not complete the study, the results of which must be considered only suggestive.

After 6 months of dietary treatment, *Olsson et al* (21) treated 20 hypercholesterolaemic and hypertriglyceridaemic but asymptomatic middle-aged men with nicotinic acid and fenofibrate and 25 non-randomized controls with placebo for 1 year. Treatment reduced total and LDL cholesterol significantly by 28% and 36% respectively, and treatment raised HDL cholesterol significantly by 23%. Visual assessment of 4 segments of the femoral angiogram suggested significantly more regression (29% of treated patients vs. 0% of control patients) and somewhat less progession of lesions in the drug treated group.

Four trials with adequate, randomized control groups have been reported. In an early study by *Cohn et al* (22), 40 patients were randomized to treatment with either clofibrate (n=16) or placebo (n=24) for 1 year. Coronary angiograms, evaluated visually, showed no significant difference in rates of lesion progression between the 2 groups. Clofibrate caused a significant but modest fall in triglycerides of 14% and a non-significant fall in cholesterol of only 3%.

Duffield et al (13) used diet, cholestyramine, nicotinic acid and clofibrate in 10 men and 2 women and compared femoral angiograms by both visual and computerised image analysis with those of 11 male and 1 female control subjects after 18 to 20 months. During the trial, cholesterol and triglycerides were respectively 19 and 37% lower and HDL was 41% higher in the treated group than in the controls. There was significantly less progression in the treated group by both methods of angiographic evaluation. Radiological improvement suggestive of regression occurred in twice as many 1 cm arterial segments in the treated as in the control group, but the figures were small.

The American NHBLI study by *Brensike et al* (14) was a larger study of patients with type II hyperlipidaemia randomized to a control or intervention group treated with cholestyramine, which caused reductions in total and LDL cholesterol of 17 and 26%, respectively. Coronary angiograms 5 years apart were visually evaluated. Lesions progressed definitely or probably in 49.1% of controls (n=57) and in 32.2% of treated patients (n=59) (one tailed p=0.03). Most of the several other classifications of angiographic changes provided non-significant but suggestive evidence of less progression and some regression of lesions in the cholestyramine group.

The largest angiograhic study published to date was the Cholesterol Lowering Atherosclerosis Study by *Blankenhorn et al* (15). The authors randomized 188 non-smoking men with previous coronary artery bypass surgery to a control group or a group treated with diet, nicotinic acid and colestipol. Eighty men in the treated group and 82 men in the control group completed the study. Large differences in lipid values between the groups were obtained. Coronary angiograms taken 2 years apart were evaluated visually. The percentage of subjects with new lesions was significantly reduced by treatment from 22 to 10 in grafts and from 30 to 18 in native arteries. A "global change score" combining lesion changes in both grafts (average 2.7 grafts/angiogram) and native arteries (average 11.1 lesions/angiogram) was 0.3 in the drug group and 0.8 in the control group, indicating significantly less progression in the former. Moreover, the global change score suggested a statistically significant difference in lesion regression: 16.2% of drug treated subjects and 2.4% of controls. A notable finding was that benefits of treatment were about the same in treated men with low (4.81–6.24 mmoles/l) and high (6.26–9.10 mmoles/l) levels of serum cholesterol at entry into the trial.

The Familial Atherosclerosis Treatment Study (FATS) trial has at present been published only in preliminary form (23). Results of quantitative coronary arteriography before and after 2 years were compared in 37 control men, 34 men treated with colestipol and lovastatin, and 32 men treated with colestipol and nicotinic acid. LDL reduction was especially pronounced in the colestipol/lovastatin group, and HDL elevation was particulary marked in the colestipol/nicotinic acid group. There was significant evidence of lesion regression in both of the treatment groups, especially in the colestipol/nicotinic acid group.

Angiographic studies have been performed on patients whose lipids have been reduced by partial ileal bypass surgery or by extracorporeal removal of plasma LDL. Although partial ileal bypass effectively lowers serum cholesterol (24), there is no convincing evidence of clinical or angiographic benefit in patients with established coronary heart disease (25). Extracorporeal removal of LDL by plasma exchange seems to retard the development of aortocoronary atheromatous lesions and reduce mortality in patients with homozygous familial hypercholesterolaemia (25). In a small study, data have been obtained with the more selective procedure of LDL apheresis suggesting regression of coronary lesions (26). Publication of results of a larger, apparently uncontrolled, coronary angiographic study employing LDL apheresis is expected in the near future (27).

Trials with clinical end-points

Several trials of dietary or pharmacological lipid reduction have been performed with use of clinical end-points. In dietary studies, the most convincing evidence of clinical benefit was obtained by *Paul Leren* (28), who demonstrated a 33% lower incidence of coronary heart disease events in 206 middle-aged male survivors of MI treated by diet compared to a randomized control group of the same size. Other dietary studies provided less persuasive evidence of benefit (29).

In the Coronary Drug Project (30), male survivors of MI were treated with 4 different drugs including nicotinic acid and clofibrate. The latter did not reduce total mortality, and a small reduction in coronary heart disease mortality was not statistically significant. In contrast, nicotinic acid significantly reduced the combined incidence of non-fatal MI and coronary heart disease death. Nine years after termination of the trial, total mortality was significantly lower in the group that had been treated with nicotinic acid compared to the control group (31). The authors speculated that the reduction in long-term mortality was due to the within-trial reduction in non-fatal MI.

In a small, partly primary preventive trial, there was a highly significant reduction in both cardiac and total mortality in men and women treated with colestipol compared to placebo (32). However, benefit was essentially limited to younger men or men with preexisting coronary heart disease.

In the Stockholm Ischaemic Heart Disease Secondary Prevention Study (33), *Carlson and Rosenhamer* randomized 555 men and women to placebo (n=276) or combined treatment with clofibrate and nicotinic acid (n=279). Treatment reduced serum cholesterol and triglycerides by 13 and 19%, respectively. After 5 years, the incidence of major non-fatal cardiovascular events was significantly reduced by 33% and total mortality by 26% (82 vs. 61 deaths) in the treatment group as compared to the control group.

A major trial of simvastatin in secondary prevention, scheduled for termination in 1993, has been initiated in Scandinavia (Scandinvian Simvastatin Survivial Study). Probucol is a lipid lowering drug with antioxidant properties, and a study of the effect of probucol on femoral atherosclerosis is in progress in Sweden (Probucol Quantitative Regression Swedish Trial).

Biochemical mechanisms

Does it make any difference how lipids are lowered pharmacologically? The major classes of lipid lowering or lipid modulating drugs are anion exchange resins, fibrates, nicotinic acid or nicotinic acid derivatives, probucol and statins (HMG-coA reductase inhibitors). Drugs representative of these classes have been employed in one or more of all the drug trials reviewed here. In our view, there is at present no conclusive evidence that a particular drug or drug combination is especially advantageous. It should be noted, however, that the clinical or angiographic benefits obtained in several studies could in part have been determined by a choice of drugs tailored to the type of lipid disorder in the trial subjects (12, 13). Anion exchange resins were used in patients with elevation of cholesterol only and nicotinic acid or fibrates in patients with combined elevations of cholesterol and triglycerides.

A better understanding of lipid disorders will hopefully help clinicians to use lipid lowering drugs more specifically. For example, gemfibrozil and particularly nicotinic acid raise HDL effectively. This may be important, since HDL is inversely correlated to the development of atherosclerosis, and this class of lipoproteins is thought to play a role in the transport of cholesterol from non-hepatic tissues to the liver for excretion in the bile or conversion to bile acids.

To take another example, nicotinic acid is the only drug that lowers Lp(a) (34). Lp(a) is a low density lipoprotein molecule to which a protein, apo(a) is attached, presumably by difulfide linkage. Lp(a) was discovered by *Kaare Berg* in 1963 (35). Several studies have shown that levels of Lp(a) greater than about 30 mg/dl are related to atherosclerosis (36), MI (37) and development of stenoses in venous grafts used for coronary bypass surgery (38). The gene for apo(a) contains a number of nucleotide sequences closely homologous to sequences in the gene for plasminogen (39). Lp(a) research in progess may therefore lead to an understanding of the interaction between lipoproteins and fibrinolysis that could become clinically important within the near future.

Conclusion

In patients with ischaemic heart disease, modulation of serum lipids and treatment with beta blockers, antiplatelet drugs and calcium antagonists have to varying degrees been shown to reduce the incidence of MI and cardiac and total mortality. A review of studies published to date indicates that the best evidence of regression or inhibition of progession of coronary or femoral artery lesions, as assessed by angiographic techniques, has been obtained by lipid modulation, especially by drugs, and, in a smaller number of studies, by the use of calcium antagonists.

Addendum

In the recently reported INTACT study (40), significantly fewer new coronary lesions (103 vs. 144) developed in a nifedipine group of 134 patients compared to a control group of 148 patients with mild coronary artery disease studied by quantitative angiopgraphy 3 years apart. There was no significant effect on progression or regression of established lesions. Clinical events were also unaffected, although there was a non-significant tendency to more deaths (12 vs. 2) and non-fatal cardiac events (52 vs. 44) in the nifedipine group.

References

1. Cruickshank JM, Smith JC. The betareceptor, atheroma and cardiovascular disease. Pharmacol Ther 1989; 42: 385-404.
2. Loaldi A, Polese A, Montorsi P, et al. Comparison of nifedipine, propranolol and isosorbide dinitrate on angiographic progression and regression of coronary arterial narrowing in angina pectoris. Am J Cardiol 1989; 64: 433-9.
3. Chesebro JH, Webster MWI, Smith HC, et al. Antiplatelet therapy in coronary disease progression reduced infarction and new lesion formation. Circulation 1989; 80 (suppl II): II-266.
4. Brown BG, Bolson EL, Dodge HT. Arteriographic assessment of coronary atherosclerosis. Arterioclerosis 1982; 2: 2-15.

5. Reiber JHC, Serruys PW, Kooijman CJ, et al. Assessment of short, medium, and longterm variations in arterial dimensions from computerassisted quantitation of coronary cineangiograms. Circulation 1985; 71: 280-8.
6. Overturf M, Smith S. Are calcium antagonists effective inhibitors of atherogenesis? In: Dal Palu C, Ross R, eds. Hypertension and atheroslcerosis. Amsterdam: Excerpta Medica, 1989: 98-106.
7. Kober G, Schneider W, Kaltenbach M. Can the progession of coronary sclerosis be influenced by calcium antagonists? J Cardiovasc Pharmacol 1989; 13 (suppl 4): S2-S6.
8. Waters D, Lesperance J, Theroux P, Francetich M, Reitman M, Havel RJ. Prevention of progression of minimal coronary lesions with a calcium channel blocker. J Am Coll Cardiol 1990; 15 (suppl A): 116A.
9. Gottlieb SO, Brinker JA, Mellits ED, et al. Effect of nifedipine on the development of coronary bypass graft stenoses in highrisk patients: a randomized, doubleblind, placebocontrolled trial. Circulation 1989; 80 (suppl II): II-228.
10. Gibson RS. Current status of calcium channelblocking drugs after Q wave and nonQ wave myocardial infarction. Circulation 1989; 80 (suppl IV): IV-107-19.
11. The Danish Study Group on Verapamil in Myocardial Infarction: Verapamil in acute myocardial infarction. Eur Heart J 1984; 5: 516-28.
12. Nikkil EA, Viikinkoski P, Valle M, Frick MH. Prevention of progession of coronary atherosclerosis by treatment of hyperlipidaemia: a seven year prospective angiographic study. Br Med J 1984; 289: 220-3.
13. Duffield RGM, Lewis B, Miller NE, Jamieson CW, Brunt JNH, Colchester ACF. Treatment of hyperlipidaemia retards progession of symptomatic femoral atherosclerosis. Lancet 1983; 2: 639-42.
14. Brensike JF, Levy RI, Kelsey SF, et al. Effects of therapy with cholestyramine on progression of coronary arteriosclerosis: results of the NHBLI type II coronary intervetion study. Circulation 1984; 69: 313-24.
15. Blankenhorn DH, Nessim SA, Johnson RL, Sanmarco ME, Azen SP, CashinHemhil L. Beneficial effects of combined colestipolniacin therapy on coronary atheroslcerosis and coronary venous bypass grafts. JAMA 1987; 257: 3233-40.
16. Moise A, Theroux P, Taeymans Y, et al. Clinical and angiographic factors associated with progression of coronary artery disease. J Am Coll Cardiol 1984; 3: 659-67.
17. Blankenhorn DH. Regression of atherosclerosis. In: Braunwald E, ed. Heart disease. Philadelphia: WB Saunders, 1988; Update: 73-82.
18. Malinow MR. Atherosclerosis: progression, regression and resolution. Am Heart J 1989; 108: 1523-36.
19. Kuo PT, Hayase K, Kostis JB, Moreyra AE. Use of combined diet and colestipol in longterm (77 years) treatment of patients with type II hyperlipoproteinemia. Circulation 1979; 59: 199-211.
20. Nash DT, Gensini G, Esente P. Effect of lipidlowering therapy on the progession of coronary atherosclerosis assessed by scheduled repetitive coronary arteriograhy. Int J Cardiol 1982; 2: 43-55.
21. Olsson AG, Ruhn G, Erikson U. The effect of serum lipid regulation on the development of femoral atherosclerosis in hyperlipidaemia: a nonrandomized controlled study. J Int Med (in press).
22. Cohn K, Sakai FJ, Langston MF. Effect of clofibrate on progression of coronary disease: a prospective angiographic study in man. Am Heart J 1975; 89: 591-8.
23. Brown BG, Lin JT, Schaefer SM, Kaplan CA, Dodge HT, Albers JJ. Niacin or lovastatin, combined with colestipol, regress coronary atherosclerosis and prevent clinical events in men with elevated apolipoprotein B. Circulation 1989; 80 (suppl II): II-266.

24. Færgeman O, Meinertz H, Hylander E, Fischerman K, Jarnum S, Nielsen OV. Effects and side effects of partial ileal bypass surgery for familial hypercholesterolaemia. Gut 1981; 23: 558-63.
25. Thompson GR. Nondietary, nonpharmacological treatment of hyperlipoproteinaemia. In: Olsson AG, ed. Atherosclerosis. Biology and clinical science. Edinburgh: Churchill Livingstone, 1987; 431-6.
26. Hombach V, Borberg H, Gadzowski A, et al. Regression der koronarsklerose bei familiarer hypercholesterolinamie IIa durch specifische LDLapherese. Deutsch Med Woch 1986; 11: 1709-15.
27. Help Study Group. The Help LDLapheresis Multicentre Study. European Atherosclerosis Society 25th Anniversary Meeting. Linköping: 1989; 58.
28. Leren P. The Oslo diet heart study. Circulation 1970; 40: 935-42.
29. Yusuf S, Furberg CD. Single factor trials: control through lifestyle changes. In: Olsson AG, ed. Atherosclerosis. Biology and clinical science. Edinburgh: Churchill Livingstone, 1987: 489-91.
30. Coronary Drug Project Research Group. Clofibrate and nicacin in coronary heart disease. JAMA 1975; 231: 360-81.
31. Canner PL, Berge KG, Wenger NK, et al. Fifteen year mortality in Coronary Drug Project patients: longerterm benefit with niacin. J Am Coll Cardiol 1986; 8: 1245-55.
32. Dorr AE, Gundersen K, Schneider, Jr JC, Spencer TW, Martin WB. Colestipol hydrochloride in hypercholesterolemic patients effect on serum cholesteol and mortality. J Chron Dis 1978; 31: 514.
33. Carlson LA, Rosenhamer C. Reduction of mortality in the Stockholm Ischaemic Heart Disease Prevention Study by combined treatment with clofibrate and nicotinic acid. Acta Med Scand 1988; 223: 405-18.
34. Carlson LA, Hamsten A, Asplund A. Pronounced lowering of serum levels of lipoprotein Lp(a) in hyperlipidemic subjects treated with nicotinic acid. J Int Med 1989; 226: 271-6.
35. Berg K. A new serum system in man the Lp system. Acta Pathol Microbiol Scand 1963; 59: 369-82.
36. Dahlen GH, Guyton JR, Attar M, Farmer JA, Kautz JA, Gotto Jr AM. Association of levels of lipoprotein Lp(a), plasma lipids, and other lipoproteins with coronary artery disease documented by angiography. Circulation 1986; 74: 758-65.
37. Rhoads GG, Dahlen G, Berg K, Morton NE, Dannenberg AL. Lp(a) lipoprotein as a risk factor for myocardial infarction. JAMA 1986; 256: 2540-4.
38. Hoff HF, Beck GJ, Skibinski CI, et al. Serum Lp(a) level as a predictor of vein graft stenosis after coronary bypass surgery in patients. Circulation 1988; 77: 1238-44.
39. McLean JW, Tomlinson JE, Kuang WJ, et al. cDNA sequence of human apolipoprotein(a) is homologous to plasminogen. Nature 1987; 300: 132-7.
40. Lichtlen PR, Hugenholtz PG, Rafflenbeul WR, Hecker H, Jost S, Deckers JW. Retardation of angiographic progression of coronary artery disease by nifedipine. Lancet 1990; 335: 1109-13.

41

Training and group intervention after myocardial infarction

JOHN GUNNAR MÆLAND

Despite evidence of a recent decline, myocardial infarction (MI) is still one of the leading causes of hospitalization, disability, and death in the industrialized countries. In Norway alone (4.2 mill. inhabitants), more than 10,000 persons are admitted to hospital each year due to a recent MI (1).

Of MI patients surviving the acute phase, about half are under the age of 70 years. Compared with the normal population, this group has a 5-fold increased risk of dying during the first year and a 2-3 times higher mortality risk during the succeeding years (2). This means that one in four MI patients is dead within five years. Of the surviving patients, every fourth suffers a non-fatal reinfarction and every second is readmitted to hospital during the same period (1, 3).

MI patients face other problems too. About one in four patients does not return to work; one-third to one-fifth of the patients show long-term emotional disturbances; and a majority of patients restrict their social and leisure activities compared with before the MI (1, 4). Subjective complaints such as breathlessness and chest pain are common and not always due to somatic factors. Nearly half of the patients restrict their physical activity due to fear of what might happen during exercise (1, 5).

Thus, there is a clear need for rehabilitative measures in a substantial number of MI patients. The aim of the rehabilitation is to restore maximal physical, psychological, and social functioning and quality of life. Hopefully, such activities may also improve the long-term prognosis after the heart attack.

The rehabilitation means can be divided into three broad categories: (1) exercise training; (2) patient education; and (3) psychosocial intervention. Although each type of intervention has its own theoretical background and clinical tradition, the various applications share a lot of common ground and are in practice most effectively combined in comprehensive group rehabilitation programmes.

Exercise training

The rationale for physical training after a MI is partly physiological, partly psychological. Early mobilization is now recognized as crucial for the prevention of complications during the acute phase of the disease. Although maximal physical capacity is clearly reduced immediately after the MI, spontaneous improvement usually occurs during the following weeks, reflecting the healing process in the myocardium (6).

However, many post-infarction patients complain of feelings of weakness, breathlessness on exertion, and chest pain even months after the acute event (1, 4, 5). Angina pectoris is present in about one-third of the patients (5, 7). However, maximal physical work capacity has been found 15-20% lower even in post-MI patients not limited by chest pain compared with healthy persons (5). The main reason seems to be the deconditioning produced by the initial immobilization and a prolonged physical inactivity during the convalescense period. Only a small minority of patients are left with permanently impaired physical capacity due to persisting left ventricular dysfunction (6).

A number of randomized controlled trials have uniformly demonstrated significant increases in maximal work capacity in post-MI patients as a result of aerobic training (5, 8-12). The peripheral training effects (Table 1) are the most important factors for this result but some studies have also

Table 1. *Physiological effects of aerobic training in patients with coronary heart disease.*

	Level of effort	
	Submaximal	Maximal
Central haemodynamic parameters:		
Heart rate	↓	=
Systolic blood pressure	↓	=
Stroke volume	↑	↑
Cardiac output	=/↓	↑
Ejection fraction	=?	=?
Peripheral parameters:		
Skeletal muscle blood flow	↓	↑
Peripheral A-V oxygen extraction	↑	↑
Total body oxygen consumption	=	↑
Myocardial parameters:		
Coronary blood flow	↑?	=
Myocardial A-V oxygen extraction	=	=?
Myocardial oxygen consumption	↓	=/↑

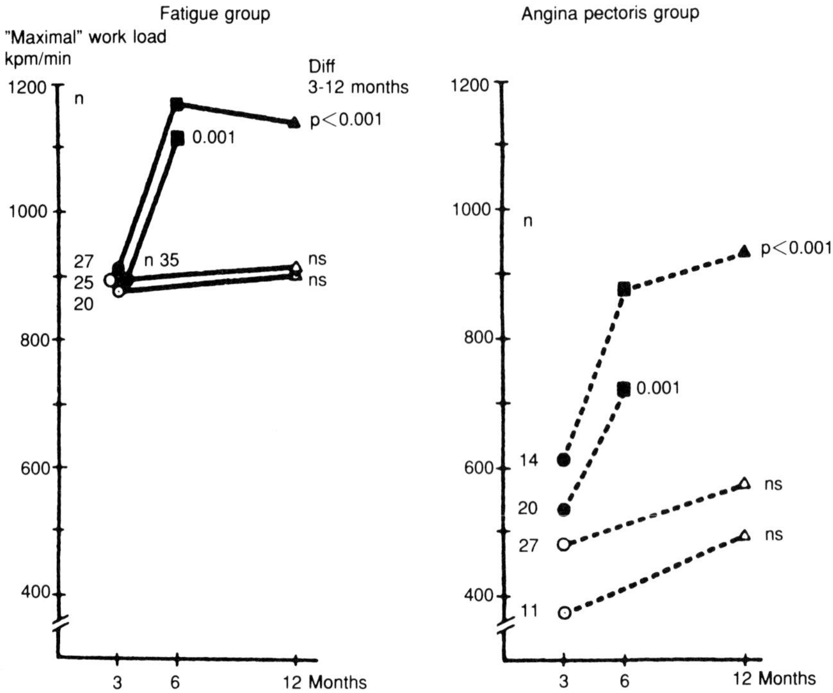

Fig. 1. *Mean (symptom-limited) maximal workload 3, 6 and 12 months after MI in non-selected patients randomized to either control or exercise training from 3 months post MI. Results are shown separately for patients who initially could exercise to fatigue and patients limited by angina pectoris. Dark symbols – training groups. Open symbols – control groups. Open punctuated symbols – training patients who did not start or discontinued. From (5).* *or discontinued. From (5).*

suggested that cardiac changes play a part in some patients (6, 11, 13, 14). In sum, these physiologic changes lower the relative aerobic requirements of submaximal workloads.

For MI patients limited by chest pain, aerobic training results in relatively greater improvement in functional capacity. *Sanne* (5) demonstrated a 38% increase in symptom-limited workload in MI patients with angina pectoris during a three months training period (Fig. 1). In comparison, MI patients who could exercise to fatigue increased their exercise tolerance by 24% during the same training period. Furthermore, angina pectoris patients who continued to exercise obtained further improvement during the next six months, whereas the fatigue group only maintained their exercise capacity.

The main explanation for improved exercise tolerance in angina pectoris patients after a training period is found in the peripheral muscular and circulatory adjustments which in turn reduce both heart rate and systolic blood pressure at a given external workload (Table 1). The resulting lower rate-pressure product implies less demand for oxygen in the myocardium, allowing the patient to sustain higher external workloads before myocardial ischaemia develops (6, 15). In addition, a number of patients are able to exercise to an even higher maximal rate-pressure product after a training period, suggesting increased myocardial oxygen supply (5, 6, 13). The exact mechanism for this cardiac effect has not been established.

The question whether aerobic training affects survival in post-MI patients is still open to debate. No single trial has documented a statistically significant reduction in mortality as a result of exercise training alone. However, the great majority of studies have suggested an improved prognosis for exercising patients but have all lacked sufficient statistical power, due to a limited number of participating patients. In a carefully conducted meta-analysis on the combined results of ten randomized clinical trials, including over 4,000 patients, statistically significant reductions for all-cause (24% reduction) and cardiovascular (25% reduction) death were demonstrated (16). In comparison, physical training did not affect the incidence of non-fatal reinfarction.

Exercise training may reduce some of the known risk factors for coronary heart disease. Physical inactivity is an established risk factor in itself. Regular aerobic training results in favourable changes in blood lipids, mainly a reduction in triglycerides and an increase in HDL-cholesterol (6, 8, 10, 12). In comparison, total cholesterol level is minimally affected. Training also reduces systolic blood pressure to some extent and helps control body weight. However, exercise training alone has not been shown to change smoking habits (10).

The psychological effects of physical training after a MI are usually striking. Paradoxically, only a few studies have addressed this important aspect with sufficient methodological sophistication. In an early controlled study, *McPherson et al* (17) found more positive changes in the sense of well-being among exercising cardiac patients as compared to both cardiac controls and normal exercising persons. A randomized clinical trial compared a 12 week exercise programme with group counselling or usual care (9). At follow-up, patients in the exercise group were less depressed and anxious than the controls and also expressed more independence and sociability.

The psychological benefits are seemingly not related to the magnitude of physical improvement. Thus, positive psychosocial changes were reported during a 6-week low-level exercise programme, whereas a subsequent long-term, more intensive training period did not result in any further psychosocial improvements (18, 19). Some patients may even experience increased distress initially during training. However, when the physical effects of the

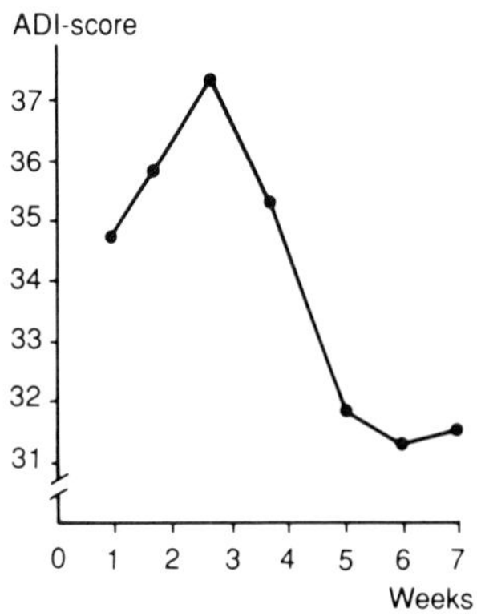

Fig. 2. *Mean level of emotional distress (anxiety, depression and irritability) in coronary heart patients (N=20) participating in an out-patient group training programme. Changes are significant (P<0.05) according to one-way analysis of variance. From (20).*

training become noticable, the great majority of patients report a "breakthrough" in self-perception and mood (Fig. 2) (20).

Organization of exercise training

The physiological effects of physical training depend on the intensity, the frequency, and the duration of the training programme.

In interval training, peak exercise intensity should generally not exceed 85% of maximal heart rate, corresponding to about 75-80% of maximal oxygen uptake, due to an increased risk of complications at higher levels of exercise (21). An alternative training model is continuous low-level exercise, corresponding to about 60% of maximal heart rate (45-50% of maximal oxygen uptake) for at least 30 minutes (22).

Most training programmes are organized as out-patient group sessions but shorter, more intensive in-patient programmes are also feasible and effective. Training five days a week over a four week period seems to give approximately the same results as a 3-months 3-days a week programme. Both approaches typically result in about 15% increase in maximal work capacity (5, 6, 23).

The duration of cardiac exercise training programmes has varied from a few weeks to several years. *Sanne* (5) found no increase in physical capacity after the first three months of training except for patients limited by angina pectoris (Fig. 1). One reason is a considerable drop in exercise compliance over time. The general experience is that less than half of the patients still participate in organized training after six months (5, 19, 24).

Although *Palatsi* (25) in an early study found only modest gains from a home-based training programme, more recent studies have suggested that home-based training may produce comparable results for low risk patients than more formal training groups (26, 27). In a comparison study of medically directed at-home training with supervised group exercise soon after a MI, the two modes of training resulted in equally large improvements in functional capacity (27).

The selection of patients for a physical training programme obviously depends on the type and intensity of the exercise. In low-intensity training, even patients with depressed left ventricular function are able to obtain increased functional capacity (28). Likewise, patients with severe angina can improve their exercise tolerance by a daily walking programme.

Before entering a group training programme, all MI patients should be maximally exercise tested and medically examined for possible contra-indications. Absolute contra-indications include manifest congestive heart failure, unstable angina pectoris, severe aortic stenosis, uncontrolled hypertension, recent thrombo-embolism and ventricular dysrhythmias and conduction disturbances related to physical exercise (29). If necessary clinical precautions are taken, exercise training programmes for MI patients can be considered safe (5, 30).

Patient education

A central determinant for the course and outcome of an acute somatic illness, such as a MI, is the patient's perceived illness (Fig. 3). Various aspects of MI patients' knowledge and beliefs about their disease have been found related to a wide range of outcome indicators, such as return to work, use

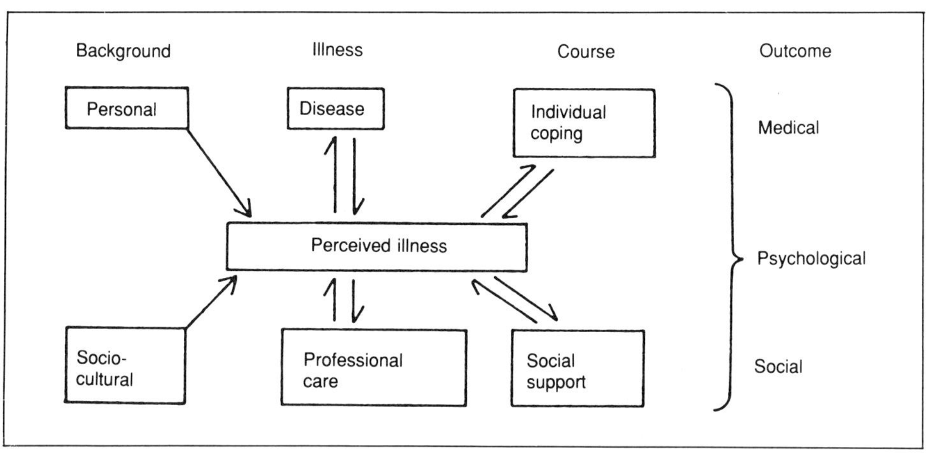

Fig. 3. *The determinants for outcome of a somatic illness. From (1).*

of health services, self-assessed health, emotional reactions, and changes in smoking behaviour (1).

The overwhelming feelings of harm and threat experienced by many MI patients during the acute phase of the illness in part reflects erroneous knowledge about the disease. Accordingly, such reactions can to some extent be counteracted if the patients are presented early with the fact that most MI patients are able to resume a normal life. Description of the "typical" course and outcome will make the recovery process more predictable and less ambiguous, factors that are related to efficient coping in threatening situations (31). In addition, increased illness knowledge will foster personal control and counteract sick role behaviour and feelings of helplessness. A better understanding of the disease mechanisms should also increase compliance with medical advice and fascilitate correct response to future medical symptoms (1, 32).

A number of studies confirm that most MI patients would like to learn more about their disease and that they are able to increase their illness knowledge even during the acute phase (33). However, the general opinion is that patient education is more effective when given at a later point of time, i.e. during the convalescence period.

The educational content can either be standardized or individualized. Whereas the latter approach seems to be more effective, standardized educational interventions have been shown to have a positive influence on outcome, too (34). Patient education given by personnel is generally more effective than use of written materials or audio-visual aids; however, the latter educational techniques are more advantagous from a cost-effectiveness perspective.

Group education offers possibilities for efficient learning and emotional support through social learning processes. In a small scale randomized clinical trial of post-hospital discussion groups, *Rahe et al* (35) found less recurrences among experimental patients over a 3-4 year follow-up. Although other studies have not confirmed group education after a MI to affect morbidity or mortality, most have shown some improvements in psychosocial functioning (9, 36-38). Educational approaches that focus on emotional support generally show better results than factual information alone.

Today, MI patients typically stay in hospital for only about one week after a MI, limiting the opportunities for in-patient education, as do the somatic and psychological disturbances commonly present at this point of time. Despite these limitations, patient education should be started already in the hospital, preferably by use of simple, standardized educational programmes supplemented with individual advice (33). At this point of time, the primary educational goal is to give the patient a correct understanding of the nature of the disease and the typical course and outcome. The natural healing process in the myocardium should be emphazised. Furthermore, the patient should be taught the principal differences between symptoms of angina pectoris and MI; the appropriate steps in physical reactivation during the first post-hospital weeks; and the general rules for resumption of daily activities.

This preparatory information should be repeated and elaborated upon in a formal group education programme after discharge from hospital. Patients should be encouraged to bring their spouses or other family members to the group sessions. The post-hospital discussion groups should be led by health professionals with experience in group processes. During each session, a core curriculum should be provided, with ample opportunities for discussion and exchange of individual experiences.

Among the various topics, the group discussions should focus on the patients' physical and emotional reactions during the convalescense; their expectations for the future; family roles; sexual life; and life-style changes. The educational programme can be supplemented with exercises in relaxation techniques or physical activities. Written or audiovisual educational materials can be used for additional learning. A series of 4-6 weekly sessions during the first post-hospital period should be sufficient.

Psychosocial intervention

In a psychological sense, the recovery process after a MI can be understood as a series of psychosocial transitions that follow the initial acute crisis, each presenting critical tasks and demands that must be managed and resolved to achieve an adaptive outcome (1).

Psychosocial readjustment after a MI involves the restoration of previous functioning within different areas of life: emotional status, work, sexual activity, family and social life, and leisure activities. It also involves changes in life-styles that represent increased risk for recurrences and death, such as smoking, unhealthy dietary habits, physical inactivity, and the so-called type-A behavioural pattern, i.e. an action-emotion syndrome characterized by chronic striving for achievement, easily aroused hostility, and a sense of time urgency (39).

Systematic psychosocial interventions for MI patients have employed various strategies, ranging from brief individual consultation during the initial illness to group activities over several years. The various group approaches can be broadly divided into two categories: (1) psychotherapeutic groups; (2) type A behaviour modification groups.

Psychotherapeutic groups

The theoretical background for this type of intervention stems largely from crisis theory. The purpose is to bring patients with similar experience together for verbal exchange of feelings and thoughts, thereby alleviating emotional reactions and fascilitating efficient coping behaviour. Also, such meetings provide an opportunity for patient education and behavioural therapy.

Only a few clinical trials of such programmes have been reported. In a randomized study, *Ibrahim et al* (40) studied the effects of weekly group meetings led by a clinical psychologist during the first year after a MI. Although no statistically significant changes were found in either physiological or psychological factors, a tendency towards improved survival, especially among the more severely ill patients, was noted. *Stern et al* (9) compared a programme of post-hospital group counselling with exercise training and usual care and found less depression and increased sociability among the group counselling participants compared with controls. The programme did not affect mobidity, mortality or return to work. A Swedish study also found some psychological benefits of a post-hospital group programme but no effects on morbidity or risk behaviour (38). In comparison, *Horlich et al* (41) noted no medical or psychological effects of post-hospital discussion groups among unselected MI patients.

Type A behaviour modification groups

In 1981, an expert panel at the U.S. National Heart Lung and Blood Institute recognized the type A behavioural pattern as an independent risk factor for coronary heart disease (42). Although recent reports have cast serious doubts whether type A is a secondary risk factor after a MI (43, 44), a meta-analysis of five studies indicated significant and consistent reductions in recurrences as a result of psychological treatments for reducing type A behaviour after a MI (45).

The largest and most convincing of these studies is the Recurrent Coronary Prevention Project (RCPP), in which 862 post-MI patients were randomly selected either to a cardiac group counselling programme or to a type A behaviour and cardiac group counselling programme (46). The type A behavioural modification programme employed a variety of techniques to help the participants identify and progressively modify type A behaviour.

Among these were: progressive muscle relaxation, self-monitoring, cognitive restructuring, self-reinforcement, and behavioural contracting. In all, the experimental patients were invited to attend a total of 62 sessions over 4.5 years (actual attendance: 61%).

The final results after 4.5 years showed that the psychological treatment was effective in reducing type A behaviour. Furthermore, the cumulative recurrence rate of fatal and non-fatal major coronary events was significantly lower (12.9%) in the psychological treatment group than in the cardiac treatment group (21.2%). However, total cardiac deaths in the follow-up period were not significantly different in the two groups (5.2% vs 7.2%) (46).

When evaluating these results, it is important to bear in mind that the participants in this study were highly selected: they were all non-smokers; they were recruited to the study by means of advertisements; 95% were classified as exhibiting type A behaviour; and at least six months had passed since the MI before they entered the study. Thus, the results from this study cannot be directely extrapolated to other MI populations.

Comprehensive rehabilitation programmes

A number of studies have used more than one intervention strategy for rehabilitation after a myocardial infarction. Typically, comprehensive rehabilitation programmes combine systematic medical surveillance, exercise training, patient education, and some form of psychosocial counselling.

In 1970, WHO initiated an international multicentre controlled study of comprehensive rehabilitation programmes for MI patients (47). The study comprised over 3,000 patients from 24 centres in Europe. The intervention programmes varied between the centers, but generally consisted of close medical monitoring; risk factor modification through health education; vocational and psychosocial guidance; and physical training. Due to wide variation between the centres regarding patient characteristics and the rehabilitation programmes, pooling of the results was not considered appropriate. Furthermore, the results regarding mortality, morbidity and return to work were not consistent among the centres, again reflecting the lack of standardization in this study. Thus, conclusions regarding the effects of comprehensive cardiac rehabilitation can regrettably not be drawn from this huge international study.

The results from the two participating Finnish centres, based upon 375 MI patients followed for three years, have been published separately (48). During follow-up, the experimental patients had, on average, lower blood pressure and lower levels of blood lipids, and also smoked fewer cigarettes than the controls. Although neither total mortality nor the incidence of non-fatal reinfarctions were significantly affected, the experimental group experienced significantly fewer sudden deaths (5.8% vs. 14.4%, $p < 0.01$) and coronary deaths (18.6% vs. 29.4%, $p < 0.02$) compared with controls.

In a comparison study, *Hedbäck et al* (49) evaluated the effects of an in- and posthospital comprehensive rehabilitation programme for MI patients. After five years, significantely fewer non-fatal reinfarctions had occurred in the rehabilitation group compared with a reference group. Also, the rehabilitated patients more often stopped smoking, less often used sedatives, and more often maintained vocational activity during follow-up. Furthermore, rehabilitated patients had somewhat fewer and significantly shorter readmissions compared to the reference group. The economical costs of the rehabilitation programme were found to be compararable to that of the usual care. However, the higher rate of return to work resulted in considerable economical savings. The net result of the rehabilitation programme was calculated to a cost-reduction of approximately 10.000 U.S.$ per rehabilitated patient over the five year period (50).

Summary and conclusion

After twenty years of research, the true effects of rehabilitation efforts after a MI have not conclusively been established. The various studies have produced conflicting results to some extent. Most investigations are subject to methodological weaknesses, either in the study design, specification of intervention programme, or choice of outcome indicators. Randomized clinical trials of behavioural interventions are notoriously difficult to undertake. It is hard to obtain sufficient funding. The study period usually extends for years, requiring devotion and disipline to complete the experiment. In order to obtain a sufficient number of participants, multicentre design has sometimes been used; however, this type of study poses other problems in the selection of patients and standardization of procedures.

One explanation for the general lack of significant effects of rehabilitation programmes may be that most studies have been concerned with unselected post-infarction patients. The non-specific tendency towards clinical improvement in the post-infarction phase tends to dilute any specific effect of rehabilitation programmes.

Although a MI in general constitutes a major life crisis with concommitant risk for later disability, the general lesson from past research does not support the earlier call for extensive rehabilitation measures for all MI

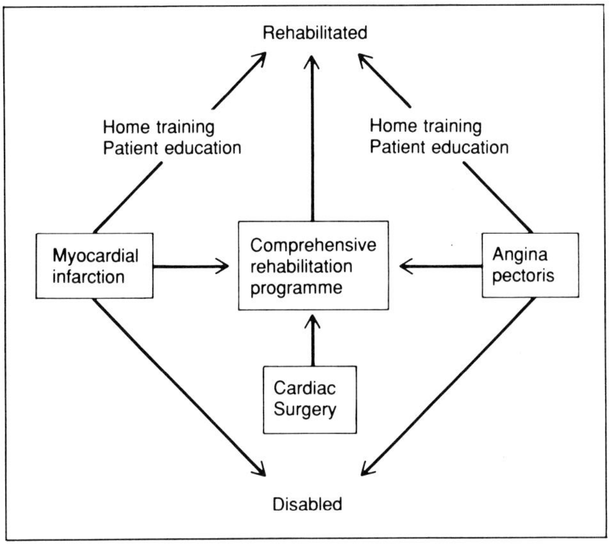

Fig. 4. *A model for the organization of cardiac rehabilitation.*

patients. The majority of patients are able to cope with the post-infarction problems with only limited professional help.

On the other hand, a number of patients are clearly in need of more formal rehabilitation efforts. Some of these patients are characterized by undue fear and uncertainty, excessive preoccupation with their disease, or unwarranted limitation in physical or social activities. Other patients have exeptional physical or mental strain at work. A few patients are severely limited by chest pain or breathlessness or posess medical factors indicating a poor prognosis.

On the basis of previous research, it can be estimated that about 30% of the total number of MI patients below 70 years of age belong to these categories. It is important that these patients are identified as early as possible in the post-MI period, before unwarranted chronic disability has been established. *Wiklund* (4) showed that a physician's assessment of requirement for rehabilitation 5-8 weeks after the MI provides a good prediction of vocational outcome one year after the MI. Another strategy would be to identify patients with rehabilitation needs from standardized psychological questionnaires. A Norwegian study showed patients' expectations for future functioning to be the best predictors for later psychosocial readjustment (1).

Thus, a stepped-up strategy for rehabilitation after a MI should be chosen, in which all patients receive a basic programme of education and psychosocial support in the hospital and during the first post-hospital weeks (Fig. 4). On the basis of systematic evaluation either before or shortly after discharge, patients with increased risk for rehabilitation failure should then be identified and offered a comprehensive rehabilitation programme, consisting of exercise training, patient education, and psychosocial intervention. The rehabilitation programme should also be open for other groups of coronary patients. By concentrating the rehabilitation efforts to the patients most in need for them, group-based comprehensive cardiac rehabilitation would undoubtly prove to be effective and worth-while.

References

1. Mæland JG, Havik OE. After the myocardial infarction. A medical and psychological study with special emphasis on perceived illness. Scand J Rehab Med 1989; (suppl. 22).
2. Mæland JG, Meen K. Predicting long-term mortality after a myocardial infarction from routine hospital data. Acta Med Scand 1988; 224: 539-47.
3. Ulvenstam G, Åberg A, Bergstrand R, et al. Recurrent myocardial infarction. 1. Natural history of fatal and non-fatal events. Eur Heart J 1985; 6: 294-302.
4. Wiklund I. Readjustment after a first myocardial infarction with special reference to emotional reaction and coping. Gøteborg: University of Gøteborg, 1984. (Thesis).
5. Sanne H. Exercise tolerance and physical training of non-selected patients after myocardial infarction. Acta Med Scand 1973; (suppl 551).
6. Widimsky J, Broustet JP. Cardiopulmonary function after myocardial infarction: effects of bed-rest, disease and training. In: Kallio V, Cay E, eds. Rehabilitation after myocardial infarction. The European experience. Public health in Europe 24. Copenhagen: World Health Organization, Regional Office for Europe, 1985: 9-21.

World Health Organization, Regional Office for Europe, 1985: 9-21.

7. Schlant RC, Forman S, Stamler J, Canner PL. The natural history of coronary heart disease: Prognostic factors after recovery from myocardial infarction in 2789 men. Circulation 1982; 66: 401-14.
8. Carson O, Phillips R, Lloyd M, et al. Exercise after myocardial infarction: a controlled trial. J Royal Coll Phys 1982; 16: 147-51.
9. Stern MJ, Gorman PA, Kaslow L. The group counseling v exercise therapy study. A controlled intervention with subjects following myocardial infarction. Arch Intern Med 1983; 143: 1719-25.
10. Oberman A, Cleary O, Larosa JC, Hellerstein HK, Naughton J. Changes in risk factors among participants in a long-term exercise rehabilitation program. Adv Cardiol 1982; 31: 168-75.
11. Froelicher V, Jensen D, Genter F, et al. A randomized trial of exercise training in patients with coronary heart disease. JAMA 1984; 252: 1291-7.
12. Marra S, Paolillo V, Spadaccini F, Angelino PF. Long-term follow-up after a controlled randomized post-myocardial infarction rehabilitation programme: effects on morbidity and mortality. Eur Heart J 1985; 6: 656-63.
13. Ehsani AA, Heath GW, Hagberg JM, Sobel BE, Holloszy JO. Effects of 12 months of intense exercise training on ischemic ST-segment depression in patients with coronary artery disease. Circulation 1981; 64: 1116-24.
14. Grodzinski E, Jette M, Blümchen G, Borer JS. Effects of a four-week training program on left ventricular function as assessed by radionuclide ventriculography. J Cardiopulmonary Rehab 1987; 7: 517-24.
15. Dressendorfer R, Amsterdam EA, Mason DT. Therapeutic effects of exercise training in

angina pectoris. In: Cohen LS, Mock MB, Ringquist I, eds. Physical conditioning and cardiovascular rehabilitation. New York: John Wiley and Sons, 1981: 121-38.
16. Oldridge NB, Guyatt GH, Fisher ME, Rimm AA. Cardiac rehabilitation after myocardial infarction. Combined experience of randomized clinical trials. JAMA 1988; 260: 954-60.
17. McPherson BD, Paivio A, Yuhasz MS, Rechnitzer PA, Pickard HA, Lefcoe NM. Psychological effects of an exercise program for post-infarct and normal adult men. J Sports Med 1967; 7: 95-102.
18. Stern MJ, Cleary P. National Exercise and Heart Disease Project. Psychosocial changes observed during a low-level exercise program. Arch Intern Med 1981; 141: 1463-7.
19. Stern MJ, Cleary P. The National Exercise and Heart Disease Project. Long-term psychosocial outcome. Arch Intern Med 1982; 142: 1093-7.
20. Mæland JG, Havik OE, Bolstad A. Rehabiliteringskurs for hjertepasienter. Psykologiske effekter. (A rehabilitation programme for heart patients: The psychological effects). Tidsskr Nor Lægeforen 1983; 103: 1637-9.
21. Hellerstein HK, Franklin BA. Exercise testing and prescription. In: Wenger NK, Hellerstein HK, eds. Rehabilitation of the coronary patient. New York: John Wiley and Sons 1978: 149-202.
22. Blumenthal JA, Rejeski WJ, Walsh-Riddle M, et al. Comparison of high- and low-intensity exercise training early after acute myocardial infarction. Am J Cardiol 1988; 61: 26-30.
23. Nordrehaug JA, Bjørkhaug A, Danielsen R, Vik-Mo H, Aam I. Økning av aerob arbeidskapasitet ved kortvarig trening av hjertepasienter (Increase in aerobic work capacity after short-term exercise training for patients with coronary heart disease). Tidsskr Nor Lægeforen 1989; 109: 687-9.
24. Oldridge NB. Compliance and exercise in primary and secondary prevention of coronary heart disease: A review. Prev Med 1982; 22: 257-62.
25. Palatsi, I. Feasibility of physical training after myocardial infarction and its effect on return to work, morbidity and mortality. Acta Med Scand 1976; (suppl 599).
26. Stevens R, Hanson P. Comparison of supervised and unsupervised exercise training after coronary bypass surgery. Am J Cardiol 1984; 53: 1524-8.
27. De Busk RF, Haskell WL, Miller NH, et al. Medically directed at-home rehabilitation soon after clinically uncomplicated acute myocardial infarction: a new model for patient care. Am J Cardiol 1985; 55: 251-7.
28. Conn EH, Williams RS, Wallace AG. Exercise responses before and after physical conditioning in patients with severely depressed ventricular function. Am J Cardiol 1982; 49: 296-300.
29. König K, Denolin H, Dorossiev D, eds. Myocardial infarction. How to prevent. How to rehabilitate. 2nd. ed. International Society and Federation of Cardiology, 1983.
30. Haskell WL. Cardiovascular complications during exercise training of cardiac patients. Circulation 1978; 57: 920-4.
31. Lazarus RS, Folkman S. Stress, appraisal, and coping. New York: Springer Publ. Co., 1984.
32. Wenger NK. Patient and family education after myocardial infarction. Postgrad Med 1975; 57: 129-34.
33. Mæland JG, Havik OE. The effects of an in-hospital educational programme for myocardial infarction patients. Scand J Rehab Med 1987; 19: 57-65.
34. Mazzuca SA. Does patient education in chronic disease have therapeutic value? J Chron Dis 1982; 35: 521-9.
35. Rahe RH, Ward HW, Hayes V. Brief group therapy in myocardial infarction rehabilitation: three- to four-year follow-up of a controlled trial. Psychosom Med 1979; 41: 229-42.

36. Ott CR, Sivarajan ES, Newton KM, et al. A controlled randomized study of early cardiac rehabilitation: The Sickness Impact Profile as an assessment tool. Heart Lung 1983; 12: 162-70.
37. Mayou R, Mac Mahon D, Sleight P, Florencio MJ. Early rehabilitation after myocardial infarction. Lancet 1981; 2, 1399-1401.
38. Theorell T. Psychosocial intervention as a part of the rehabilitation after a myocardial infarction. Int Rehab Med 1984; 5: 185-8.
39. Friedman M, Rosenman RH. Type A behavior and your heart. New York: Alfred A. Knopf, 1974.
40. Ibrahim MA, Feldman JG, Sultz HA, Staiman MG, Young LJ, Dean D. Management after myocardial infarction: a controlled trial of the effect of group psychotherapy. Int J Psychiatry Med 1974; 5: 253-68.
41. Horlich L, Cameron R, Firor W, Bhalerao U, Baltzan R. The effects of education and group discussion in the post myocardial infarction patient. J Psychosom Res 1984; 26: 485-92.
42. The Review Panel on Coronary-Prone Behavior and Coronary Heart Disease: A critical review. Circulation 1981; 63: 1199-215.
43. Case RB, Heller SS, Case NB, Moss AJ, and The Multicenter Post-Infarction Research Group. Type A behavior and survival after acute myocardial infarction. N Engl J Med 1985; 312: 737-41.
44. Ragland DR, Brand RJ. Type A behavior and mortality from coronary heart disease. N Engl J Med 1988; 318: 65-9.
45. Nunes E, Frank KA, Kornfield DS. Psychologic treatment for the type A behavior pattern and for coronary heart disease: A meta-analysis of the literature. Psychosom Med 1987; 48: 159-73.
46. Friedman M, Thoresen CE, Gill JJ, et al. Alteration of type A behavior and its effect on cardiac recurrences in post myocardial infarction patients: Summary results of the recurrent coronary prevention project. Am Heart J 1986; 112: 653-65.
47. Dorossiev D, ed. Rehabilitation and comprehensive secondary prevention after acute myocardial infarction. WHO Euro Reports and Studies 84. Copenhagen: World Health Organization, Regional Office for Europe, 1983.
48. Kallio V, Hämäläinen H. Reduction in sudden deaths by a multifactorial intervention programme after acute myocardial infarction. Lancet 1979: 2: 1091-4.
49. Hedbäck B, Perk J. 5-year results of a comprehensive rehabilitation programme after myocardial infarction. Eur Heart J 1987; 8: 234-42.
50. Perk J. Cardiac rehabilitation. Medical and socioeconomic results of a comprehensive programme. Linköping: Linköping University, 1989. (Thesis).

42

Ischaemic heart disease and family intervention

SYNNØVE FØNNEBØ KNUTSEN

Coronary heart disease (CHD) is known to aggregate in families (1-6) and atherosclerotic changes have been found already in childhood (7) and youth (8). The family therefore emerges as a very good setting for early prevention of ischaemic heart disease. Even if the risk of CHD is minimal both in children/youth and in premenopausal women, early intervention has the potential for greater incidence reduction than intervention started later in life. It is during childhood, the formative years, that the basis for later habits is laid. In line with this, there seems to be a general consensus of opinion, at least among pediatricians, that prevention of CHD should begin in childhood and that a more prudent diet starting at an early age can influence the risk of CHD in later life (9).

As expected, studies have shown that different lifestyle characteristics are shared to a greater extent by family members than by others. Hunter et al (10) found a positive correlation between smoking habits of teenagers and the smoking habits of their parents. Others have found that dietary habits (11, 12), physical fitness (13) and exercise habits (14) are similar within families. *Garn and Clark* (15) showed that fatness runs in families. Children of lean parents are most often lean, whereas children of obese parents are most often obese. The same was true for spouses. These similarities seemed to be due to similarities in caloric intake and caloric expenditure. Even for coronary-prone behavior, *Matthews et al* (16) found family resemblance. Traditional coronary risk factors also aggregate in families. *Knutsen and Knutsen* found that both wives (17) and children (18) of men identified as at high risk for CHD had approximatey 20% higher risk of coronary heart disease compared to same-aged married women and children in the normal population (Table 1 and 2). The wives and children were found to differ from those in the general population with regard to dietary habits also. In

Table 1. *The Family Intervention Study. Age-adjusted mean levels of serum lipids, blood pressure, BMI and percentage of daily smokers in wives of high-risk men, compared to the same age married women in the general population. 25-49 years.*

Variable	Wives of high-risk men N=911	Married women in gen. pop. N=4271
Total cholesterol mmol/l	5.98	5.78***
HDL-cholesterol mmol/l	1.74	1.77
HDL-chol/tot chol %	30.01	31.58***
Triglycerides mmol/l	1.13	1.10
Systolic BP mmHg	122.5	121.6
Diastolic BP mmHg	78.9	78.5
Body Mass Index g/cm^2	2.31	2.28*
Coronary risk score	4.55	3.81**
Per cent daily cigarette smokers[1])	47.3	42.1**

Differences tested using the two-tailed t-test. *** $p<.001$. ** $p<.01$. * $p<.05$.
1) Differences tested using the Chi-square statistic.

Table 2. *The Family Intervention Study. Age-adjusted mean levels of coronary risk factors among children of high-risk men and children in the general population. Age 12-19.*

Variable	High-risk children N=367	Children in the gen. pop. N=389
Total cholesterol mmol/l	4.50	4.25***
HDL-cholesterol mmol/l	1.36	1.03*
HDL-chol/tot chol %	30.9	33.7***
Triglycerides mmol/l	1.22	1.03***
Systolic BP mmHg	117.8	117.1
Diastolic BP mmHg	61.1	61.3
Body Mass Index g/cm^2	2.11	2.09*
Per cent daily smokers	25	23

Age-adjustment and statistical analysis done using analysis of variance with age as covariate.
*** $p<.001$. ** $p<.01$, * $p<.05$.

the Framingham Study, *Kannel* (19) found that risk factor levels among wives varied according to their husband's risk status as shown in Table 3. In the Muscatine Study also, *Schrott et al* (20) found that risk factor levels among relatives varied according to the risk status of their school-aged children (Table 4). This study also reported an increased frequency of cardiovascular disease mortality in the relatives of children belonging to the highest risk group. Most studies find parent-child correlation of serum lipids (21-27) and eight (13, 25-31) have also found a spouse correlation, indicating that coronary risk factors are also influenced by factors other than heredity and most likely by common environmental factors. Family correlations have been found for blood pressure also (13, 22, 32).

Table 3. *The Framingham Heart Study*[1]*) - correspondence of risk factors among spouses: Married couples, aged 30-62. Risk factor levels in wives of husbands with low, medium, and high risk factor levels.*

	Level of risk factors in wives							
	Tot chol		Systolic BP		Obesity		Cigarettes	
Risk status of husbands	N	Mean	N	Mean	N	%	N	% smokers
Low	402	214	604	120	165	9	151	24
Medium	804	227	242	131	132	17	138	37
High	310	235	110	136	23	22	960	47

1) (*Kannel* 1976)
*Definitions:

	Tot cholesterol mg/dl	Systolic BP mmHg
Low	< 200	< 120
Medium	200-259	120-147
High	>259	> 147

	Obesity Rel Wt	Smoking status
Low	< 100	Never smoked
Medium	100-119	Former smoker
High	> 119	Cigarette smoker

Table 4. *The Muscatine Study*[1]*) – Values of cholesterol and triglycerides among siblings, parents, aunts/uncles and grand-parents of school children, aged 5-16, with age- and sex-adjusted low, medium and high levels of total cholesterol.*

	Risk level* among children					
	Tot Cholesterol			Triglycerides		
	Low	Medium	High	Low	Medium	High
Siblings	138	157	179	66	72	82
Parents	172	188	232	116	117	135
Aunts/Uncles	188	192	218	119	120	119
Grandparents	210	213	235	153	129	146

1) (*Schrott et al.* 1979)
* Definition: Risk according to cholesterol levels
Low – < 5th percentile at two consecutive screenings
Medium – 5th-95th percentile at two consecutive screenings
High – > 95th percentil at two consecutive screenings

For lifestyle intervention, the family therefore stands out as a natural unit for CHD intervention, but few studies have been reported using this method. The family approach to intervention can be looked upon in two different ways:

1. The family members are considered useful in giving support to a person who needs to change their lifestyle because of increased coronary risk.
2. The whole family is considered as having increased coronary risk and thus the whole family becomes the unit of intervention.

These two approaches will be discussed separately and studies where these two approaches have been used, will be reviewed.

1. The family as support for a coronary high-risk person

Until recently, the family has been utilized mainly as a support network for the family member identified as needing intervention. *Epstein* (33) used the family as support for children who needed weight reduction. *Witschi* (34) used family-cooperation in implementing a cholesterol-reducing diet. With regard to ischaemic heart disease, *Baranowski et al* (35) used the family as support for cardiovascular risk reduction. *Leren* (36) and *Hjermann* (37) both invited wives together with their coronary high risk husbands to sessions where dietary instruction was given. The favorable long-term results reported by *Hjermann* is partly ascribed to the inclusion of the wives (38). Also in the Gothenborg Trial (39), wives were invited to dietary information sessions together with their high-risk husbands. The same was done in MR-FIT (40) and among the high-risk groups of the WHO Collaborative trial (41). In the WHO trial the spouses were also invited to cooking classes. In an attempt to control blood pressure, *Earp et al* (42) studied the effect of involving family members in the measurements and monitoring of blood pressure during home visits as opposed to standard hypertensive care. No significant differences were found, but blood pressure was lowered more in the groups who received home-visits. Also in Finland (43), spouses were recruited to aid in the changes necessary to obtain risk reduction among high-risk persons. Of the studies mentioned, the Oslo Trial (37) and the Belgian part of the WHO Collaborative trial (44) have reported the largest effects on risk factor levels after intervention.

2. The entire family is identified as the unit of intervention

This approach has been given more attention lately. Persons who are told that they are at increased risk for CHD, will most probably be more motivated for lifestyle changes than if they only serve as support for another family member who is identified as at high risk. Three studies using the family as the unit of intervention have been reported. The Family Heart Study (45) investigated the feasibility of changing dietary habits using the family approach in 233 randomly selected families who volunteered to participate for at least 5 years. A family was included if it contained at least two persons between the ages of 6 and 65. Monthly group sessions for adults as well as for children were arranged as well as cooking classes. In addition, field trips and potlucks were used to further enhance dietary changes. The 5-year results of this study, which aimed at changing to a hypocholesterolaemic diet, have not yet been published. The second study, which also used the family approach, was the San Diego Family Health Project (46). 206 families were recruited through elementary schools and followed for 2 years. These families were Anglo-American or Mexican-American families. They volunteered to participate and were motivated for follow-up by being payed $ 50 for each measuring session that the family attended. The intervention in this study was broader and included both diet, smoking and exercise. Significant differences were found in dietary habits between the control and intervention families at evaluation. Favorable changes were also found in blood pressure. But for serum lipids, only Anglo-American parents showed lower levels than the control group and the difference was due to the fact that the control group had increased its levels whereas the intervention group remained stable. Both of these family studies were done in random families, without any defined risk of CHD.

The first study identifying the whole family as having increased coronary risk is The Family Intervention Study in Tromsø (47). Following the second Tromsø survey in 1979/80, 1,373 men were identified as at high risk for CHD on the basis of low relative-HDL (HDL-chol/tot chol <17.6%) and/or high total cholesterol (>7.86 mmol/l). In addition to elevated serum lipids and blood pressure, it was found that a greater proportion of them were daily cigarette smokers, were inactive during leisure, were heavy coffee drinkers, and used butter/hard margarine as spreadfat more often than other men. They also used fruits/vegetables less frequently than men in the general population. Also the wives and children had increased risk factor levels (17, 18). The families were randomized to intervention and control. The men in the intervention group were informed of their increased risk in a letter and told that also their family (those living together with them) had increased risk due to shared lifestyle. The whole family was asked to be present during two home-visits where new blood tests, blood pressure and dietary information was collected as well as intervention given. Of the 673 families randomized to intervention, 608 were visited.

In addition to the two home-visits, the families were sent quarterly newsletters and offered stop-smoking clinics and dietary information meetings with food samples. The men were offered new blood tests 1.5 years after the home visit. The families in both the intervention and control group were rescreened at the third Tromsø Survey in 1986/87. At rescreening, all family members in the intervention group reported significantly more favorable dietary habits for spreadfat, cooking fat and type of milk as well as for coffee consumption, use of fruits and vegetables and use of salt as compared to the control group (48). Significantly lower serum cholesterol was found among men and wives in the intervention group, but no differences were found in the children.The results so far indicate that the high-risk men have reduced their risk of CHD by 10% as compared to those in the control group. The risk reduction among the wives and children is more difficult to evaluate. The experience from this study shows that a family approach to CHD intervention which involves identifying even children as at high risk, is both feasible and well received. The design was such that it can also be adopted in the clinical setting. Although the changes obtained are relatively small, further studies should be pursued to find more effective ways of using the family approach in prevention of CHD.

Conclusion

There is general agreement that a lowering of coronary risk factors in the whole population would lead to fewer new cases of ischaemic heart disease (49, 50). The natural experiment in Norway during World War II gives us an indication of what can be obtained through dietary and smoking changes in a whole population. Not only did the incidence of CHD decrease (51), but also the incidence of other lifestyle-related diseases, such as diabetes, was reduced (52).

Although such dramatic changes are not conceivable today, it is important to find intervention methods than can influence as large a proportion of the population as possible. Family intervention is one way, and has been shown to be both feasible and well accepted. However, our experience also shows that this method alone will not make large impacts on the population incidence of ischaemic heart disease. Implementing the family approach through the already existing mother-care and school-health clinics in Scandinavia could possibly yield additional effects since these clinics reach all families with children. Even if these clinics do not have a tradition in prevention of CHD, they are used to giving dietary advice for other reasons. It would therefore probably be both feasible and relatively easy to incorporate specific lifestyle intervention with the aim of reducing the risk of CHD in the families.

However, even if family intervention is the most logical approach to intervention on ischaemic heart disease, additional measures such as political decisions involving economic, agricultural and smoking policies are probably needed in order to obtain major changes in the population risk of CHD.

References

1. Thomas CB, Cohen BH. The familial occurrence of hypertension and coronary artery disease with observations concerning obesity and diabetes. Ann Intern Med 1955; 42: 90-127.
2. Rose G. Familial patterns in ischaemic heart disease. Br J Prev Soc Med 1964; 17: 537-42.
3. Sack J, Evans KA. The increased risk of death from ischaemic heart disease in first degree reatives of 121 men and 96 women with ischaemic heart disease. J Med Genet 1966; 3: 239-57.
4. Deutscher S, Ostrander LD, Epstein FH. Familial factors in premature coronary heart disease – a preliminary report from the Tecumseh community health study. Am J Epidemiol 1970; 91: 233-7.
5. Phillips RL, Lilienfeld AM, Diamond EL, Kagan A. Frequency of coronary heart disease and cerebrovascular accidents in parents and sons of coronary heart disease index cases and controls. Am J Epidemiol 1974; 100: 87-100.
6. Rissanen AM, Nikkila EA. Coronary artery disease and its risk factors in families of young men with angina pectoris and in controls. Br Heart J 1977; 39: 875-83.
7. McGill HD. Morphologic development of the atherosclerotic plaque. In: Lauer RM, Shekell RB, eds. Childhood prevention of atherosclerosis and hypertension. New York: Raven Press, 1980: 41.
8. McNamara JJ, Molot MA, Stremple JF, et al. Coronary artery disease in combat causalities in Vietnam. JAMA 1971; 216: 1185-7.
9. Wynder EL, Berenson GS, Strong WB, et al. Coronary heart disease prevention: Cholesterol, a pediatric perspective. Prev Med 1989; 18: 323-409.
10. Hunter S, Baugh JC, Webber L, et al. Social learning effects on trial and adoption of cigarette smoking in children: The Bogalusa Heart Study. Prev Med 1982; 11: 29-42.
11. Patterson TL, Rupp J, Sallis J, et al. Aggregation of dietary calories, fats, and sodium in Mexican-American and Anglo-American families. Am J Prev Med 1988; 4: 75-82.
12. Perusse L, Tremblay A, Leblanc C, et al. Familial resemblance in energy intake: contribution of genetic and environmental factors. Am J Clin Nutr 1988; 47: 629-35.
13. Perusse L, Leblanc C, Tremblay A, et al. Familial aggregation in physical fitness, coronary heart disease risk factors, and pulmonary function measurements. Prev Med 1987; 16: 607-15.
14. Sallis JF, Patterson TL, Buono MJ, Atkins CJ, Nader PR. Aggregation of physical activity habits in Mexican-American and Anglo families. J Behav Med 1988; 11: 31-41.
15. Garn SM, Clarke DC. Trends in fatness and the origins of obesity. Pediatrics 1976; 57: 443-56.
16. Matthews KA, Krantz DS. Resemblances of twins and their parents in Pattern A behavior. Psychosom Med 1976; 38: 140-4.
17. Knutsen SF, Knutsen R. Wives of coronary high-risk men - are they also at higher risk? The Tromsø Heart Study. J Intern Med 1990; in press.
18. Knutsen SF, Knutsen R. Children of coronary high-risk men. Do they need to worry? Submitted 1990.
19. Kannel WB. Recent highlights from the Framingham Study. Aust NZJ Med 1976; 6: 373-86.
20. Schrott HG, Clarke WR, Wiebe DA, et al. Increased coronary mortality in relatives of hypercholesterolemic school children: The Muscatine Study. Circulation 1979; 59: 320-6.
21. Van Natta PA, Jenkins JA, Chase GA, et al. The East Baltimore Study – Familial aggrega-

tion of plasma lipid levels in juveniles in a black inner-city population. Am J Epidemiol 1981; 114: 385-97.
22. Laskarzewski PM, Morrison JA, Kelly K, et al. Parent-child coronary heart disease risk factor associations. Am J Epidemiol 1981; 114: 827-35.
23. Greenberg RA, Green PP, Roggenkamp KJ, et al. The constancy of parent-offspring similarity of total cholesterol throughout childhood and early adult life. J Chron Dis 1984; 37: 833-8.
24. Namboodiri KK. The collaborative lipid research clinics program family study. Familial associations of plasma lipids and lipoproteins. Am J Epidemiol 1985; 119: 975-96. 975-96.
25. Godfrey RC, Stenhouse NS, Cullen KJ, et al. Cholesterol and the Child: Studies of the cholesterol levels of Busselton school children and their parents. Aust Paediat J 1972; 8: 72-8.
26. Mjøs OD, Thelle DS, Førde OH, Vik-Mo H. Family study of high density lipiprotein cholesterol and the relation to age and sex. Acta Med Scand 1977; 201: 323-9.
27. Garrison RJ, Castelli WP, Feinleib M, et al. The association of total cholesterol, triglycerides and plasma lipoprotein cholesterol levels in first degree relatives and spouse pairs. Am J Epidemiol 1979; 110: 313-21.
28. Rao DC, Morton NE, Gulbrandsen CL, et al. Cultural and biological determinants of lipoprotein concentrations. Ann Hum Genet 1979; 42: 467-77.
29. Barrett-Connor E, Suarz L, Criqui M. Spouse concordance of plasma cholesterol and triglycerides. J Chron Dis 1982; 35: 333-40.
30. Cheraskin E, Ringsdorf WM. Familial biochemical patterns. Atherosclerosis 1970;II: 247-50.
31. Sackett DL, Anderson GD, Milner R, et al. Concordance for coronary risk factors among spouses. Circulation 1975; 52: 589-95.
32. Patterson TL, Kaplan RM, Sallis JF, Nader PR. Aggregation of blood pressure in Anglo-American and Mexican-American families. Prev Med 1987; 16: 616-25.
33. Epstein LH, Wing RR, Koeske R, et al. Long term effects of family based treatment of childhood obesity. J Consult Clin Psychol 1987; 55: 91-5.
34. Witschi JC, Singer M, Wu-ee M and Stare FJ. Family cooperation and effectiveness in a cholesterol-lowering diet. J Am Diet Ass 1978; 72: 384-9.
35. Baranowski T, Nader PR, Dunn K, Vanderpool N. Family self-help: promoting changes in health behavior. J Communic 1982; 32: 161-72.
36. Leren P. The Oslo Diet-Heart Study: Eleven-year report. Circulation 1970; 42: 935-42.
37. Hjermann I, Holme I, Velve Byre K, Leren P. Effect of diet and smoking intevention on the incidence of coronary heart disease. Report from the Oslo Study group of a randomised trial in healthy men. Lancet 1981; ii: 1303-10.
38. Hjermann I, Holme I, Leren P. Oslo Study: Diet and antismoking trial. Results after 102 months. Circulation 1986; 80 (suppl 2A): 7-11.
39. Wilhelmsen L, Berglund G, Elmfeldt D, et al. The multifactor primary prevention trial in Goteborg, Sweden. Eur Heart J 1986; 7: 279-88.
40. Multiple Risk factor intervention trial group. Multiple risk factor intervention trial. Risk factor changes and mortality results. JAMA 1982; 248: 1465-77.
41. WHO. WHO European Collaborative trial in the multifactorial prevention of coronary heart disease. Copenhagen: WHO Regional Office for Europe, 1989.
42. Earp JA, Ory MG, Strogatz DS. The effects of family involvement and practitioner home visits on the control of hypertension. Am J Public Health 1982; 72: 1146-53.
43. Puska P, Salonen J, Nissinen A, Tuomilehto J. The North Karelia Project. Prev Med 1983; 12: 191-5.

44. Kornitzer M et al. Begian Heart Disease Prevention project. Incidence and mortality results. Lancet 1983;i: 1066-70.
45. Carmody TP, Istvan J, Matarazzo JD, et al. Applications of social learning theory in the promotion of heart-healthy diets: The Family Heart Study dietary intervention model. Health Ed Res 1986; 1: 13-27.
46. Nader PR, Sallis JF, Patteerson TL, et al. A family approach to cardiovascular risk reduction: Results from the San Diego Family Health Project. Heath Educ Q 1989; 16: 229-44.
47. Knutsen SF, Knutsen R. The Tromsø Heart Study: Family approach to intervention on CHD. Feasibility of risk factor reduction in high-risk persons – project description. Scand J Soc Med 1989; 17: 109-19.
48. Knutsen SF, Knutsen R. The Tromsø study: The Family Intervention Study. Effect of intervention on some coronary risk factors and dietary habits. 6-year follow-up. 1990; submitted.
49. Khaw KT, Rose G. Cholesterol screening programmes: how much potential benefit? Br Med J 1989; 299: 606-7.
50. Goldman L, Weinstein MC, Williams LW. Relative impact of targeted versus population-wide cholesterol interventions on the incidence of coronary heart disease. Projections of the coronary heart disease policy model. Circulation 1989; 80: 254-60.
51. Westlund K. Hjerteinfarktets insidensvariasjoner. Nord Med 1971; 15: 458-65.
52. Westlund K. Incidence of diabetes mellitus in Oslo, Norway 1925 to 1954. Br J Prev Soc Med 1966; 20: 105-16.

Epidemiological aspects

43

Ischaemic heart disease and risk factors

DAG S. THELLE

Human Characteristics and Aetiological Factors

A risk factor for ischaemic heart disease (IHD) may be defined as any factor which has been shown in an epidemiological study to be associated with the incidence of ischaemic heart disease. This rather wide definition includes characteristics like sex, age, and family history, or more socially determined variables such as religious affiliations and social class. Table 1 gives a summary of the more important risk factors identified so far. In addition to these factors a number of background conditions may be listed which have been shown to determine the IHD risk like civil status, length of education, occupation, religious affiliation, ethnic origin and poverty during childhood.

One may distinguish between two major types of risk factors; individual traits and external exposure. Both types of factors may, to some extent, be amenable, but obviously some more than others. Direct causal factors are factors, which if changed would result in subsequent changes in the incidence of IHD.

The indirect factors on the other hand exert their influence via other and more direct factors. Vegetarian diet is protective so far as it is low in saturated fat which is a direct causal factor. Stress at the working site may increase the risk of IHD, but mainly as a promoter of increased cigarette-smoking or other habits.

The most important risk factors from a preventive point of view are those factors which are necessary for the occurrence of IHD and which are amenable. In the Nordic countries those factors would be nutrition and blood lipids, blood pressure and smoking habits. Obviously age, sex and heritage are factors which cannot be affected, but they carry important information which will influence the risk assessment based upon other factors.

Table 1.

Individual traits and characteristics	*External factors (exposure)*
Age	*A) Probably direct causal factors:*
Sex	*Nutrition*
Family history	– *High saturated fat intake*
Blood lipids	– High cholesterol intake
– total cholesterol	– High salt intake
– LDL cholesterol	
– HDL cholesterol	
– Fatty acids	
– Triglycerides	
Sedimentation rate, haemoglobin, uric acid, leucocytes, thrombosis and coagulation factors	*Cigarettes*
Diabetes mellitus	Alcohol abuse
Blood pressure	*Physical inactivity*
Overweight: waist/hip ratio	Coffee
Menopause	Anti-contraceptives
Tissue type antigen	Tolbutamine
Non-specific ECG changes	Phenormin
	B) Probably indirect associations:
	Vegetarianism (protective)
	Life-events (stress)
	Soft water

The word risk implies the probability for having a IHD event within a defined time period, or before a certain age. Our knowledge is very limited when it comes to assessing the IHD risk of a 20-year old with a certain risk factor profile, or on the other hand a 65-year old. The longitudinal studies done so far have almost exclusively adressed middle-aged men.

Family history of ischaemic heart disease

A large number of studies have demonstrated the importance of a positive family history of IHD as a risk factor (1). This applies in particular to the occurrence of IHD at young age, e.g. before 55-60 years in men and 60-65 years in women. This excess risk can only partly be explained by the occurrence of familial hypercholesterolaemia which was first described by *Carl Muller* in 1939 (2). His conclusion, that the triade xantomathosis, IHD and hypercholesterolaemia was an autosomal dominant inherited disorder has later been confirmed, and is an outstanding example of how IHD may be inherited.

However, as only a minor part of the family transferred risk in a population is via this disorder, and as no laboratory test which may quantify this risk is available yet, a thorough family history is needed to give an estimate of this risk. In the Norwegian National Health Screening Service (NHSS) the family history is recorded during the screening for IHD in high risk subjects. Based upon the Norwegian material a combined risk score of blood lipids, blood pressure and cigarette smoking is multiplied by 1.5 if the examined subject has a positive family history (3). This may seem a low figure, but it is important to realize that part of the familial risk is already taken care of by the other factors included in the risk score.

An important genetic risk factor which is independent of the blood lipids and blood pressure is Lp (a) lipoprotein (4).

This lipoprotein will probably be included in the future among the laboratory tests aimed at identifying high risk subjects.

Sex

Before menopause IHD is predominantly a male disease with a relative risk of 4-8 for men compared to women of the same age.

This age related protection of the female sex cannot be explained by differences in risk factor levels.

It is difficult to get a clear picture of the importance of the risk factors when reviewing the epidemiological studies assessing risk factors for IHD in women. This may partly be due to the low number of hard coronary events among women. In many studies different diagnostic categories have been lumped together to achieve sufficient numbers for reasonable calculations. It may well be that some of these categories have different risk-factor associations and the lumping has weakened true relationships. Also the different studies differ with regard to which factors that have been examined. To ommit a factor which is aetiologically directly related to IHD, and correlated to any of the examined variables will imply that one or more of these variables will get more attention as a causal factor than it deserves.

From the different studies in women, disregarding design and selection procedures there seems to emerge a pattern of risk factors, slightly different from those identified in men. Firstly, in all studies which have included diabetes mellitus and blood pressure or a history of hypertension, these two factors turn out to be the most important ones, closely followed by cigarette smoking. But this latter factor may behave differently according to age group, being more important in the very young (premenopausal) women, than in the elderly. Triglycerides seem to play a larger role in the female gender than they do in men (5). This, in connection with the relative importance of diabetes mellitus, casual blood glucose, and the relationship

Table 2. *Total cholesterol and relative risk for IHD.*

Total cholesterol mg/dl	Population at risk	IHD n (%)	RR
– 199	268	4 (1.5)	1
200-249	1090	30 (2.8)	1.9
250-299	1450	81 (5.6)	3.7
300-349	688	60 (8.7)	5.8
350-399	179	28 (15.6)	10.4
400+	50	10 (20.0)	13.3
	3725	213 (5.7)	

between triglycerides and factor VII (6) suggests the existence of a metabolic syndrome or a combination of factors which carries an increased CHD risk. Such a syndrome may be more important (relatively) than environmentally induced hypercholesterolaemia in women. This does not mean that total cholesterol is not a coronary risk factor also in women, but the relationship is weaker than for men.

The protection which premenopausal women have against atherosclerosis is a challenge for future research, and the answers to this question may carry with them consequences for preventive cardiology in men also.

Blood lipids

Total cholesterol

Total cholesterol is the classical IHD risk factor, repeatedly shown to be operating both in low and high incidence areas (7).

Table 2 shows the increase in relative risk with increasing total cholesterol in a longitudinal study of 3,725 men in Oslo aged 40-49 years followed for 10 years (8).

This relationship is very similar to that observed in other and larger populations (9). The large relative risk observed for the few men with total cholesterol above 400 mg/dl (10.4 mmol/l) is striking. A preventive effort aiming only at those with 350 mg/dl or above would, even with a high therapeutic yield of e.g. 50%, only result in the avoidance of 19 IHD cases, or a decrease in IHD incidence from 5.7 to 5.2%.

A more recent study is the mortality follow-up of more than 44,000 Norwegian men aged 35-49 years by *Tverdal* (10). The screening took place in 1972-1977 and the very high cholesterol levels usually resulted in dietary intervention. Fig. 1 shows the standardized mortality ratios at different cholesterol levels for IHD (including sudden death of unknown cause). The

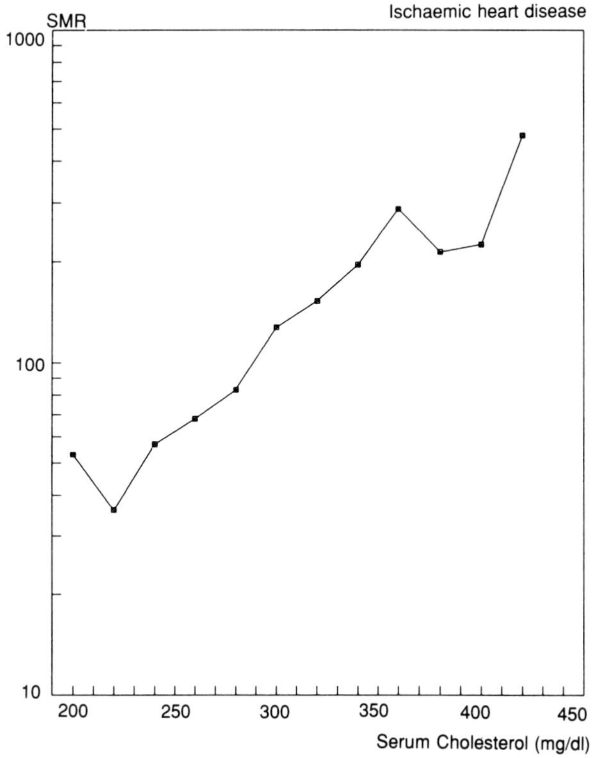

Fig. 1. *IHD standardized mortality ratio (SMR) by serum cholesterol, men age 35-49 (10).*

cholesterol values were obtained by methods which give about 8% higher levels than the presently used enzymatic methods. The cholesterol levels in this chapter have been adjusted accordingly. The lowest cholesterol category (< 193 mg/dl or 5.02 mmol/l) has a higher mortality ratio than the second lowest category (193-210, or 5.02-5.46 mmol/l), and there is a deflection at the upper end. For the category 340-376 (8.83-9.78 mmol/l) the ratios are lower than in 322-339 mg/dl (8.37-8.82 mmol/l). However, for the group at 377 mg/dl or above the ratio is very high indeed.

The most probable explanation for the deflection at the upper end of the cholesterol curve is the intervention which was aimed at the high cholesterol subjects (11, 12).

The increase at the lower end is not explained. International data indicate that IHD risk continues to decline to at least below 4.0 mmol/l (7).

Triglycerides

The role of triglycerides as IHD risk factors is still under debate. In most studies of middle-aged men, triglycerides have not been shown to be independent of the other risk factors. One of the problems in assessing the role of triglycerides may be that the diagnostic category IHD is too wide, and that triglycerides are less important risk factors for angina pectoris than myocardial infarction as has been suggested by *Åberg et al* (13). In an extensive review *M. Austin* concludes that it is too early to dismiss triglycerides as an independent risk factor (14). Her arguments are mainly that methodological problems have been too large to assess the true relationship between triglycerides and IHD. For practical preventive purposes, however, at present triglycerides do not seem to provide additional information on IHD risk when total cholesterol and other risk factors have been taken into account (15).

HDL cholesterol

In contrast to total cholesterol no ecological correlation has been established between HDL cholesterol and the incidence of IHD. This was used as an argument against the possible protective role of HDL cholesterol (16) which was suggested from some early studies (17). Later studies rediscovered alphaliprotein as a protective factor even though there are results still deviating from these findings (18-21).

Only a few studies have taken HDL-cholesterol into consideration as a selection factor (22, 23), and until *Frick et al* published their results no studies have shown that an increase in HDL cholesterol level would be followed by a reduced IHD risk.

An analysis of the impact of changes in different lipoprotein classes including the other risk factors, revealed that both HDL cholesterol and LDL cholesterol were independently associated with the IHD incidence. Thus when one lipid fraction was controlled, the other still had an effect.

A mean decrease of 6% in LDL cholesterol was associated with an 11% decrease in IHD incidence. The average HDL cholesterol increase of 11% was associated with 18% decrease in CHD risk.

To what extent this is also valid for subjects with higher HDL cholesterol levels is not known. From the mortality follow-up data of NHSS there seems to be a threshold value suggesting that an increase above 1.0-1.49 mmol/l does not carry any further beneficial effect for men (Table 3, 4) (24).

Body mass index

Body mass index (BMI) is an important determinant for the blood lipids and blood pressure, and it may seem surprising that the univariate relationship

Table 3. *HDL-cholesterol and mortality 22,734 men aged 40-54 followed for 6 years.*

HDL-C	Deaths/1,000 obs. years CHD	total
< 1.0	3.55	6.85
1.0-1.49	2.02	4.86
1.5-1.99	1.64	5.59
2.0+	2.11	10.62

Table 4. *HDL-cholesterol and mortality 22,574 women aged 40-54 followed for 6 years.*

HDL-C	Deaths/1,000 obs. years CHD	total
< 1.0	.95	4.06
1.0-1.49	.33	2.16
1.5-1.99	.13	2.02
2.0 +	–	2.24

with BMI is relatively weak. As is seen in Fig. 2 only the very high BMI category of 3.2 g/cm^2 or above carries a sizeable risk above that of the other categories (10).

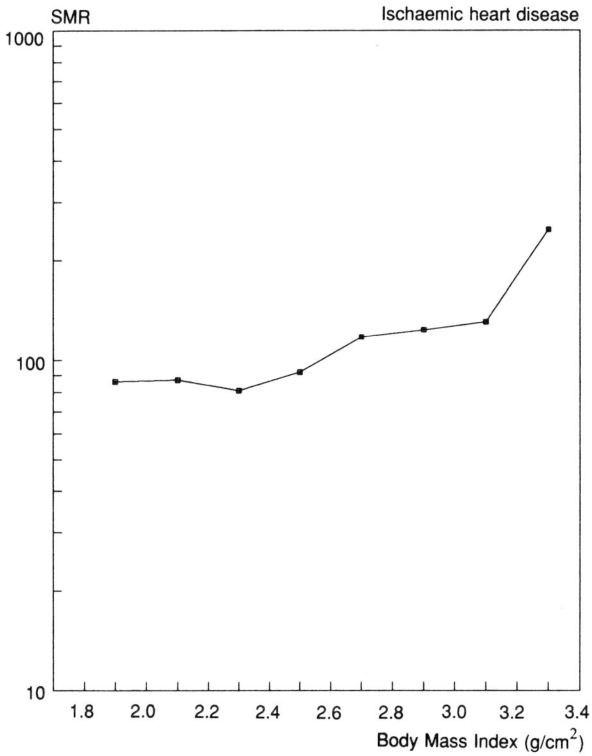

Fig. 2. *IHD standardized mortality ratio (SMR) by body mass index, men age 35-49 (10).*

Physical activity

Physical activity in leisure time is a determinant for many of the risk factors (25), and it is not always easy to single out an independent contribution from this life-style characteristic. The problem of self-selection is also present when this variable is included in a longitudinal analysis. Still, when adjusting for the effect of total cholesterol, a 20% lower IHD risk is observed for those who regularily take part in recreational exercise compared to the more sedentary part of the population (10). Within each exercise category, however, the cholesterol gradient is similar to that observed in the general population.

Thus, when assessing the evidence which has been accumulating the last 20-30 years, a consistently strong protective effect is emerging (26, 27).

Cigarette smoking

The Norwegian NHSS data provides new evidence of the relationship between IHD and cigarette-smoking (10). The risk curve (Figure 3) differs from that of total cholesterol especially by not showing an increased SMR

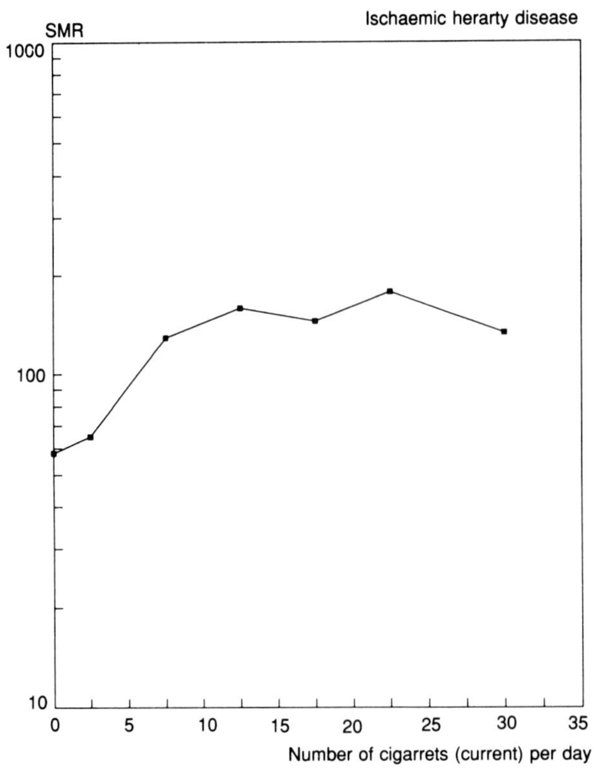

Fig. 3. *IHD standardized mortality ratio (SMR) by number of cigarettes per day, men age 35-49 (10).*

beyond the category 15 cigarettes or more. In the no smoking category, the SMR exceeding 200, giving a relative risk of 3-4 for smokers as compared to non-smokers. This is in accordance with other reports on the IHD risk associated with cigarette-smoking (28).

The fate of the ex-smokers may be of more interest from a preventive point of view. The Norwegian material shows a decline in relative risk for IHD including sudden death (SD) in men with increasing time since quitting smoking (10).

		Time since quitting			
Cause of death		< 3 months	3-12 months	1-5 years	5+years
IHD+SD	RR	2.6	1.8	1.6	1.0
All deaths	RR	1.7	1.8	1.5	1.0

One cannot conclude that this decline is solely due to quitting smoking. Other risk factors may also have changed, but the decline in relative risk for all causes indicates that the smoking induced risk is really reversible.

Population attributable risk of total cholesterol, cigarette smoking and blood pressure

Population attributable risks obviously depend upon what is chosen as a base value of the risk factor. The value of 210 mg/dl (5.46 mmol/l) as a cut-off for total cholesterol would give a population attributable risk of 56% (10). The corresponding figure for systolic blood pressure above 130 mmHg is 38%, whereas the population attributable risk for cigarette-smoking would be 42%. The high attributable risk for smoking, even if the relative risk may seem low, is due to the high prevalence of this habit in the Norwegian population. BMI on the other hand gives an attributable risk of 5%, demonstrating the low importance of this factor as an IHD risk factor in the population.

When the three risk factors: blood pressure, total cholesterol and cigarette smoking are put together, a potential preventive proportion may be calculated, using the mentioned values as base levels. If we assume total independence and reversibility of risk, (which obviously is not true) the fraction of non-preventable IHD deaths would be (1-0.56) (1-0.38) (1-0.42) = 0.16, implying that more than 80% of IHD deaths might be postponed until after the age of sixty. A similar calculation based upon the Framingham data gave a lower preventive fraction, 48% (29). The main reason for this difference is the somewhat older population in Framingham compared to the

Norwegian sample, the use of higher cut-off points for the risk factors and the decreasing strength of these three risk factors with increasing age. Still, the high figures for preventable fractions both in Norway and USA illustrate the potential preventability of IHD.

References

1. Berg K. Genetics of coronary heart disease In: Steinberg AG, Motulsky AG, Childs B, eds. Progress in Medical Genetics. Vol V. Philadelphia: WB Saunders 1983; 35-90.
2. Muller C. Angina pectoris in hereditary xanthomatosis. Arch Intern Med 1939; 64: 675-700.
3. Håndbok for hjertekarundersøkelsen. Statens helseundersøkelser. Oslo 1987.
4. Rhoads GG, Dahlen G, Berg K, Morton NE, Dannenberg AL. Lp (a) lipoprotein as a risk factor for myocardial infarction. JAMA 1986; 256: 2540-4.
5. Carlson LA, Böttiger LE. Risk factors for ischaemic heart disease in men and women. Results from the 19-year follow-up of the Stockholm prospective study. Acta Med Scand 1985; 218: 481-9.
6. Meade TW, Mellows S, Brozovik M, et al. Haemostatic function and ischaemic heart disease: principal results of the Northwick Park Heart Study. Lancet 1986; 2: 533-7.
7. Westlund K, Nicolaysen R. Ten-year mortality and morbidity related to serum cholesterol. A follow-up of 3,751 men aged 40-49. Scand J Clin Lab Invest 1972; (suppl 127): 1-24.
8. Keys A, ed. Coronary heart disease in seven countries. Circulation 1970; 41 (suppl 1): 1-121.
9. Martin MJ. Serum cholesterol, blood pressure, and mortality: implications from a cohort of 361 662 men. Lancet 1986; ii: 933-6.
10. Tverdal A. A mortality follow-up of persons invited to a cardiovascular disease study in five areas in Norway. National Health Screening Service, Oslo 1989.
11. Bjartveit K, Foss OP, Gjervig T. The Cardiovascular disease study in Norwegian counties. Results from first screening. Acta Med Scand 1983; (suppl 675): 1-184.
12. Hjermann I, Velve Byre K, Holme I, Leren P. Effect of diet and smoking intervention on the incidence of coronary heart disease. Lancet 1981; 2: 1303-10.
13. Åberg H, Lithell H, Selinus I, Hedstrand H. Serum triglycerides are a risk factor for myocardial infarction but not for angina pectoris. Atherosclerosis 1985; 54: 89-97.
14. Austin MA. Plasma triglyceride as a risk factor for coronary heart disease. Am J Epidemiol 1989; 129: 249-59.
15. Tverdal A, Foss OP, Leren P, Holme I, Lund-Larsen PG, and Bjartveit K. Serum triglycerides as an independent risk factor for death from coronary heart disease in middle-aged Norwegian men. Am J Epidemiol 1989; 129: 458-65.
16. Stamler J. Epidemiology of coronary heart disease. Med Clin North Am 1973; 57: 5-46. 1973
17. Keys A, Blackburn H. Background of the patient with coronary heart disease. Progr Cardiovasc Dis 1963; 6: 14-44.
18. Miller GJ, Miller NE. Plasma-high-density-lipoprotein concentration and development of ischaemic heart-disease. Lancet 1975; i: 16-9.
19. Miller NE, Førde OH, Thelle DS, Mjøs OD. The Tromsø Heart Study. High-density lipoprotein and coronary heart disease: a prospective case-control study. Lancet 1977; i: 965-8.

20. Castelli WP, Doyle JT, Gordon T, et al. HDL cholesterol and other lipids in coronary heart disease. Circulation 1977; 55: 767-72.
21. Pocock SJ, Shaper AG, Phillips AN, Walker M, Whitehead TP. High density lipoprotein cholesterol is not a major risk factor for ischaemic heart disease in British men. Br Med J 1986; 292: 515-9.
22. Frick MH, Elo O, Haapa K, et al. Helsinki heart study: Primary-prevention trial with gemfibrozil in middle-aged men with dyslipidemia. N Engl J Med 1987; 317: 1237-45.
23. Knutsen SF, Knutsen R. The Tromsø heart study: Family approach to intervention on CHD. Feasibility of risk factor reduction in high risk persons - project description. Scand J Soc Med 1989; 17: 109-19.
24. National Health Screening Service, Health Services of Finnmark, Sogn og Fjordane, and Oppland counties, Ullevål Hospital, Central Laboratory, Oslo. The cardiovascular disease study in Norwegian counties. Results from second screening. National Health Screening Service 1988.
25. Blair SN, Cooper KH, Gibbons LW, Gettman LR, Lewis S, Goodyear N. Changes in coronary heart disease risk factors associated with increased treadmill time in 753 men. Am J Epidemiol 1983; 118: 352-9.
26. Morris JN, Everitt MG, Pollard R, Chave SP, Semmence AM. Vigorous exercise in leisure-time: protection against coronary heart disease. Lancet 1980; 2: 1207-10.
27. Paffenbarger RS Jr, Hyde RT, Wing AL, Hsieh CC. Physical activity, all cause mortality, and longevity of college alumni. N Engl J Med 1986; 314: 605-13.
28. Surgeon General (USA) : The health consequences of smoking: Cardiovascular disease. Washington DC 1983.
29. Sturmans F, Mulder PGH, Valkenburg HA. Estimation of the possible effect of interventive measures in the area of ischemic heart diseases by the attributable risk percentage. Am J Epidemiol 1977; 105: 281-89.

44

Blood pressure and coronary heart disease

KNUT WESTLUND

Blood pressure as a risk factor in asymptomatic persons

The shape of the risk curve connecting blood pressure (BP) with risk of a first myocardial infarction (MI) is not well defined. This contrasts with the straight line relationship of the logarithm (or the logit) of infarction incidence or mortality to serum cholesterol. Possibly, there is a difference between incidence and mortality where BP is concerned, although such a

Table 1. *Incidence of first MI related to BP. 10-year follow-up of Oslo men aged 40-49.*

	Number of		10 year incidence per cent age-adjusted
	Men	First MI	
Systolic (mmHg)			
<115	424	25	6.0
115-124	1051	40	3.9
125-134	1113	47	4.3
135-144	568	36	6.2
145-154	273	28	9.9
155-164	114	13	10.8
165-184	91	13	13.7
185+	33	8	21.6
	3667	210	5.7
Diastolic (mmHg)			
<75	530	27	5.3
75-84	1753	71	4.1
85-94	945	64	6.6
95-104	312	28	8.6
105-114	89	14	15.2
115+	36	6	15.0
	3665	210	5.7

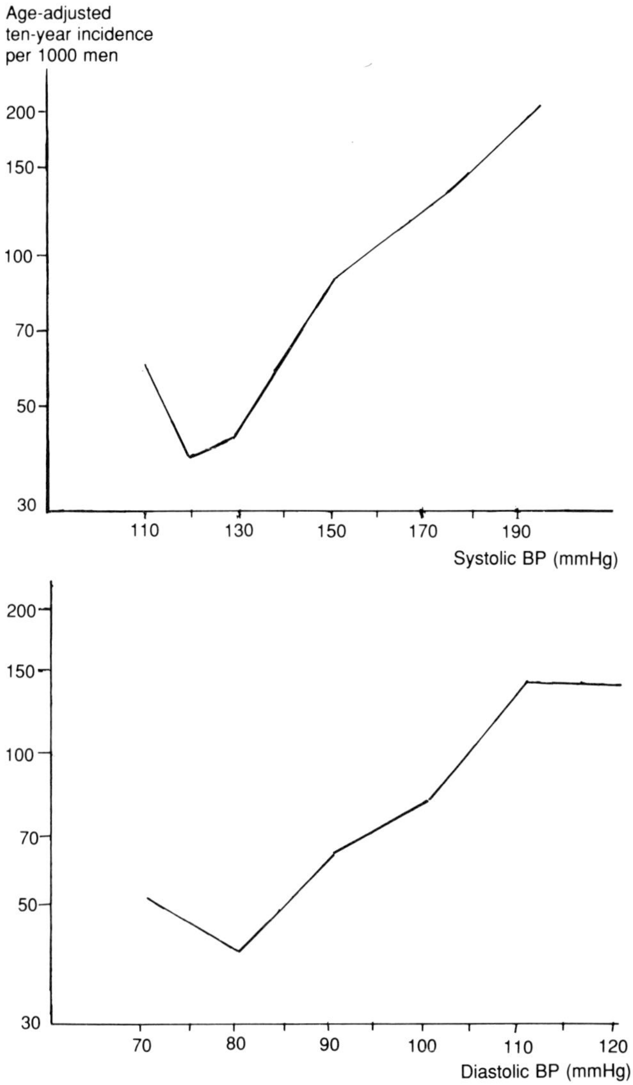

Fig. 1. *Age-adjusted incidence of first MI, per 1000 men at baseline, related to BP. 10-year follow-up of Oslo men aged 40-49 years.*

conclusion is difficult to justify from the bewildering number of studies of different age groups, different length of follow-up, different base line BP distributions, and different number of subjects.

Table 1 is an example of an incidence study (1), which shows first MI's in a 10-year follow-up of 3,667 Oslo men aged 40-49. Fig. 1 shows the risk curves. Two points may be noted: a) The upturn of the curve at low pressure, resulting in an incidence in the lowest group (under 115 mmHg systolic or 75 mmHg diastolic) similar to that of the total group; and, b) the population attributable risk is quite modest: 24% for systolic pressure 135 mmHg or above and 25% for diastolic pressure 85 mmHg or above.

Table 2. *44,300 men, age 35-49, followed for 6-11 years. Standardized mortality rates for CHD and stroke. Five areas in Norway.*

	Deaths from CHD			Deaths from stroke		
Systolic blood BP (mmHg)	Obs	Exp	SMR	Obs	Exp	SMR
-109	8	13.1	61	–	1.47	
110-119	41	73.4	56	4	8.28	32
120-129	107	163.9	65	5	18.45	
130-139	171	180.4	95	29	20.19	
140-149	121	127.9	95	10	14.18	112
150-159	93	71.3	130	8	7.76	
160-169	68	33.8	201	3	3.68	230
170-179	37	14.3	260	9	1.54	
180-189	22	7.4	296	5	.76	625
190+	24	6.4	373	4	.68	
	692	691.9	100	77	76.99	100

Another feature, which is visible primarily in the diastolic curve, is the suggestion of a deflection at high pressure. The observation period in this study started in the late 1950's, and treatment of BP is unlikely to have had much effect. Rather, the bending of the curve may reflect the old clinical

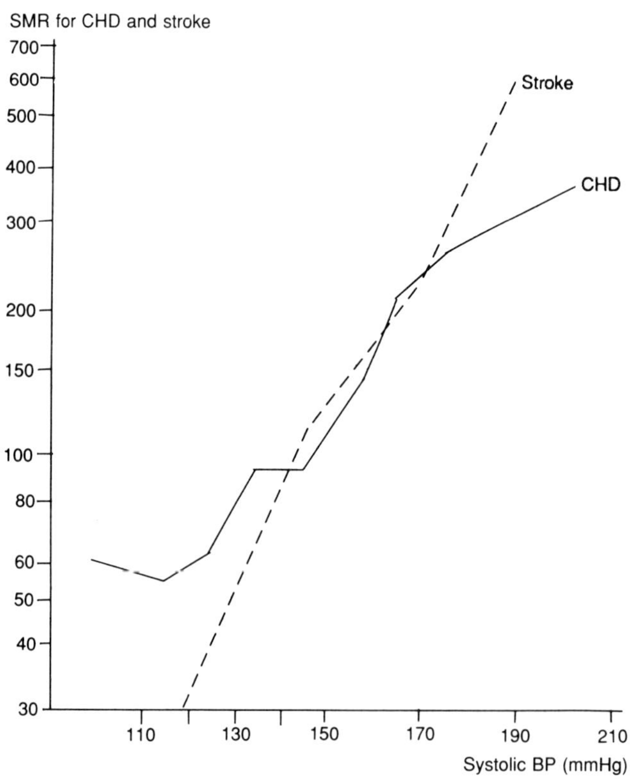

Fig. 2. *Standardized mortality ratios (SMR) for CHD and stroke, related to systolic BP; Norwegian men aged 35-49 years, followed for 6-11 years.*

saying that it takes a strong heart (with open coronaries) to sustain a high BP. That this phenomenon is seen so irregulary in present-day prospective studies may perhaps be ascribed to the fact that there are few really high BP available for follow-up.

Recently, *Tverdal* (2) has published a mortality follow-up of more than 44,000 Norwegian men aged 35-49. The screening took place during 1972-1977 and high BP in most cases resulted in follow-up examinations and, if indicated, drug treatment (3). Table 2 and Fig. 2 show standardized mortality ratios at different systolic pressures for coronary heart disease (CHD) (including sudden death of unknown cause) and stroke. The risk curve for CHD has a slightly sigmoid shape, similar to the curves (Fig. 1) from a time when treatment was much less common than in 1972-77. It is hardly justified to deduce a mortality-lowering effect of treatment from the shape of the CHD curve. Perhaps more disturbing is the absence of a clear effect of intervention on stroke mortality.

Serum cholesterol apparently looses most of its predictive power after the age of 60. Not so with BP. A five-year mortality follow-up of a large number of persons screened in Bergen (4) showed a very clear gradient of CHD mortality to systolic BP at ages 60-69 and 70-79 in both men and women. The gradient became less steep (on a logarithmic scale) with increasing age, however, and at age 80 and over the trend was irregular. With diastolic pressure the gradient was hardly discernible at age 70-79. The CHD-mortality predictive power of BP at age 60-69 and 70-79 is evident even in a 20-year follow-up of the Bergen material (5).

Roughly, the CHD-risk in men equals the risk in women with 50 mmHg higher systolic or 35 mmHg higher diastolic pressure (4).

A topic of much debate has been whether systolic or diastolic pressure is the better predictor. *Holme and Waaler* (4) found that systolic pressure predicted CHD mortality slightly better than diastolic. *Tverdal* (6), following up men under the age of 50, found an age-dependence. At age 35-39 diastolic pressure appeared to be the better predictor, whereas there was practically no difference at age 45-49. It should be noted that in both these studies the BP was measured by mercury sphygmomanometers. Even with the best of training of observers, it is difficult to avoid bias in the reading of diastolic pressure. Electronic devices are now being widely used in population surveys, and we can look forward to follow-up studies where heart rate is combined with mean arterial pressure, or with a combination of systolic and an unbiased diastolic pressure, into a predictive index. Possibly, the best index may be different, not only for different age groups but for different causes of death, in particular CHD and stroke.

Even with the best of instruments the difficulties in standardizing the measuring situation will always set limits to the accuracy obtainable in population surveys. In particular, the resting time prior to taking the readings is critical.

Blood pressure shows some correlation with serum cholesterol, but practically none with cigarette smoking. The three risk factors can be combined in various ways to provide a powerful predictive index for MI incidence or CHD deaths.

No correlation has been established between population BP means and population incidence or mortality rates from CHD. Apparently, BP is a less fundamental risk factor for CHD than serum cholesterol.

The incidence of angina pectoris is related to BP in a manner similar to the incidence of MI (7).

Blood pressure as a prognostic factor in persons with symptomatic CHD

a) Acute attack of myocardial infarction

The 10-year follow-up of Oslo men aged 40-49 (1) showed a slight, nonsignificant increase in case fatality of first MI with increasing diastolic pressure, but no suggestion of an association with systolic pressure.

b) Prognosis of survivors of myocardial infarction

In general, the risk factors for CHD death are the same in MI patients as in symptom-free men, but the risk for MI patients is of course much higher, given a certain risk factor combination (2). More specifically, the prognostic importance of BP was examined in the Beta-Blocker Pooling Project (8). The total number of infarction patients randomized to placebo was 6,706. In the placebo group the following total mortality percentages were observed in a one-year follow-up:

Systolic BP (mmHg)	Mortality %	Diastolic BP (mmHg)	Mortality %	Heart rate	Mortality %
<110	7.0	<70	6.5	<70	4.5
110-139	6.5	70-89	6.7	70-89	6.7
140+	7.1	90+	7.1	90+	13.6

A slight increase in mortality is seen with increasing diastolic pressure, whereas the systolic trend is irregular. In contrast, the mortality rise with increasing heart rate is strong. The blood pressures are measured at baseline, i.e. after the infarction.

As a group, MI patients have a lower BP than others of comparable age.

Thus, in surveys carried out by the National Health Screening Service of Norway during 1985-88 more than 700 men aged 40-62 with a previous MI attended. Age-adjusted systolic pressure was 3.9 mmHg lower and diastolic 1.6 mmHg lower than in other men (5). The findings were similar when the comparison was made separately for men with and without drug treatment for high BP. This reversal of what must have been the situation prior to the MI, is in strong contrast to what was seen for serum cholesterol. The MI men (and women) had a serum cholesterol mean as much above the others as they were likely to have had prior to the MI. Thus, at least in middle-aged MI patients, serum cholesterol is a much greater problem than BP. Hopefully, non-pharmacological treatment of serum cholesterol will also influence the BP in a favourable direction.

Effect of blood pressure treatment on CHD incidence

One of the unpleasant surprises of recent times is the lack of reversibility of CHD risk when high BP is lowered by drugs. A review of findings in randomized trials has been given by *Holme* (9). The incidence of CHD for all trials with untreated control group is given as:

Active treatment: .... 374/12,976 = 28.8 per 1,000 persons randomized
Control: .... 397/12,924 = 30.7 per 1,000 persons randomized

Among the trials with a treated control group, the Hypertension Detection and Follow-up Program (HDFP)(10) deserves special mention. Participants were recruited by population-based screening of 159,000 people aged 30 to 69 in 14 communities throughout the United States. Nearly 11,000 persons with elevated BP were randomized to either Stepped care (SC) (n=5,485) or Referred care (RC) (n=5,455). SC was a systematic antihypertensive programme offered in special centres, whereas RC patients were referred to their usual sources of care, "with special referral efforts for those with more severe hypertension or organ system damage." The five-year mortality findings were:

Diseases	SC	RC
Myocardial infarction	51	69
Other ischaemic heart disease	80	79
Cerebrovascular diseases	29	52
Other cardiovascular diseases	35	40
Total cardiovascular deaths	195	240
Total non-cardiovascular deaths	154	179
Total deaths	349	419

It is difficult to be certain how much of this difference can be ascribed to better BP control in the SC group. However, taking the results at face value, we note that the savings involve 23 deaths due to cerebrovascular diseases and 17 deaths due to ischaemic heart disease – rather similar for the two causes.

The HDFP enrolled a representative sample of hypertensives. However, the study was conducted under academic auspices, involving control of the patient selection. The total effect of drug treatment in the community may be a different story. In Norwegian follow-up studies (2, 3) the variable "Under treatment for high BP" is statistically associated with an increased risk of CHD, even in multiple regressions with BP and a number of other independent variables included. The effect of treatment on blood lipid levels does not appear to explain the higher mortality in the treated group (3). In an observational setting, it is impossible to completely exclude an unknown confounding factor. However, an analysis of the characteristics of persons on BP treatment in Norway (5) showed that the selection to treatment is not in accordance with recommended criteria. At a given BP relatively more women than men are being treated, more elderly than middle-age, more fat than lean, more non-smokers than smokers. Apparently, sound indications for drug treatment of BP have not yet penetrated the community, and it is uncertain how many lives, if any, are being saved. The recent swing towards non-pharmacological treatment is wholly to be recommended.

Summary

Coronary heart disease incidence is strongly dependent on BP, but the shape of the risk curve differs from that of serum cholesterol. In particular, there may be an upturn of risk at low BP, a phenomenon which may be related to the difficulty of reducing CHD incidence by the lowering of BP. Blood pressure has little predictive power for case fatality in attacks of first MI or for CHD deaths in the follow-up of MI survivors. Drug treatment of elevated BP, even in well controlled trials with careful selection of patients, has not consistently shown a reduction in CHD mortality. In the general population the results of drug treatment may be even less satisfactory.

References

1. Westlund K, Nicolaysen R. Ten-year mortality and morbidity related to serum cholesterol. Scand J Clin Lab Invest 1972; 30 (suppl 127).
2. Tverdal A. A mortality follow-up of persons invited to a cardiovasular disease study in five areas in Norway. Oslo, National Health Screening Service, 1989.

3. National Health Screening Service. The cardiovascular disease study in Norwegian counties. Results from second screening. Oslo 1988.
4. Holme I, Waaler HT. Five-year Mortality in the City of Bergen, Norway, according to age, sex and blood pressure. Acta Med Scand 1976; 200: 229-39.
5. National Health Screening Service. Unpublished data.
6. Tverdal A. Systolic and diastolic blood pressures as predictors of coronary heart disease in middle aged Norwegian men. Br Med J 1987; 294: 671-3.
7. Natvig H, Borchgrevink CF, Dedichen J, et al. A controlled trial of the effect of linolenic aacid on incidence of coronary Heart Disease. Scand J clin Lab Invest 1968; 22 (suppl 105).
8. The Beta-Blocker Pooling Project Research Group. The Beta-Blocker Pooling Project (BBPP): subgroup findings from randomized trials in post infarction patients. Eur Heart J 1988; 9: 8-16.
9. Holme I. Drug treatment of mild hypertension to reduce the risk of CHD: is it worthwhile? Stat Med 1988; 7: 1109-20.
10. Hypertension Detection and Follow-up Program Cooperative Group. Five-Year findings of the hypertension detection and follow-up program. I. Reduction in mortality of persons with high blood pressure, including mild hypertension. JAMA 1979; 242: 2562-71.

45

Dynamics in the epidemiology of ischaemic heart disease: Effect of treatment and prevention

GORM JENSEN

Ischaemic heart disease (IHD) and its index disease event, acute myocardial infarction (AMI), is a leading cause of morbidity and mortality in the Nordic countries. Consequently, prevention and treatment of IHD is a major concern of the Health Care System of the Nordic countries. In this review, the effect of prevention and treatment on the natural history and occurrence of IHD in Denmark will be analyzed. Although be dealing with the morbidity and the mortality in Denmark, the same type of reasoning may be applied to data from other countries. It must be emphasized that very little hard data exists, and that the conclusions are based on estimates, suppositions and extrapolations.

Contribution to morbidity and mortality from IHD and AMI in Denmark

Heart disease is a leading cause of death, responsible for approximately one third of the deaths of middle-aged and elderly males, and elderly females (Fig. 1) (1). The vast majority of deaths from heart disease are due to IHD. Fiftyfive per cent of IHD deaths are caused by AMI, the remainder by chronic IHD and symptomatic IHD. Although IHD is a disease of the elderly, 33% (n=2,972) and 12% (n=921) deaths in males and females respectively, occur in subjects below the age of seventy.

The annual risk of incurring a fatal or non-fatal AMI for a middle-aged man is approximately 5.5‰ and for a middle-aged female approximately 1.0‰ (2). Angina pectoris (AP) occurs with a prevalence of approximately 2% in 50-59 year old males, 4% among males above 60 years of age and 2% among females aged 60 years or more (3). The prevalence of chronic IHD (inclusive AP) has been assessed to be approximately 3% (150,000 individuals, approximately), but firm figures are not available (4).

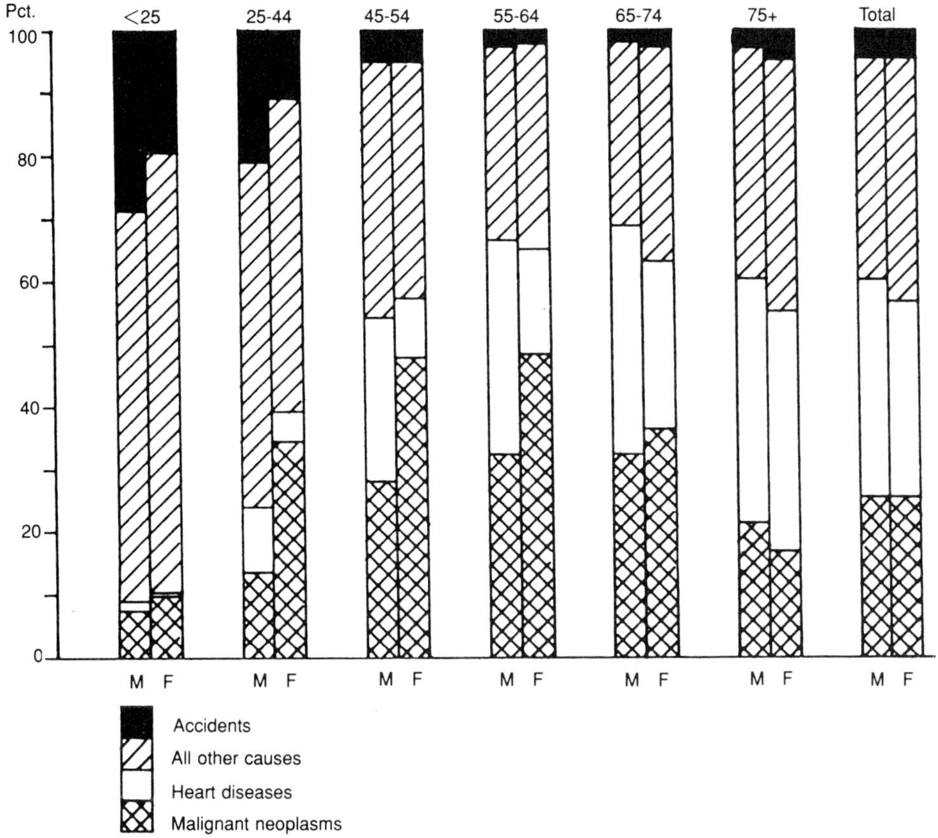

Fig. 1. *Percentage distribution of deaths from 4 causes, sex and age.*

Development in the mortality from IHD and AMI

There are good reasons for believing that the mortality from IHD, as well as from AMI, peaked between 1975 and 1981, and that the mortality has slightly decreased since then – by approximately 10% (5, 6) (Fig. 2). Thus Denmark may be experiencing the same features as seen in the United States and Finland, where the mortality has decreased by approximately 25-40%. A possible explanation will be discussed later.

IHD and the Health Care System

IHD (including AMI) is the most common diagnosis on discharge. They comprise 16.5% of all patients discharged from somatic hospitals; further, these patients occupy 18.5% of the beds (34,344 out of a total of 207,473

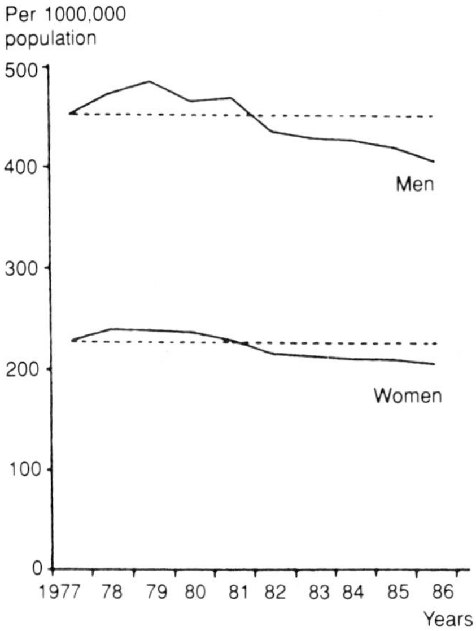

Fig. 2. *Age-standardized mortality rates for IHD per 100,000, males and females 1977-86 (6).*

discharges, and 313,073 out of a total of 1,667,069 bed-days) (7). The average duration of hospitalization for AMI decreased from 1983 from 11.7 to 9.5 days, probably reflecting changes in medical practice. A remarkable development has occurred regarding admissions for AMI and symptomatic heart disease (Table 1). The admittance rate for AMI has increased slightly, but that for symptomatic IHD has increased dramatically. Unfortunately, we do not have access to age-standardized discharge rates for AMI and symptomatic heart disease. However, the slight increase in AMI-discharges may reflect a slightly increasing mean age in the population. On the other hand, the increase in discharges of patients with symptomatic heart disease is greater than may be reasonably explained from a slight change in age-distribution. The profile of discharges of chronic IHD is similar to that for AMI.

Approximately 12,000 patients are discharged after suffering non-fatal AMI, and a few thousand patients experience other forms of symptoms, such as AP or arrhythmia; altogether approximately 15,000 patients may annually join a subpopulation of chronic IHD patients. As the average an-

Table 1. *Discharges from somatic hospitals 1983-87.*

Discharges, heart disease	1983	1985	1987
AMI	16,584	17,678	17,860
Symptomatic heart disease	13,124	14,832	16,484
Chronic IHD	9,722	9,642	9,495

nual mortality is approximately 10%, this subpopulation is roughly 150,000 persons (Fig. 3). This estimate is supported by statistics of pharmaceutical sales (8), showing a sale of approximately 55,000 DDD's of cardiac glucosides, 5,000 DDD's of antiarrhythmic drugs, and 35,000 DDD's of nitrates, corresponding roughly to 60-80,000 symptomatic IHD patients.

What can be deduced from the mortality and hospital statistics?

There are several possible explanations for the reduction of the mortality from IHD.

Firstly, the reduction in mortality may reflect decreased case-fatality rates, and secondly, it may reflect decreasing incidence rates of IHD and AMI. At this time, unfortunately, no reliable incidence data over a period of time are available, in particular no data regarding the incidence of first AMI.

IHD is a chronic relapsing condition. A patient suffering a non-fatal AMI is very likely to suffer relapses, until he succumbs to the disease. The first AMI is the index event; succeeding AMI's should not be counted, when considering the true frequency of the disease in the population. If, therefore, the case-fatality rate of the first AMI decreased, the proportion of surviving patients with an increased risk of (relapsing) AMI's, and consequently AMI incidence and frequencies, would tend to increase. It must be recognized that increased therapeutic efficiency has the effect of creating a larger subpopulation of patients suffering from chronic IHD, and in turn giving rise to an increasing number of relapsing cases of acute exacerbations of IHD. This is a direct consequence of the chronic relapsing nature of IHD (Fig. 3).

Is therapeutic efficiency increasing?

No age-standardized population data are available concerning case-fatality rates, but it seems likely from the mortality and discharge rates that case-fatality rates have decreased significantly. This could be expected from clinical studies. Thrombolytic treatment, commenced in 1985-6 and becoming standard treatment from 1988, should reduce the over-all mortality of AMI by perhaps 10-15%. However, this will not be reflected in present day statistics. On the other hand, the effect of secondary prophylaxis with beta-blockers, ACE-inhibition treatment of severe heart failure, improved treatment of unstable angina, might have a similar impact on the fatality rate.

It is not known whether adequate symptomatic medical treatment of chronic AP has an effect on mortality, but it seems likely. In respect of surgical treatment of IHD, the number of patients selected for surgery during the period in question was insufficient to influence the national mortality data, irrespective of just how well the survival effect appears to be documented.

However, most cardiologists would agree that in recent years a "silent revolution" has taken place in the treatment of IHD; smaller and larger improvements in therapy and diagnosis have contributed to this. Hard data, confirming this development, are urgently needed.

Has the incidences of IHD changed?

There are no acceptable data available to elucidate this important question. The frequency of AMI remains more or less unchanged; as argued previously, this possibly reflects a decreased incidence of first AMI, a decreased fatality rate and an increased relapse rate – the latter two factors cancelling each other. Coronary risk factor distribution in the population shows a dissimilar development. While total-cholesterol levels have decreased on the average by approximately 8% during the period 1978 to 1983 (9), blood pressure has increased by 1-2% in the same period. The first factor would lead to a decrease in the incidence of about 15%, while the increase in blood pressure presumably increases the incidence by approximately 4%. New data are urgently needed concerning this important aspect of cardiovascular epidemiology.

Future developments in treatment, and possible population effects

Firstly, the effect of the standard use of thrombolysis in AMI will become apparent in the coming years. Case-fatality rates for AMI could decrease to below 10%, and the late mortality could also be significantly reduced, if present day technologies were employed in full measure. This would tend to increase the subpopulation previously mentioned with chronic IHD requiring medical supervision and care.

The very success in the therapy of IHD has the paradoxiccal effect of *increasing* the number of patients with chronic IHD, and *increasing* the need for health care facilities for the treatment and control of IHD.

Future developments in prevention, and possible population effects

Increasing efforts from government agencies and professional and voluntary health organizations have been directed at promoting healthy life-style habits in the population. One can only hypothesise about the effect.

Rose & Shipley (11) have made an interesting analysis concerning the effect on mortality of lowering the cholesterol level and lowering the occurrence of cigerette smoking. Both measures would prolong life, but cessation of smoking would – by decreasing the risk of cancer, actually increase the life-time risk of heart attacks, while lowering cholesterol would decrease the life-time risk of heart attacks, its place being taken by a typical mixture of other causes of death. The effect of treatment of high blood pressure is discussed in another chapter of this book. An increase in the risk of AMI has been observed in treated hypertensives in observational studies (12).

Conclusion

The treatment of IHD has become increasingly efficient, decreasing fatality rates and decreasing mortality, prolonging life and thus increasing the number of chronic cases of IHD. Prevention of IHD also prolongs life, but may, by exposing more subjects to the higher morbidity rates of the elderly, also result in a higher number of patients with acute and chronic heart disease. These seemingly paradoxical dynamic changes in the epidemiology of IHD should be considered when planning future Health Care.

References

1. Causes of death in Denmark 1987. Vital Statistics I: 24: 1989. National Board of Health 1989.
2. Nyboe J, Jensen G, Appleyard M. Schnohr P. Risk factors for acute myocardial infarction in Copenhagen I: Hereditary, educational and socioeconomic factors. Eur Heart J 1989; 10: 910-6.
3. Jensen G. Epidemiology of chest pain and angina pectoris, with special reference to treatment needs. Acta Med Scand 1984; 682. (Thesis).
4. Jensen G. Akut myokardieinfarkt – Epidemiologiske aspekter. I: Thygesen K, Kjekshus JK, eds. Hjerteinfarkt. København: FADL's forlag, 1985: 31-42.
5. Kamper-Jørgensen F, et al. Hjertedødelighed i Danmark ved et vendepunkt? Ugeskr Læg 1984; 146: 1006-8.
6. Mosbech J, Kristensen FB, Otzen J. Dødsårsagsmønsteret i ti-året 1977-86 i Danmark for lungelidelser, iskæmisk hjertesygdom og cerebrovaskulære sygdomme. Ugeskr Læg 1989; 151: 1395-6.
7. Sygdomsmønsteret for indlagte patienter 1987. Hospital statistics II: 43: 1989. National Board of Health 1989.
8. Lægemiddelforbruget i Danmark 1988. Dansk lægemiddelstatistik. Herlev 1989.
9. Appleyard M. The Copenhagen City Heart Study. A book of tables with data from the first examination (1976-78) and a five year follow-up (1981-83). Scand J Soc Med 1989; 170 (suppl 41): 1-160.

10. Clausen J, Jensen G. Is the blood pressure in Denmark increasing? J Int Med. In press.
11. Rose G. Shipley M. Effects of coronary risk reduction on the pattern of mortality. Lancet 1990; 335: 275-7.
12. Jensen G, Nyboe J, Appleyard M, Schnohr P. Risk factors for acute myocardial infarction in Copenhagen. II: Smoking, alcohol intake. oral contraception, obesity, diabetes, physical activity, blood pressure and lipids. Eur Heart J. In press.

Index